General Medicine

First, second and third edition authors:

Rachael Hough

Iftikhar Ul Haq

Robert Parker

Asheesh Sharma

4th Edition

CRASH COURSE

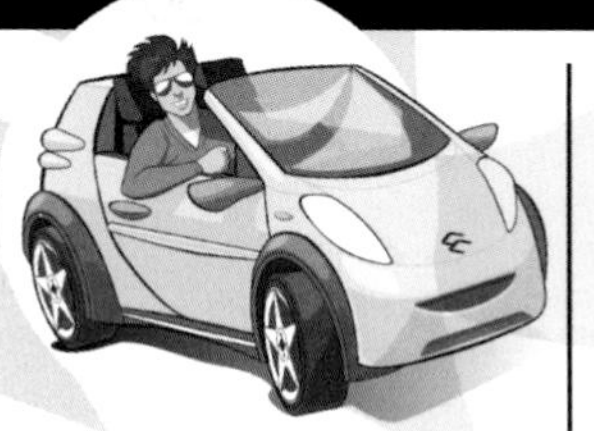

SERIES EDITOR:
Dan Horton-Szar
BSc(Hons), MBBS(Hons), MRCGP
Northgate Medical Practice,
Canterbury,
Kent, UK

FACULTY ADVISOR:
Richard Makins
BSc(Hons), MBBS, MD, FRCP
Consultant Gastroenterologist,
Cheltenham General Hospital,
Cheltenham, UK

General Medicine

Oliver A. Leach
BSc, MBChB, MRCP
Clinical Fellow,
Nuffield Department of Clinical Neurosciences,
Radcliffe Hospitals NHS Trust,
Oxford, UK

Gijs I. van Boxel
BMBCh, PhD, MRCS
Specialty Registrar General Surgery
Oxford Deanery, Oxford, UK

MOSBY

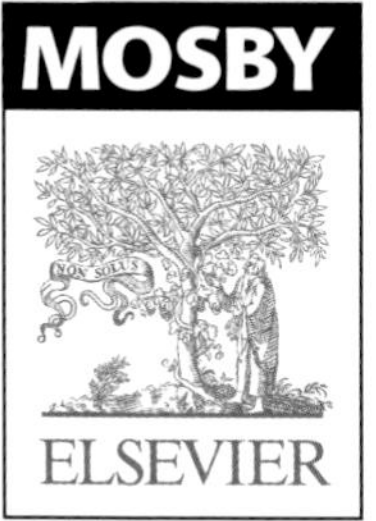

Edinburgh London New York Oxford Philadelphia St Louis Sydney Toronto 2015

ELSEVIER
MOSBY

Commissioning Editor: Jeremy Bowes
Development Editor: Helen Leng
Project Manager: Andrew Riley
Designer: Christian Bilbow
Illustration Manager: Jennifer Rose

First edition 1999

Second edition 2005

Third edition 2008

Fourth edition 2013

Updated Fourth edition 2015

Reprinted 2015

ISBN: 978-0-7234-3864-9

British Library Cataloguing in Publication Data
A catalogue record for this book is available from the British Library

Library of Congress Cataloging in Publication Data
A catalog record for this book is available from the Library of Congress

Notices
Knowledge and best practice in this field are constantly changing. As new research and experience broaden our understanding, changes in research methods, professional practices, or medical treatment may become necessary.

Practitioners and researchers must always rely on their own experience and knowledge in evaluating and using any information, methods, compounds, or experiments described herein. In using such information or methods they should be mindful of their own safety and the safety of others, including parties for whom they have a professional responsibility.

With respect to any drug or pharmaceutical products identified, readers are advised to check the most current information provided (i) on procedures featured or (ii) by the manufacturer of each product to be administered, to verify the recommended dose or formula, the method and duration of administration, and contraindications. It is the responsibility of practitioners, relying on their own experience and knowledge of their patients, to make diagnoses, to determine dosages and the best treatment for each individual patient, and to take all appropriate safety precautions.

To the fullest extent of the law, neither the publisher nor the authors, contributors, or editors, assume any liability for any injury and/or damage to persons or property as a matter of products liability, negligence or otherwise, or from any use or operation of any methods, products, instructions, or ideas contained in the material herein.

The Publisher's policy is to use **paper manufactured from sustainable forests**

Printed in China

Last digit is the print line: 10 9 8 7 6 5 4 3 2

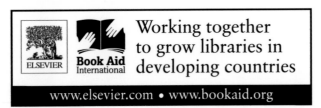

Series editor foreword

The *Crash Course* series first published in 1997 and now, 16 years on, we are still going strong. Medicine never stands still, and the work of keeping this series relevant for today's students is an ongoing process. These fourth editions build on the success of the previous titles and incorporate new and revised material, to keep the series up to date with current guidelines for best practice, and recent developments in medical research and pharmacology.

We always listen to feedback from our readers, through focus groups and student reviews of the *Crash Course* titles. For the fourth editions, we have completely re-written our self-assessment material to keep up with today's 'single-best answer' and 'extended matching question' formats. The artwork and layout of the titles has also been largely re-worked to make it easier on the eye during long sessions of revision.

Despite fully revising the books with each edition, we hold fast to the principles on which we first developed the series. *Crash Course* will always bring you all the information you need to revise in compact, manageable volumes that integrate basic medical science and clinical practice. The books still maintain the balance between clarity and conciseness, and provide sufficient depth for those aiming at distinction. The authors are medical students and junior doctors who have recent experience of the exams you are now facing, and the accuracy of the material is checked by a team of faculty advisors from across the UK.

I wish you all the best for your future careers!

Dr Dan Horton-Szar

Series Editor

Authors

The last five to ten years have seen many exciting discoveries and developments in medicine. Some of these have remained in the laboratory and have not yet filtered their way through to clinical medicine, but in other areas the rewards of research are plainly obvious; take, for instance, the proliferation of monoclonal antibodies that are now available to treat a wide range of conditions. The growth of evidence-based medicine has provided a vast database to draw on, which is often distilled into guidelines such as those provided by the National Institute for Health and Clinical Excellence (NICE). Furthermore, this evidence has led to a plethora of scoring systems used to calculate risk and to aid treatment. However, what must be remembered is that taking an accurate history, being able to trust your examination findings and communicating well with patients remain of the utmost importance.

The ever-increasing depth of knowledge has led to even greater specialization, and the volume of material is often daunting. In this edition we have tried to include developments from the last few years without becoming overwhelmed by minutiae. Where guidelines are available we have included them in the further reading section, so that more detail can be found if required. In addition we have included some of the more recent review papers written in the major journals. The practice exam questions should be enjoyable as well as testing, and we hope that this book will serve students well as a revision guide from the start of their studies to the end.

Oliver A. Leach and Gijs I. van Boxel

Faculty Advisor

The *Crash Course in General Medicine* is an invaluable revision aid for students approaching their final medical exams. The rate of change in modern medicine is staggering and to keep up to date with all aspects of such changes is virtually impossible. This 4th edition, like earlier versions, provides a concise account of a broad range of general medicine from the salient features of history taking and clinical examination to investigations and further management. Useful links to current national guidelines allow readers to ensure their knowledge is as complete as possible. *Crash Course* will also be of great help to junior doctors in their first years of clinical practice leading up to preparation for higher professional exams.

Richard Makins

Acknowledgements

First and foremost we would like to thank Richard for his guidance, expertise and patience in the preparation of this fourth edition. We could not have asked for a better faculty advisor. We would like to thank all the staff at Elsevier in the preparation of the manuscript, in particular Andrew, Helen and Nicola. We are grateful to Dan for giving us the opportunity to be part of the institution that is the Crash Course series.

I would like to thank Dr Paul Dennis and Dr Tim Lancaster for all their educational hard work; this is a product of their passion for teaching medicine. Thank you to Magdalen College Oxford, and in particularly Mr Simon Kreckler. Dr Mark Pobjoy and Louise Robson, for their faith and support in my role as a tutor. Lastly, I would like to thank my students, past and present, for keeping me on my toes. It is said the best way to learn material is to teach it. This has certainly been the case for me; the atrial waveform will haunt me for life.

Gijs I. van Boxel

Firstly, thanks to Tom for thinking of me for the Crash Course review, without which I would not have had this opportunity. I would also like to thank Dr Jane Norman for offering her expert advice on the haematology chapter. Finally, thanks to all those teachers and students who over the past few years have provided advice, inspiration, and challenge.

Oliver A. Leach

Dedication

Thanks to Rose for putting up with me during the writing of this edition.

Thanks to my parents who have been a great source of help and advice.

Oliver A. Leach

Thanks to my wonderful wife for her patience, love and guidance.

Thanks to my Pa, Ma and Jojo without whom I would never have been in this position.

Last, but by no means least, thank you Otto for your relentless persistence in trying to stop me from finishing this project.

Gijs I. van Boxel

Contents

Series editor foreword . . . v
Prefaces . . . vii
Acknowledgements . . . ix
Dedication . . . xi

1. Taking a history . . . 1
General principles: the bedside manner . . . 1
The history . . . 1
Presenting complaint (PC) . . . 2
History of the presenting complaint (HPC) . . . 2
Past medical history . . . 2
Medications and allergies (DHX) . . . 2
Family history (FHX) . . . 3
Social history (SHX) . . . 3
Systems review . . . 3
Conclusion of history taking . . . 9

2. Examination of the patient . . . 11
Introduction . . . 11
First things first . . . 11
Visual survey . . . 11
The face and body habitus . . . 12
The hands . . . 13
The cardiovascular system . . . 14
The respiratory system . . . 17
The abdomen . . . 18
The nervous system . . . 22
The limbs . . . 27
The joints . . . 29
The skin . . . 30
Lymphadenopathy . . . 31
Breast examination . . . 31
Neck examination . . . 31

3. The clerking . . . 33
Introduction . . . 33
Medical sample clerking . . . 34

4. Chest pain . . . 37
Introduction . . . 37
Differential diagnosis of chest pain . . . 37
History in the patient with chest pain . . . 37
Examining the patient with chest pain . . . 38
Investigating the patient with chest pain . . . 39

5. Shortness of breath . . . 43
Introduction . . . 43
History in the patient with breathlessness . . . 43
Examining the patient with breathlessness . . . 44
Investigating the patient with breathlessness . . . 46

6. Palpitations . . . 49
Introduction . . . 49
Differential diagnosis by description of the rhythm . . . 49
History . . . 49
Consequences of palpitations . . . 50
Examining the patient with palpitations . . . 50
Investigating the patient with palpitations . . . 51

7. Cough and haemoptysis . . . 53
Introduction . . . 53
Differential diagnosis of cough and/or haemoptysis . . . 53
History in the patient with cough and haemoptysis . . . 53
Examining the patient with cough and haemoptysis . . . 54
Investigating the patient with cough and haemoptysis . . . 54

8. Pyrexia of unknown origin . . . 57
Introduction . . . 57
Causes of PUO . . . 57
History in the patient with PUO . . . 57
Examining the patient with PUO . . . 57
Investigating the patient with PUO . . . 58

9. Dyspepsia . . . 61
Introduction . . . 61
Causes of dyspepsia . . . 61
History and examination in the patient with dyspepsia . . . 61
Investigating the patient with dyspepsia . . . 61

10. Haematemesis and melaena 65
Introduction 65
Differential diagnosis of haematemesis and melaena 65
History in the patient with haematemesis and melaena 65
Examining the patient with haematemesis and melaena 65
Investigating the patient with haematemesis and melaena 67

11. Change in bowel habit 71
Introduction 71
Differential diagnosis of a change in bowel habit 71
History in the patient with a change in bowel habit 71
Examining the patient with a change in bowel habit 71
Investigating the patient with a change in bowel habit 72

12. Weight loss 75
Introduction 75
Differential diagnosis of weight loss 75
History in the patient with weight loss . . . 75
Examining the patient with weight loss . . 76
Investigating the patient with weight loss . 77

13. Jaundice 79
Introduction 79
Differential diagnosis of jaundice 79
History in the patient with jaundice 79
Examining the patient with jaundice 79
Investigating the patient with jaundice . . . 81

14. Abdominal pain 85
Introduction 85
Differential diagnosis of abdominal pain . . 85
History in the patient with abdominal pain . .85
Examining the patient with abdominal pain . .87
Investigating the patient with abdominal pain 88

15. Urinary symptoms 91
Introduction 91
Differential diagnosis of urinary symptoms . .91
History in the patient with urinary symptoms 91
Examining the patient with urinary symptoms 93
Investigating the patient with urinary symptoms 93

16. Haematuria and proteinuria 97
Introduction 97
Differential diagnosis of haematuria and proteinuria 97
History in the patient with haematuria and proteinuria 98
Examining the patient with haematuria and proteinuria 99
Investigating the patient with haematuria and proteinuria 99

17. Hypertension 103
Introduction 103
Differential diagnosis of hypertension 103
History in the patient with hypertension . .103
Examining the patient with hypertension. .104
Investigating the patient with hypertension 104
Management of the hypertensive patient. . 106

18. Headache and facial pain. 109
Introduction 109
Differential diagnosis of headache and facial pain 109
History in the patient with headache and facial pain 109
Examining the patient with headache and facial pain 111
Investigating the patient with headache and facial pain 112

19. Joint disease 115
Differential diagnosis of joint disease . . .115
History in the patient with joint disease . .115
Examining the patient with joint disease . .116
Investigating the patient with joint disease 118

20. Back pain 121
Introduction 121
Differential diagnosis of back pain. 121
History in the patient with back pain . . .121
Examining the patient with back pain . . .123
Investigating the patient with back pain . .123

21. Skin lesions and rash. 125
Differential diagnosis by appearance. . . . 125
History in the patient with skin rashes . . . 127
Examining the patient with a skin rash. . . 128
Investigating the patient with skin rashes. . 129

22. Loss of consciousness 131
Introduction 131
Differential diagnosis of loss of consciousness. 131
History in the patient with loss of consciousness. 131
Examining the patient with loss of consciousness. 133
Investigating the patient with loss of consciousness. 134

23. Confusional states 137
Introduction 137
Differential diagnosis of confusional state 137
History in the confused patient 137
Examining the confused patient 139
Investigating the confused patient. 140

24. Stroke and transient ischaemic attack . . . 141
Introduction 141
Differential diagnosis of stroke 141
History in the stroke patient 141
Examining the stroke patient 141
Investigating the stroke patient 143

25. Lymphadenopathy and splenomegaly . . . 147
Introduction 147
Differential diagnosis of lymphadenopathy and splenomegaly . . . 147
History in the patient with lymphadenopathy or splenomegaly . . . 148
Examining the patient with lymphadenopathy or splenomegaly . . . 149
Investigating the patient with lymphadenopathy or splenomegaly . . . 150

26. Sensory and motor neurological deficits 153
Introduction 153
Differential diagnosis of sensory and/or motor neurological deficits. 153
History in the patient with sensory and/or motor neurological deficits. 153
Examining the patient with sensory and/or motor neurological deficits. 156
Investigating the patient with sensory and/or motor neurological deficits 159

27. Vertigo and dizziness 161
Introduction 161
Differential diagnosis in the patient with vertigo or dizziness 161
History in the patient with vertigo. 161
Examining the patient with vertigo 162
Investigating the patient with vertigo . . . 163

28. Excessive bruising and bleeding 165
Introduction 165
Differential diagnosis of bruising and bleeding 165
History in the patient with bruising and bleeding 166
Examining the patient with bruising and bleeding 167
Investigating the patient with bruising and bleeding 167

29. Anaemia 171
Introduction 171
Differential diagnosis of anaemia 171
History in the anaemic patient 171
Examining the anaemic patient 173
Investigating the anaemic patient 174

30. Cardiovascular system 179
Ischaemic heart disease. 179
Acute coronary syndromes 183
ST-segment elevation myocardial infarction (STEMI) 184
Non-ST-segment elevation myocardial infarction and unstable angina 186
Arrhythmias 190
Heart failure 196
Hypertension 200
Valvular heart disease and heart murmurs 204
Miscellaneous cardiovascular conditions 209

31. Respiratory disease 217
Respiratory failure 217
Asthma 219
Chronic obstructive pulmonary disease . . 221

Pneumonia 226
Pulmonary embolism 228
Lung cancer 229
Tuberculosis 232
Pneumothorax 235
Pleural effusion 237
Cystic fibrosis 238
Bronchiectasis 239
Interstitial lung diseases 239
Hypoventilation syndromes and sleep-related respiratory disorders 241
Acute respiratory distress syndrome 242

32. Gastrointestinal and liver disease 245
Oesophageal disorders 245
Gastroduodenal disorders 247
Small bowel disorders 250
Inflammatory bowel disease 252
Colorectal disease 256
Infective enteritis 259
Irritable bowel syndrome and non-ulcer dyspepsia 260
Diseases of the gallbladder 261
Diseases of the pancreas 262
Diseases of the liver 265

33. Genitourinary disease 273
Acute kidney injury 273
Chronic kidney disease 275
Glomerular disease 278
Urinary tract infections 281
Renal calculi 282
Urinary tract malignancies 283
Miscellaneous conditions 284
Fluid and electrolyte balance 284

34. Central nervous system 289
Cerebrovascular disease 289
Headache syndromes 293
Movement disorders 295
Multiple sclerosis 298
Central nervous system infection 300
Epilepsy 302
Intracranial tumours 306
Disorders affecting muscle and the neuromuscular junction 307
Disorders of the peripheral nerves 309
Disorders of the spinal cord 310
Miscellaneous neurological disorders 311
Dementia 312

35. Metabolic and endocrine disorders 313
Diabetes mellitus 313
Obesity and metabolic syndrome 320
Thyroid disorders 321
Lipid disorders 326
Metabolic bone disease 328
Hypercalcaemia 332
Hyperparathyroidism 332
Hypoparathyroidism 334
Pituitary disorders 335
Disorders of the adrenal glands 339
Miscellaneous endocrine conditions 343

36. Musculoskeletal and skin disorders 345
Rheumatoid arthritis 345
Osteoarthritis 348
Spondyloarthropathies 349
Crystal arthropathy 351
Systemic lupus erythematosus 352
Antiphospholipid syndrome 354
Polymyalgia rheumatica and giant cell arteritis 354
Vasculitis 356
Other connective tissue disorders 357
Skin disease 360
Skin manifestations of systemic disease . . 364
Skin tumours 365
Skin infection 365

37. Haematological disorders 367
Anaemia 367
Myelodysplastic syndromes 375
Leukaemia 375
Multiple myeloma 379
Lymphoma 380
Myeloproliferative disease 383
Bleeding disorders 384
Disseminated intravascular coagulation . . 386
Thrombotic disorders and thromboembolism 386
Thrombotic thrombocytopenic purpura and haemolytic uraemic syndrome 388

38. Infectious diseases. 391
Introduction 391
HIV and AIDS 391
Malaria .396
Drug-resistant bacteria 398

39. Drug overdose and abuse 399
Epidemiology 399
Aetiology 399
Presentation 399
Investigations 401
Management 401
Illegal drugs 402
Alcohol misuse and withdrawal 402

Self-assessment 405
Single best answer questions (SBAs) 407
Extended-matching questions (EMQs). 419
SBA answers. 429
EMQ answers 439
Index 443

Taking a history

Objectives

The key learning points for this chapter:

- Take a history from a patient.
- Use open questions initially, followed by more specific questions based on your developing differential diagnosis.
- Ask relevant questions for each organ system.

GENERAL PRINCIPLES: THE BEDSIDE MANNER

Medical students are often told that '90% of the diagnosis is in the history'. Although there is a large amount of truth in this statement, this is only the case if your history-taking skills are accurate and relevant. This, in turn, is largely dependent on your bedside manner and the ability to build up a good rapport with your patient. There is no easy recipe for developing a good bedside manner but courtesy, patience and letting the patient express their ideas, concerns and expectations are essential ingredients. The mnemonic 'PEAS' (Pause, Empathize, Acknowledge, Summarize) can be used to remember the basis of good communication.

Whenever you meet a patient, introduce yourself politely and do not forget relatives or friends who may also be present. Try to put the patient at ease, as visiting the doctor is very stressful for most people, particularly if they think that they have a serious illness. If you cannot speak the same language, try to get an interpreter. If a patient has hearing difficulties, sit closer, write things down or speak louder!

The aims of the history are as follows:

- To establish rapport with the patient.
- To obtain an accurate, sequential account of the patient's symptoms through open questions and create a differential diagnosis.
- To ask specific questions to focus on the most likely diagnoses.
- To determine risk factors for these possible diagnoses.
- To put this problem or problems into the context of the patient's life.

This chapter provides a framework for taking a comprehensive history. However, the important thing is that you develop an approach with which you are comfortable and then practise it again and again. In this way you will not miss things out and you will be able to concentrate more on what the patient is telling you rather than what comes next. With experience you will recognize patterns and explore different avenues in the history.

Make sure not to miss out on non-verbal clues, as facial expression and body posture can sometimes tell you more than the words themselves. If you are looking up, they will also feel that you are genuinely listening to what they are saying. It is important to strike a good balance between recording the history accurately and maintaining eye contact.

As a general principle, start the consultation by asking very open-ended questions, such as 'How are you?' or 'What symptoms have made you come to the clinic today?' This gives the patient the opportunity to say what they want. Then ask more specific questions to clarify important aspects.

Try to take the history and then write it down afterwards; it enables you to listen and appear to be listening without distraction, plus you can organize your thoughts before committing them to paper. However, when you are learning it may be easier to make notes as you go along; you can also have prompts on your paper to enable you to fill in all sections. As you gain experience, you will find it easier to memorize the patient's history and write it down later.

THE HISTORY

At the start of every history you should always:

- Document the date, time and place of consultation. This should be done on both sides and each subsequent sheet of paper. (Remember that the clerking is a legal document.)
- Record the age, sex and occupation of the patient.

- Document who referred the patient and if they were seen as an emergency.
- Document your name, grade and role (e.g. CT1 van Boxel, Gen Surg SHO on call)

PRESENTING COMPLAINT (PC)

This is a sentence or short list explaining the reason the patient has seen you today. Resist the temptation to write the entire history in this section, particularly when there are multiple symptoms; however, mentioning an obvious background condition can be helpful (e.g. 'One week increasing shortness of breath and productive cough. Background: 10-year history of COPD').

HISTORY OF THE PRESENTING COMPLAINT (HPC)

This is where the presenting complaint is explored in great detail. It is impossible to describe a system that will work for all complaints in every situation. You will need to develop your own techniques, likes and dislikes. Inadequate relevant detail in this section is the commonest problem in medical student histories:

- Aim to obtain a coherent, sequential chronological description of the events leading to the consultation.
- Ask the relevant questions to the symptoms (e.g. for pain, 'Where is it?', 'What is its character?')
- Keep the differential diagnoses for a symptom in your mind and seek evidence to confirm or refute them.
- Use the review of symptoms questions for the system you suspect to fill in extra detail (e.g. if the complaint is a cough, ask about dyspnoea, pain, sputum, etc., and record it in the presenting complaint).
- Ask about the relevant risk factors (e.g. if pulmonary embolus is suspected ask about immobility, travel, etc.).
- Recapitulate the history back to the patient, as this helps cement the story in your mind and reassures the patient that you are listening.
- If the history is long, or vague, using the opening question 'So when did you last feel well?' gives a platform to begin from.
- Seek collateral history from witnesses, friends or family where necessary (e.g. after a seizure). It is always worth asking the patient first whether they mind you speaking to family or friends.
- With chronic complaints, it is vital to ask about how the symptoms are affecting the patient's life.
- Document relevant negative findings (e.g. headache, but no photophobia or neck stiffness).

Finally, ask if they have any thoughts or worries as to what the diagnosis might be; this can be very enlightening and will help you build a good working relationship as you will be addressing their concerns. What the doctor is interested in and what the patient is interested in can be diametrically different.

HINTS AND TIPS

If the patient presents with pain, the SOCRATES principle is a useful framework for remembering to ask all the relevant information: Site, Onset, Character, Radiation, Associated features, Timing, Exacerbating/relieving factors, Severity.

PAST MEDICAL HISTORY

Ask the patient if they have had any previous operations or medical problems. It is prudent to probe a little about each illness and how the diagnosis was made. Lists of past history are commonly and sometimes wrongly carried forward from one hospital visit to the next. Record the history in chronological order and, where possible, record the year, hospital and consultant involved for each episode. Many patients may forget past illnesses, particularly if anxious, and it is worth developing a routine to ask them specifically about diabetes, hypertension, angina or heart disease, rheumatic fever, tuberculosis, epilepsy, asthma/emphysema/bronchitis, jaundice, stroke or transient ischaemic attacks.

HINTS AND TIPS

MJTHREADS is a useful mnemonic for remembering to ask about specific medical conditions: Myocardial infarction, Jaundice, Tuberculosis, Hypertension, Rheumatic fever, Epilepsy, Asthma, Diabetes, Stroke.

MEDICATIONS AND ALLERGIES (DHX)

Record which medications the patient is currently taking, how often and at what dose. If the prescribed medications are not being taken, ask why. Ask if there have been any recent changes in medication. Always ask what drugs the patient has taken in the past. For example, a patient with pulmonary fibrosis as a consequence of amiodarone may well have stopped taking it years before! Finally, ask about any non-prescription medications that may be obtained from a chemist or health food shop.

Does the patient have any allergies to any medications or anything else at all, no matter how trivial? If yes, what was the exact nature of the reaction? Was it anaphylaxis or did they experience a rash? It is worth asking about penicillin directly as many patients state they have a penicillin allergy but on closer questioning, they may describe a non-specific symptom and a beta-lactam antibiotic can be given safely if the need is there.

If the patient says they have no allergies it is traditional to write 'No known drug allergies' (NKDA).

FAMILY HISTORY (FHX)

Do any diseases 'run' in the patient's family – in particular ischaemic heart disease, cancer, diabetes and autoimmune disorders? Record illnesses in close relatives, including age of death where relevant. Generally speaking, family members affected before the age of 60 are deemed to be relevant. Drawing a family tree can be helpful in some patients.

SOCIAL HISTORY (SHX)

The importance of this part of the history is to establish how the illness affects the patient's life and how they are coping at home. Ask about:

- Who is at home? If they have a partner, are they fit and well?
- What is the home like? If the patient is elderly, is there a warden?
- If the patient is disabled, have appropriate modifications been made?
- Do they need help with daily tasks, such as washing, dressing, feeding, cleaning or shopping?
- Do they have dependent children? Who is looking after them at the moment?
- Is there a nearby relative who helps or does the patient have meals-on-wheels, a home help or a district nurse?
- What is their occupation? Details of their past and present occupation can be important (e.g. industrial lung disease).
- Are they still able to work despite the current problem?
- Some diagnoses can be particularly important in relation to work, such as heavy goods vehicle drivers and epilepsy.
- Do they, or did they, smoke? Smoking is a significant cause of many diseases. Record smoking in pack/years
- Alcohol past and present. Record as units per week (Fig. 1.1).

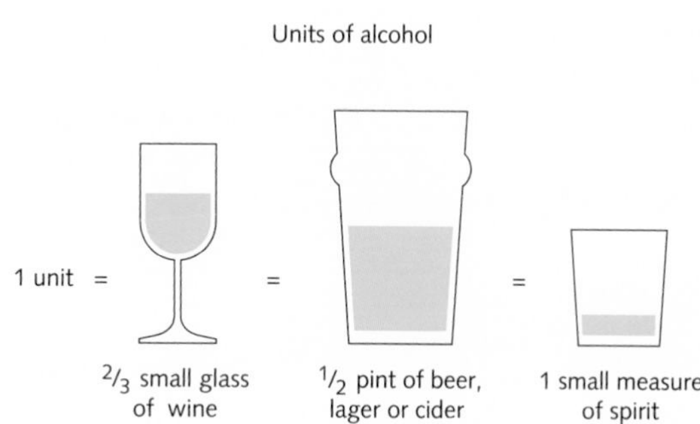

Fig. 1.1 Units of alcohol. These refer to a standard pub measure of wine (12% alcohol by volume), a small pub measure of spirits (40% alcohol by volume) and standard strength beer (3–4% alcohol by volume). An easy way to work out the units for a drink is to remember that the alcohol percentage is equivalent to the number of units in one litre of the drink (e.g. a litre of 40% whiskey contains 40 units and a 330-mL bottle of 6% lager contains 2 units).

- Do they use 'recreational' drugs? These have health, social and financial implications.
- Have they recently been abroad? They may have been exposed to different infective agents.
- Do they have pets (particularly budgerigars, pigeons and parrots)?
- Sexual history is not appropriate in every history but may be important (e.g. for hepatitis or human immunodeficiency virus (HIV)).

SYSTEMS REVIEW

Patients occasionally focus on one minor symptom while omitting to tell you of another more significant symptom. In fact, this can be a deliberate act, asking the doctor to deal with a simple problem (e.g. sore throat) while deciding whether to ask for help with the real worry such as impotence or rectal bleeding. Performing a quick systems review will prevent you from missing other important diseases.

Alternatively, if the symptoms are multiple and non-specific, a review of systems can shine light on the consultation and aid a differential diagnosis.

The symptoms to ask about in each system are outlined below. This list cannot be exhaustive and some symptoms are repeated as they cross organ systems though with different emphasis.

General symptoms

Fatigue

This is a non-specific symptom that can accompany many organic as well as psychiatric diseases. Look particularly for evidence of anaemia or hypothyroidism.

Appetite

Anorexia is a feature of many diseases, again organic and psychiatric; increased appetite despite weight loss is seen in hyperthyroidism. Distinguish between reduced appetite, nausea or dysphagia

Weight change

Weight loss can be deliberate (dieting) or due to chronic disease. The causes are discussed in detail in Ch. 12.

Weight gain is seen in pregnancy, hypothyroidism, Cushing's syndrome, polycystic ovarian disease and 'comfort eating' due to anxiety or depression.

Sweats

Drenching sweats occurring at night are seen in lymphoma, chronic leukaemia and tuberculosis. This is commonly referred to as B-symptoms (and addition to weight loss and fever).

Pruritus (itching)

Pruritus can be due to local skin disease or systemic disease, as shown in Fig. 1.2.

Sleep pattern

If there is difficulty in sleeping, ask if the problem is in going to sleep or in waking early. Difficulty in getting off to sleep is often due to worry or anxiety, whereas early morning wakening is a feature of depression. Sleep apnoea is common and can be debilitating as hypersomnolence limits daytime function. The commonest medical condition affecting sleep is obstructive sleep apnoea (see Ch. 30). Ask about snoring, whether sleep is refreshing, morning headaches and restless leg movements. The patient's partner is often the best source of information.

Fig. 1.2 Causes of pruritus.

Cause	Examples
Skin disease	Scabies, eczema, lichen planus, urticaria, dry skin (elderly, hypothyroidism)
Systemic disease	Hepatic (biliary obstruction, pregnancy) Malignancy (particularly lymphoma) Haematological (polycythaemia, iron deficiency) Chronic renal failure Drugs (sensitivity, opiates) Endocrine (diabetes mellitus, hyper/ hypothyroidism, carcinoid syndrome) Parasitic (trichinosis) Neurological (multiple sclerosis) Psychogenic

Cardiovascular symptoms

Chest pain

Establish the site, radiation, character, exacerbating and relieving factors, and severity; discussed in detail in Ch. 4.

Shortness of breath (dyspnoea) and exercise tolerance

Exertional dyspnoea can be due to poor left ventricular function, pulmonary oedema, arrhythmia or valvular disease (see Ch. 30).

Orthopnoea is breathlessness on lying flat, usually from increased pulmonary venous congestion. This symptom can be present in diaphragm palsy and even in chronic obstructive pulmonary disease, as diaphragmatic input to ventilation is less efficient when the patient is lying flat.

Paroxysmal nocturnal dyspnoea (PND) is waking during the night due to severe breathlessness (pulmonary oedema).

Sudden onset of breathlessness, irrespective of body position or exercise, is often due to arrhythmia, pneumothorax or pulmonary embolism (see Ch. 5).

Taking a relevant exercise tolerance history is important. Ask the patient whether they can walk up a set of stairs (in one go, without being out of breath once upstairs) and how far they can walk on the flat. Remember that joint problems may be the limiting factor rather than cardiorespiratory reserve.

Blackouts (syncope)

Syncope is the transient loss of consciousness and motor tone, which may be due to arrhythmia, valvular heart disease, postural hypotension or vertebrobasilar insufficiency (see Ch. 22).

Palpitations

Palpitations mean different things to different people and they should be explored carefully as they may be insignificant or they may be life-threatening. Most commonly they refer to awareness of one's heart beating (see Ch. 6).

Ankle and calf swelling

This can be due to right ventricular failure, low plasma oncotic pressure (e.g. decreased albumin levels) or drugs (e.g. calcium channel blockers), or it can be gravitational.

Calf swelling can be due to:

- Deep vein thrombosis: recent travel, immobility or surgery, pregnancy, combined oral contraceptive pill, family history, malignancy.
- Ruptured Baker's cyst: in the elderly, secondary to osteoarthritis of the knee.

- Muscle trauma.
- Cellulitis.
- Tumour: sarcoma (rare).

Calf, thigh or buttock pain on exertion (claudication)

Intermittent claudication due to peripheral vascular disease causes calf, thigh or buttock pain on exercise. The amount of exercise required to cause pain tends to be consistent although it often deteriorates slowly. It is relieved within a predictable period of time on rest.

Spinal claudication due to spinal stenosis also causes calf, thigh or buttock pain on exertion, possibly by causing occlusion of the spinal arteries. However, the claudication distance tends to be variable.

Respiratory symptoms

Dyspnoea

Clarify the degree of dyspnoea and its consequences for everyday tasks; try and separate respiratory dyspnoea from cardiac causes though there is much overlap (see Ch. 5).

Cough

The causes of cough are multiple. Associated features will help in developing a sensible differential diagnosis (see Ch. 7).

Sputum

How much sputum is produced? Ask about its colour, texture and time course:

- Yellow/green: usually infection, acute asthma (due to eosinophils).
- Frothy: pulmonary oedema.
- Rusty: lobar pneumonia (pneumococcal).
- Blood: pulmonary embolism, lung cancer, pneumonia (see Ch. 7).
- Taste: foul in bronchiectasis and abscess.
- Smell: foul in bronchiectasis.

Chest pain

Needs a careful assessment of character, position, timing, precipitating factors, etc. Chest pain is usually pleuritic in respiratory disease (Ch. 4) and is potentially due to pneumonia, pneumothorax or pulmonary embolus.

Wheeze

Patients with airways obstruction sometimes notice an audible expiratory wheeze.

Hoarse voice

This may be caused, for example, by recurrent laryngeal nerve palsy in bronchial carcinoma.

Gastrointestinal disease

Abdominal pain

Establish the site, radiation, character, exacerbating and relieving factors, and severity. This is discussed in detail in Ch. 14.

Dysphagia

Dysphagia means difficulty in swallowing. Ask about:

- The onset and progression of symptoms
- Where do things get stuck? This may give a clue as to the site of the lesion.
- Is there difficulty with solids, fluids or both? Neuromuscular disorders tend to present with dysphagia for fluids at onset, whereas mechanical obstruction results in dysphagia for solids at onset.

The causes of dysphagia are outlined in Fig. 1.3.

Fig. 1.3 Causes of dysphagia.

Disorder	Examples
Oropharyngeal lesions	Pharyngitis, quinsy, lymphoma
Intrinsic oesophageal and gastric lesions	Peptic stricture Carcinoma of oesophagus or gastric fundus Foreign body Oesophageal web (Paterson–Brown–Kelly or Plummer–Vinson syndrome) Infection (*Candida albicans*) Pharyngeal pouch Schatzki's ring (lower oesophageal narrowing) Leiomyoma of oesophageal muscle
Extrinsic oesophageal compression	Goitre with retrosternal extension Intrathoracic tumours (lymphoma, bronchial carcinoma) Enlarged left atrium
Neuromuscular disorders	Achalasia Scleroderma Diffuse oesophageal spasm Diabetes mellitus Myasthenia gravis Myotonia dystrophica Bulbar or pseudobulbar palsy, e.g. motor neurone disease or stroke Diphtheria
Psychological	Globus hystericus

Nausea and vomiting

What does the vomitus look like?

- Yellow-green: upper gastrointestinal (GI) contents plus bile.
- Brown (faeculant): lower small bowel contents.
- Bright-red blood: active upper GI bleeding (Ch. 10).
- 'Coffee grounds': 'old' upper GI bleeding.

How 'violent' was the vomiting? Projectile vomiting indicates pyloric stenosis, most commonly seen in infants, but may arise as a consequence of duodenal ulceration in adults.

Indigestion

'Heartburn' or 'dyspepsia' is due to reflux of the gastric contents into the oesophagus. Be aware that heartburn can easily be confused with cardiac chest pain. Always explore these symptoms carefully.

Change in bowel habit or stools

Has there been a change? Ask about diarrhoea and constipation, or the presence of one alternating with the other (see Ch. 11).

Is there any rectal bleeding? Is the bleeding with or without mucus? The causes of rectal bleeding are summarized in Fig. 1.4. Anal and rectal lesions result in fresh blood on the outside of the stool, on the paper on wiping, or in the pan. Higher lesions result in blood intermixed with the stool. Melaena implies upper GI bleeding and the passage of altered blood originating proximal to the hepatic flexure.

Inquire about tenesmus. Tenesmus is the painful desire to defecate when there is no stool in the rectum. This is due to a lesion in the lumen or wall of the rectum mimicking faeces.

Jaundice and itch

Jaundice can be insidious or acute and the patient may therefore not have noticed it. Ask family or friends whether they have noticed a change in skin colour. Itching is caused by build-up of bile salts in the skin and is a feature of obstructice jaundice (see Ch. 13). It can be asked about directly and may even be evident on clinical examination through scratch marks. Jaundice may indicate liver impairment and bruising and should therefore be asked about directly as clotting factor biosynthesis may be impaired.

Fig. 1.4 Causes of rectal bleeding.

Haemorrhoids
Anal fissure
Carcinoma (anus, rectum or colon)
Polyps
Diverticulitis (including Meckel's diverticulum) but not diverticulosis
Colitis (infective, ulcerative, Crohn's, ischaemic)
Angiodysplasia

Abdominal swelling

Ask whether the patient has noticed a change to the size of their abdomen (be careful not to offend patients by assuming they have an acutely distended abdomen!). Remember the 7 F's: Foetus, Flatus, Fat, Fluid, Flipping great mass, Faeces and Full bladder.

Genitourinary symptoms

Dysuria

This is discomfort during or after micturition due to urinary tract infection or recent urethral instrumentation (catheter or cystoscope).

Change in urine appearance

What does the urine look like?

- Cloudy: infection, precipitated urates or phosphates.
- Frothy: proteinuria.
- Orange: very concentrated urine, bilirubin, rifampicin.
- Red/smoky: haematuria, haemoglobinuria, myoglobinuria, rifampicin, 'black water fever' due to haemolysis in *Plasmodium falciparum* malaria, eating beetroot.
- Dark on standing: porphyria.
- Green: drugs containing methylene blue (commercial analgesics).

See Ch. 16 for the causes of haematuria and proteinuria.

Frequency and nocturia

Increased frequency of micturition can be due to:

- Bladder irritation: infection, stones, tumour.
- Outflow obstruction: prostatic hypertrophy, urethral stricture.
- Neurological: multiple sclerosis, cauda equina syndrome.

Note that, in polyuria, there is an increased volume of urine as well as frequency of micturition.

Nocturia can be due to any of the causes of polyuria (see Ch. 15) and increased frequency.

Hesitancy

Hesitancy followed by a poor stream with terminal dribbling are features of prostatic enlargement. These symptoms are often associated with benign prostatic hypertrophy, but could indicate carcinoma of the prostate.

Loin pain

This can be associated with renal disease (Ch. 14).

Incontinence

This can be either urge incontinence (e.g. detrusor instability) or stress incontinence (e.g. weak pelvic musculature following childbirth). It can be functional, as people with mobility problems may not be able to get to the loo quickly enough.

Menstruation

Determine the pattern of the normal cycle. Then ask about flow (heavy or light), intermenstrual bleeding, postcoital bleeding or dysmenorrhoea.

Discharge

Vaginal or penile discharge can indicate infection.

Neurological symptoms

Headache

This is a difficult symptom for the doctor, with the diagnosis ranging from the trivial to the fatal. Ask about red flag symptoms (see Ch. 18).

Dizziness

This can also be unsteadiness (Chs 22 and 26).

Blackouts

See Ch. 22.

Visual disturbance

Vision can be affected by lesions of the optic pathway, of the nerves controlling eye movements (third, fourth, sixth) or conjugate gaze.

Altered hearing

Ask about deafness, tinnitus and vertigo (Ch. 27).

Altered smell

Anosmia can result from head injury, nasal polyps, following viral upper respiratory tract infections or frontal lobe tumours.

Speech disturbance

There are three types of disordered speech:

- Dysarthria: difficulty in articulating speech but language content is completely normal.
- Dysphonia: difficulty in voice production.
- Dysphasia: difficulty in understanding or expressing language, caused by lesions affecting the dominant cerebral hemisphere (usually the left).

Fig. 1.5 shows the characteristic speech abnormalities that result from lesions at specific anatomical sites.

Limb weakness, paraesthesiae and sensory loss

These are covered in detail in Ch. 34.

Metabolic and endocrine symptoms

Symptoms associated with metabolic and endocrine problems are varied and multiple – these symptoms are described in detail in Ch. 35. The two most common endocrine conditions to consider and ask about are disorders of the thyroid (Fig. 1.6) and diabetes (Fig. 1.7).

Musculoskeletal symptoms

Weakness

This is covered in detail in Ch. 34.

Pain

Pain can arise in the muscles (Ch. 24), joints (Ch. 19), or bones (Fig. 1.8).

Stiffness

Stiffness, particularly after inactivity (e.g. early morning stiffness), is a feature of inflammation.

Joint swelling

This can be caused by infection, inflammation, blood (haemarthrosis) or crystal deposition.

Disability

How do the symptoms affect lifestyle? This is extremely important in patients with rheumatological diseases.

Skin symptoms

Rash

The distribution may be very helpful in determining the diagnosis (Ch. 21).

Pruritus

For the causes of pruritus, see Fig. 1.2.

Precipitants

Has there been any recent change in detergents, soap, shampoo, etc.?

Fig. 1.5 Causes and features of abnormalities of speech arising from lesions at specific anatomical sites.

Site of lesion	Causes	Features of speech
Dysarthria		
Mouth	Ulcers, macroglossia	Slurred
Lower cranial nerve lesions (9th to 12th)	Bulbar palsy (stroke, poliomyelitis, motor neurone disease, syringobulbia, malignancy)	Nasal quality, slurred Associated features such as dysphagia
Upper cranial nerve lesions (9th to 12th)	Pseudobulbar palsy (stroke, motor neurone disease, multiple sclerosis)	Spastic speech, like 'Donald Duck' Associated features such as dysphagia and emotional lability
Cerebellum	Multiple sclerosis, stroke, tumour, hereditary ataxias, alcohol, hypothyroidism	Scanning ('staccato') speech Flow is broken Syllables explosive
Extrapyramidal	Parkinsonism	Difficulty initiating speech Monotonous and slightly slurred
Toxic	Acute alcohol intoxication	Slurred
Dysphonia		
Neuromuscular junction	Myasthenia gravis	Weak, nasal speech Deteriorates on repetition
Vocal cord disease	Tumour, viral laryngitis, tuberculosis, syphilis	Weak volume, husky quality
Vocal cord paralysis	Recurrent laryngeal nerve palsy (mediastinal carcinoma, intrathoracic surgery or trauma, aortic aneurysm)	Weak volume, husky quality
Dysphasia		
Broca's area (inferior frontal gyrus)	Infarction, bleeding, space-occupying lesion	Expressive dysphasia Comprehension intact Difficulty in finding appropriate words and so speech non-fluent
Wernicke's area (superior temporal gyrus)	Infarction, bleeding, space-occupying lesion	Receptive dysphasia Fluent speech but words are disorganized or unintelligible Comprehension impaired
Frontotemporoparietal lesion	Infarction (left middle cerebral artery), bleeding, space-occupying lesion	Global dysphasia Marked receptive and expressive dysphasia
Posterior part of superior temporal/ inferior parietal lobe	Infarction, bleeding, space-occupying lesion and raised intracranial pressure, dementia	Nominal aphasia Unable to name specific objects Other aspects of speech preserved

Fig. 1.6 Differences in the history between hyperthyroidism and hypothyroidism.

Symptom	Hyperthyroidism	Hypothyroidism
Temperature intolerance	Heat	Cold
Weight	Decreased	Increased
Appetite	Increased	Decreased
Bowel habit	Diarrhoea	Constipation
Psychiatric	Anxiety, irritability	Poor memory, depression
Menstruation	Oligomenorrhoea	Menorrhagia
Others	Palpitations, sweating, eye changes, pretibial myxoedema, acropachy	Dry skin, brittle hair, arthralgia, myalgia

Fig. 1.7 Symptoms of diabetes mellitus.

Mechanism	Symptoms
Due to hyperglycaemia	Polyuria Polydipsia Fatigue Blurred vision Recurrent infections, e.g. *Candida* Weight loss (type I)
Due to complications	Peripheral neuropathy Retinopathy Vascular disease

Haematological symptoms

These can be summarized as follows:

- Symptoms of anaemia: low haemoglobin (Ch. 29).
- Recurrent infections: low white cell count.

Fig. 1.8 Causes of bone pain.

Cause	Example
Tumour	Primary tumour (benign or malignant), metastases
Infection	Osteomyelitis (*Staphylococcus*, *Haemophilus influenzae*, *Salmonella*, tuberculosis)
Fracture	Traumatic, pathological
Metabolic	Paget's disease, osteomalacia

- Bleeding or bruising: low platelets (Ch. 28).
- Any recent glandular swelling?

CONCLUSION OF HISTORY TAKING

The way to become skilled in history taking for both clinical practice and examinations is to try and clerk as many patients as you can with the range of listed presentations. It is important to write these up with a list of diagnoses and a plan, then practise presenting to other people. Then ask yourself how you could do it better next time.

HINTS AND TIPS

At the end of the history ask two questions:

'Is there anything else you are worried about or want to tell me?' It is possible that the patient may now feel ready to tell you about their main concern.

'Is there anything that you are worried this might be?' There is often visible relief when this question is asked and it enables you to address the patient's real feelings about their illness.

HINTS AND TIPS

Good history taking is not easily taught or learnt the night before an examination. It is acquired through experience, lots of it!

HINTS AND TIPS

Be careful not to label a patient's symptoms as 'functional'. All organic causes must be ruled out before making this diagnosis – it is a diagnosis of exclusion.

Examination of the patient

Objectives

The key learning points for this chapter:

- How to perform a thorough physical examination smoothly while being able to focus on the findings.
- The anatomy and pathophysiology underlying physical signs and their interpretation.

INTRODUCTION

When it comes to examining patients, practice really does make perfect. Examiners will be able to tell whether you have examined many patients or not within the first 30 seconds of seeing you in action! Therefore, take every opportunity you have to rehearse your technique. Let others watch you examine and critique. These could be your teachers, fellow students, and even patients can give you valuable feedback.

FIRST THINGS FIRST

There are four essential things you must do whenever you see a patient:

- Introduce yourself, wash your hands, shake hands and explain to the patient what you would like to do and why, thereby obtaining their consent for the examination.
- Ask the patient to move into the position required for the system you are looking at, expose the area concerned and then make sure that the patient is comfortable and that their privacy is respected and modesty maintained.
- Ask the patient if they have any pain. A good phrase to use is 'Are you in any pain currently? If I cause you any discomfort during my examination, please let me know and I will stop immediately'.
- From the moment you first see the patient, try to decide whether they look well or ill. There is plenty of time while an examiner introduces you to the patient, and while the patient undresses and gets on to the couch, for you to gain a lot of information.

You will probably find that all clinical teachers will show you a slightly different format for examination technique. The important thing is to develop an approach that you are comfortable with and then keep practising it until it becomes second nature.

In examinations you will almost always be asked to examine a particular system: 'Examine this gentleman's chest', 'What do you notice about this lady's face?' This chapter describes the technique for each system and how to interpret the clinical signs you will find. Of course, once qualified, you should do a full examination for all your patients.

VISUAL SURVEY

It is accepted practice that all clinical examinations are performed from the right-hand side of the patient. The most important thing is to decide is how well or ill the patient is, as described above. Other specific abnormalities should then be looked for.

Patient position, general behaviour and around the bed

Is the patient comfortable? Are they anxious? Are they breathless? Are they in pain? Can they see? Are they deaf? Can the patient walk? Are there any handy clues around the bed (diabetic drinks, wheelchair, nebulizer, catheter, oxygen, drains)? Taking time to assess these factors has several advantages: it will help you with the diagnosis, it helps to prioritize your approach as a practising clinician, and it will calm your nerves in clinical examinations.

Cyanosis

This is a bluish discoloration which is seen when the absolute concentration of reduced (deoxygenated) haemoglobin in the blood is greater than 5 g/dL. Central cyanosis is seen best in the tongue. It is caused by underlying respiratory or cardiovascular disease. Peripheral cyanosis can be due to either central cyanosis or reduced peripheral circulation, as poorly perfused peripheral tissue will take up oxygen more readily. Remember that a patient with central cyanosis is always peripherally cyanosed, yet peripheral cyanosis can occur in the absence of central cyanosis. Reduced peripheral circulation is seen in shock, cold weather and vascular abnormalities. Cyanosis is seen rarely in anaemia but occurs more readily in polycythaemia.

Very rarely, other forms of reduced haemoglobin, such as methaemoglobin or sulphaemoglobin, can cause cyanosis.

Jaundice

Jaundice is a yellow discoloration of the skin, sclera and mucous membranes due to serum bilirubin concentrations greater than 30 μmol/L, which becomes more obvious at concentrations greater than 50 μmol/L. Jaundice can be due to increased bilirubin production (prehepatic), abnormal bilirubin metabolism in the liver (hepatic) or reduced bilirubin excretion (posthepatic) (see Ch. 13). It is much easier to see in natural as opposed to artificial lighting.

Yellow skin (particularly palms and soles) with normal sclera can be due to carotenaemia (excessive consumption of carrots, or hypothyroidism) or uraemia.

Pallor

Generalized pallor can be racial, inherited (albinism) or due to anaemia, shock, myxoedema or hypopituitarism. Localized pallor is seen in disruption of the arterial supply, as in Raynaud's phenomenon.

Hydration

Signs of dehydration include dry mucous membranes, tachycardia, postural hypotension and reduced skin turgor. If the patient is in hospital, hydration status should be monitored more accurately using urine output, fluid balance charts and central venous pressure (if very ill).

Overhydration can sometimes result from the overenthusiastic administration of IV fluids, particularly in the elderly. Clinical signs include pulmonary or peripheral oedema, raised jugular venous pressure (JVP) and a third heart sound.

Pigmentation

Generalized pigmentation is usually of racial origin but may also arise in haemochromatosis (greyish-bronze), occupational exposure (slate-grey appearance with argyria in silver workers) and with some drugs (slate-grey with amiodarone).

Pigmentation may also be raised with increased ACTH levels, as in Addison's disease, Cushing's disease (ACTH-secreting pituitary tumour), ectopic ACTH production and Nelson's syndrome (following bilateral adrenalectomy for Cushing's disease).

Chronic illness may be associated with pigmentation, common examples being chronic liver disease, chronic uraemia or chronic haemolysis.

As well as Addison's disease, local areas of pigmentation may be seen in Peutz–Jeghers syndrome (brown lesions around the lips) and neurofibromatosis (café au lait patches).

Localized areas of depigmentation, particularly affecting the back of the hand and neck, are seen in vitiligo. It may be associated with other autoimmune diseases.

THE FACE AND BODY HABITUS

Examiners will often take you to a patient and simply ask 'What is the diagnosis in this patient?' or 'What do you notice about this patient's face?' The conditions in Fig. 2.1 are often known as 'spot diagnoses' – they have characteristic physical features and often come up in examinations.

Fig. 2.1 Common 'spot diagnoses'.

Disease	Examples
Endocrine	Hypothyroidism, hyperthyroidism, acromegaly, Cushing's syndrome, Addison's disease
Metabolic	Paget's disease, chronic liver disease, uraemia/stigmata of dialysis
Neuromuscular	Parkinson's disease, myotonia dystrophica, facial nerve palsy, Horner's syndrome, ptosis, choreoathetosis
Connective tissue	SLE, scleroderma, Marfan's syndrome, ankylosing spondylitis
Hereditary	Turner's syndrome, Down's syndrome, Klinefelter's syndrome, achondroplasia
Cardiovascular	Mitral facies Cyanotic congenital heart disease
Physiological	Chloasma of pregnancy
Haematological	Thalassaemia
Infection	Congenital syphilis
Dermatology	Pigmentation, purpura, psoriasis, neurofibromatosis, Osler–Weber–Rendu disease (hereditary haemorrhagic telangiectasia) herpes zoster, pemphigoid/pemphigus, necrobiosis lipoidica diabeticorum

All these 'spot diagnoses' have characteristic physical signs. SLE, systemic lupus erythematosus.

THE HANDS

The hands can provide a wealth of information for the alert clinician. When you are asked to examine the hands, consider the normal structures present and examine them in turn. Where appropriate, go on to examine the functional use of the hand (e.g. undoing a button or picking up a pen). This is particularly important in neurological abnormalities and destructive arthritides (e.g. rheumatoid arthritis).

Hands

- Blue: peripheral cyanosis.
- Pallor: anaemia (skin creases) and Raynaud's phenomenon.
- Pigmentation: Addison's disease (skin creases).
- Depigmentation: vitiligo.
- Palmar erythema (Fig. 2.2).

Nail

- Koilonychia: spoon-shaped nails seen in iron deficiency.
- Leuconychia: white nails due to hypoalbuminaemia (Fig. 2.3).
- Clubbing: loss of the nail bed angle. The causes are shown in Fig. 2.4.
- Splinter haemorrhages: terminal lesions usually due to trauma, proximal lesions found in infective endocarditis and vasculitis.
- Quincke's sign: capillary pulsation in the nail bed due to aortic regurgitation.
- Beau's lines: horizontal grooves in the nails caused by temporary arrest of nail growth as a result of acute severe illness.
- Onycholysis: separation of the nail from the nail bed as a result of psoriasis, trauma, fungal infection and hyperthyroidism.
- Yellow nails: yellow nail syndrome with lymphatic hypoplasia (peripheral oedema and pleural effusions).

Fig. 2.2 Causes of palmar erythema.

Causes	Examples
Physiological	Pregnancy Puberty Familial
Pathological	Chronic liver disease Rheumatoid arthritis Thyrotoxicosis Oral contraceptive pill Polycythaemia

Fig. 2.3 Causes of hypoalbuminaemia.

Causes	Examples
Reduced intake	Malnutrition
Reduced synthesis	Liver disease
Increased utilization	Chronic illness
Increased loss	Nephrotic syndrome (kidneys) Protein-losing enteropathy (gut) Severe burns (skin)

- Half-and-half nails: the proximal nail is white and the distal nail is brown or red as a result of chronic renal failure.

Tendons

- Xanthomata: hypercholesterolaemia.
- Dupuytren's contractures (thickening of the palmar fascia): associated with alcoholic liver disease, epileptics treated with phenytoin, vibrating tools and familial and idiopathic causes.

Joints

- Destructive arthropathy: e.g. rheumatoid arthritis.
- Heberden's nodes: osteophytes of the distal interphalangeal joints.
- Bouchard's nodes: osteophytes of the proximal interphalangeal joints.

Neuromuscular

- Localized wasting: ulnar or median nerve lesions.
- Generalized wasting: C8/T1 anterior horn cell, nerve root or brachial plexus damage, combined median

Fig. 2.4 Causes of clubbing.

Causes	Examples
Respiratory	Tumour: bronchial carcinoma, mesothelioma Chronic suppuration: abscess, bronchiectasis, empyema Fibrosis: from any cause Vascular: arteriovenous malformation
Cardiovascular	Congenital cyanotic heart disease Subacute bacterial endocarditis Atrial myxoma
Gastrointestinal	Inflammatory bowel disease Lymphoma Cirrhosis
Endocrine	Thyrotoxicosis (acropachy)
Familial	Autosomal dominant

and ulnar nerve damage, disuse atrophy in severe arthritis, profound cachexia.
- Myotonia: failure to relax after voluntary contraction. It is seen in myotonic dystrophy, for instance, after shaking the patient's hand.

Other signs

- Sclerodactyly (tightening of the skin causing tapering of the fingers): look also for calcinosis, Raynaud's phenomenon, oesophageal dysmotility (ask the patient if they have difficulty on swallowing) and telangiectasia – hence CREST syndrome.
- Large hands with doughy swelling: acromegaly (often called spade-like hands).
- Asterixis: a coarse flapping tremor seen when the hand is outstretched with the wrist extended and fingers apart. It is caused by metabolic encephalopathy (e.g. liver failure, carbon dioxide retention, uraemia).
- Action tremor: this is rapid and fine in amplitude. It is worsened by holding the hands in a particular posture (e.g. hands outstretched) or by movement. It is characteristic of benign essential tremor, thyrotoxicosis and excessive caffeine intake and is an exaggeration of physiological tremor.
- Resting tremor: the thumb moves across the tips of the fingers. This 'pill-rolling' tremor is worst at rest and is characteristic of parkinsonism.
- Intention tremor: this is absent at rest, present on maintaining a posture and exaggerated by movement. It is characteristic of disorders of the cerebellum and its connections.

HINTS AND TIPS

When examining the hands, always look at the elbows for a psoriatic rash, rheumatoid nodules or gouty tophi.

THE CARDIOVASCULAR SYSTEM

General inspection

- Does the patient look well or ill?
- Are they lying flat?
- Are they cachectic (cardiac cachexia)?
- Is there evidence of a congenital syndrome associated with cardiac abnormalities such as Marfan's syndrome or Down's syndrome?

Position

Help the patient to adopt a comfortable position at 45° with the chest exposed. In women, cover the chest until ready to examine the praecordium.

Hands

- Clubbing: subacute bacterial endocarditis (SBE) and congenital cyanotic heart disease.
- Cyanosis: peripheral vasoconstriction, pulmonary oedema and right-to-left shunt.
- Splinter haemorrhages: SBE.
- Janeway's lesions: non-tender macules in the palms due to SBE.
- Osler's nodes: painful nodules on the pulps of the fingers due to SBE.
- Quincke's sign: aortic regurgitation.
- Xanthomata: hypercholesterolaemia (vascular disease).

Radial pulse

- Rate: normally between 60 and 100 bpm (see Ch. 6).
- Rhythm: regular or irregular (see Ch. 6).
- Radioradial delay: dissecting thoracic aortic aneurysm.
- Radiofemoral delay: coarctation of the aorta.
- Character: best determined by palpation of a larger artery (e.g. brachial or carotid arteries).

Blood pressure

- Level: hypertension is a risk factor for vascular disease.
- Lying and standing: postural hypotension.
- Right and left: left may be lower than right in aortic dissection.
- Wide pulse pressure: in the elderly and aortic regurgitation.
- Narrow pulse pressure: aortic stenosis.
- Pulsus paradoxus: exaggerated fall in pulse pressure during inspiration resulting in a faint or absent pulse in inspiration; caused by severe asthma or cardiac tamponade.

Brachial and carotid artery

- Character: collapsing (Fig. 2.5), slow-rising (aortic stenosis), bisferiens (mixed aortic valve disease),

Fig. 2.5 Causes of a collapsing pulse.

Causes	Examples
Physiological	Elderly Pregnancy Exercise
Pathological	Aortic regurgitation Patent ductus arteriosus Fever Thyrotoxicosis Anaemia Arteriovenous shunts

alternans (severe left ventricular failure), jerky (hypertrophic obstructive cardiomyopathy).

- Corrigan's sign: prominent carotid pulsation due to aortic regurgitation.

Jugular venous pressure

When assessing JVP, the patient should be at 45° with their head resting on a pillow (this relaxes the sternocleidomastoid muscles). Pulsation should be up to 3 cm above the sternal angle (8 cm above right atrium). Differences between JVP and carotid pulsation in normal subjects are shown in Fig. 2.6. JVP acts as a manometer for right atrial pressure and is raised when right atrial pressure is raised (Fig. 2.7). Abnormalities in the waveform result from specific underlying pathologies (Fig. 2.8).

Restrictive cardiomyopathy, constrictive pericarditis and pericardial tamponade are all associated with Kussmaul's sign (JVP rises during inspiration).

HINTS AND TIPS

If the JVP is not visible at 45°, try sitting the patient upright, laying the patient flat and eliciting the hepatojugular reflux, as it may be either too high or too low to be seen.

Face

- Central cyanosis: right-to-left shunt.
- Anaemia: possible high-output cardiac failure.
- Malar flush: mitral valve disease.
- Jaundice: haemolysis due to mechanical valves.

Fig. 2.6 Differences between jugular venous pressure and carotid pulsation.

Feature	Carotid pulsation	JVP
Palpable	Yes	No
Number of visible peaks	One	Two
Occlusion by gentle pressure	No	Yes (fills from above)
Sitting upright	No change	Height falls
Lying flat	No change	Height rises
Gentle pressure on liver	No change	Height rises (hepatojugular reflux)
Deep inspiration	No change	Height rises

Fig. 2.7 Causes of a raised jugular venous pressure.

Right ventricular failure
Volume overload (over-enthusiastic IV fluids)
Superior vena caval obstruction (JVP is non-pulsatile)
Tricuspid valve disease (stenosis and regurgitation)
Pericardial effusion causing tamponade
Constrictive pericarditis

- Xanthelasmata: hypercholesterolaemia (vascular disease).
- Mouth: high-arched palate in Marfan's syndrome.
- De Musset's sign: head nodding due to aortic regurgitation.
- Roth's spots in the retina: bacterial endocarditis.

Praecordium

Look for scars and deformities, including:

- Sternotomy scar: arterial bypass grafts and valve replacements.
- Mitral valvotomy scar under the left breast: always look for it, as it indicates a previously closed mitral valvotomy.
- Skeletal deformities: can cause an ejection systolic flow murmur.

Apex beat

The apex beat should be at the mid-clavicular line in the fifth left intercostal space.

- Lateral displacement: left or severe right ventricular dilatation. Lung pathology may also cause displacement.
- Impalpable: obesity, pleural effusion, pericardial effusion, chronic obstructive airways disease and dextrocardia (palpable on the right!).
- Tapping: mitral stenosis (palpable first heart sound).
- Heaving: 'pressure overload' in aortic stenosis or hypertension.
- Thrusting: 'volume overload' in aortic regurgitation, mitral regurgitation (ventricle usually markedly displaced).
- Diffuse: left ventricular dilatation.
- Double impulse: left ventricular aneurysm or hypertrophic cardiomyopathy.

Palpation

Parasternal heave is caused by the enlargement or hypertrophy of the right ventricle.

A thrill is a palpable murmur and indicates significant valve disease; it can be systolic or diastolic and therefore its position in the cardiac cycle should be

Fig. 2.8 Abnormalities of jugular venous waveform.

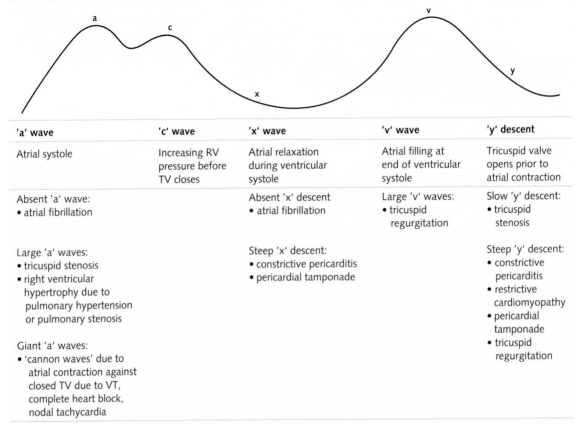

'a' wave	'c' wave	'x' wave	'v' wave	'y' descent
Atrial systole	Increasing RV pressure before TV closes	Atrial relaxation during ventricular systole	Atrial filling at end of ventricular systole	Tricuspid valve opens prior to atrial contraction
Absent 'a' wave: • atrial fibrillation		Absent 'x' descent • atrial fibrillation	Large 'v' waves: • tricuspid regurgitation	Slow 'y' descent: • tricuspid stenosis
Large 'a' waves: • tricuspid stenosis • right ventricular hypertrophy due to pulmonary hypertension or pulmonary stenosis		Steep 'x' descent: • constrictive pericarditis • pericardial tamponade		Steep 'y' descent: • constrictive pericarditis • restrictive cardiomyopathy • pericardial tamponade • tricuspid regurgitation
Giant 'a' waves: • 'cannon waves' due to atrial contraction against closed TV due to VT, complete heart block, nodal tachycardia				

RV, right ventricular; TV, tricuspid valve; VT, ventricular tachycardia.

assessed by timing its relation to a central pulse. Palpate in all valve areas (Fig. 2.9).

Auscultation

- Listen in all four areas with the bell and diaphragm (Fig. 2.9).
- Roll the patient to the left-hand side to listen with the bell at the axilla for mitral stenosis.
- Sit the patient forward to listen with the diaphragm at the left sternal edge in expiration (with breath held) for aortic regurgitation.
- Listen to the first and second sounds, then for third and fourth sounds.
- Are there any murmurs? (See Ch. 30.)
- Listen for additional sounds including opening snap, ejection click, pericardial knock or rub, and mechanical valves.
- Time any abnormalities against the carotid pulsation.
- Listen to the carotid arteries for bruits (atheroma) or radiation of aortic stenotic murmur.

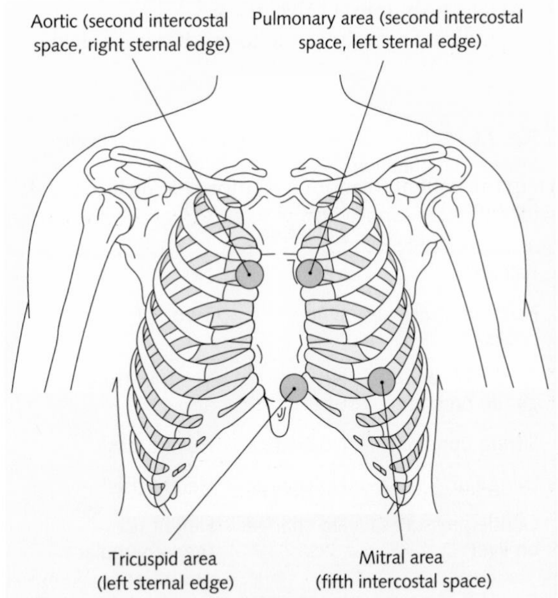

Fig. 2.9 Positions of auscultation of the cardiac valves.

To conclude...

- Examine the lung bases for pulmonary oedema and pleural effusions indicating left ventricular failure.
- Look for sacral oedema.
- Palpate for hepatomegaly, which occurs in right ventricular failure.
- Look for pitting oedema and note the level (e.g. to knees).
- Palpate the peripheral pulses: pulses in the legs may be diminished in peripheral vascular disease. Systolic and diastolic murmurs may be heard in the femoral arteries that are due to aortic regurgitation (pistol shots and Duroziez's sign).
- Full set of observations and ECG.
- Dip the urine for haematuria (endocarditis).

THE RESPIRATORY SYSTEM

Visual survey

- Does the patient look well or ill? Is the patient alert?
- Respiratory rate: normally around 12–16 breaths per min.
- Cachexia: COPD or underlying malignancy.
- Sputum pot: note contents.
- Nebulizer and medications.
- Distress: breathless at rest and moving around in the bed.
- Pursed lip breathing: chronic small airways obstruction.
- Voice: hoarse in bronchial carcinoma (recurrent laryngeal nerve palsy).
- Chest drain and contents.

Position

Help the patient to adopt a comfortable position at 45° with the chest exposed. In women, cover the chest until you are ready to examine it.

Hands

- Clubbing: see Fig. 2.4.
- Cyanosis: respiratory failure.
- Wasting of small muscles: infiltration of T1 by bronchial neoplasm (Pancoast's tumour).
- Tar-stained fingers: increased likelihood of malignancy and obstructive airways disease.
- Asterixis (flap): carbon dioxide retention.
- Evidence of conditions which may involve the lungs (e.g. systemic sclerosis, rheumatoid arthritis) (see Ch. 31).

Pulse

- Tachycardia: severe respiratory disease (e.g. pulmonary embolism, acute asthma or pneumonia).
- Bounding: carbon dioxide retention.
- Atrial fibrillation: e.g. sepsis secondary to pneumonia.

Blood pressure

Pulsus paradoxus is seen in severe acute asthma.

Jugular venous pressure

- Right ventricular failure: chronic respiratory disease with pulmonary hypertension.
- Superior vena caval obstruction: bronchial carcinoma.
- Large 'a' waves: cor pulmonale.

Face

- Central cyanosis: respiratory failure.
- Anaemia: chronic respiratory disease, particularly malignancy.
- Horner's syndrome: apical carcinoma (Pancoast's tumour) involving cervical sympathetic nerves (see Ch. 34).
- Fine tremor: beta-agonists.
- Plethoric facies: secondary polycythaemia.

Trachea

Warn the patient before you palpate the trachea! Note the following:

- Tracheal deviation reflects pathology in the upper mediastinum (Fig. 2.10).
- Feel for tracheal tug in acute respiratory distress.
- The distance from the cricoid cartilage to the suprasternal notch should be 2–3 cm – this distance reduces in hyperinflation.

COMMUNICATION

Always take care to explain what you are doing to the patient when you are examining the trachea. If done badly, it may be uncomfortable, and if you hurt the patient you are likely to fail.

Fig. 2.10 Causes of tracheal deviation.

Towards lesion	Away from lesion
Collapse	Tension pneumothorax
Apical fibrosis	Massive pleural effusion
Pneumonectomy	Large mass (e.g. thyroid)

Thorax

Perform inspection, palpation, percussion and auscultation on the front of the chest first. Then sit the patient forward, palpate for lymphadenopathy and then repeat the examination on the back of the chest. Typical patterns of respiratory abnormalities are shown in Fig. 2.11.

Inspection

On inspecting the chest, assess the following:

- Respiration: use of accessory muscles (respiratory distress).
- Recession: intercostal and subcostal (respiratory distress).
- Scars: including previous surgery and chest drains.
- Deformity: barrel chest (seen in long-standing airways obstruction as a result of hyperinflation), pectus excavatum, pectus carinatum.
- Radiotherapy: tattoos or skin changes indicate previous treatment for malignancy.

Expansion

- Ask the patient to take a deep breath in and note symmetry and comfort.
- The chest circumference should expand by at least 5 cm on deep inspiration.
- Any significant pulmonary disease will reduce expansion.
- In unilateral disease, the affected side will move less than the other.
- Note any chest wall tenderness, which is usually caused by musculoskeletal abnormalities.

Vocal fremitus

Ask the patient to say '99' and palpate with the ulnar border of the hand. Increased vocal fremitus indicates consolidation; decreased indicates pleural effusion or collapse. This part of the examination has been largely superseded by auscultating for vocal resonance.

Percussion

Compare one side with the other and remember the axillae. The following signs are important:

- Hyper-resonance: pneumothorax.
- Dull: solid organ (liver or heart), consolidation, collapse, pleural thickening, peripheral tumours, severe fibrosis, previous old pneumonectomy.
- Stony dull: pleural effusion.

Auscultation

- Normal breath sounds are termed 'vesicular'.
- Bronchial breathing, whispering pectoriloquy, increased vocal resonance: consolidation (sometimes fibrosis and above pleural effusion).
- Wheeze: small airways obstruction (polyphonic), large airway obstruction (e.g. bronchial carcinoma (monophonic or localized)) and cardiac failure.
- Fine crackles: pulmonary fibrosis, pulmonary oedema.
- Coarse crackles: infection.
- Absent breath sounds: pleural effusion.
- Pleural rub: pleural irritation due to pneumonia or pulmonary embolus.

To conclude...

- Pitting oedema indicates right ventricular failure.
- Sputum inspection, peak flow, oxygen saturation, temperature and chest X-ray: these can be remembered by the mnemonic SPOT-X.

HINTS AND TIPS

The upper border of the liver is normally at the 6th intercostal space in the right midclavicular line. If the percussion note remains resonant below this, the lungs are hyperinflated.

THE ABDOMEN

Visual survey

- Appearance: does the patient look well or ill?
- Is the patient in pain?
- Patient's position: think of peritonism if very still, appendicitis (psoas irritation) if knees flexed and renal colic if rolling around in agony.
- Cachexia: chronic disease, particularly malignancy.
- Drowsy: encephalopathy (hepatic or uraemia).
- Hydration status.

Position

The patient can initially be assessed sitting at 45°. For examination of the abdomen itself, the patient should be as flat as can be tolerated comfortably (this relaxes the abdominal muscles). Exposure should be from 'nipples to knees' but bear in mind the patient's dignity.

Hands

- Clubbing: cirrhosis, inflammatory bowel disease.
- Leuconychia: liver failure, nephrotic syndrome, protein-losing enteropathy.

Fig. 2.11 Findings on clinical examination of common respiratory diseases.

Pathology	General signs	Tracheal deviation	Palpation	Percussion note	Breath sounds	Causes
Pneumothorax	Tachycardia and hypotension in tension pneumothorax	Away from affected side if tension	Reduced expansion, reduced TVF	Normal or hyper-resonant	Reduced or absent	Spontaneous (particularly tall healthy males and Marfan's syndrome), trauma, airways obstruction, cystic fibrosis, pulmonary abscess
Consolidation	Pyrexia, tachycardia	None	Reduced expansion, increased TVF	Dull	Increased vocal resonance, whispering pectoriloquy, bronchial breath sounds	Pneumococcus, *Haemophilus influenzae, Staphylococcus aureus, Klebsiella, Pseudomonas, Mycoplasma, Legionella,* influenza type A, *Aspergillus*
Pleural effusion		Away from affected side if large	Reduced expansion, reduced TVF	Stony dull	Absent	Transudate (<30 g/L protein): cardiac failure, liver failure, nephrotic syndrome, Meigs' syndrome, myxoedema Exudate (>30 g/L protein): malignancy, pneumonia, pulmonary embolus, rheumatoid arthritis, SLE, subphrenic abscess, pancreatitis, trauma, Dressler's syndrome
Collapse		Towards affected side	Reduced expansion, reduced TVF	Dull	Reduced or absent	Foreign body or mucous plugs (asthma, aspergillosis) within the bronchial lumen, bronchial carcinoma arising from the bronchus itself, extrinsic compression by enlarged lymph nodes (malignancy, tuberculosis)
Fibrosis	Clubbing	Towards affected side if apical disease	Reduced expansion, increased TVF	Normal or dull	Fine inspiratory crepitations	Cryptogenic fibrosing alveolitis, sarcoidosis, drugs (amiodarone, bleomycin), radiation, inhalation of dusts (asbestos, coal), extrinsic allergic alveolitis, ankylosing spondylitis, rheumatoid arthritis, systemic sclerosis, tuberculosis
Bronchiectasis	Clubbing, purulent sputum	Normal	Normal or reduced expansion, normal or increased TVF	Normal or dull	Coarse inspiratory crepitations, occasional polyphonic wheeze	Congenital (cystic fibrosis, Kartagener's syndrome, hypogammoglobulinaemia), idiopathic, bronchial obstruction (foreign body, carcinoma, lymphadenopathy), infection (childhood measles or whooping cough, tuberculosis, aspergillosis, postpneumonia)
Bronchospasm	Hyperexpanded chest, tremor (if on beta-agonist), Harrison's sulci, pectus carinatum	Normal	Reduced expansion, normal TVF	Normal, hyper-resonant over bullae, reduced liver dullness	Polyphonic wheeze, crepitations in chronic obstructive airways disease	Anaphylaxis

TVF, tactile vocal fremitus.

- Koilonychia: chronic iron deficiency, consider occult neoplasm, particularly in the stomach and caecum.
- Palmar erythema: cirrhosis.
- Asterixis: hepatic encephalopathy and uraemia.
- Dupuytren's contracture: alcoholic liver disease.
- Half-and-half nails: renal failure.

Arms

- Scratch marks: obstructive jaundice (particularly primary biliary cirrhosis) and lymphoma.
- Needle track marks: viral hepatitis.
- Muscle wasting: proximal myopathy due to alcohol, steroid excess or underlying malignancy (paraneoplastic).
- Bruising: hepatic impairment.

Face

- Jaundice: prehepatic, hepatic or posthepatic (see Ch. 13).
- Anaemia: from any cause (see Ch. 29).
- Xanthelasmata: hypercholesterolaemia (primary biliary cirrhosis or nephrotic syndrome).
- Kayser–Fleischer rings: Wilson's disease (best seen by slit-lamp examination).

Mouth

- Hydration.
- Glossitis and stomatitis: iron deficiency and megaloblastic anaemia.
- Pigmentation: Addison's disease, chronic liver disease, chronic renal failure and Peutz–Jeghers syndrome.
- Telangiectasia: hereditary haemorrhagic telangiectasia (Osler–Weber–Rendu disease).
- Crohn's disease: lip swelling and mucosal ulceration.
- Gingival hypertrophy.

Neck

Look for left supraclavicular lymphadenopathy – caused by metastasis from underlying gastrointestinal carcinoma (Virchow's node or Troisier's sign).

HINTS AND TIPS

Always palpate the neck from behind the patient with the neck slightly flexed to relax the sternocleidomastoid muscles.

Trunk and back

Spider naevi arise in the distribution of the superior vena cava – five or more suggest underlying chronic liver disease, pregnancy or hyperthyroidism.

Gynaecomastia and sexual hair loss indicate chronic liver disease.

The abdomen

Inspection

Observe closely, looking for the following:

- Scars: previous surgery or trauma.
- Distension (Fig. 2.12).
- Obvious mass: including movement with respiration.
- Bruising: Cullen's (para-umbilical) and Grey Turner's (flanks) signs in acute pancreatitis (these are rare).
- Dilated veins and caput medusae: portal hypertension or inferior vena cava obstruction (venous flow is upwards).
- Expansile pulsation: abdominal aortic aneurysm.
- Striae: pregnancy or Cushing's syndrome.
- Node: umbilical nodule (Sister Mary Joseph's nodule) is a metastasis from intra-abdominal malignancy.
- Peristalsis: if visible this indicates an obstruction, though it may be normal in a thin or elderly patient.

Palpation

HINTS AND TIPS

Always look at the patient's face when palpating the abdomen to ensure that you know immediately if you are causing discomfort.

Before you touch the patient, ask if they are tender anywhere and start palpation away from that area. Feel gently in each of the four quadrants, noting tenderness

Fig. 2.12 Causes of generalized abdominal swelling.

Cause	Aetiology
Fluid	Ascites
Faeces	Constipation
Fetus	Pregnancy
Flatus	Bowel obstruction
Fat	Obesity
Fibroids	And any other tumour or organomegaly

Fig. 2.13 Features to determine for any mass.

Site
Shape
Size, including upper, lower and lateral limits
Consistency
Tenderness
Fluctuance
Fixation to underlying or overlying structures
Transillumination (where appropriate)
Local lymph node involvement
Bruit

or masses. Then feel more deeply in each quadrant to determine the characteristics of any mass found (Fig. 2.13).

If a mass is present, consider what structures normally lie at that site and what disease processes might affect that structure (see Ch. 14). Next, palpate for hepatomegaly and splenomegaly, starting in the right iliac fossa. Examine for renal masses by bimanual palpation. If hepatomegaly or splenomegaly is present, comment on consistency (smooth or irregular) and size in centimetres (not finger breadths) beneath the costal margin (the causes of hepatomegaly are shown in Fig. 2.14; the causes of splenomegaly are discussed in detail in Ch. 25). A palpable liver must also be assessed for pulsatility (tricuspid regurgitation), tenderness and bruits.

Fig. 2.14 Causes of hepatomegaly.

Cause	Examples
Cirrhosis	Any cause,* particularly primary biliary cirrhosis and haemochromatosis
Tumour	Benign, malignant, primary (hepatocellular carcinoma) and metastases
Venous congestion	Right ventricular failure, Budd–Chiari syndrome, tricuspid disease
Infection	Viral hepatitis,* abscess, syphilis, Weil's disease,* hydatid disease, brucellosis
Cysts	Polycystic disease
Haematological	Lymphoproliferative disease,* myeloproliferative disease*
Metabolic	Storage diseases,* amyloidosis*
Inflammatory	Sarcoidosis*

Remember the 'C's for common causes: Cirrhosis, Carcinoma and Cardiac failure. Note that the liver may appear large in the absence of true hepatomegaly when it is pushed down by a hyperinflated lung (as in acute asthma or chronic obstructive airways disease) and when a Riedel's lobe is present (normal anatomical variation of the right hepatic lobe).
**Denotes the causes of hepatosplenomegaly.*

Fig. 2.15 Causes of unilateral and bilateral palpable kidneys.

Type	Cause
Unilateral	Tumour (hypernephroma, nephroblastoma) Hydronephrosis, pyonephrosis Hypertrophy of single functioning kidney Perinephric abscess or haematoma Polycystic disease (only one kidney palpable)
Bilateral	Polycystic kidneys (autosomal dominant in adults, autosomal recessive in children) Amyloidosis Bilateral hydronephrosis

Do not forget the distinguishing features of the spleen and kidney (see Fig. 25.2); the causes of a renal mass are summarized in Fig. 2.15.

Finally, palpate for abdominal aortic aneurysm and examine the groins for lymphadenopathy and herniae.

Percussion

Always percuss from resonance to dullness. Use percussion to determine the size of the liver and spleen, starting at the chest, moving inferiorly. Percuss over any masses to determine their consistency. Always assess for ascites by looking for a fluid thrill and shifting dullness. Fig. 2.16 summarizes the causes of ascites. Look for tenderness on percussion; this is a useful clinical sign that may indicate peritoneal irritation.

Auscultation

- Bowel sounds may be normal, increased or decreased: increased in bowel obstruction (high-pitched and tinkling) and absent in the ileus (functional motor paralysis of the bowel) of any cause (Fig. 2.17).

Fig. 2.16 Causes of ascites.

Type	Cause
Transudate (protein <25 g/L)	Cardiac failure Liver failure Hypoproteinaemia Meigs' syndrome Myxoedema Constrictive pericarditis (rare) Cirrhosis with portal hypertension
Exudate (protein >25 g/L)	Intra-abdominal malignancy Infection (tuberculosis, perforation, spontaneous) Pancreatitis Budd–Chiari syndrome Lymphatic obstruction (chylous)

Fig. 2.17 Causes of ileus.

Following intra-abdominal surgery where the gut has been handled
Peritonitis
Pancreatitis
Hypokalaemia
Uraemia
Diabetic ketoacidosis
Intra-abdominal haemorrhage
Retroperitoneal haematoma
Retroperitoneal trauma, e.g. surgery for aortic aneurysm
Anticholinergic drugs

- Arterial bruits: may be heard over stenosed vessels such as renal arteries.
- Succussion splash: any cause of gastric outlet obstruction.

To conclude...

- Digital rectal examination often provides useful clinical information and in some circumstances is essential, such as rectal bleeding, iron deficiency or change in bowel habit. Genital examination may also be needed in some circumstances. In the clinical examinations, if you say that you would also like to examine the genitalia and perform a rectal examination, you will usually be taken to the next case.
- If there is hepatosplenomegaly, go on to examine all lymph node sites, bearing in mind the multitude of potential causes (see Ch. 25).
- Look at the legs for pitting oedema (Fig. 2.18).
- Examine hernial orfices.

Fig. 2.18 Causes of lower limb oedema.

Cause	Examples
Pitting	Unilateral: • deep vein thrombosis • unilateral compression of veins (nodes, tumour) Bilateral: • right ventricular failure • tricuspid stenosis • constrictive pericarditis • hepatic failure • nephrotic syndrome • protein-losing enteropathy • inferior vena cava obstruction (thrombosis, nodes, tumour) • immobility • kwashiorkor
Lymphatic (non-pitting)	Obstruction by nodes, tumour or infection (filariasis) Congenital hypoplasia (Milroy's disease) Myxoedema

THE NERVOUS SYSTEM

All medical short case examinations will involve at least one neurology case.

Although it is true that neuroanatomy is complicated and many different diseases can affect each part, the end result is a limited repertoire of patterns of signs. The best approach is to identify which signs are present using a well-rehearsed technique and consider where the lesion is likely to be. You can then think of which diseases affect that part of the nervous system and look for additional evidence to support the diagnosis.

The clinical signs and common diseases associated with different parts of the nervous system are discussed in detail in Ch. 26. This section covers a practical approach to the examination technique itself. It is particularly important to practise this routine over and over again.

Visual survey

- Appearance: does the patient look well or ill?
- Conscious level: is the patient alert, drowsy or unresponsive?
- Age: for instance a young patient is more likely to have multiple sclerosis or an inherited disease; an elderly patient is more likely to have had a stroke.
- General clues: such as the need of a wheelchair or diabetic drinks?
- Posture: how is the patient sitting? Is the patient leaning towards one side (hemiparesis)? Is there a tremor at rest (parkinsonism)?
- Speech: when the patient speaks does the speech sound normal? (See Fig. 1.5.)

Cranial nerves

Features and examinations of the cranial nerves include the following.

First cranial nerve (olfactory)

- Sensory only.
- This is not routinely tested but ask the patient if they have noticed anything abnormal about their sense of smell.
- Sense of smell can be tested using bottles containing essences, although this test is rarely performed. (Note that ammonia should not be used as it also stimulates the trigeminal nerve.)
- Anosmia can result from head injury (fracture of the cribriform plate), upper respiratory tract infection, tumour (olfactory groove meningioma or glioma) or Kallmann's syndrome (anosmia with hypogonadotrophic hypogonadism).

Second cranial nerve (optic)

The order of examination can be remember with AFRO.

- Sensory only.
- Visual **A**cuity: ask the patient to read some print or Snellen's chart (with spectacles if normally worn). Test each eye separately. Any lesion from the cornea, lens, retina, optic nerve, optic chiasm, optic radiation or occipital cortex can result in reduced acuity.
- Visual **F**ields: test each eye individually. Make sure your eyes are on the same level as the patient's. Move your fingers from beyond your visual field inwards and ask the patient to tell you when they can see them. Check each quadrant. Use a red hatpin to determine the blind spot. Typical field defects are shown in Fig. 2.19. Vision can be formally assessed using perimetry. If the visual fields are intact, look for inattention by simultaneously stimulating both the left and right.
- Pupillary **R**eflexes: the pupillary reactions to light and accommodation should be tested. It is essential to understand the sympathetic and parasympathetic innervation of the pupils as well as the neurological pathways involved in the light and convergence reflexes if pupillary abnormalities are to be understood (see *Crash Course: Nervous System*). Pupillary abnormalities in coma patients are described in Fig. 22.5. Other clinical abnormalities include:
  - physiological anisocoria: slight difference in size.
  - senile miosis: small, irregular pupils in old age.
  - total afferent pupillary defect (complete lesion of optic nerve): if for instance the left eye is affected, shining a light in it fails to cause pupillary constriction in either eye – absent direct and consensual reflexes. However, if light is shone in the right eye the left pupil constricts (i.e. the right eye consensual reflex is intact).
  - relative afferent pupillary defect (RAPD) occurs if there is incomplete damage to the afferent pathway (e.g. previous retrobulbar neuritis due to multiple sclerosis). The swinging light test is performed (i.e. the light is moved from one eye to the other alternately). If the left eye has a RAPD, there will be reduced conduction along its afferent pathway. Therefore, if the light is initially shone in the left eye, both pupils will constrict; on moving the light to the right eye, bilateral constriction occurs again; when the light returns to the left eye, the pupil dilates because of its reduced afferent conduction. This is diagnostic of a RAPD.
  - Horner's syndrome: see Ch. 34
  - Argyll Robertson pupil: a small, irregular pupil that 'accommodates but does not react' (i.e. fixed to light but constricts on convergence). Almost diagnostic of neurosyphilis (occasionally occurs in diabetes mellitus).
  - myotonic pupil (Holmes–Adie pupil): a dilated pupil that reacts very slowly to light and constricts incompletely to convergence. Most common in young females and, if combined with absent tendon reflexes, this is Holmes–Adie syndrome.
- **O**phthalmoscopy: common abnormalities on ophthalmoscopy are papilloedema (Fig. 2.20), optic atrophy (Fig. 2.21), diabetic retinopathy (Fig. 2.22), hypertensive retinopathy (see Fig. 30.22) and, in exams, retinitis pigmentosa. Pigmentary retinal degeneration may also occur in other conditions such as Refsum's disease and Laurence–Moon–Biedl syndrome.

COMMUNICATION

Prolonged gazing with an ophthalmoscope can be uncomfortable for the patient. Be aware of this – giving the patient a short break can be helpful.

Fig. 2.19 Visual field defects.

Defect	Site of lesion	Causes
Tunnel vision	Retina	Glaucoma, retinitis pigmentosa, laser therapy for diabetic retinopathy
Enlarged blind spot	Optic nerve	Papilloedema (due to any cause)
Central scotoma	Macula, optic nerve	Optic atrophy, optic neuritis, retinal disease affecting macula
Monocular visual loss	Eye, optic nerve	Extrinsic compression, toxic optic neuropathy
Bitemporal hemianopia	Optic chiasm	Pituitary tumour, craniopharyngioma, sella meningioma
Quadrantic hemianopia	Temporal lobe (superior) Parietal lobe (inferior)	Stroke, tumour
Homonymous hemianopia	Occipital cortex, optic tract	Stroke, tumour

Fig. 2.20 Causes of papilloedema.

Cause	Examples
Raised intracranial pressure	Tumour, abscess, hydrocephalus, haematoma, benign intracranial hypertension, cerebral oedema (trauma)
Venous occlusion	Central retinal vein thrombosis, cavernous sinus thrombosis
Malignant hypertension	Grade IV hypertensive retinopathy
Acute optic neuritis	Multiple sclerosis, sarcoidosis
Metabolic	Hypercapnia, hypoparathyroidism
Haematological (rare)	Severe anaemia, acute leukaemia

Third, fourth and sixth cranial nerves

- Ask the patient to follow your finger with their eyes and tell you if they 'see double'.
- Look for nystagmus. This is involuntary rhythmic eye oscillation. It may be pendular, with equal movement in all directions, or more commonly 'jerk nystagmus' with a slow drift away from the point of fixation and a fast corrective phase. It occurs physiologically at the extremes of lateral gaze and >2 beats are required for it to be significant. It may be due to peripheral lesions (affecting the labyrinth or 8th nerve), central vestibular or brainstem lesions, or cerebellar lesions. As a general rule, peripheral lesions cause unidirectional nystagmus that is horizontal or torsional, has a fast phase away from the side of the lesion and improves with fixation. In nystagmus due to central lesions, the fast phase is toward the side of the lesions, it may occur in more than one direction and does not improve with fixation. Brainstem lesions may cause unusual patterns including upbeat or downbeat nystagmus. Congenital causes and early loss of central vision (e.g. albinism) may cause pendular nystagmus.
- Assess conjugate gaze by asking the patient to look at your hand and then to a finger on your other hand, and then from one to the other as quickly as possible. If there is an internuclear ophthalmoplegia (a lesion in the medial longitudinal fasciculus), there will be slow movement in the adducting eye and nystagmus in the abducting eye. If one eye is covered, or if convergence is attempted, adduction is normal, as this is a disorder of conjugate gaze. Internuclear ophthalmoplegia is usually caused by multiple sclerosis but may occasionally result from vascular lesions.
- Diplopia in all directions of gaze may result from myasthenia gravis, ocular myopathy or disease in the surrounding tissue of the eye, such as Graves' disease, tumour or orbital cellulitis.

Fig. 2.21 Causes of optic atrophy.

Cause	Examples
Pressure on optic nerve	Tumour, glaucoma, aneurysm, Paget's disease
Demyelination	Multiple sclerosis
Vascular	Central retinal artery occlusion
Metabolic	Diabetes mellitus, vitamin B_{12} deficiency
Toxins	Methyl alcohol, tobacco, lead, quinine
Trauma	Including surgery
Consecutive	Due to extensive retinal disease such as choroidoretinitis
Hereditary prolonged papilloedema	Friedreich's ataxia, Leber's optic atrophy

Fig. 2.22 Stages of diabetic retinopathy.

Stage	Features
Background	Dot haemorrhages (microaneurysms), blot haemorrhages, hard exudates
Preproliferative	All of the above, plus multiple soft exudates (cotton wool spots), flame haemorrhages, venous beading and loops, IRMAs
Proliferative	All of the above, plus new vessel formation on retina or iris (rubeosis iridis), retinal detachment, preretinal or vitreous haemorrhage, glaucoma (with rubeosis iridis)
Maculopathy	Hard exudates (possibly in a ring – 'circinate') within a disc width of the macula; decreased acuity not correcting with a pinhole suggestive of macular oedema (therefore must check acuity)

Note that cataracts are also more common in diabetes, and that retinopathy may have been treated by laser photocoagulation (burns around the periphery of the retina, destroying ischaemic tissue and thus reducing the drive for new vessel formation). IRMA, intraretinal microvascular abnormality.

Third cranial nerve (oculomotor)

- Motor supply to levator palpebrae superioris, all orbital muscles except the superior oblique and lateral rectus muscles, and parasympathetic tone to pupillary reflex.

- Controls pupillary reflexes, in addition to the second cranial nerve. Test the reaction to light and accommodation (as above).
- Lesion of this nerve results in ptosis and a dilated pupil with no reaction to light or accommodation. The eye looks 'down and out' at rest and is unable to look upwards or inwards.
- Causes of 3rd cranial nerve lesions are infarction, posterior communicating artery aneurysm (which is painful), mononeuritis multiplex (see Ch. 26), demyelination, tumour and neurosyphilis. Medical, as opposed to mechanical, compression causes of 3rd nerve palsy often spare the parasympathetic nerve fibres (i.e. there is 'pupillary sparing'). Conversely, compressive lesions are associated with relatively less ophthalmoplegia. This is because the parasympathetic fibres run on the surface of the nerve.

Fourth cranial nerve (trochlear)

- Motor supply to the superior oblique muscle.
- Patient may have the head tilted away from the lesion.
- Diplopia on looking down and away from the lesion with one image at an angle to the other.
- Lesions of the 4th cranial nerve are usually associated with 3rd cranial nerve lesions and have a similar aetiology.
- Patients with a 4th cranial nerve palsy have difficulty with vision when walking downstairs or reading a book.

Sixth cranial nerve (abducens)

- Motor supply to the lateral rectus.
- There is diplopia on abduction of the affected eye with two images side by side.
- Lesions of the 6th cranial nerve are caused by mononeuritis multiplex, diabetes mellitus, demyelination, tumour, infarction, thiamine deficiency (Wernicke's encephalopathy), raised intracranial pressure (false localizing sign) and neurosyphilis.

Fifth cranial nerve (trigeminal)

- Sensation to the face (ophthalmic, maxillary and mandibular branches).
- Motor supply to the muscles of mastication (temporalis, masseter and pterygoid muscles).
- Test sensation in the distribution of each division comparing one side with the other.
- Remember the corneal reflex, which requires intact motor function of the 7th cranial nerve (as well as intact sensory function of the trigeminal nerve) for blinking.
- Ask the patient to clench the teeth.
- Ask them to hold the mouth open while you try to push it shut.
- Test jaw jerk, which is increased in pseudobulbar palsy and reduced or absent in bulbar palsy.
- The causes of 5th cranial nerve lesions are shown in Fig. 2.23.

Seventh cranial nerve (facial)

- Sensation of taste from the floor of the mouth, the soft palate and anterior two-thirds of the tongue.
- Motor supply to the muscles of facial expression and the stapedius muscle.
- Parasympathetic supply to the salivary and lacrimal glands.
- Ask the patient to wrinkle the forehead, screw the eyes tightly shut, show the teeth and blow the cheeks out.
- In lower motor neurone lesions all the muscles are affected.
- In upper motor neurone lesions, the upper half of the face and emotional expressions are spared (e.g. normal eye closure and wrinkling of the forehead).
- Taste is not usually examined formally but ask if the patient has noticed any recent change. Involvement of the nerve to stapedius causes hyperacusis (increased sensitivity to high-pitched or loud sounds).
- Fig. 2.24 summarizes the causes of facial nerve palsies.

HINTS AND TIPS

Crossed signs – cranial nerve abnormalities contralateral to limb abnormalities – should alert you to the possibility of a brainstem lesion.

Eighth cranial nerve (vestibulocochlear)

- Sensory to the utricle, saccule and semicircular canals (vestibular), and to the organ of Corti (cochlea).

Fig. 2.23 Causes of a trigeminal nerve lesion.

Anatomical site	Examples
Brainstem	Tumour, infarction, demyelination, syringobulbia
Cerebellopontine angle	Acoustic neuroma, meningioma
Petrous temporal bone	Trauma, tumour, middle ear disease, herpes zoster
Cavernous sinus	Tumour, thrombosis, aneurysm of internal carotid artery
Peripheral	Meningeal tuberculosis, syphilis, lymphoma, carcinoma, sarcoid

Fig. 2.24 Causes of facial nerve palsies.

Anatomical site	Examples
Upper motor neurone central	Stroke, tumour
Lower motor neurone pons angle	Stroke, tumour, demyelination, motor neurone disease
Cerebellopontine angle	Acoustic neuroma, meningioma
Petrous temporal bone	Bell's palsy, herpes zoster (Ramsay Hunt)
Middle ear disease	Infection, tumour
Peripheral	Trauma, parotid disease, mononeuritis multiplex, sarcoid, Guillain–Barré syndrome

- Ask if the patient has noticed any difficulty with hearing.
- Assess the ability of the patient to hear whispered numbers with the other ear covered.
- Rinne's test: place a vibrating tuning fork on the mastoid process and then at the external auditory meatus – the test is positive if the sound is louder when the fork is held at the external auditory meatus (i.e. air conduction) than when placed on the mastoid process (i.e. bone conduction). This is normal. An abnormal test (Rinne negative) indicates conductive deafness.
- Weber's test: place a vibrating tuning fork at the centre of the forehead; the sound will be heard towards the normal ear in sensorineural deafness or towards the affected ear in conductive deafness.
- The causes of vestibular disease are shown in Fig. 27.1.
- The causes of conductive and sensorineural deafness are described in Fig. 2.25.

Fig. 2.25 Causes of deafness.

Type	Examples
Conductive	Wax, foreign body, otitis externa, injury to tympanic membrane, otitis media, otosclerosis (e.g. Paget's disease), middle ear tumour (e.g. cholesteatoma)
Sensorineural	Presbycusis (due to old age), noise-induced, drugs (aminoglycosides, aspirin overdose), infection (meningitis, syphilis, measles), congenital (maternal rubella, cytomegalovirus, toxoplasmosis), Ménière's disease, acoustic neuroma, trauma, Paget's disease

Fig. 2.26 Causes of glossopharyngeal, vagus and accessory nerve palsies.

Anatomical site	Examples
Central (brainstem)	Tumour, infarction, syringobulbia, motor neurone disease
Peripheral	Tumour or aneurysm near the jugular foramen, trauma of skull base, Guillain–Barré syndrome, poliomyelitis

Ninth and tenth cranial nerves

- Look at palatal movement (ask the patient to say 'Aah').
- Lesions cause reduced palatal elevation on the affected side, with the uvula pulled towards the normal side.
- Check the gag reflex (9th, sensory; 10th, motor).
- The causes of 9th and 10th nerve lesions are summarized in Fig. 2.26.

Ninth cranial nerve (glossopharyngeal)

- Sensory to pharynx and carotid sinus and taste to the posterior third of the tongue.
- Motor supply to the stylopharyngeus muscle.
- Parasympathetic to the parotid gland.

Tenth cranial nerve (vagus)

- Sensory to the larynx.
- Motor supply to the cricothyroid and the muscles of the pharynx and larynx.
- Parasympathetic to the bronchi, heart and gastrointestinal tract.

Eleventh cranial nerve (accessory)

- Cranial root provides the motor supply to some muscles of the soft palate and larynx.
- Spinal root provides the motor supply to the trapezius and sternocleidomastoid muscles.
- Ask the patient to shrug the shoulders and test against resistance.
- Ask the patient to turn his or her head against your resisting hand and test the sternocleidomastoid muscle bulk.

Twelfth cranial nerve (hypoglossal)

- Provides the motor supply to the styloglossus, hyoglossus and all intrinsic muscles of the tongue.
- Ask the patient to open the mouth. Look for wasting and fasciculation, indicating a lower motor neurone lesion of the tongue.

- Then ask the patient to protrude the tongue. If there is a unilateral lesion the tongue will deviate towards the side of the lesion.
- Upper motor neurone lesions are due to stroke, tumour or motor neurone disease.
- Lower motor neurone lesions are due to diseases in the posterior fossa, skull base and neck, including tumour, motor neurone disease, syringobulbia, trauma and poliomyelitis.

THE LIMBS

Inspection

- Wasting: lower motor neurone lesion, muscle disease and disuse.
- Fasciculation: lower motor neurone lesion.
- Scars: particularly from surgery.
- Deformity: may cause mononeuropathy by entrapment, and contractures may be the result of neurological disease.
- Tremor (Fig. 2.27).
- Pes cavus: Charcot–Marie–Tooth disease, (hereditary motor and sensory neuropathy) Refsum's disease.

Tone

Reduced tone is a feature of a lower motor neurone lesion or cerebellar lesion. Hypertonia may manifest as either spasticity or rigidity. Spasticity describes the sudden build up of increased tone during the first few degrees of passive movement. The resistance lessens as the movement is continued and this is characteristic of upper motor neurone lesions. This is often described as the 'clasp-knife' phenomenon. Rigidity describes the sustained resistance to passive movement seen in extrapyramidal conditions (e.g. parkinsonism). This may be described as 'lead pipe' rigidity and when associated with a tremor gives rise to 'cogwheel' rigidity. Test for clonus (usually at ankle, but can also do at patella), signifying an upper motor neurone lesion.

Fig. 2.27 Causes of tremor.

Type	Features	Causes
Resting	Seen when patient relaxed with hands at rest	Parkinsonism
Postural	Seen when hands held outstretched	Benign essential tremor Anxiety Thyrotoxicosis Beta-2-agonists
Intention	Seen when patients try to touch examiner's finger with their own finger	Cerebellar disease

Fig. 2.28 Grading muscle power.

Grade	Features
0	No movement at all
1	Flicker of movement only
2	Movement only when gravity excluded
3	Movement against gravity only
4	Movement against gravity and some additional resistance
5	Normal power

Power

All muscle groups should be tested and scored (Fig. 2.28). You will need to learn the root value for each movement (Fig. 2.29). Remember to compare muscle power of one side to the other for each group.

Look for pronator drift by asking the patient to hold their arms outstretched, palms upward, and close their eyes. Marked weakness will be easily apparent. If an upper motor neurone lesion affecting the parietal lobe is present, the arm will drift downwards and the hand will pronate.

Coordination

Ask the patient to alternately touch their nose and your finger. In cerebellar disease, there will be an intention tremor and past pointing (i.e. the patient overshoots the examining clinician's finger consistently towards the side of the lesion). Ask the patient to tap one palm with alternating sides of the other hand as quickly as possible (demonstrate to the patient what you would like them to do). In cerebellar disease, this will be slow, poorly coordinated and the action of the moving hand has a high amplitude – this is dysdiadochokinesis.

To check coordination in the lower limbs, ask the patient to lift the leg, place the heel on the knee of the opposite leg and gently run it down the shin and repeat this motion. In cerebellar disease, this will be slow and clumsy.

Reflexes

Practise as often as you can. Learn the root value of each reflex (Fig. 2.30). Reflexes can be reduced, normal or increased. They will be reduced or absent in lower motor neurone lesions, sensory neuropathy and severe muscle disease (disruption of reflex arc), and will be

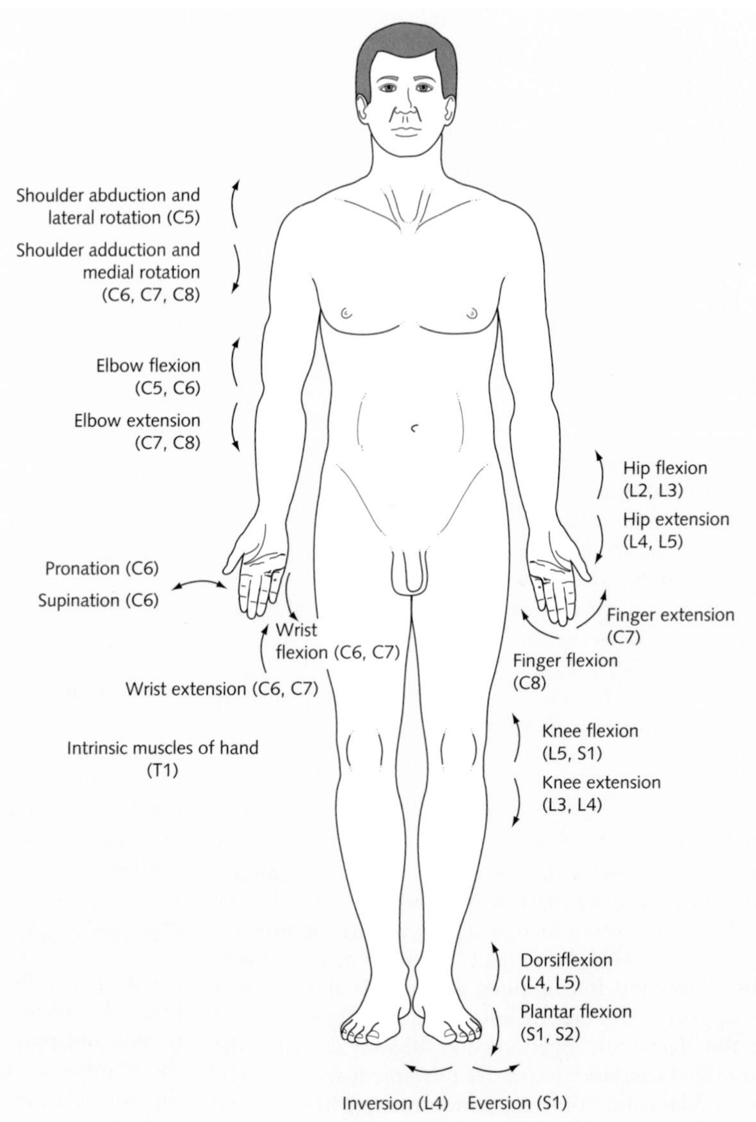

Fig. 2.29 Nerve roots for each muscle group movement.

exaggerated in upper motor neurone lesions. Check plantar response, which is normally downgoing but will be upgoing in upper motor neurone lesions.

Sensation

Test each dermatome (Fig. 2.31) for the sensation of light touch, pinprick (and temperature). Then, starting distally, check vibration and joint position sense. Remember the different pathways these senses take (Fig. 2.32). The tests for the various sensory modalities are shown in Fig. 2.33.

Gait

- Ask the patient to walk for 2–3 m, turn and walk back, then walk heel to toe (cerebellar ataxia) and finally stand on toes and on heels (any muscle weakness will now manifest itself).
- Make sure you walk with the patient so you can catch them if they fall.
- An immense amount of information can be gained by careful study of these aspects of gait (see Fig. 26.3).
- Romberg's test: this assesses posterior column function (proprioception).

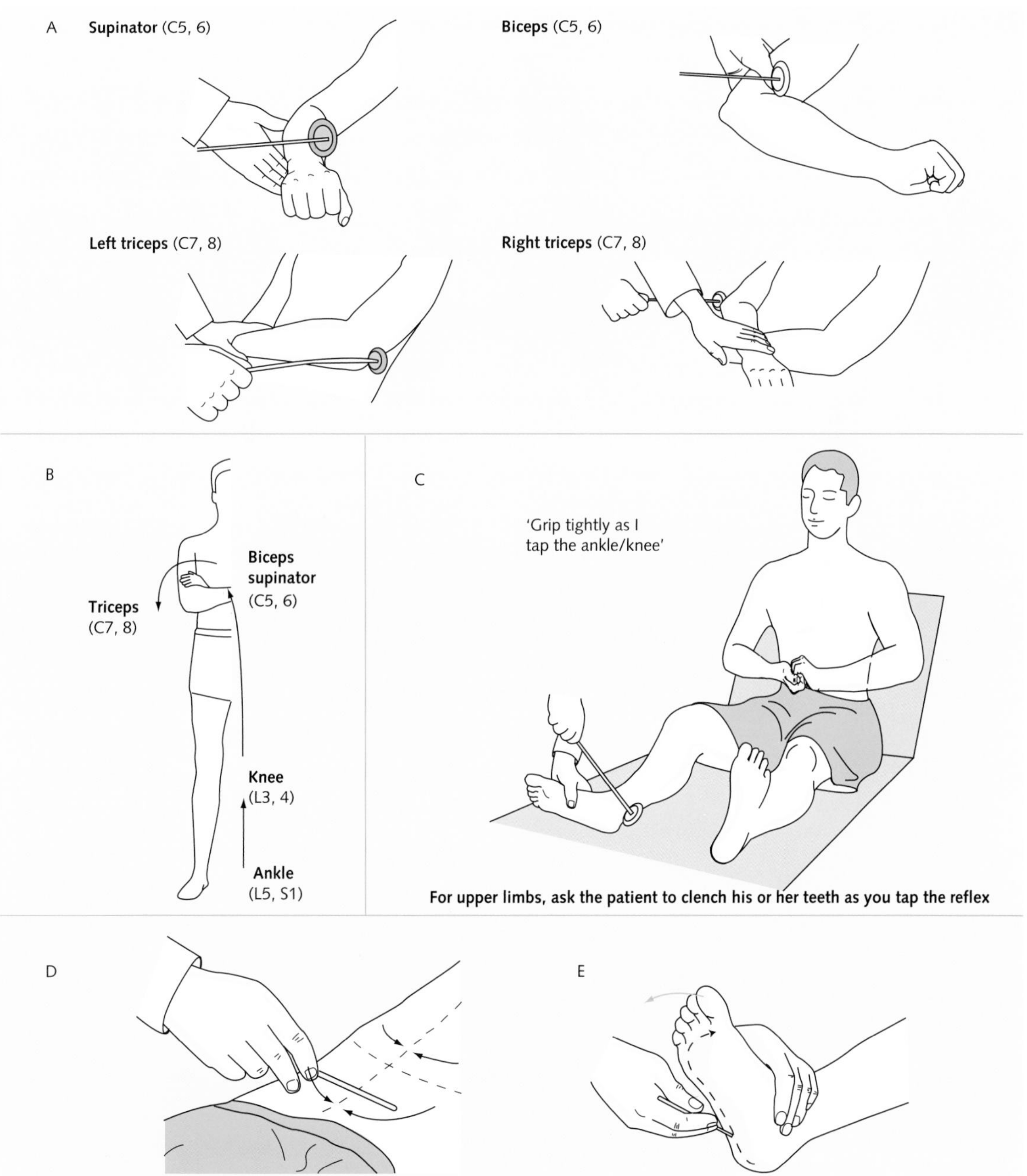

Fig. 2.30 Eliciting reflexes. (A) Upper limb tendon reflexes. (B) A simple way to remember root values of reflexes. (C) Testing ankle jerk with reinforcement. (D) Abdominal reflexes: test in four quadrants shown. (E) The normal response is a downgoing hallux. In an upper motor neurone lesion, the hallux dorsiflexes and other toes fan out (the Babinski response).

HINTS AND TIPS

Sensory testing is difficult and subjective. A thorough inspection and examination of tone, power, coordination and reflexes may help to predict which sensory abnormality should be expected.

THE JOINTS

Diseases affecting the musculoskeletal system and how to distinguish between different disease processes on clinical examination have been discussed in detail in Ch. 19. However, remember the following broad components to the examination of joints.

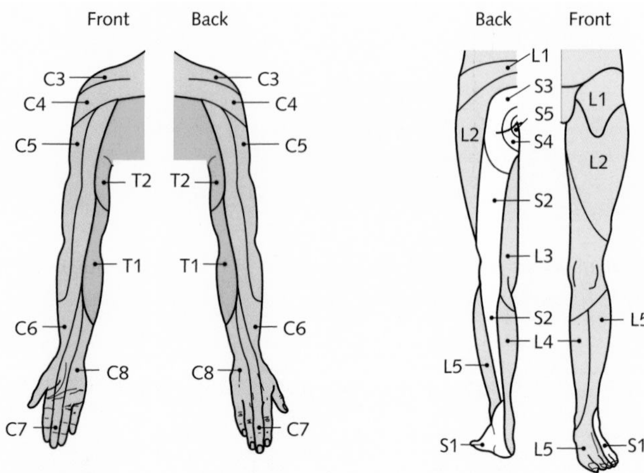

Fig. 2.31 Dermatomes of the upper and lower limbs.

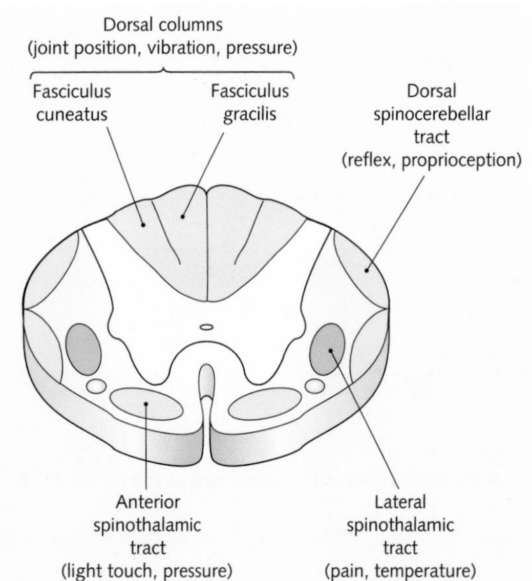

Fig. 2.32 Anatomy of sensory pathways within the spinal cord.

Visual survey

- Does the patient look well or ill?
- Anaemia: chronic disease, blood loss (peptic ulcer due to non-steroidal anti-inflammatory drug use), bone marrow suppression (immunosuppressive therapy), haemolysis (autoimmune associated with systemic lupus erythematosus) and hypersplenism (Felty's syndrome in rheumatoid arthritis).
- Face: scleroderma, systemic lupus erythematosus, cushingoid facies (long-term steroid therapy).
- Stooped: ankylosing spondylitis and osteoporosis.
- Psoriatic rash.
- Subcutaneous rheumatoid nodules: particularly at the elbow.
- Gouty tophi: on the pinna and elbow.
- Look for evidence of long-term steroid treatment (see Fig. 35.18).

Look

- Deformity.
- Scars: previous surgery.
- Erythema: acute inflammation or infection.
- Swelling: osteophytes, synovial hypertrophy and acute inflammation.
- Muscle wasting: disuse, nerve entrapment, mononeuritis multiplex or long-term steroid therapy.

Feel

- Increased temperature: acute inflammation or infection.
- Tenderness.
- Effusions.
- Crepitus on movement.

Move

- Active and passive movement.
- Is pain associated with movement?
- Is the joint stable? Are there intact ligaments and supporting musculature?

Assessment of disability

It is very important to get an impression of how limiting the joint problem is. For example, in a patient with rheumatoid arthritis, ask the patient to undo some buttons or write their name with a pen.

THE SKIN

The clinical approach to skin rashes will be discussed in detail in Ch. 36. When asked to look at a rash, you will be awarded marks for giving a good description, even if

Fig. 2.33 Tests for different sensory modalities.

Sensation	Tested using	Pathway	Level of decussation
Pain	Neurotip	Lateral spinothalamic tract	At level of sensory root within one spinal segment
Temperature	Tuning fork for cold	Lateral spinothalamic tract	At level of sensory root within one spinal segment
Light touch	Cotton wool	Anterior spinothalamic tract	At level of sensory root within several spinal segments
Vibration	Tuning fork	Posterior columns (fasciculus gracilis and fasciculus cuneatus)	Medulla oblongata
Joint position sense	Move fixed joints	Posterior columns (fasciculus gracilis and fasciculus cuneatus)	Medulla oblongata
Two-point discrimination	Orange stick	Posterior columns (fasciculus gracilis and fasciculus cuneatus)	Medulla oblongata

you are unable to make a diagnosis. Remember to describe the following:

- Distribution: this can be diagnostic in itself.
- Shape.
- Size.
- Colour.
- Consistency.
- Temperature.
- Tenderness.
- Margins.
- Relation to the surface: raised, flat, or ulcerated.
- Fixation to underlying structures.

COMMUNICATION

Remember that patients with skin lesions and rashes are often very sensitive about their appearance.

LYMPHADENOPATHY

Examine all lymph node sites (Fig. 2.34). Always examine the cervical lymph nodes standing behind the patient. The causes of generalized and localized lymphadenopathy are discussed in Ch. 25. If lymphadenopathy is present, pay special attention to examination of the spleen and liver.

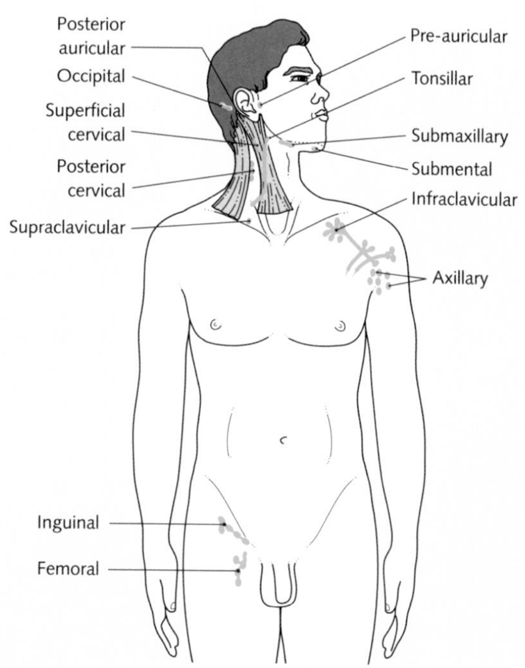

Fig. 2.34 Examination of lymph node sites.

BREAST EXAMINATION

Breast examination should be performed in women who have symptoms of breast disease or when an underlying malignancy is suspected. Do not forget that breast tissue extends into the axillae. Breast examination must be approached sensitively with a full explanation. Male students and doctors should have a female chaperone to help put the patient at ease (and to protect themselves from accusations of inappropriate behaviour).

NECK EXAMINATION

In clinical exams, when asked to examine the neck there will usually be a thyroid mass or lymphadenopathy. However, do not forget the salivary glands, branchial cyst, pharyngeal pouch, cervical rib, carotid body

Fig. 2.35 Causes of thyroid gland enlargement.

Form of enlargement	Causes
Diffuse enlargement (goitre)	Idiopathic Physiological: puberty, pregnancy Autoimmune: Hashimoto's and Graves' diseases Iodine deficiency: endemic, e.g. Derbyshire neck Thyroiditis: de Quervain's (viral), Riedel's (autoimmune) Drugs: carbimazole, lithium, sulphonylureas Genetic: dyshormonogenesis (Pendred's syndrome)
Solitary nodule	Thyroglossal cyst Prominent nodule in multinodular goitre Adenoma Cyst Carcinoma (papillary, follicular, anaplastic, medullary) Lymphoma

tumour and cystic hygroma. Causes of lymphadenopathy are described in Ch. 25. Fig. 2.35 lists the causes of thyroid enlargement.

First, look very carefully at the neck, lifting the hair out of the way if necessary. Look for obvious masses, scars, skin changes or deformity. If there is a mass in the region of the thyroid gland, ask the patient to take a sip of water into their mouth and then swallow – a goitre will move upwards on swallowing. In addition, ask the patient to open the mouth and then watch as the tongue protrudes – a thyroglossal cyst will move upwards. If a mass is present, assess its properties as described in Fig. 2.13. Percussion is useful to determine retrosternal extension of a goitre. Bruits may be audible in the thyroid gland (thyrotoxicosis) or carotid artery (atheroma). If you find a thyroid mass, you should go on to assess thyroid status as shown in Fig. 2.36.

HINTS AND TIPS

If the neck is normal, examine the JVP, listen to the carotid artery for bruits and re-examine for cervical rib.

Fig. 2.36 Examination of thyroid status.

	Hyperthyroidism	Hypothyroidism
Mood	Irritability, anxiety	Depression, slowness
Weight	Thinness	Overweight
Hands	Fine tremor, palmar erythema, sweaty palms, acropachy*	Puffiness, anaemia, Tinel's sign (carpal tunnel syndrome)
Pulse	Tachycardia, atrial fibrillation	Bradycardia
Face	Lid lag, lid retraction, exophthalmos,* ophthalmoplegia,* chemosis*	Loss of outer third of eyebrow, puffy eyes and face causing characteristic appearance, xanthelasmata
Skin	Pretibial myxoedema (shins)*	Dry, thin hair
Neuromuscular	Proximal myopathy	Slow-relaxing ankle jerks, cerebellar signs

**Denotes features that are specific to Graves' disease.*

The clerking 3

Objectives

The key learning points for this chapter:

- Structure your clerking in a logical manner.
- Appreciate factors in the clerking that make it easier for colleagues to review.
- Vary the clerking according to the patient's symptoms.
- Know how to conclude the clerking and the purpose that this serves.

INTRODUCTION

The doctor's 'clerking' is a written summary of the patient's history and examination. It is a legal document and should be precise, complete and legible. Avoid using abbreviations – although the meaning may be obvious to you, they may be interpreted very differently in a different speciality or hospital. However, in real life, abbreviations litter the medical notes and you ought to be familiar with the most common ones.

The 'history of presenting complaint' section is a useful place to document the most relevant positive and negative historical points. Less relevant details can be recorded in their appropriate subsection. For example, in the case presented here, the relevant negative historical points have been included in the 'history of presenting complaint' rather than elsewhere in the clerking.

At the end of the clerking, the salient points should be emphasized in a summary statement. You should then, always, compile a 'problem list'. This is often forgotten by students and junior doctors alike, but is invaluable in planning appropriate investigations and management. In some patients, it will not be appropriate, or even possible, to take a full history and perform a full clinical examination (e.g. in an emergency situation). We have outlined a clinical example.

As a student, it is good practice to be very thorough as it helps you to learn the relevant questions and to avoid missing anything important. However, with practice, you will learn to tailor carefully the clinical approach to each patient based on their individual, and often very different, needs.

MEDICAL SAMPLE CLERKING

Hospital No. X349282

BLOGGS, Joe DOB 29/4/54
66 year old man

01/01/12 07.20 Referred by General practitioner

PC Shortness of breath

1. Presenting complaint should be brief, but it is helpful to mention relevant background information.

HPC 4-day history of worsening dyspnoea. Gradual onset over hours.
Initially noted while climbing stairs at home. Over the last 12 hours has become short of breath at rest. No periods of relief sinc onset.
Relieving/exacerbating factors:
Relieved by rest. Exacerbated by exertion.
Associated symptoms:
Cough productive of green sputum for 3 days.
Sharp left sided posterior chest pain worsened by coughing and inspiration.
Feels 'feverish'.
Relevant direct questions:
Usually unlimited exercise tolerance
Lifelong non-smoker
No asthma, tuberculosis exposure, occupational exposure to chemicals or asbestos.
No pets or travel abroad
No haemoptysis, worsening of chest pain on exertion, ankle swelling, calf pain palpitations, trauma to chest wall, orthopnoea or paroxysmal nocturnal dyspnoea.

2. Mention only the relevant negatives.

3. A useful way of recording important negatives on one line.

PMH
1971 appendectomy
1980 duodenal ulcer (no symptoms since)

No diabetes, hypertension, rheumatic heart disease, epilepsy, jaundice, cerebrovascular disease

S/E
General - fatigue lately, appetite unchanged, weight stable, no sweats or pruritus
CVS - as above
RS - As above
GIT - No current indigestion. No symptoms like previous duodenal ulcer. No vomiting/dypnoea/abdominal pain
GUS - No urinary symptoms
NS - No headache/syncope. No dizziness/limb weakness/sensory loss. No disturbed vision/hearing/smell/speech
MS - No joint pain/stiffnrss/swelling. No disability
Skin - No rash/pruritus/bruising

DH No regular or over the counter medication.
Penicillin allergy - facial swelling and rash as young child

4. Always record the dose and frequency of any drugs – remember you'll be writing the drug chart later! Always document that you have asked about drug allergies.

Fam Hx Father died of 'heart attack' aged 60
Mother died of 'old age' at 96

Social Hx Lives with wife who is fit and well
Own house. Stairs
Completely independent
Never smoked
Alcohol: 24 units per week
Sexual history: not appropriate
No recent overseas travel
No pets
Occupation: hotel porter

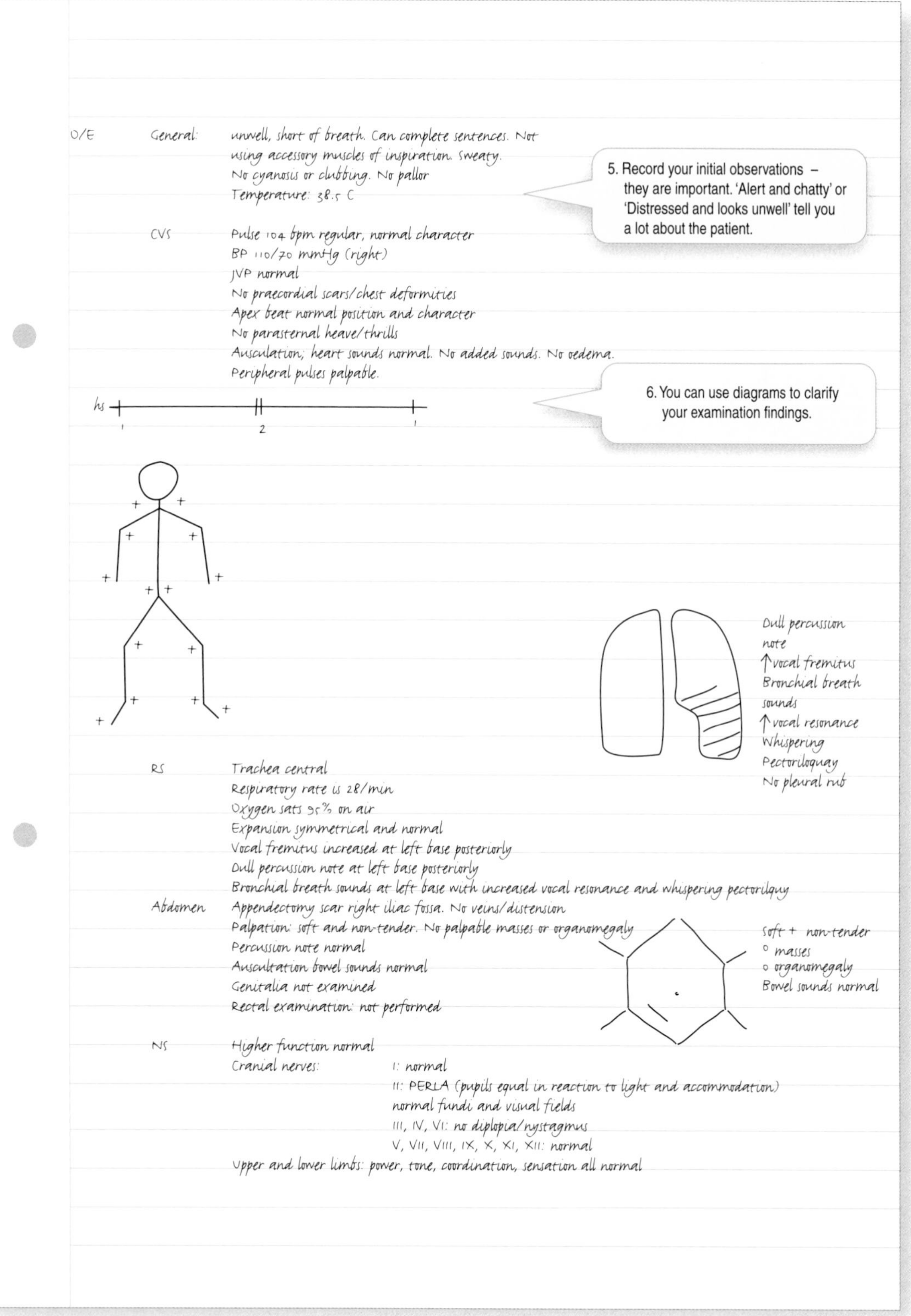

O/E General: unwell, short of breath. Can complete sentences. Not using accessory muscles of inspiration. Sweaty.
No cyanosis or clubbing. No pallor
Temperature: 38.5 C

5. Record your initial observations – they are important. 'Alert and chatty' or 'Distressed and looks unwell' tell you a lot about the patient.

CVS Pulse 104 bpm regular, normal character
BP 110/70 mmHg (right)
JVP normal
No praecordial scars/chest deformities
Apex beat normal position and character
No parasternal heave/thrills
Ausculation; heart sounds normal. No added sounds. No oedema.
Peripheral pulses palpable.

hs 1 2 1

6. You can use diagrams to clarify your examination findings.

Dull percussion note
↑vocal fremitus
Bronchial breath sounds
↑vocal resonance
Whispering Pectoriloquay
No pleural rub

RS Trachea central
Respiratory rate is 28/min
Oxygen sats 95% on air
Expansion symmetrical and normal
Vocal fremitus increased at left base posteriorly
Dull percussion note at left base posteriorly
Bronchial breath sounds at left base with increased vocal resonance and whispering pectoriloquy

Abdomen Appendectomy scar right iliac fossa. No veins/distension
Palpation: soft and non-tender. No palpable masses or organomegaly
Percussion note normal
Auscultation bowel sounds normal
Genitalia not examined
Rectal examination: not performed

soft + non-tender
° masses
° organomegaly
Bowel sounds normal

NS Higher function normal
Cranial nerves: I: normal
II: PERLA (pupils equal in reaction to light and accommodation)
normal fundi and visual fields
III, IV, VI: no diplopia/nystagmus
V, VII, VIII, IX, X, XI, XII: normal
Upper and lower limbs: power, tone, coordination, sensation all normal

Reflexes	Right	Left
Biceps	++	++
Supinator	++	++
Triceps	++	++
Knee	++	++
Ankle	+	+
Plantar	↓	↓

Joints and skin — Normal

Summary — 58 year old male non-smoker presents with a 4 day history of worsening exertional dyspnoea associated with a productive cough, pleuritic left sided chest pain and symptoms of fever.
On examination he is short of breath and tachypnoeic. He has a pyrexia and signs of consolidation at the left base. The most likely diagnosis is left-sided community acquired poneumonia.

Problem list — Dyspnoea? Left basal pneumonia.
Penicillin allergy.

Plan — Full blood count, Urea and Electrolytes, C-Reactive protein
Blood and sputum for microscopy and culture
Chest X-ray
CURB-65 score when blood results available
Antibiotics as per local protocol
Arterial Blood Gas
Urine for pneumococcus/legionella antigens
Intravenous access and fluid
Senior Review

Oliver Leach,
ST2 medicine
Bleep 1234

7. Sign your notes, including printed surname and bleep number.

Chest pain 4

Objectives

The key learning points for this chapter:

- Understand the causes of chest pain.
- Have a systematic approach to assessing a patient presenting with chest pain.
- Understand the sequence of investigations in a patient with chest pain.

INTRODUCTION

Chest pain is a common cause for both referral and admission to hospital – ranging from a simple musculoskeletal strain to a life-threatening myocardial infarction (Fig. 4.1). The many possible aetiologies therefore need to be elucidated. Taking a clear history is essential in making the correct diagnosis.

DIFFERENTIAL DIAGNOSIS OF CHEST PAIN

Pleuritic chest pain

This is a sharp pain caused by irritation of the pleura that is worse on deep inspiration, coughing or movement. The differential diagnosis includes the following:

- Pneumothorax.
- Pneumonia.
- Pulmonary embolus.
- Pericarditis: retrosternal.

Central chest pain

The differential diagnosis of central pain includes the following:

- Angina: crushing/tightness.
- Myocardial infarction: angina-like but commonly more severe, long-lasting and with associated symptoms.
- Dissecting aortic aneurysm: tearing interscapular pain.
- Oesophagitis: burning.
- Oesophageal spasm.

Chest wall tenderness

The differential diagnosis of chest wall tenderness includes the following:

- Rib fracture.
- Shingles (herpes zoster): pain precedes rash.
- Costochondritis (Tietze's syndrome).

Atypical presentations

The differential diagnosis in atypical presentations (or in any of the above) includes anxiety and referred pain from vertebral collapse causing nerve root irritation or intra-abdominal pathology (e.g. pancreatitis, peptic ulcer or biliary tree disorders).

HISTORY IN THE PATIENT WITH CHEST PAIN

A careful history of the chest pain will generally be suggestive of the likely underlying problem. The SOCRATES principle (Site, Onset, Character, Radiation, Associated features, Time course, Exacerbating/relieving factors and Severity) is particularly suited to chest pain and will allow for the formation of a sensible differential diagnosis. The focus should then turn to specific risk factors.

What type of chest pain does the patient have?

Onset and progression of pain

Cardiac ischaemic pain typically builds up over a few minutes and may be brought on by exercise, emotion or cold weather. In angina, the pain resolves on resting or with nitrate (GTN) usage. It is often reproducible with consistent effort. In unstable angina, the pain may come on at rest or be of increasing frequency or severity. In myocardial infarction (MI), the pain is severe, often associated with systemic symptoms such as nausea, vomiting and sweating, often lasts for at least 30 min and is not usually fully relieved by GTN. The terms angina and MI now all fall under the umbrella term 'acute coronary syndrome' or 'ACS'. Spontaneous pneumothorax and pulmonary embolism usually cause sudden onset of

Fig. 4.1 Differential diagnosis in chest pain.

Cardiovascular	Respiratory	GI	Musculoskeletal
Angina	Pneumonia	Gastritis	Rib fracture
Myocardial infarction	Pulmonary embolism	Pancreatitis	Varicella zoster
Pericarditis	Pneumothorax	Gastro-oesophageal reflux disease (GORD) and spasm	Costochondritis
Dissecting aortic aneurysm		Bilary colic/cholecystitis	Vertebral

pleuritic pain and dyspnoea (the patient often remembers exactly what they were doing at the time).

Site and radiation of pain

Cardiac ischaemia and pericarditis cause retrosternal pain. With ischaemia, the pain is tight and 'crushing', band like, etc., often radiating to the neck, jaw or arms. Pericarditis is pleuritic and may be worse on lying flat but relieved by sitting forward. A dissecting aortic aneurysm causes tearing pain radiating through to the back. Pulmonary disease may cause unilateral pain, which the patient can often localize specifically. Oesophageal disease can also cause retrosternal pain and may mimic cardiac pain. Referred pain from vertebral collapse or shingles will follow a dermatomal pattern.

Nature of pain

The precise nature of the pain gives important clues as to the underlying diagnosis. Most commonly the pain is dull/tight or sharp/stabbing. Asking patients to point with one finger to the site of the pain can help in distinguishing between the different types of chest pain.

Are there any associated symptoms?

Important associated symptoms include:

- Dyspnoea: pulmonary embolism, pneumonia, pneumothorax, pulmonary oedema in cardiac ischaemia, hyperventilation in anxiety (these patients will often complain of tingling in their extremities which is due to the fact that they blow off too much carbon dioxide).
- Cough: purulent sputum in pneumonia, haemoptysis in pulmonary embolism, frothy pink sputum in pulmonary oedema, dry in pneumothorax.
- Rigors: pneumonia (particularly lobar pneumococcal pneumonia).
- Calf swelling: has a pulmonary embolism (PE) arisen from deep vein thrombosis (DVT)?
- Palpitations: arrhythmia, e.g. new-onset atrial fibrillation, can cause angina or result from cardiac ischaemia, PE or pneumonia.
- Clamminess, nausea, vomiting and sweating are features of myocardial infarction or massive pulmonary embolism.

Are risk factors present?

Important risk factors include:

- Ischaemic heart disease: smoking, family history, hypercholesterolaemia, hypertension, diabetes.
- PE: recent travel, immobility, surgery, family history, pregnancy, malignancy, contraceptive pill.
- Pneumothorax: spontaneous (young, thin men, more commonly smokers), trauma, emphysema, asthma, malignancy.

EXAMINING THE PATIENT WITH CHEST PAIN

The examination should focus on determining the cause of the pain, then looking for risk factors and consequences of the underlying problem. A schematic guide to examining the patient with chest pain is given in Fig. 4.2.

What is the cause of the pain?

Pay particular attention to:

- Pulse: tachycardia/bradycardia or arrhythmia.
- Blood pressure: discrepancy between left and right arms in aortic dissection (the pulse volumes may also be unequal). Shock in tension pneumothorax, massive pulmonary embolism, MI.
- Chest wall tenderness: rib fracture, costochondritis, anxiety, shingles.
- Chest examination: pneumothorax, consolidation, pleural rub, pulmonary oedema, third heart sound.
- Cardiac examination: rub (pericarditis), murmur of aortic regurgitation in aortic dissection.

HINTS AND TIPS

Patients who have a median sternotomy scar are common in finals. Always check the legs for vein harvesting scars and listen out for a metallic heart sound.

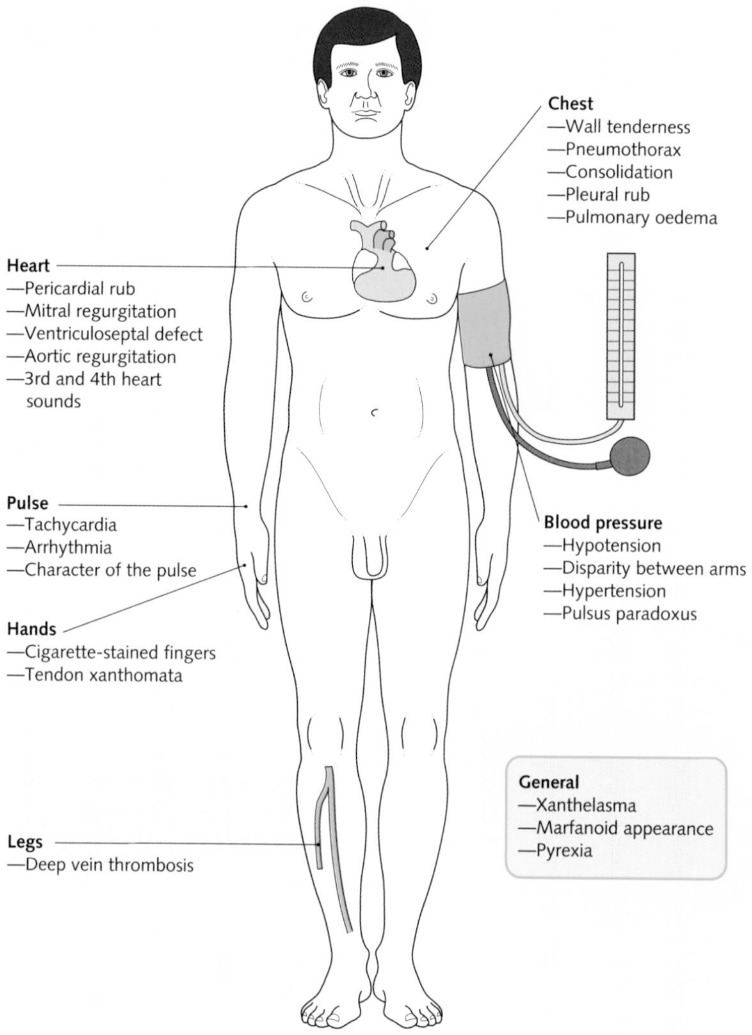

Heart
—Pericardial rub
—Mitral regurgitation
—Ventriculoseptal defect
—Aortic regurgitation
—3rd and 4th heart sounds

Pulse
—Tachycardia
—Arrhythmia
—Character of the pulse

Hands
—Cigarette-stained fingers
—Tendon xanthomata

Legs
—Deep vein thrombosis

Chest
—Wall tenderness
—Pneumothorax
—Consolidation
—Pleural rub
—Pulmonary oedema

Blood pressure
—Hypotension
—Disparity between arms
—Hypertension
—Pulsus paradoxus

General
—Xanthelasma
—Marfanoid appearance
—Pyrexia

Fig. 4.2 Examining the patient with chest pain.

Are there risk factors?

The following risk factors may be present:

- Abnormal lipids: xanthelasma, tendon xanthoma.
- Tar-stained fingers: predisposition to ischaemic heart disease.
- Hot, oedematous, tender calf suggesting deep vein thrombosis.
- Hypertension, ischaemic heart disease, features of Marfan's syndrome or of diabetes.

INVESTIGATING THE PATIENT WITH CHEST PAIN

All patients with chest pain should have an electrocardiogram (ECG) and chest radiograph (CXR). Further investigation will be directed by findings in these tests in conjunction with the history and clinical examination.

The acute phase

Blood tests

Patients will have a full blood count, urea and electrolytes and glucose performed as routine. Other tests may include cardiac enzymes, troponin I or T (see Ch. 30) at 6–12 h after symptom onset, inflammatory markers or D-dimers, as guided by history and examination. Aspartate transaminase and lactate dehydrogenase are now largely redundant in acute ischaemic chest pain.

HINTS AND TIPS

While troponin is a useful enzyme to investigate potential myocardial ischaemia, it may also be raised (although often to a lesser extent) in the following conditions: renal impairment, heart failure, sepsis, PE, acute pericarditis.

Electrocardiogram

New-onset left bundle branch block, T-wave changes, ST depression and elevation (Fig. 4.3) on ECG are suggestive of an acute coronary syndrome. It is vital to recognize those patients who would benefit from thrombolysis, or more commonly these days, angioplasty (percutaneous coronary intervention – PCI) as soon as possible. The management of myocardial infarction with and without ST segment elevation is discussed later (see Ch. 30). Changes suggestive of PE are shown in Fig. 4.4. Arrhythmia may also be detected on ECG. Serial or continuous ECGs may be needed as all the disease processes can be dynamic.

HINTS AND TIPS

Although not always possible, it is very useful to compare the ECG done in the acute setting with an old ECG. Changes such as LBBB and T-wave inversion may indeed be long-standing, which would alter your management.

HINTS AND TIPS

Grace score: a scoring system to predict outcome for those patients presenting with acute coronary syndrome (ACS). It calculates a score based on (at presentation): age, heart rate, systolic blood pressure, creatinine, class of CCF, troponin rise and ECG changes. The score predicts subsequent chance of death or MI during admission and at 6 months. All patients with ACS should be Grace scored as a matter of routine (see Ch. 30 for details).

Fig. 4.3 Causes of ST elevation on ECG.

Cause	Distribution of ST elevation
Myocardial infarction	Inferior aVF, II, III Anteroseptal V_{1-4} Lateral I, aVL, V_{4-6}
Pericarditis	Across all leads (saddle-shaped ST change)
Prinzmetal's angina	Leads of affected coronary artery (spasm)
Aortic dissection	Only if coronary artery involved
Left ventricular aneurysm	Persistent elevation for 6 months following infarct

Fig. 4.4 ECG changes associated with pulmonary embolus.

Sinus tachycardia
Atrial arrhythmia, e.g. atrial fibrillation
Right heart strain
Right axis deviation
Right bundle branch block
S_1 Q_3 T_3, i.e. deep S wave in I, Q wave in III, T-wave inversion in III

Note that sinus tachycardia may be the only abnormality present.

Chest X-ray

Pneumothorax, consolidation (pneumonia), widened mediastinum (aortic dissection), pulmonary oedema (myocardial ischaemia/infarction), wedge infarct (PE) and fractured ribs may be detected on CXR.

Arterial blood gases

The assessment of arterial blood gases is useful in determining the severity of PE (although a normal gas certainly does not rule this diagnosis out!), pneumonia or pulmonary oedema, showing hypoxia and occasionally hypocapnia. In hyperventilation related to anxiety, the Po_2 may be mildly elevated while there will be hypocapnia and a respiratory alkalosis. Always remember to note the inspired oxygen concentration at the time of obtaining the arterial blood sample.

Echocardiogram

Echocardiography can be used acutely to demonstrate cardiac dysfunction, valvular pathology, pericardial effusions and aortic dissection (particularly transoesophageal echocardiography). Computed tomography (CT) is an alternative in aortic dissection.

Percutaneous coronary intervention

Angioplasty and coronary artery stenting can be used to reopen occluded arteries in acute myocardial infarction instead of thrombolysis. Coronary angiography allows direct visualization of the coronary arterial anatomy. It is used in angina to determine whether elective angioplasty or coronary artery bypass grafting might be beneficial.

The subacute phase

Imaging for pulmonary embolism

Ventilation–perfusion ($\dot{V}/\dot{Q}$) scan was the standard imaging used to diagnose PE. However, interpretation of this test can be difficult, so a CT pulmonary angiogram is now preferred to a $\dot{V}/\dot{Q}$ scan in many centres, especially if underlying lung disease is present. Pulmonary angiography via cannulation of the pulmonary arteries remains the definitive investigation when there are doubts regarding the diagnosis.

Exercise test

An exercise test may be diagnostic when angina is suspected. It is mainly used in risk stratification post MI or in the outpatient clinic when investigating chest pain. It is *contraindicated* in acute coronary syndromes.

Upper gastrointestinal endoscopy

Upper gastrointestinal endoscopy will confirm oesophagitis and should be considered when the cause of chest pain is unclear.

Shortness of breath

Objectives

The key learning points for this chapter:

- Understand the causes of shortness of breath.
- Have a systematic approach to assessing a patient presenting with shortness of breath.
- Understand the sequence of investigations in a patient with shortness of breath.

INTRODUCTION

Shortness of breath (dyspnoea) is the subjective sensation of breathlessness which is excessive for a given level of activity. Dyspnoea may be due to any of the following:

- Pulmonary disease: disorders of the airways, lung parenchyma, pleura, pulmonary vasculature and right ventricle, respiratory muscles or chest wall.
- Cardiac disease: left ventricular systolic and diastolic dysfunction, arrhythmias or ischaemic heart disease.
- Systemic disease: e.g. anaemia, thyrotoxicosis or ketoacidosis.
- Non-organic causes: e.g. anxiety or chronic hyperventilation syndrome.

HISTORY IN THE PATIENT WITH BREATHLESSNESS

Severity

Quantify the severity by exercise capacity (e.g. distance walked on the flat or on hills, while dressing or climbing stairs). Has this changed in recent times? Does it affect daily activities?

Onset of dyspnoea

The onset of breathlessness and rate of decline give clues to its aetiology:

- Acute onset may indicate a sudden new change such as aspiration of a foreign body, pneumothorax, pulmonary embolism, acute asthma or acute pulmonary oedema.
- Subacute onset is more suggestive of parenchymal disease, pleural effusion, pneumonia and carcinoma of the bronchus or trachea.
- Chronic onset and progressive decline is associated with chronic obstructive pulmonary disease (COPD), interstitial lung disease and some non-respiratory causes, e.g. progressive heart failure.

Aggravating and precipitating factors

- Precipitating factors: exercise increases the demand for oxygen and as such many pulmonary and cardiac causes of dyspnoea are aggravated by exercise. Cold and airborne material (such as pollen) can irritate the airways and can cause dyspnoea in the context of asthma. Dyspnoea that improves at weekends or on holiday may imply a trigger factor at work.
- Aggravating factors: position can affect dyspnoea; orthopnoea is the term used for shortness of breath on lying flat and often indicates underlying cardiac dysfunction. Paroxysmal nocturnal dyspnoea is breathlessness that wakes the patient from their sleep and, again, is generally a symptom of cardiac disease.

HINTS AND TIPS

When clarifying the duration of symptoms, asking 'When were you last well?' and then 'Take me through what has happened since' often opens the consultation better than the more direct 'How long has this been going on?'

Associated features

In addition to the above, assess the following in patients with breathlessness:

- Cough: a chronic persistent cough has many causes, e.g. underlying lung disease, asthma, gastro-oesophageal reflux, postnasal drip or drugs (especially angiotensin-converting enzyme (ACE) inhibitors where patients may suffer with a dry cough). How long has the cough

been present? Is the cough worse at any particular time of day? (Asthma, for example, typically has a nocturnal cough, whereas chronic bronchitis associated cough is particularly bad in the morning.)
- Sputum: how much? What does it look like?
- Haemoptysis: This is coughing up blood, either frank blood or blood-tinged sputum. It needs to be distinguished from haematemesis and nasopharyngeal bleeding (see Ch. 7).
- Stridor: a harsh sound caused by turbulent airflow through a narrowed airway. Inspiratory stridor suggests upper airway obstruction and may indicate impending airway compromise. Inspiratory and expiratory stridor can indicate fixed obstruction.
- Wheeze: a wheeze is a whistling noise in expiration caused by turbulent airflow through narrowed intrathoracic airways. The commonest causes are asthma and COPD.

Other factors

- Occupational history, including exposure to asbestos and dusts. Occupational lung disease is important as changing the working environment may improve symptoms or the patient may benefit from financial compensation.
- Known lung disease: current, such as asthma or previously such as tuberculosis?
- History of atopy: asthma, seasonal allergic rhinitis (hayfever) or eczema?
- Pets: can exacerbate asthma or cause chronic lung diseases (extrinsic allergic alveolitis, e.g. 'pigeon fanciers' lung').
- Current medications: non-cardioselective beta-blockers may exacerbate wheeze.
- Previous medications: e.g. amiodarone, can cause interstitial lung disease.
- Angina or previous myocardial infarction: symptoms of cardiac dyspnoea.
- General health: e.g. weight loss, appetite, etc., for a non-respiratory cause for the dyspnoea.
- Full smoking history.

EXAMINING THE PATIENT WITH BREATHLESSNESS

The examination findings of common respiratory conditions are listed in Fig. 5.1 and the examination approach in the patient with breathlessness is summarized in Fig. 5.2. For more detailed description of examination findings in respiratory disease see Ch. 31.

Inspection

Observe the patient from the end of the bed – note the respiratory rate or surreptitiously do it while feeling the pulse. Assess work of breathing, use of accessory muscles and any audible sounds. Then proceed to a systematic examination looking for:

- Central cyanosis (a bluish colour in the mouth and tongue due to excess deoxygenated haemoglobin (Hb), i.e. >5 g Hb/100 mL of blood): commonly associated with respiratory and cardiac disease. Cyanosis is an unreliable guide to hypoxaemia and is difficult to appreciate in anaemic patients. Peripheral cyanosis can be due to poor peripheral circulation (e.g. cardiac failure, peripheral vascular disease, or physiological due to cold).

Fig. 5.1 Findings on examination of common respiratory conditions.

Condition	Movement on side of lesion	Position of trachea	Percussion	Tactile vocal fremitus	Breath sounds
Pleural effusion	↓	Central or deviated away from effusion if massive	↓ ('stony dull')	↓	↓ with bronchial breathing at top of effusion
Pneumothorax	↓	Central or deviated away	↑	↓	↓
Pneumonia	↓	Central or deviated towards if associated with collapse	↓	↑	Increased vocal resonance Bronchial breathing (absent if obstruction of bronchus) Coarse crepitations
Pulmonary fibrosis	↓	Central or deviated towards if upper lobe involvement	↓	↑	Fine crepitations

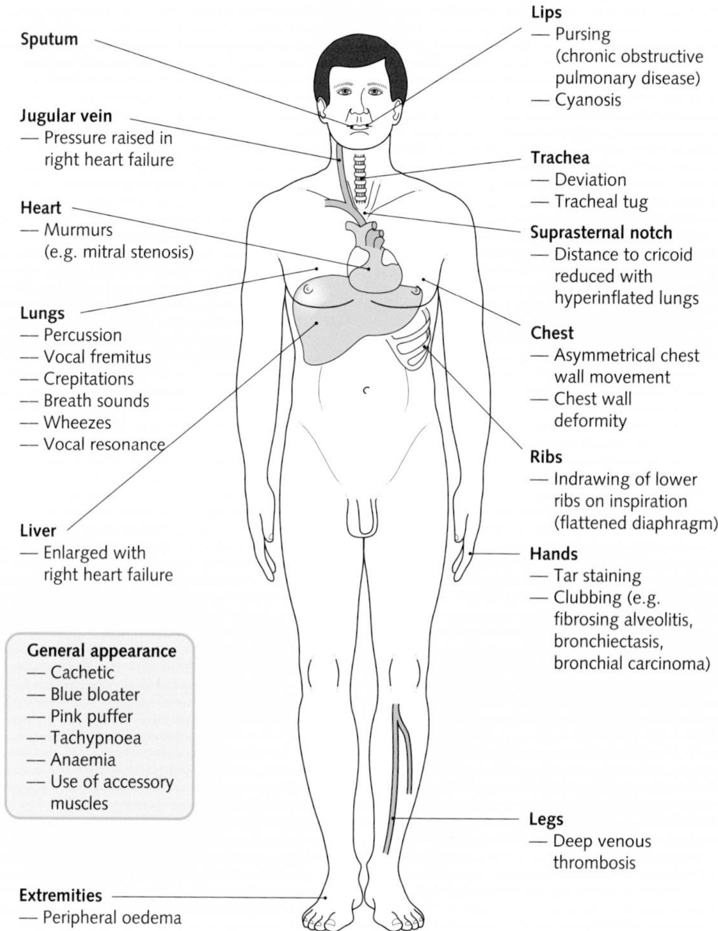

Fig. 5.2 Examining the patient with breathlessness.

- Anaemia: pale conjunctivae.
- Tar staining of the fingers.
- Clubbing: respiratory causes include carcinoma of the bronchus; suppurative lung disease (e.g. empyema, lung abscess, bronchiectasis, cystic fibrosis); fibrosing alveolitis; chronic suppurative pulmonary tuberculosis; mesothelioma.
- Chest movements on inspiration and expiration: the pathology is normally found on the side with diminished movement. Expiration should last about twice as long as inspiration.
- Lip pursing: this is common in patients with severe obstructive airways disease and associated alveolar air trapping. By pursing the lips, the patient can achieve positive end expiratory pressure (auto-PEEP) which will ease the work of breathing.
- Barrel-shaped chest: emphysema.
- Kyphoscoliosis: can decrease chest size and expansion.
- Use of accessory muscles of respiration.
- Paradoxical abdominal movement: diaphragmatic weakness.
- Pattern of breathing: Cheyne–Stokes respiration describes cyclical variation in depth of breathing with periods of rapid and deep inspiration followed by periods of apnoea due to depression of the $P\text{CO}_2$ below the apnoeic threshold. It can be seen in neurological disease, severe left ventricular failure and healthy people when at high altitude (so unlikely to be seen in an exam!)

Palpation

- Cervical lymphadenopathy: malignant disease or infection.
- Trachea: deviation may indicate underlying chest or cardiac disease.
- Expansion of the rib cage.
- Tactile vocal fremitus.
- Compare both sides anteriorly and posteriorly.

HINTS AND TIPS

Always look in the sputum pot:
- Purulent, moderate quantity – bronchitis or pneumonia.
- Purulent, copious quantity – bronchiectasis or pneumonia.
- Pink and frothy – pulmonary oedema.
- Blood-stained – causes of haemoptysis.
- Rust-coloured – pneumococcal lobar pneumonia.

Percussion

- Percuss both anteriorly and posteriorly in a systematic manner.
- Increased resonance: indicates increased air beneath – acutely in pneumothorax or chronically in emphysema.
- Decreased resonance: indicates increased solid matter beneath – infection or effusion (classically 'stony dull').

Auscultation

- Expiration: may be prolonged in COPD.
- Bronchial breathing: consolidation, cavitation or at the top of an effusion.
- Breath sounds: diminished over an effusion, pneumothorax and in the obese.
- Rhonchi or wheeze: partially obstructed bronchi; found in asthma, COPD and occasionally left ventricular failure. If polyphonic, usually suggests multiple small-airway narrowing. If monophonic and fixed, it can indicate a fixed single obstruction, e.g. a central malignant lesion.
- Crepitations or crackles (sudden opening of small closed airways): pulmonary congestion (fine crepitations in early inspiration); fibrosing alveolitis (fine crepitations in late inspiration); bronchial secretions (coarse crepitations).
- Friction rub: pleural disease.
- Assess vocal resonance: ask the patient to say and then whisper '99'. It provides the same information as vocal fremitus but is often easier to detect. Consolidation leads to increased and easily heard speech due to solid lung tissue conducting the sounds to the chest wall.

HINTS AND TIPS

To simulate bronchial breathing, place the stethoscope over your own trachea and listen.

INVESTIGATING THE PATIENT WITH BREATHLESSNESS

The following investigations should be performed. It is worth making the distinction between appropriate investigations in the acute and chronic setting.

Acute

- Full blood count: anaemia, leucocytosis in pneumonia.
- Urea, electrolytes and bicarbonate: renal failure producing breathlessness due to acidosis or fluid overload.
- Blood glucose: diabetic ketoacidosis may present with acute dyspnoea.
- Chest X-ray: examine methodically.
- Electrocardiogram (ECG): examine systematically looking for evidence of acute or chronic cardiac and respiratory disease. Remember that pulmonary embolism may simply show a sinus tachycardia.
- Arterial oxygen saturation: easy to perform and may obviate the need for blood gas analysis.
- Arterial blood gases: pH, Po_2 and Pco_2, base excess, bicarbonate concentration and lactate level (see Respiratory failure, Ch. 31). If possible, these should be taken with the patient breathing room air. This investigation must be performed if there is any concern regarding oxygenation or ventilation.
- CT scanning: used to assess both acute and chronic dyspnoea (e.g. to investigate PE and to diagnose and quantify interstitial lung disease and bronchiectasis). Prior to requesting this scan you would be required to perform a Well's score to assess the probability of the patient having a PE (Fig. 5.3).
- Ventilation–perfusion scan: suspected pulmonary embolism (PE), although more likely to have CTPA these days.

Fig. 5.3 Well's score for assessment of pulmonary embolism.

Clinical signs and symptoms of DVT	+3
Pulmonary embolism most likely diagnosis, or equally likely	+3
Tachycardia (HR >100)	+1.5
Immobilization for at least 3 days, or surgery in the past 4 weeks	+1.5
Previous objective diagnosis of PE or DVT	+1.5
Haemoptysis	+1
Active cancer	+1

Score: >6.0, high probability of PE; 2.0–6.0, moderate probability of PE; <2.0, low probability of PE.

HINTS AND TIPS

Remember that nail varnish, in particular red nail varnish, will interfere with pulse oximetry measurements and should be removed.

Chronic

- Spirometry: distinguish between obstructive and restrictive lung pathology. This is best done for diagnosis when the patient is well. Lying and standing vital capacity will screen for diaphragm weakness.
- Peak expiratory flow rate: useful for assessing acute decline especially in asthmatic patients who often know their best results.
- Full pulmonary function tests: transfer factor, flow–volume loop and lung volumes.
- Bronchoscopy: if an endobronchial lesion is suspected.
- Echocardiogram: assess cardiac structure and function including pulmonary hypertension.

HINTS AND TIPS

People commonly say that they stop walking because of their breathing. Never just accept this, as they often mean something different. On closer questioning, they may report other symptoms such as chest pain, palpitations, muscle fatigue, tiredness ('just run out of steam'). These are important, as they may point to a different diagnosis or different treatment.

HINTS AND TIPS

Remember, the upper lobes of the lungs are best heard on the anterior chest wall.

Palpitations 6

Objectives

The key learning points for this chapter:

- Understand the differential diagnosis of palpitations.
- Have a logical approach to assessing the patient with palpitations.
- Direct investigations in a patient with palpitations.

INTRODUCTION

Always check what the patient means by 'palpitations', or clarify what you mean by them, because the word means different things to different people. It is usually understood as an awareness of the heartbeat. The most common cause is an arrhythmia or dysrhythmia, as it is also often called, although other causes include conditions causing an increase in stroke volume (e.g. regurgitant valvular disease) or conditions causing an increase in cardiac output, often non-cardiac causes (e.g. exercise, thyrotoxicosis, anaemia or anxiety). If an arrhythmia is suspected, determine whether there is an underlying cause.

DIFFERENTIAL DIAGNOSIS BY DESCRIPTION OF THE RHYTHM

Regular rhythm

The differential diagnosis of regular palpitations (Fig. 6.1) includes the following:

- Heavy heartbeats with normal rate: most often cardiac consciousness with sinus rhythm. It tends to be worse at rest, especially when in bed at night and during periods of stress.
- Fast heart rate: sinus tachycardia, atrial flutter with block, supraventricular tachycardia or ventricular tachycardia.
- Bursts of fast beats: paroxysmal atrial tachycardia. There is often a very long history dating back years with a single attack followed by a long interval before the next attack. Other causes include atrial flutter, junctional rhythm or ventricular tachycardia.
- Slow heart rate: sinus bradycardia, atrioventricular block.

Irregular rhythm

The differential diagnosis of irregular palpitations (Fig. 6.1) includes the following:

- Missed beats, 'thumps': multiple ectopics from the atrium or ventricle. The symptoms are more troublesome at rest and may disappear during exercise.
- Fast (or normal if treated): atrial flutter with variable block, atrial fibrillation (persistent irregularity with exercise), and multiple premature beats with sinus tachycardia.

HISTORY

A careful history of the palpitations will often lead to the correct diagnosis, especially as between episodes examination and investigations may be unremarkable. Are they continuous or intermittent? Are they fast, normal rate or slow? Are they regular or irregular? When did the palpitations start? This can vary from a few minutes to decades. Generally, if the onset dates back years and there have been no serious complications (e.g. syncope) the palpitations are usually benign.

How often do the palpitations occur and how long do they last for? They may last for days or seconds, with intervals between episodes of a few hours to years. Has the patient learned any manoeuvres to terminate the attacks? Enquire about the patient's concerns as they may fear serious underlying cardiac disease, although there is often a benign cause. Are there any associated features? These may be related to the underlying cause (e.g. angina, features of hyperthyroidism) or be a consequence of the palpitations (e.g. dizziness or syncope).

HINTS AND TIPS

Ask the patient to tap out their heart rhythm on the desktop. This will often give a good guide to diagnosis.

Fig. 6.1 Differential diagnosis of palpitations.

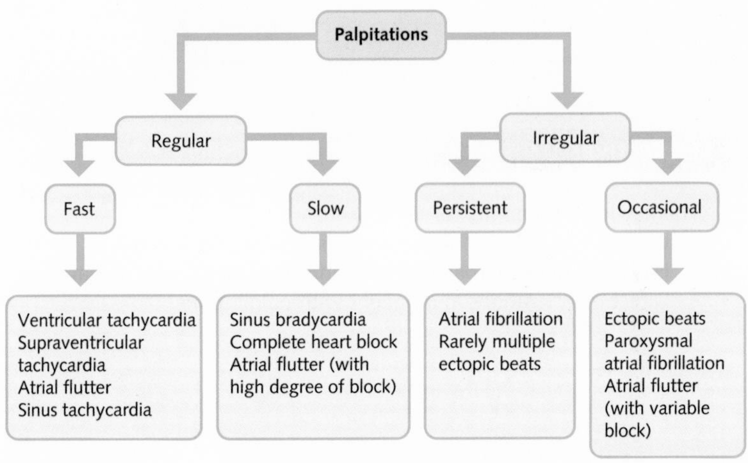

Causes and contributing factors

Ask about smoking, alcohol, work, stress, caffeine (tea, coffee, cola) intake and any illegal drug use. These may contribute to extrasystoles.

A history of ischaemic and valvular heart disease (including previous rheumatic fever) should be sought. This needs to be made prominent in the PMH as structural heart problems will predispose to pathological arrhythmias.

A family history of palpitations or sudden cardiac death may be important (e.g. hypertrophic obstructive cardiomyopathy or long QT syndromes).

A full drug history of both prescribed and over-the-counter medications is essential. Remember, many drugs, both cardiac and non-cardiac, can promote palpitations. Most anti-arrhythmic drugs are also potentially pro-arrhythmic.

Non-cardiac causes of sinus tachycardia and causes of sinus bradycardia are outlined in Figs 6.2 and 6.3, respectively.

Non-cardiac causes of palpitations include the following:

- Thyrotoxicosis: may cause sinus tachycardia, paroxysmal atrial tachycardia, and atrial flutter/fibrillation.
- Hypothyroidism (myxedema): may be responsible for sinus bradycardia.
- Anxiety: a very common cause of palpitations.

Fig. 6.2 Non-cardiac causes of sinus tachycardia.

Exercise
Fever
Anaemia
Thyrotoxicosis
Pregnancy
Arteriovenous fistulae
Anxiety of pain
Cigarettes, alcohol, caffeine
Sympathomimetic drugs (e.g. cocaine)

CONSEQUENCES OF PALPITATIONS

Palpitations can cause a range of problems, from minor anxiety to syncope or sudden death. This accounts for much of the patient's concern. If a benign arrhythmia is present, reassurance that the condition is not serious is often all that is required. Changes in rate may be more serious, compromising coronary blood supply and leading to symptoms of myocardial ischaemia or cardiac failure.

Tachycardia or bradycardia may lead to a reduction in cardiac output and cause dizziness or collapse (e.g. Stokes–Adams attacks in complete heart block). Ventricular tachycardia is potentially life-threatening.

EXAMINING THE PATIENT WITH PALPITATIONS

A guide to examining the patient with palpitations is given in Fig. 6.4. Look for signs of systemic diseases. Next feel the pulse. Note the following:

Fig. 6.3 Causes of sinus bradycardia.

Athletes (physiological)
Hypothyroidism
Obstructive jaundice
Raised intracranial pressure
Hypopituitarism
Hypothermia
Cardiac causes include ischaemia, drugs (e.g. digoxin and beta-blockers), inflammation, degeneration/fibrosis

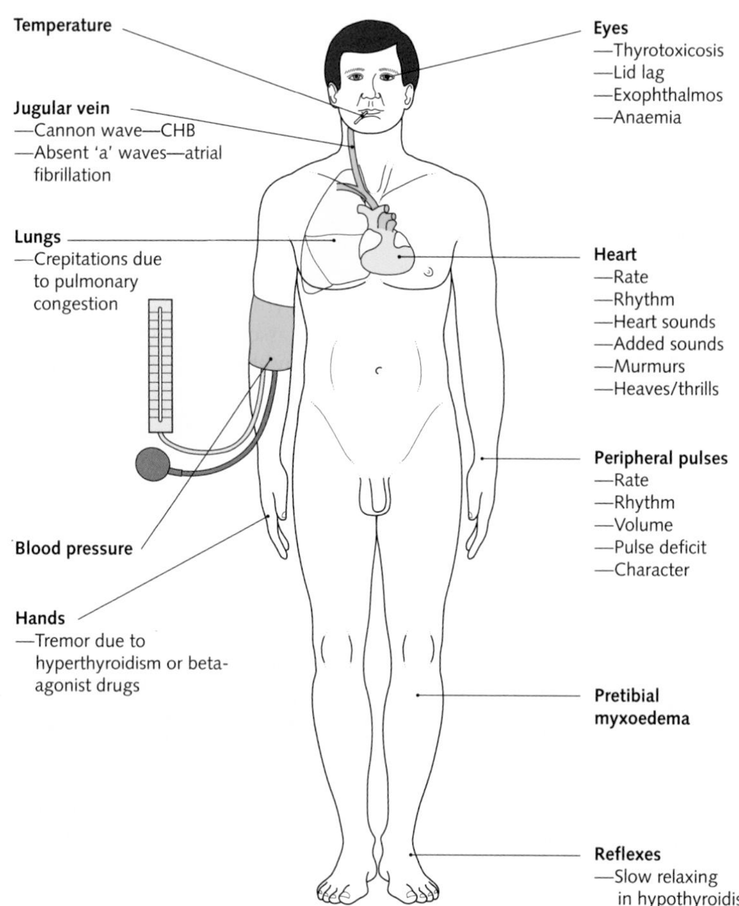

Fig. 6.4 Examining the patient with palpitations. CHB, complete heart block.

- Rate: beats per minute.
- Rhythm: regular, regularly irregular (e.g. Wenckebach second-degree heart block), irregularly irregular: e.g. multiple ectopic beats or atrial fibrillation.
- Volume/character: e.g. a collapsing pulse of hyperdynamic circulation or a low-volume pulse of shock or aortic stenosis. Remember this may be positional, so raising the arm above the heart may exaggerate a collapsing pulse.

If the patient is symptom-free at the time of examination, the pulse may be normal.

The blood pressure will be low if the arrhythmia leads to a reduction in cardiac output. Hypertension may predispose to atrial fibrillation.

The jugular venous pressure may be elevated if cardiac failure is present. Irregular cannon 'a' waves are visible with complete heart block, and 'a' waves are absent in atrial fibrillation.

A displaced apex may indicate cardiomyopathy. Feel for heaves and thrills with associated right ventricular enlargement and valvular heart disease. Assess the rate and rhythm by auscultation. The pulse rate felt at the radial artery may be slower than the apical rate in atrial fibrillation (pulse deficit). Listen for cardiac murmurs (e.g. evidence of mitral valve disease, mitral valve prolapse). Focus on any abnormal findings (see Ch. 30).

HINTS AND TIPS

An irregularly irregular pulse (atrial fibrillation) is irregular in BOTH rhythm AND volume.

INVESTIGATING THE PATIENT WITH PALPITATIONS

The following tests should be performed.

Vital signs

- Pulse, blood pressure, respiratory rate and saturations.
- Pulse oximetry.

Blood tests

- Full blood count: anaemia.
- Urea and electrolytes: disturbances of potassium or, less commonly, magnesium and calcium may contribute to refractory arrhythmias.
- Thyroid function tests: hypo/hyperthyroidism.
- Drug concentration if appropriate (e.g. digoxin levels in suspected toxicity).

Other tests

- 12-lead electrocardiogram (ECG): although mandatory for everyone with palpitations, this test rarely provides the diagnosis as it is unlikely that they will be caught on a resting 12-lead ECG. Wolff–Parkinson–White syndrome will be seen at rest, as will atrial fibrillation. Ectopic beats may be seen. Careful analysis of the QRS morphology and QT interval, etc., may be important.
- 24-h ECG: for intermittent symptoms. It should be carried out with a diary of symptoms to see if they correlate with any rhythm disturbances found.
- Echocardiogram: to exclude any underlying structural heart disease.
- 'Cardiomemo': if symptoms do not occur every day, a 'cardiomemo' can record the heart rhythm at the press of a button.
- Exercise test: the induction of symptoms under controlled conditions with ECG monitoring may be appropriate.
- Electrophysiological studies: more rarely, patients may be referred for specialized studies. These can be used to induce arrhythmias, locate the origin of any arrhythmic foci, assess the response to drug treatment or destroy any aberrant pathway via radiofrequency ablation.

HINTS AND TIPS

Atrial fibrillation with a fast ventricular response ('fast AF') is easily confused with a regular tachycardia when assessing the pulse.

Cough and haemoptysis

Objectives

The key learning points for this chapter:

- Know the classification and causes of cough and haemoptysis.
- Have a systematic approach to assessing a patient presenting with cough or haemoptysis.
- Have a logical approach to investigating patients with cough or haemoptysis.

INTRODUCTION

Cough is a non-specific reaction to irritation anywhere in the respiratory tract from the pharynx to the alveoli. The most common cause is infection, bacterial or viral. 'Acute cough' is defined as cough of <3 weeks' duration and if it persists for >8 weeks it becomes a 'chronic cough' and subacute if somewhere in between. As most viral upper respiratory tract infections will have resolved within 3 weeks, any cough lasting >8 weeks or >3 weeks with other symptoms warrants systematic investigation.

DIFFERENTIAL DIAGNOSIS OF COUGH AND/OR HAEMOPTYSIS

Cough

The differential diagnosis of cough includes:

- Postnasal drip: rhinitis, sinusitis.
- Upper respiratory tract infections: viral or bacterial, causing laryngitis, tracheobronchitis, etc.
- Pressure on the trachea: e.g. from a goitre; this may be associated with stridor.
- Lower respiratory tract causes: almost any lung pathology may be associated with cough, in particular asthma (classically a nocturnal cough), chronic obstructive pulmonary disease (COPD), pneumonia, bronchiectasis, interstitial lung disease and carcinoma.
- Left ventricular failure.
- Drugs: especially angiotensin-converting enzyme (ACE) inhibitors and irritants, e.g. occupational agents.
- Psychogenic/habitual cough.
- Gastro-oesophageal reflux disease (GORD): reflux is a common cause of chronic cough and may not be obvious from symptoms.

Haemoptysis

Common causes of haemoptysis include the following:

- Acute infections: e.g. pneumonia, exacerbations of COPD.
- Bronchiectasis: can be responsible for massive haemoptysis.
- Bronchial carcinoma: secondary malignancies and benign tumours can also lead to haemoptysis but are less common.
- Pulmonary tuberculosis (TB): a common cause worldwide.
- Other chronic infection: e.g. lung abscess, pulmonary aspergillosis.
- Pulmonary embolus: due to lung infarction.
- Left ventricular failure: typically pink, frothy sputum.
- Alveolar haemorrhage: usually due to a systemic vasculitis, e.g. Goodpasture's syndrome and Wegener's granulomatosis.
- Trauma: e.g. contusions to the chest, inhalation of foreign bodies or after intubation.

Rare causes of haemoptysis include the following:

- Bleeding diatheses.
- Interstitial lung disease.
- Mitral stenosis.
- Idiopathic pulmonary haemosiderosis.
- Arteriovenous malformations: Osler–Weber–Rendu disease (hereditary haemorrhagic telangiectasia), a favourite in exams but rare in practice.
- Eisenmenger's syndrome.
- Pulmonary hypertension.
- Cystic fibrosis.

In up to 15% of cases, no cause for haemoptysis is found.

HISTORY IN THE PATIENT WITH COUGH AND HAEMOPTYSIS

The nature of the cough may help in diagnosis (Fig. 7.1). Assess the following in patients with cough or haemoptysis:

- How severe is the cough and how disabling has it become to the patient's life?

Fig. 7.1 Conditions with characteristic cough.

Pressure on trachea	'Brassy' cough – hard and metallic
Tracheitis	'Hot poker' cough – often associated with retrosternal pain
Laryngeal nerve paralysis (e.g. secondary to tumour)	'Bovine' cough – often associated with hoarse voice
Laryngitis (e.g. croup)	'Seal' cough – barking, hoarse cough
Pharyngitis	'Hacking' cough – frequent, irritating
Small airways (e.g. asthma)	'Wheezy' cough – often associated with shortness of breath

- How long has the cough been present? The longer a cough is present, the less likely it is to be due to infection and other diagnoses should be sought.
- Is the cough worse at night? Cough can be the only symptom of asthma.
- Weight loss or other systemic symptoms? Think of carcinoma or lung abscess.
- Has the patient been in contact with any person with infection? Think of TB, especially in at-risk patient groups.
- History of chest trauma?
- Post-nasal drip: the sensation of dripping in the back of the throat causing a 'throat clearing' cough.
- Any prior medical history, e.g. cystic fibrosis, rheumatic fever–haemoptysis or lung transplantation needing immunosuppressive drugs.
- GORD: the lack of overt indigestion or waterbrash doesn't exclude reflux as a cause of chronic cough.
- Family history of bleeding disorders?
- Drug history, in particular ACE inhibitors. Of people taking ACE inhibitors, 10–20% will have a dry, tickly cough. It is thought to be related to increased levels of bradykinin. It is more common in women than in men. Angiotensin receptor antagonists are better tolerated as they do not interact with the bradykinin activation pathway.
- A travel history may suggest more rare diagnoses.
- Cigarette smoking? This can cause a cough in its own right by acting as an irritant but is strongly associated with bronchial malignancy.
- Occupational agents or exposure to dusts that might account for the cough?

HINTS AND TIPS

Be sure what the patient means by 'coughing up blood'. It is confused with epistaxis and haematemesis more times than you would believe!

EXAMINING THE PATIENT WITH COUGH AND HAEMOPTYSIS

A full general and respiratory examination should be carried out (Fig. 7.2 and see Ch. 31). Assess the following:

- If the patient is breathless, assess the severity by observing respiratory rate and the work of breathing (e.g. using accessory muscles).
- Anaemia: if present, think of malignancy, connective tissue diseases or chronic infection.
- Finger clubbing: suspect bronchial carcinoma, lung abscess, mesothelioma, bronchiectasis, cystic fibrosis or fibrosing alveolitis. Whilst looking at the nails, always look for tar staining
- Cyanosis: hypoxaemia, acute (e.g. pneumonia) or chronic (e.g. COPD, interstitial lung disease).
- Lymphadenopathy: infection or malignancy.
- Look in the sputum pot if the cough is productive.
- Examine for a goitre. Is there retrosternal extension?
- Signs of bronchial carcinoma: e.g. Horner's syndrome, paraneoplastic syndromes.
- Examine the legs for deep vein thromboses: pulmonary embolus (PE) causing haemoptysis.
- Skin: systemic vasculitides may have skin manifestations.
- Facial pain in sinusitis.
- Full respiratory examination: auscultate for bronchial breathing in lobar consolidation, fine crepitations with left ventricular failure or interstitial lung disease and the coarser crepitations of bronchiectasis. A pleural rub may indicate pulmonary infarction.
- Full cardiac examination: auscultate for murmurs, especially mitral stenosis or a pericardial rub.
- Pulmonary hypertension: loud pulmonary component of the second heart sound, a right ventricular heave, a pulmonary systolic murmur and prominent 'a' waves in the jugular venous pressure.
- A localized monophonic wheeze, not disappearing on coughing, suggests a blocked major airway from a carcinoma or a foreign body.

HINTS AND TIPS

Never forget tuberculosis. It is not a historical disease and is easily overlooked.

INVESTIGATING THE PATIENT WITH COUGH AND HAEMOPTYSIS

The following investigations are often used in patients with cough or haemoptysis.

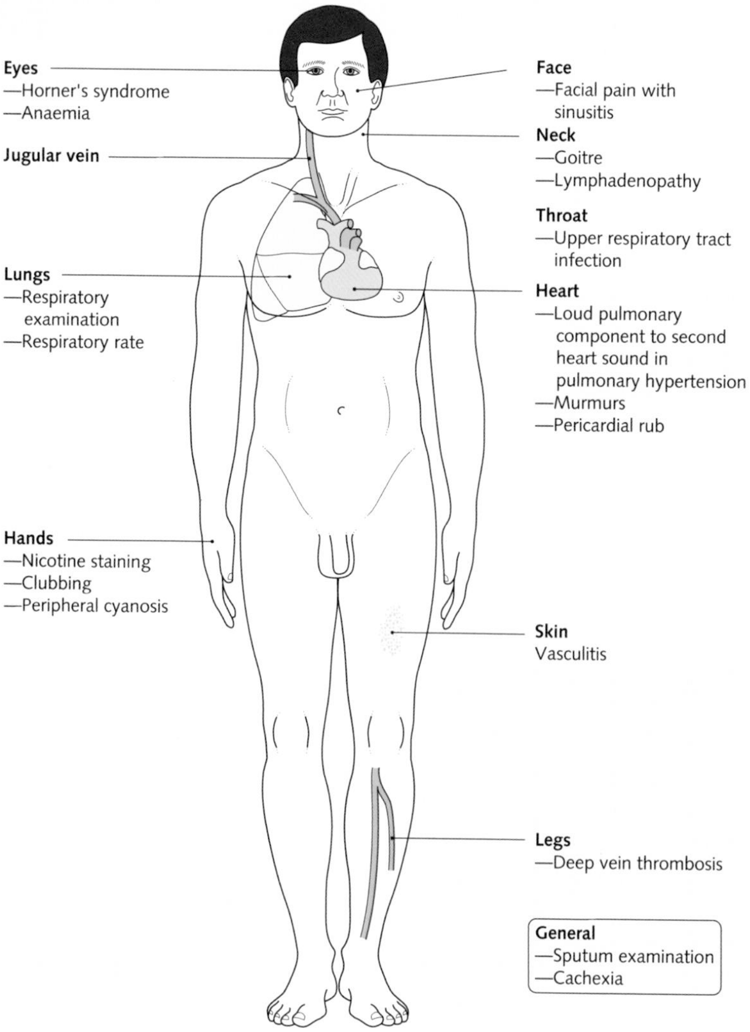

Eyes
—Horner's syndrome
—Anaemia

Jugular vein

Lungs
—Respiratory examination
—Respiratory rate

Hands
—Nicotine staining
—Clubbing
—Peripheral cyanosis

Face
—Facial pain with sinusitis

Neck
—Goitre
—Lymphadenopathy

Throat
—Upper respiratory tract infection

Heart
—Loud pulmonary component to second heart sound in pulmonary hypertension
—Murmurs
—Pericardial rub

Skin
Vasculitis

Legs
—Deep vein thrombosis

General
—Sputum examination
—Cachexia

Fig. 7.2 Examining the patient with cough and haemoptysis.

Bedside

- Vital signs: heart rate, respiratory rate, oxygen saturations, temperature.
- Peak expiratory flow rate.
- Sputum: acid-fast bacillus test (AFBs) for TB, microscopy, culture and cytology.

Blood tests

- Full blood count: anaemia with malignancies, white cell count with infection, pulmonary eosinophilia.
- Urea and electrolytes: check renal function if vasculitis suspected. Electrolytes may be deranged in malignancy (e.g. small cell carcinoma releasing ADH).
- Arterial blood gas analysis.

Imaging

- Chest radiograph: may reveal the pulmonary cause of the cough (e.g. pneumonia, carcinoma, interstitial lung disease, bronchiectasis, bilateral hilar lymphadenopathy in sarcoidosis or tuberculosis).
- CT (sometimes HRCT): to assess malignancy, interstitial lung disease and bronchiectasis.
- CT pulmonary angiogram: if a PE is suspected.
- Sinus X-rays or computed tomography (CT).

Further tests

- Pharyngoscopy: if an upper respiratory cause is suspected.

- Bronchoscopy with or without washings, brushings or biopsies.
- Endobronchial ultrasound ± FNA.
- Peak flow diary: asthma.
- Simple spirometry: if airways disease is suspected.
- Specific lung function tests: if the cause has not been found after the above tests have been carried out (see Ch. 31).
- Gastroscopy, barium swallow or 24-h oesophageal pH recording: to investigate possible GORD.

Pyrexia of unknown origin

Objectives

The key learning points for this chapter:

- The causes of pyrexia of unknown origin (PUO).
- How to assess a patient with PUO thoroughly.
- The pattern of investigation in a patient with PUO.

INTRODUCTION

Fever is a common symptom and a cause is often obvious, such as viral respiratory tract infection. Pyrexia of unknown origin (PUO), also called fever of unknown origin, is defined as a persistent and unexplained fever lasting at least three weeks where a diagnosis has not been reached despite three days of investigation in hospital or three outpatient visits.

CAUSES OF PUO

There is a wide differential diagnosis; the causes can be broadly classified as in Fig. 8.1. The most common malignancy to cause fever is lymphoma, although PUO can also be attributed to solid tumours, particularly renal cell and gastrointestinal carcinoma.

HISTORY IN THE PATIENT WITH PUO

This must be thorough. The systemic enquiry must be rigorous and every symptom explored in detail. Pay particular attention to

- Past medical history, particularly recurrent infection and immunosuppression.
- Surgical history, including complications, and any history of accidents.
- Travel: has there been exposure to endemic diseases (e.g. malaria, histoplasmosis)? The incubation period of many tropical diseases may mean that the symptoms start after arrival back home.
- Contact with animals, both domestic and wild, which may suggest zoonoses, e.g. leptospirosis, Q fever (coxiellosis), salmonellosis, cat-scratch disease (bartonellosis), psittacoses and ornithoses, toxoplasmosis, hydatid disease, toxocariasis, meningitis, anthrax.
- Is there clear exposure to disease-carrying vectors: ticks (e.g. borreliosis, tick typhus), mosquitoes (e.g. malaria, dengue), sand flies (e.g. leishmaniasis).
- Contact with infected people.
- Sexual history: specifics of sexual practice may be helpful.
- IV drug use and sharing of needles.
- Drug history, including over-the-counter medication and any drugs recently started.
- Alcohol intake.
- Immunization history.
- Family history: may point to inherited disorders such as familial Mediterranean fever.
- Symptoms: such as sweats, weight loss, itch, lumps and rash.

Further information can often be obtained by repeating the history to look for additional or missed clues which may point to the diagnosis.

COMMUNICATION

A thorough sexual history is important and becomes easier to elicit with practice.

EXAMINING THE PATIENT WITH PUO

The examination of a patient with PUO is shown in Fig. 8.2. It must be especially thorough and should be repeated frequently. Remember to pay attention to:

- Teeth and throat (e.g. periodontal disease/dental abscess).
- Joint signs and temporal artery tenderness.

Fig. 8.1 The causes of PUO.

Causes	Percentage of cases	Further information
Infections	15–30%	See Ch. 35
Connective tissue disorders	33–40%	See Ch. 33
Malignancy	10–30%	See Ch. 34
Miscellaneous, e.g. drugs, thyroid disorders	5–14%	
Undiagnosed	20–30%	

PUO, pyrexia of unknown origin.

- Eye signs (e.g. conjunctival petechiae).
- Skin lesions (e.g. rashes, petechiae, vasculitic infarction).
- Lymphadenopathy and organomegaly.
- Heart murmurs and stigmata of endocarditis.
- Rectal and vaginal examinations (abscesses, masses, retained tampon).

INVESTIGATING THE PATIENT WITH PUO

Investigations are best directed by the history and examination; for example, if the patient has recently returned from an area where malaria is endemic, thick and thin blood films should be requested. Frequently there will be few clues, and the best way to proceed is to request general non-specific screening tests, the results of which may direct further investigation.

Full blood count and differential white cell count

The full blood count may yield useful information though it is often non-specific:

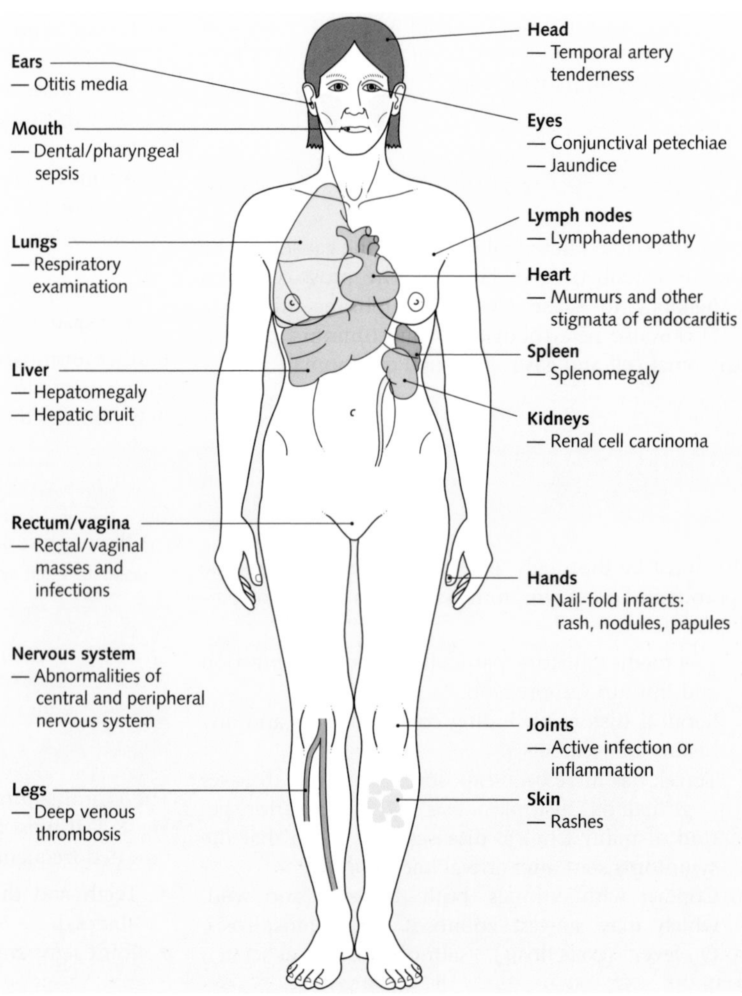

Fig. 8.2 Examining the patient with pyrexia of unknown origin (PUO).

- Neutrophilia: bacterial infections, myeloproliferative disease, malignancy (esp. fast-growing neoplasms), connective tissue disease.
- Lymphocytosis: acute viral infection, chronic intracellular bacterial infection, e.g. tuberculosis and brucellosis, protozoal infection.
- Monocytosis: subacute bacterial endocarditis, inflammatory disease such as Crohn's disease and connective tissue disease, Hodgkin's disease, brucellosis, tuberculosis.
- Atypical lymphocytosis: infectious mononucleosis (acute Epstein–Barr virus infection), cytomegalovirus infection, toxoplasmosis.
- Leukopenia: viral infections, lymphoma, systemic lupus erythematosus, brucellosis, disseminated tuberculosis, drugs.
- Eosinophilia: helminth infection (e.g. schistosomiasis, filariasis), malignancy (especially Hodgkin's disease), drug reaction, pulmonary eosinophilia.

Inflammatory markers

The erythrocyte sedimentation rate (ESR) may be raised in any condition causing inflammation. A very high ESR suggests the following:

- Multiple myeloma.
- Systemic lupus erythematosus.
- Temporal (giant cell) arteritis.
- Polymyalgia rheumatica.
- Still's disease.
- Rheumatic fever.
- Lymphoma.
- Subacute bacterial endocarditis.

Plasma viscosity provides similar information to ESR. C-reactive protein is an 'acute-phase reactant' produced by the liver which, although non-specific, is useful for monitoring disease progress as its level varies more rapidly than ESR due to its short half-life.

Urea and electrolytes

Assessment of urea and electrolytes may reveal renal impairment or electrolyte abnormalities due to the underlying disease, for instance renal impairment in vasculitis.

Liver function tests

Abnormal results suggest further investigation of the liver may be helpful. Note that alkaline phosphatase may also be raised in metabolic bone disease, Hodgkin's disease, Still's disease, polymyalgia rheumatica and patients with bony metastases; if the gamma GT is also raised it suggests the source is hepatic. Mild derangement of liver function is often seen in serious systemic illness, and any abnormality should be monitored closely.

Bacteriology, serology and viral load

Samples should be taken from any possible site and sent for microscopy and culture:

- Urine: bacteria (infections), haematuria (e.g. bacterial endocarditis, renal cell carcinoma). Early morning urine for renal tract TB.
- Blood: taking several samples from different sites at different times will increase the yield of results.
- Faeces: microscopy for ova, cysts and parasites; culture for bacteria; tests for *C. difficile* toxin.
- Vaginal and cervical swabs.
- Urethral swabs in men.
- Sputum microscopy and culture; induced sputum may be required.
- Throat swab cultures.
- Bone marrow and cerebrospinal fluid: if lumbar puncture or bone marrow aspiration is performed, samples should be sent for culture including TB.

Many specific serological tests are available, often detecting both IgG and IgM levels, and should be performed as directed by the history and examination. Raised IgM levels may indicate acute infection, but a positive IgG result may need to be repeated to look for a rising titre. Occasionally serology is performed 'blindly' if there are no clues as to the diagnosis. An HIV test should be considered in anyone presenting with PUO.

In certain circumstances it may be useful to check and monitor the viral load (e.g. CMV, EBV, HIV).

Chest X-ray

This may show, for instance, tuberculosis, abscess or lymphadenopathy.

Further investigations

These are best directed by clinical findings and the results of initial tests, but it may be necessary to proceed 'blindly'. Non-invasive tests should be performed first. In this case, the following are reasonable initial investigations:

- Autoimmune screen including rheumatoid factor, extractable nuclear antigens and ANCA.
- Immunoglobulins and protein electrophoresis.
- Interferon release assay for TB (e.g. QuantiFERON/T-spot).
- Antistreptolysin-O titre and tumour markers.
- Abdominal ultrasound or CT scan.

All non-essential drugs should be stopped on admission. It may be necessary to withhold other drugs, and the response monitored. If there is still no clue as to the cause, the system most likely to be responsible should be investigated and the following tests may be considered:

- Echocardiogram (transthoracic or transoesophageal).
- CT scan of chest with contrast, bronchoscopy and bronchoalveolar lavage.
- Bone marrow biopsy and culture.
- FDG-positron emission tomography (FDG-PET) or white cell scintigraphy.
- Temporal artery biopsy if patient aged over 55.
- Lumbar puncture, lymph node biopsy or liver biopsy.
- Exploratory laparoscopy is occasionally needed.

Rare causes should be considered including hyperthyroidism, phaeochromocytoma and familial Mediterranean fever.

Factitious fever is deliberate manipulation of the thermometer, classically said to occur in young women, and should be considered if no other cause can be found and the patient looks inappropriately well despite fever.

If all else fails, consideration should be given to blind treatment, for instance treating suspected TB with antituberculous chemotherapy, endocarditis with antibiotics and vasculitides with steroids.

HINTS AND TIPS

Remember to go over the history and examination repeatedly, even when investigations are in progress.

Dyspepsia 9

Objectives

The key learning points for this chapter:

- Understand the differential diagnosis of dyspepsia.
- Have a systematic approach to assessing a patient presenting with dyspepsia.
- Have a logical approach to investigating patients with dyspepsia.

INTRODUCTION

Dyspepsia describes a group of symptoms that relate to the upper gastrointestinal (GI) tract. These symptoms include upper abdominal discomfort, retrosternal pain, anorexia, nausea, vomiting, bloating, fullness, heartburn and early satiety. The prevalence of these symptoms have been estimated between 20 and 30%.

The approach to this common presenting complaint involves directing investigations towards those most likely to benefit (e.g. those at risk of cancer where a firm endoscopic/histological diagnosis must be made) as opposed to those in whom empirical therapy is safe and a firm diagnosis would not significantly alter their management (e.g. a young, otherwise well, patient with dyspepsia and no *Helicobacter pylori* infection).

CAUSES OF DYSPEPSIA

This chapter emphasizes that it is not always essential to make a firm diagnosis in the dyspeptic patient in order to treat them appropriately. However, a definitive diagnosis may be reached following investigation or if further investigations are performed at the discretion of the clinician, perhaps due to persistent, uncontrolled symptoms. The causes of dyspepsia are shown in Fig. 9.1.

HISTORY AND EXAMINATION IN THE PATIENT WITH DYSPEPSIA

The following features should be asked for, although the precise symptoms correlate poorly with the underlying cause:

- Heartburn: usually retrosternal and often worse with leaning forward or lying down. Suggestive of acid reflux and may be associated with 'waterbrash', a flood of saliva in the mouth as a reflex response to acid in the lower oesophagus.
- Chest pain: burning retrosternal pain, not related to exertion (unlike angina), which may radiate between the shoulder blades. This can relate to acid-provoked oesophageal spasm, which, like angina, is relieved by nitrates.
- Nocturnal cough/asthma: occasionally due to acid reflux.
- Aggravating factors for reflux:
  - increased intra-abdominal pressure: stooping/bending/obesity/pregnancy
  - spicy or fatty foods
  - alcohol ingestion: also causes gastritis
  - cigarettes, caffeine, theophylline, calcium channel blockers, beta-blockers, anticholinergic drugs: reduce lower oesophageal sphincter tone
  - non-steroidal anti-inflammatory drugs (NSAIDs) interfere with prostaglandin cytoprotection
  - hiatus hernia.
- Epigastric pain: feature of peptic ulcer disease. Aggravated by food (gastric ulcer) or fasting (duodenal ulcer), but not always.

The most important part of the assessment in these patients is to identify those who require endoscopic investigation (see below). This depends on the presence of the 'red flag symptoms or signs' listed in Fig. 9.2, which MUST be looked for specifically. These features all suggest an elevated risk of cancer and help to ensure that endoscopy is not denied to those at risk of cancer.

INVESTIGATING THE PATIENT WITH DYSPEPSIA

An approach to the dyspeptic patient is outlined in Fig. 9.3. The management of specific conditions is further explained in Ch. 32.

The investigations used are explained below. Specialized investigations are used predominantly in cases such

Fig. 9.1 Causes of dyspepsia (see Ch. 32).

Duodenal ulcer**
Gastric ulcer**
Oesophageal/gastric cancer*
Oesophagitis/GORD
Gastritis/duodenitis**
Non-ulcer dyspepsia**
Hiatus hernia
Oesophageal motility disorders
Biliary pathology

*or** *indicates the conditions associated with* Helicobacter pylori *infection. It is unclear whether it is causative in all these conditions, but some (marked**) have been shown to respond favourably to its eradication.*
GORD, gastro-oesophageal reflux disease.

Fig. 9.2 Symptoms in patients with dyspepsia which indicate that diagnostic endoscopy should be performed.

Unintentional weight loss >3 kg
Gastrointestinal bleeding
Previous gastric surgery
Epigastric mass
Previous gastric ulcer
Unexplained iron-deficiency anaemia
Dysphagia/odynophagia
Persistent vomiting
Suspicious barium meal
Age ≥55 years with recent-onset dyspepsia lasting more than 4 weeks

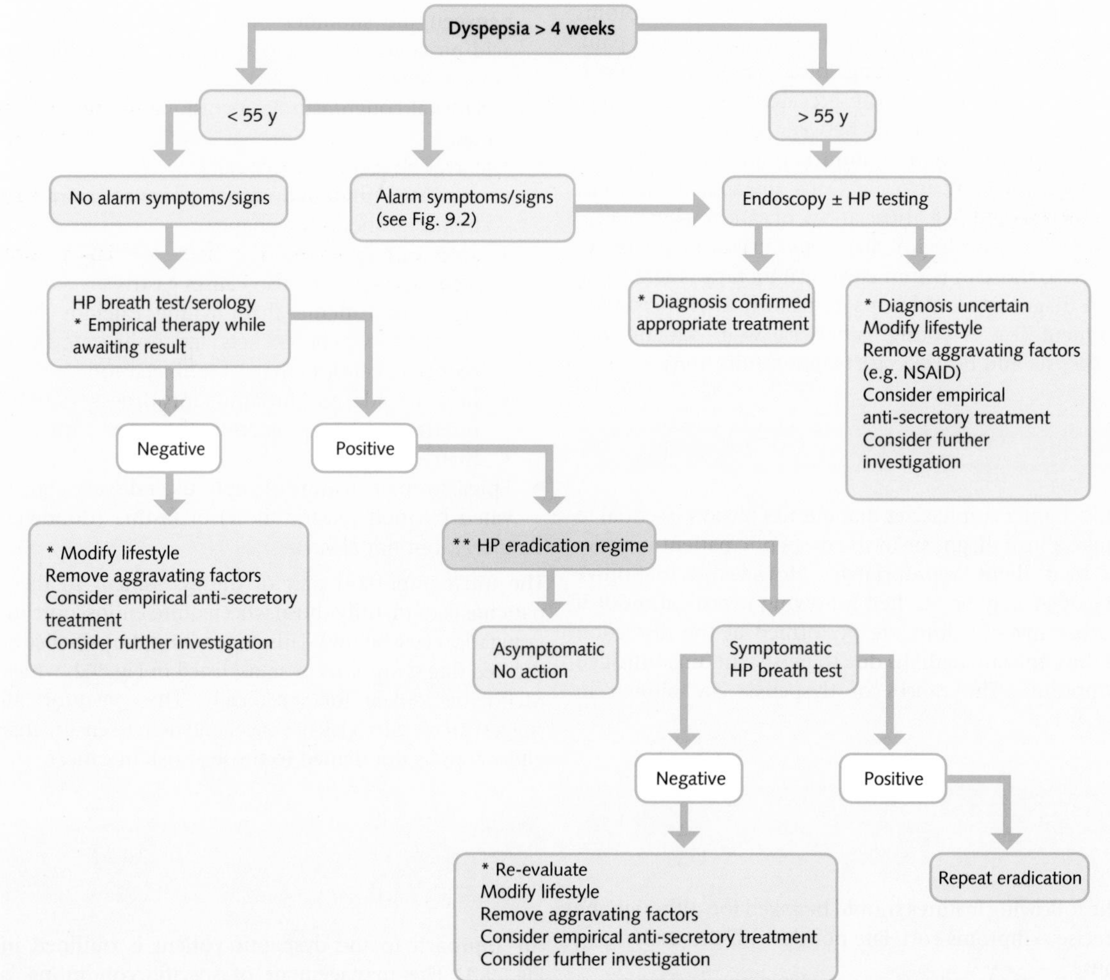

Fig. 9.3 Algorithm for the investigation and management of patients with dyspepsia. See Ch. 32. Seek local microbiological advice. Further information on the management of dyspepsia can be obtained from www.nice.org.uk/guidance (Guidance CG17, Dyspepsia: quick reference guide). HP, *Helicobacter pylori;* NSAID, non-steroidal anti-inflammatory drug.

as persistent symptoms not responding to the approach in Fig. 9.3 or atypical symptoms (e.g. laryngeal discomfort or atypical chest pain that may result from acid reflux or oesophageal dysmotility). It is important to remember that the majority of patients with dyspepsia can be managed safely without extensive investigations provided the algorithm in Fig. 9.3 is adhered to.

HINTS AND TIPS

Although dyspepsia or heartburn is usually a gastrointestinal complaint, some older patients with 'dyspepsia' turn out to have angina pectoris. Make sure you question the patient carefully to ensure that the problem is gastrointestinal in origin.

Common investigations

- Full blood count: microcytic anaemia and/or thrombocytosis may suggest gastrointestinal blood loss and needs urgent further investigation.
- Electrocardiography (ECG): if considering the diagnosis of angina in cases of atypical chest pain. Acid reflux can cause non-specific ECG changes and therefore further investigations such as exercise tolerance testing may be necessary.
- *Helicobacter pylori* testing: several tests are available. Carbon-tagged breath tests (depend on urease breakdown of urea) are the most accurate and can confirm eradication following treatment (but cannot be used in patients taking proton pump inhibitors, bismuth or within 4 weeks of antibiotic use). Immunoglobulin G serological tests confirm previous infection but cannot provide information on eradication and have a high false-positive rate and are therefore not reliable and should not be used. Urease tests can be used on endoscopic specimens and histology/culture can confirm these findings.
- Endoscopy (oesophagogastroduodenoscopy, OGD): very safe but not totally risk-free (4 in 100 000). Allows visualization of the upper gastrointestinal tract to the second part of the duodenum and biopsy and therapeutic manoeuvres if required (see Ch. 32).
- Barium meal: alternative for patients in whom endoscopy is not possible, e.g. elderly frail patients in whom sedation is dangerous.

Specialized investigations

- Oesophageal motility studies: manometry demonstrates motility disorders (e.g. achalasia, systemic sclerosis, diffuse oesophageal spasm).
- 24-h intraluminal pH monitoring: confirms acid reflux in difficult cases.
- Abdominal ultrasound: if a mass or biliary pathology is suspected (see Ch. 32).

Haematemesis and melaena

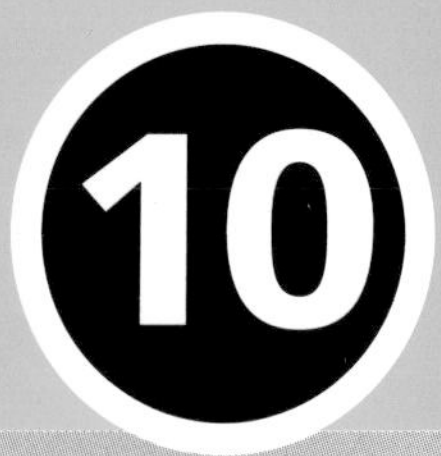

Objectives

The key learning points for this chapter:
- Know the causes of haematemesis and melaena.
- Assess a patient with haematemesis and melaena, particularly in an emergency.
- Understand the investigations of haematemesis and melaena.

INTRODUCTION

Haematemesis is the vomiting of fresh (bright red) or altered ('coffee grounds') blood. Melaena is the production of black, tarry stools, and is due to bleeding in the gastrointestinal (GI) tract usually above the hepatic flexure. Both are typical signs of an upper GI bleed. GI bleeding is an emergency, and treatment is usually initiated before a diagnosis has been made (see Ch. 32).

DIFFERENTIAL DIAGNOSIS OF HAEMATEMESIS AND MELAENA

Fig. 10.1 gives the differential diagnosis of haematemesis and melaena. It is important to note that melaena alone may be caused by pathology in the small bowel or ascending colon.

HISTORY IN THE PATIENT WITH HAEMATEMESIS AND MELAENA

The history may have to be taken after initial resuscitation procedures. It is important to determine whether the blood has been vomited or coughed. In cases of difficulty, the presence of food mixed with the blood or an acid pH is suggestive of haematemesis, although the vomitus may not be acidic in patients with carcinoma of the stomach.

Haematemesis may be due to blood swallowed from the nasopharynx or mouth. You must ask about the following.

Presenting complaint

- Non-specific symptoms of hypovolaemia: faintness, weakness, dizziness, sweating, palpitations, dyspnoea, pallor, collapse. These symptoms may precede the actual haematemesis/melaena.
- Symptoms of chronic blood loss: suggests gastric carcinoma if associated with anorexia and weight loss.
- Heartburn: oesophagitis.
- Weight loss and anorexia: carcinoma.
- Dysphagia or odynophagia (pain on swallowing): oesophageal carcinoma or oesophagitis.
- Retching, especially after an alcohol binge: Mallory–Weiss tear.
- Sudden severe abdominal pain: possible bowel perforation.
- Intermittent epigastric pain relieved with antacids: peptic ulceration.

Other important points

- Current drugs: aspirin, non-steroidal anti-inflammatory drugs, steroids or excessive alcohol are suggestive of gastric erosions; iron therapy causes black stools but this is not melaena; anticoagulation will exacerbate bleeding.
- Chronic excessive alcohol intake and other causes of liver disease (see Ch. 13): oesophageal varices.
- A past history of GI bleeds and their cause.
- Family history: inherited bleeding disorders.

EXAMINING THE PATIENT WITH HAEMATEMESIS AND MELAENA

The approach to examining the patient with haematemesis and melaena is given in Fig. 10.2. Step back from

Fig. 10.1 The differential diagnosis of haematemesis and melaena.

Cause	Notes
Peptic ulcer disease	Causes 50% of major upper GI bleeds. 10% mortality
Erosive gastritis	Causes 20% of upper GI bleeds, rarely severe
Mallory–Weiss tear	Causes 10% of upper GI bleeds. Laceration in GOJ mucosa, often following retching (e.g. after alcohol binge)
Oesophagitis	Due to GORD
Ruptured oesophageal varices	Cause 10–20% of upper GI bleeds. Mortality up to 40%. Due to portal hypertension
Vascular abnormalities	Vascular ectasias or angiodysplasias. Also cause of lower GI bleeding
Gastric neoplasm	Causes 5% of upper GI bleeds
Rare causes	Oesophageal ulcers or tumours, aortoenteric fistula after abdominal aortic surgery, pancreatic tumour, biliary bleeding, blood dyscrasias

GI, gastrointestinal; GOJ, gastro-oesophageal junction; GORD, gastro-oesophageal reflux disease.

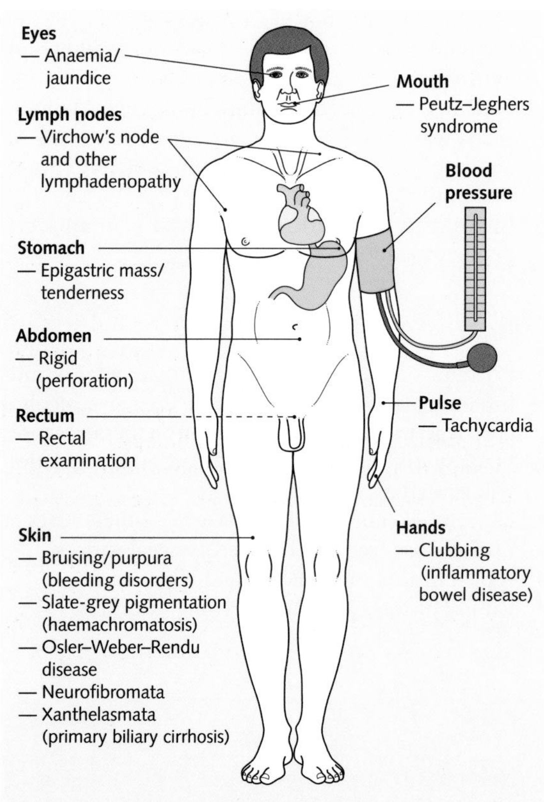

Fig. 10.2 Examining the patient with haematemesis and melaena.

the patient for a few seconds. Do they look well, or pale and clammy? An initial commonsense impression affects the immediacy of subsequent management. The first priority in a patient with active bleeding is to follow the ABC principles, which include obtaining good venous access and starting appropriate fluid replacement.

- Clubbing: inflammatory bowel disease, cirrhosis.
- Pulse and blood pressure: tachycardia is a reflex response to hypovolaemia (due to bleeding) and usually precedes a blood pressure fall. A young and healthy patient may lose more than 500 mL of blood before a rise in heart rate or fall in blood pressure occurs. If the patient is hypotensive, IV fluid resuscitation is imperative, as is frequent monitoring of pulse and blood pressure to assess haemodynamic trends.
- Skin: bruises, purpura (bleeding disorders); telangiectasia (Osler–Weber–Rendu disease (hereditary haemorrhagic telangiectasia – autosomal dominant)); neurofibromata; pale (shut down)
- Jaundice: may indicate portal hypertension and clotting abnormality.
- Anaemia: mucous membranes. If clinically anaemic, this may indicate chronic blood loss.
- Lymphadenopathy: especially Virchow's node (left supraclavicular lymph node) associated with gastric carcinoma (Troisier's sign).
- Mouth: pharyngeal lesions; pigmented macules (Peutz–Jeghers syndrome).

- Cachexia.
- A rigid abdomen suggests bowel perforation.
- Epigastric tenderness suggests peptic ulcer disease, oesophagitis, hiatus hernia or gastric carcinoma.
- Epigastric mass: gastric carcinoma.
- If malignancy is suspected, examine for metastases.
- Signs of chronic liver disease and portal hypertension support the possibility of oesophageal varices (see Ch. 13).

INVESTIGATING THE PATIENT WITH HAEMATEMESIS AND MELAENA

HINTS AND TIPS

A large upper GI bleed may cause the passage of fresh blood per rectum rather than melaena; in this setting the patient is likely to be haemodynamically unstable.

An algorithm for the investigation of the patient with haematemesis and melaena is given in Fig. 10.3. The following investigations should be carried out which will aid in diagnosis as well as contribute to predicting associated mortality (Figs 10.4 and 10.5)

Bedside

- Heart rate, blood pressure, respiratory rate and oxygen saturations.

Blood tests

- A full blood count should be performed. The haemoglobin may be normal in the acute phase, despite a large GI bleed, as it takes some hours for haemodilution to occur. A low haemoglobin on initial presentation and/or a low mean corpuscular volume (MCV) suggests chronic blood loss, and the white cell count may be raised after a GI bleed. Platelet count may be reduced after an acute bleed or increased after chronic blood loss. A very low platelet count should raise suspicion of a bleeding diathesis.
- Group and save even if there is only a small GI bleed and the patient is haemodynamically stable. Blood should be cross-matched for more significant bleeding.
- A clotting screen should also be performed, as the prothrombin time is raised in liver disease. More specific investigations may be indicated (e.g. in patients with haemophilia or von Willebrand's disease).
- Urea is raised because of the absorption and subsequent breakdown of protein when blood reaches the small bowel. Intravascular volume depletion causing prerenal impairment also contributes.

Further investigations

- On erect chest X-ray, the presence of gas under the right hemidiaphragm indicates bowel perforation.
- Endoscopy (gastroscopy) is usually performed within 24 h if the patient is shocked or has significant co-morbidity, immediately if variceal bleeding is suspected. It allows direct visualization of the pathology and provides a diagnosis in around 90% of cases. This will determine the most appropriate form of medical therapy. The risk of rebleeding (the major cause of mortality) may be estimated. Treatment may be given endoscopically (e.g. banding or sclerosing a bleeding varix, or adrenaline (epinephrine) injection of a bleeding vessel). If the endoscopy is negative, a colonoscopy should be performed to rule out a proximal colonic bleed.
- Barium examinations are becoming less common as endoscopy is becoming more widely available.

Most patients do not require further tests but occasionally these are performed under the guidance of a specialist when the diagnosis remains uncertain (see Fig. 10.3):

- Isotope studies: abdominal gamma scanning can detect extravasation of radioisotope-labelled red blood cells if active bleeding is present. These are now very rarely undertaken.
- Mesenteric angiography again requires active bleeding to localize the source. It can also be used to visualize the portal venous system.
- CT/MRI $\pm$ capsule endoscopy are modern means of investigating small intestinal pathology.
- Diagnostic laparoscopy before laparotomy and surgically assisted enteroscopy are occasionally performed.

Despite extensive investigation, a small minority of patients will remain undiagnosed. If bleeding is severe, laparotomy may be required but if it is not severe the patient may attend for repeat 'top-up' transfusions or iron infusions as required.

HINTS AND TIPS

Elevated blood urea with normal serum creatinine suggests gastrointestinal blood loss.

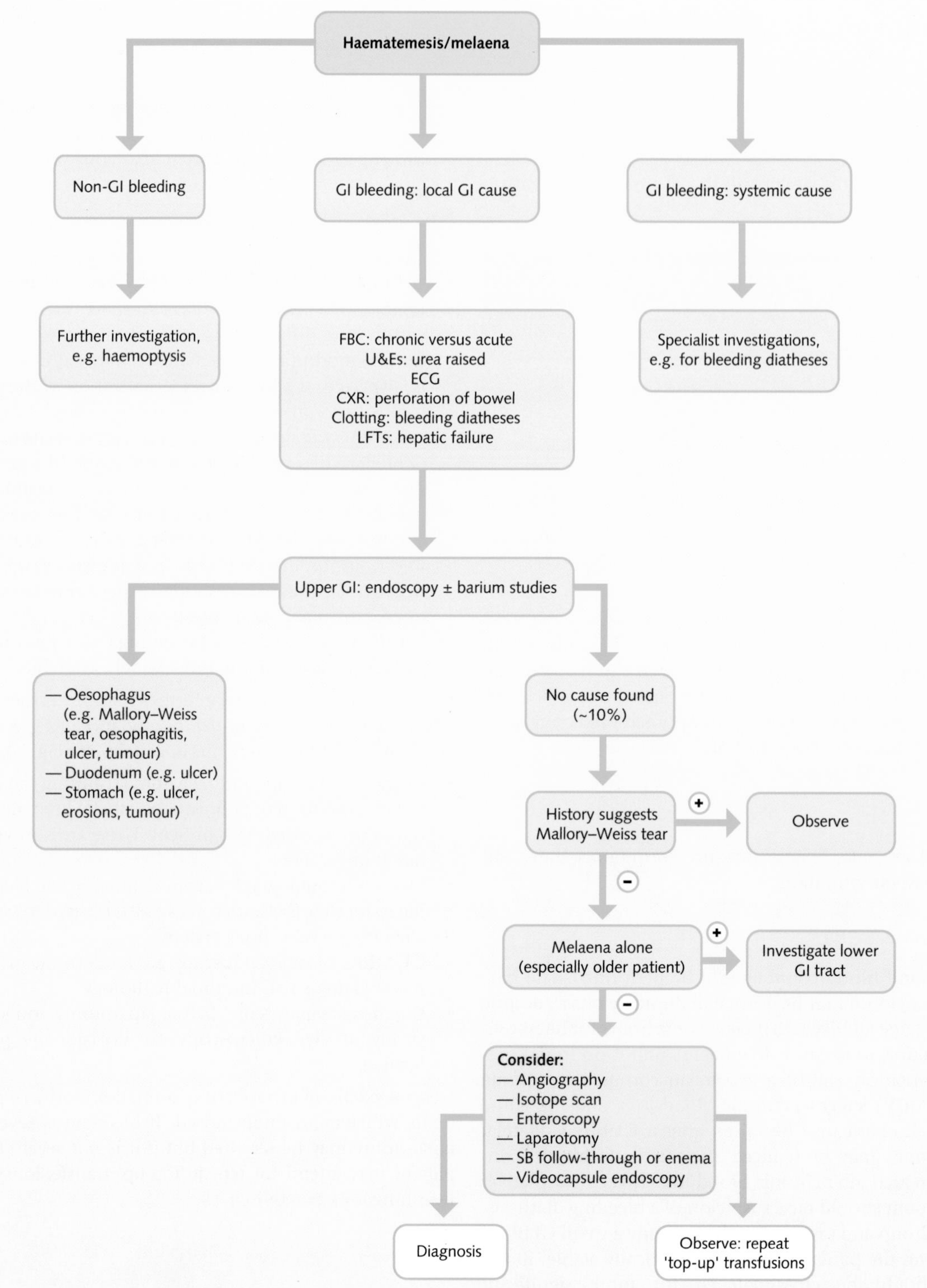

Fig. 10.3 Algorithm for the investigation of the patient with haematemesis and melaena. ECG, electrocardiogram; CXR, chest X-ray; FBC, full blood count; GI, gastrointestinal; LFTs, liver function tests; SB, small bowel; U&Es, urea and electrolytes.

Fig. 10.4 Rockall score. The score is used to predict mortality (pre and post endoscopy) for patients presenting with a GI bleed.

Variable	Score 0	Score 1	Score 2	Score 3
Age	<60	60–79	80	
Shock	No shock	Pulse >100 SBP >100	SBP <100	
Co-morbidity	Nil major		CCF, IHD, major morbidity	Renal or liver failure, metastatic cancer
Diagnosis	Mallory–Weiss tear	All other diagnosis	GI malignancy	
Evidence of bleeding	None		Blood, adherent clot, spurting vessel	

SBP, systolic blood pressure.

Fig. 10.5 Prediction of rebleeding and mortality from the Rockall score.

	Mortality	
Score	**Initial score (%)**	**Final score after endoscopy (%)**
0	0.2	0
1	2	0
2	6	0.2
3	11	3
4	25	5
5	40	11
6	50	17
7	50	27
8+	–	41

Change in bowel habit

Objectives

The key learning points for this chapter:

- Know the causes of diarrhoea and constipation.
- Assess patients with altered bowel habit.
- Understand the pattern of investigation for patients with altered bowel habit.

INTRODUCTION

Always ask about the patient's normal bowel habit because there are considerable differences between people, usually varying from three times a day to once every 3 days. Changes in a patient's usual bowel habit are important and may suggest an underlying pathology. Constipation is defined as abnormally delayed or infrequent passage of dry hardened stool. Diarrhoea is defined as abnormally frequent intestinal evacuations with more or less fluid stools. Figs 11.1 and 11.2 summarize the causes of diarrhoea and constipation, respectively.

DIFFERENTIAL DIAGNOSIS OF A CHANGE IN BOWEL HABIT

HINTS AND TIPS

Make sure that by 'constipation' and 'diarrhoea' you and the patient mean the same thing.

HINTS AND TIPS

Note the features of acute GI obstruction: absolute constipation, vomiting, pain and abdominal distension.

HISTORY IN THE PATIENT WITH A CHANGE IN BOWEL HABIT

Ask about the following.

Presenting complaint

- Normal bowel habit and diet.
- Onset: sudden or chronic. Infectious diarrhoea is usually of acute onset.
- Frequency of defecation.
- Stool appearance: formed, loose or watery; colour – normal, red (blood from low in the gastrointestinal (GI) tract), black (melaena), yellow (mucus and slime), 'redcurrant jelly' (intussusception), putty-coloured (obstructive jaundice); volume; do the stools float? (high fat content – think of malabsorption).
- Associated features (e.g. pain, fever, vomiting, weight loss, extraintestinal manifestations of inflammatory bowel disease) (see Ch. 32).
- Nocturnal symptoms: these go against a functional disorder.
- Tenesmus (a sense of incomplete voiding).
- Smell: offensively malodorous in malabsorption; characteristic smell of melaena.
- Symptoms of thyrotoxicosis.

Other important points

- Relationship to food.
- Contact with diarrhoea sufferers.
- Stress.
- Foreign travel.
- Drugs: antacids, laxatives, cimetidine, digoxin, antibiotics, alcohol.
- Surgical history (e.g. multiple bowel resections for Crohn's disease can result in malabsorption).

EXAMINING THE PATIENT WITH A CHANGE IN BOWEL HABIT

The examination approach in the patient with a change in bowel habit is given in Fig. 11.3.

Fig. 11.1 Differential diagnosis of diarrhoea (see Ch. 32).

Causes	Examples
Infective	Bacterial: *Campylobacter* (poultry), *Salmonella* (meat, poultry and dairy), *Shigella* (faecal–oral transmission) Viral: rotavirus, Norwalk virus, cytomegalovirus Protozoa: *Giardia lamblia, Cryptosporidium, Entamoeba histolytica*
Inflammatory	Inflammatory bowel disease Malignancy Radiation enteritis
Ischaemic	Emboli or mesenteric atheromatous disease
Functional	Irritable bowel syndrome
Secretory	Infection (e.g. cholera) VIPoma/Zollinger–Ellison/carcinoid Villous adenoma Factitious diarrhoea (e.g. laxative abuse) Bile salt malabsorption (disruption of enterohepatic circulation)
Osmotic	Medications (e.g. antacids and lactulose) Disaccharidase deficiency Factitious diarrhoea
Malabsorption	See Ch. 32 for causes
Systemic illness	Hyperthyroidism, diabetes mellitus, Addison's disease (see Ch. 35)
Overflow diarrhoea	Faecal impaction in elderly
Drugs	Alcohol, digoxin, metformin, neomycin, proton pump inhibitors, bisphosphonates

Fig. 11.2 Differential diagnosis of constipation (see Ch. 32).

Causes	Examples
Congenital	Hirschsprung's disease
Mechanical obstruction	Inflammatory stricture (e.g. Crohn's disease, diverticulitis) Neoplasm Extraluminal mass (e.g. pelvic) Rectocele
Lifestyle	Diet Dehydration Immobility Lack of privacy (e.g. hospital ward)
Pain	Fissure-in-ano Thrombosed haemorrhoids Postoperative
Metabolic/ endocrine	Hypothyroidism (see Ch. 35) Hypercalcaemia Diabetic neuropathy
Drugs	Opiates, anticholinergics, diuretics
Neurological	Paraplegia (see Ch. 34) Multiple sclerosis
Functional	Irritable bowel syndrome Idiopathic megacolon/rectum

INVESTIGATING THE PATIENT WITH A CHANGE IN BOWEL HABIT

The wide range of possible diagnoses in patients with altered bowel habit is reflected by the large number of tests that may be performed. Some of these are used commonly, whereas others are used much less frequently and only under the guidance of specialists.

Common investigations

Blood tests

- Full blood count.
- Urea and electrolytes, including calcium.
- Thyroid function tests.
- Blood glucose: diabetes.
- Liver function tests.
- Albumin: decreased in malabsorption, protein-losing enteropathies, inflammatory diseases.
- In malabsorption: anaemia – vitamin B_{12}, folate, iron; hyponatraemia in profound secretory diarrhoea; reduced absorption of fat-soluble vitamins – prolonged prothrombin time (vitamin K), hypocalcaemia (vitamin D), visual impairment rarely (vitamin A).
- Anti-tissue transglutaminase antibodies if suspect coeliac disease.
- Inflammatory markers (erythrocyte sedimentation rate and C-reactive protein) – raised in infection/ inflammation. Many centres now measure plasma viscosity.

Imaging

- Abdominal X-ray: pancreatic calcification suggests chronic pancreatitis, distended intestinal loops and fluid levels suggest obstruction, and gross dilatation of the colon suggests Hirschsprung's disease (rare). Featureless colon, with loss of haustral markings, may indicate colitis.
- Abdominal ultrasound and/or computed tomography for suspected masses and pancreatitis. Or MRI

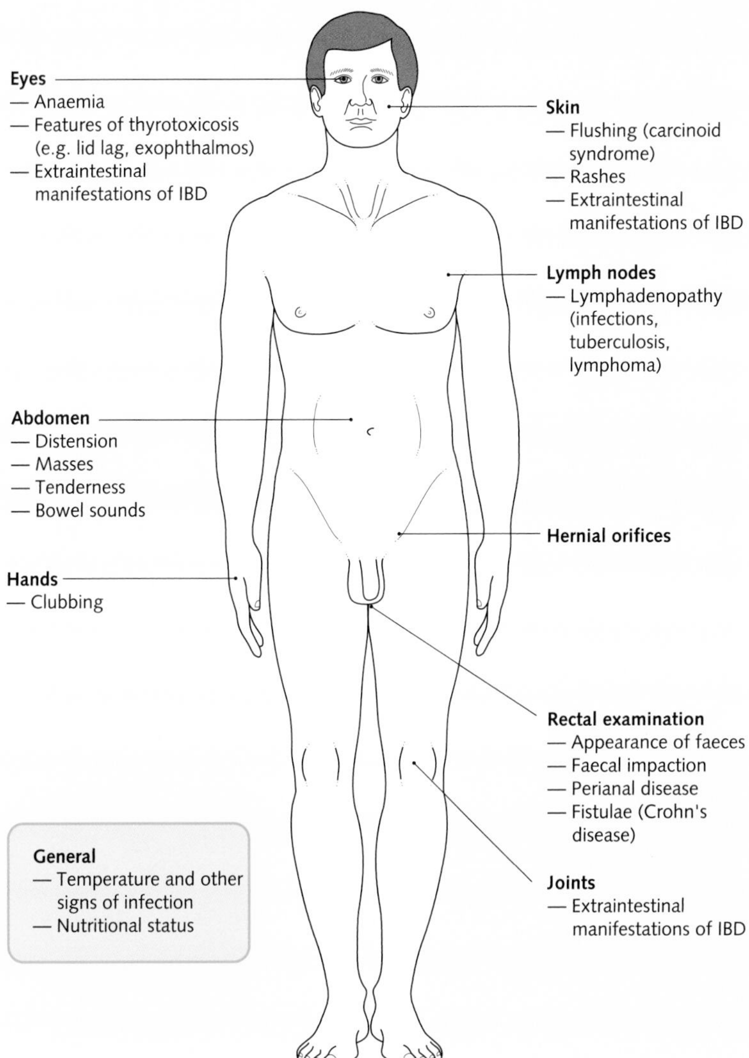

Fig. 11.3 Examining the patient with a change in bowel habit. IBD, inflammatory bowel disease.

enterography, particularly in young people, to avoid ionizing radiation.

- Videocapsule endoscopy for small bowel pathology.

Invasive investigations and direct visualization of the bowel

- Rigid sigmoidoscopy – performed without sedation (e.g. in outpatients) and allows inspection and/or biopsy of rectal mucosa.
- Flexible sigmoidoscopy/colonoscopy – examination of the large bowel and allows for biopsies even if macroscopically normal to exclude microscopic colitis.
- Oesophagogastroduodenoscopy (OGD) and D2 biopsy for malabsorption.
- Endoscopic retrograde cholangiopancreatography, magnetic resonance cholangiopancreatography and/or endoscopic ultrasound for suspected biliary and pancreatic pathology.

Further investigations

- Stool microscopy, culture and detection of *Clostridium difficile* toxin if suspect infection.
- Faecal calprotectin as a means of differentiating inflammatory from non-inflammatory diarrhoea, this is now commonly used.
- Faecal elastase test for pancreatic exocrine function.

- Xylose absorption test for mucosal function (this is a research tool only).
- Assessment of bile salt absorption using radioisotope-labelled bile acids (SeHCAT scan).
- Faecal clearance of alpha-1-antitrypsin to investigate protein-losing enteropathy.
- Laxative screen.
- Colonic transit study: to confirm constipation and measure the transit time.
- Studies of pelvic floor function: defecating proctography and anal manometry.
- Fasting gut hormones: serum vasoactive intestinal polypeptide (VIPoma); serum gastrin (Zollinger–Ellison syndrome); chromogrannin calcitonin (medullary thyroid carcinoma); cortisol (Addison's disease); 24-h urinary 5-hydroxyindoleacetic acid (carcinoid syndrome).

Weight loss 12

Objectives

The key learning points for this chapter:
- Understand the many causes of weight loss.
- Have a logical approach to assessing the patient with involuntary weight loss.
- Know how to direct investigations in a patient with weight loss.

INTRODUCTION

Weight loss is due to either a decreased energy intake or increased energy output, or both. Involuntary weight loss is a common manifestation of physical or psychological illness and always warrants further investigation. It should be confirmed objectively with records of previous weights. If this is not possible, a change in clothes size gives a useful clue. Family members may be able to give a more objective history.

DIFFERENTIAL DIAGNOSIS OF WEIGHT LOSS

Distinguish deliberate from involuntary weight loss from the outset. Fig. 12.1 summarizes the differential diagnosis of weight loss.

HINTS AND TIPS

Malignancies anywhere that produce a high metabolic rate or which lead to anorexia or dysphagia (e.g. oesophageal carcinoma) will result in weight loss. Therefore malignancy must be excluded in patients with unexplained weight loss.

HISTORY IN THE PATIENT WITH WEIGHT LOSS

Weight loss can be a complication of disease in any system.

Try to confirm weight loss objectively with records of previous weights. Ask members of the family or friends if they have noticed weight loss. Ask about the amount of weight loss, its duration and any accompanying symptoms such as anorexia or increased appetite.

Further factors to assess, if the cause is not apparent, include the following.

Presenting complaint

- How much weight has been lost? Over what time frame? Intentional?
- Diet: detailed intake and any recent changes in diet history.
- Physical activity: any changes in level.
- Careful GI history: change in bowel habit, melaena, PR bleeding, change in stool consistency.

Systems review

- Symptoms of chronic infection, inflammation or malignancy: fever and sweats, rashes, general malaise, anorexia, change in bowel habit, floating stools (malabsorption), haemoptysis, haematemesis, haematuria, obstructive urinary symptoms (prostate), melaena (or bleeding from any other site), 'lumps and bumps' (including breast), joint or muscle tenderness, contacts with infected people, dysphagia.
- Symptoms of renal insufficiency: anorexia, general malaise and lethargy, bruising, urinary symptoms (e.g. polyuria and nocturia), vomiting, hiccoughs.
- Menstrual history: in premenopausal women significant weight loss may lead to amenorrhoea, particularly in anorexia nervosa.
- Cardiorespiratory symptoms: cardiac cachexia.
- Neurological symptoms.
- Psychiatric symptoms – make sure to do a depression screen and don't forget anorexia nervosa.

Finally the symptoms of endocrinopathies include the following:

- Diabetes: polyuria and polydipsia, weakness and fatigue, blurred vision, pruritus or thrush, nocturnal enuresis.
- Adrenal insufficiency: dizziness and collapses, weakness, nausea and diarrhoea, pigmentation.

Fig. 12.1 The differential diagnosis of weight loss.

Causes	Examples
Psychiatric/ psychological	Anorexia nervosa Depression or agitation Catatonia Schizophrenia Laxative or diuretic abuse Neglect (e.g. 'tea and toast' diet in widowhood) See *Crash Course: Psychiatry*
Pathological	Endocrine Uncontrolled diabetes mellitus Hyperthyroidism and rarely hypothyroidism Adrenal insufficiency Phaeochromocytoma Hypopituitarism Severe diabetes insipidus See Ch. 35
Drugs	Alcohol, tobacco, laxatives or diuretics, opiates, amphetamines
Infections	Tuberculosis HIV (human immunodeficiency virus) Other chronic infections and infestations See Ch. 38
Chronic inflammation	Inflammatory bowel disease Connective tissue disease See Chs 32 & 36
Malignancy	
Chronic illness	Cardiac failure ('cardiac cachexia') Chronic obstructive pulmonary disease Chronic renal failure See Chs 30, 31 & 32
Gastrointestinal	Peptic ulcer disease Dysphagia Malabsorption Liver disease See Ch. 32
Neurological	Motor neurone disease Myopathies Poliomyelitis See Ch. 34

- Thyrotoxicosis: tremor, diarrhoea, irritability, heat intolerance, palpitations.
- Phaeochromocytoma: headache, sweating and tachycardia are the classic triad.
- Panhypopituitarism: pallor, dizziness, loss of body hair, loss of libido, amenorrhoea, visual field defects, symptoms of hypothyroidism.

Other important points

- Full drug history: including over-the-counter and illegal medicines.
- Alcohol intake: with and without associated liver disease.
- Smoking: if recent onset, this may lead to eating less; if chronic, assess its association with malignancies.

HINTS AND TIPS

Many patients with unexplained weight loss fear an underlying malignancy. It is important to make time to address these concerns.

EXAMINING THE PATIENT WITH WEIGHT LOSS

The causes of weight loss are multiple and may be associated with pathology of any system. As such it is crucial the clinical examination is thorough, detailed and complete to pick up any clue regarding the underlying cause.

General observation

The examination approach in the patient with weight loss is given in Fig. 12.2. Does the patient look like they have lost weight (loose skin, loose clothes)? Check the temperature. Does the patient look well or ill? The patient's weight, height and body mass index should be documented.

General examination

- Clubbing: malignancy, cirrhosis, inflammatory bowel disease and infections (chronic suppurative lung disease, infective endocarditis).
- Leuconychia and palmar erythema: liver disease (leuconychia reflects hypoalbuminaemia).
- Koilonychia: iron-deficiency anaemia.
- Pigmentation: increased in Addison's disease (particularly in palmar creases) but decreased in anaemia.
- Joint swelling and decreased range of movement: connective tissue diseases.
- Tremor, goitre and eye signs: hyperthyroidism (see Fig. 35.7).
- Jaundice and other signs of liver failure (e.g. spider naevi) (see Ch. 13).
- Muscle wasting.
- Skin rashes.

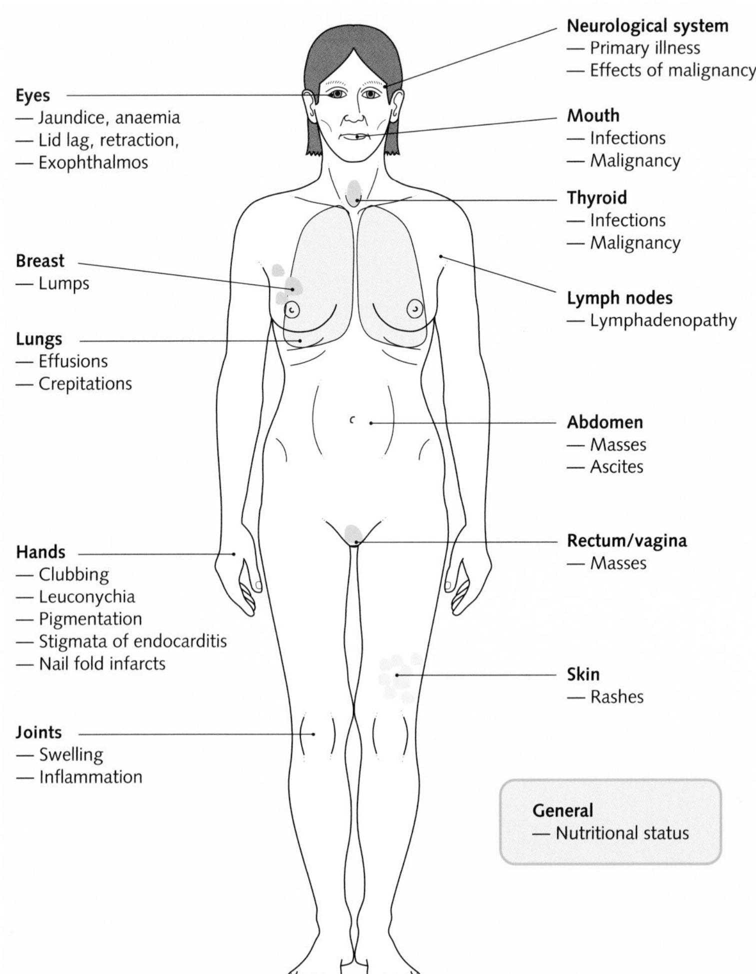

Fig. 12.2 Examining the patient with weight loss.

- Blood pressure: phaeochromocytoma.
- Mouth: infections and malignancies.
- Lymphadenopathy.

Examination of individual systems

The following individual systems should be examined:

- Respiratory system: infection or malignancy.
- Cardiac system.
- Gastrointestinal system: including careful palpation for abdominal masses, rectal examination and organomegaly (e.g. liver metastases). Always do a digital rectal examination.
- Neurological system: motor neurone disease, myopathy, paraneoplastic or metastatic manifestations of malignancy.
- Breast lumps.
- Vaginal examination: pelvic malignancy.

INVESTIGATING THE PATIENT WITH WEIGHT LOSS

As the potential causes of weight loss are multiple, investigations need to be tailored to the history and clinical examination findings. Nonetheless, the following investigations should be carried out:

Basic tests

- Full blood count: anaemia with malignancy, iron deficiency, vitamin B_{12} deficiency, or folate deficiency, with inadequate dietary intake.
- Urea and electrolytes for uraemia and chronic kidney disease.
- Liver function tests (LFTs): liver failure or metastases, although LFTs may be normal with metastases.
- Chest X-ray: infection or tuberculosis, and malignancy.
- Calcium profile: bone metastases.

Endocrinopathy

- Blood glucose: diabetes, low glucose in liver failure, Addison's disease.
- Thyroid function tests.

Infectious disease

- Inflammatory markers (erythrocyte sedimentation rate and C-reactive protein): increased in infection, inflammation, myeloma and other malignancies.
- Blood cultures.

Gastrointestinal causes

- Coeliac screen.
- If inflammatory bowel disease is suspected, consider colonoscopy.
- Stool culture and microscopy.
- Imaging modalities such as CT/MRI/ultrasound scan.

Jaundice 13

Objectives

The key learning points for this chapter:

- Understand the metabolism of bilirubin.
- Use this as a template for understanding the causes of jaundice.
- Assess the jaundiced patient.
- Understand the investigation of jaundice.

INTRODUCTION

Jaundice (icterus) is the yellow discoloration of the skin, sclera and mucosae that is detectable when serum bilirubin concentrations exceed approximately 50 μmol/L. Normal bilirubin metabolism is summarized in Fig. 13.1. Broadly speaking, jaundice can arise as a result of increased red blood cell (RBC) breakdown, disordered bilirubin metabolism or reduced bilirubin excretion.

DIFFERENTIAL DIAGNOSIS OF JAUNDICE

The causes of jaundice are outlined in Fig. 13.2. 'Prehepatic' jaundice usually results from the excessive production of bilirubin by haemolysis (see Fig. 13.1) but can also result from inherited metabolic defects, the commonest of which is Gilbert's syndrome. 'Hepatic' jaundice results from hepatocyte dysfunction causing disordered bilirubin metabolism. It is important to note that hepatocellular dysfunction usually causes some cholestasis and may also cause 'pale stools/dark urine' (see below). 'Posthepatic' jaundice is caused by reduced bilirubin excretion due to intra- or extrahepatic biliary obstruction.

HISTORY IN THE PATIENT WITH JAUNDICE

The following factors should be assessed when obtaining a history in a patient with jaundice.

Presenting complaint

- Pruritus, dark urine and pale stools: underlying cholestasis.
- Abdominal pain: the episodic, colicky, right hypochondrial pain of biliary colic will commonly be due to gallstones. A dull, persistent epigastric or central pain radiating to the back may suggest a pancreatic carcinoma.
- Fevers or rigors: cholangitis.
- Weight loss: underlying malignancy, particularly pancreatic cancer.

Other important points

- Duration of illness: a short history of malaise, anorexia and myalgia are suggestive of viral hepatitis. If there is a prolonged history of weight loss and anorexia in an elderly patient, carcinoma is more likely.
- Full recent drug history: particularly paracetamol, oral contraceptive pill.
- Alcohol consumption: acute alcoholic hepatitis, cirrhosis.
- Infectious contacts: hepatitis A.
- Recent foreign travel to areas of high hepatitis risk.
- Recent surgery: surgery for known malignancy, biliary stricture due to previous endoscopic retrograde cholangiopancreatography (ERCP) (if they had a sphincterotomy).
- IV drug abuse, tattoos, unprotected sex: increased risk of hepatitis B and C.
- Occupation: sewage workers are at increased risk of leptospirosis.
- Family history of recurrent jaundice: inherited haemolytic anaemias and Gilbert's syndrome.

EXAMINING THE PATIENT WITH JAUNDICE

The causes of jaundice are multiple and may therefore indicate underlying pathology in one of many organ systems. As such it is crucial to perform a detailed

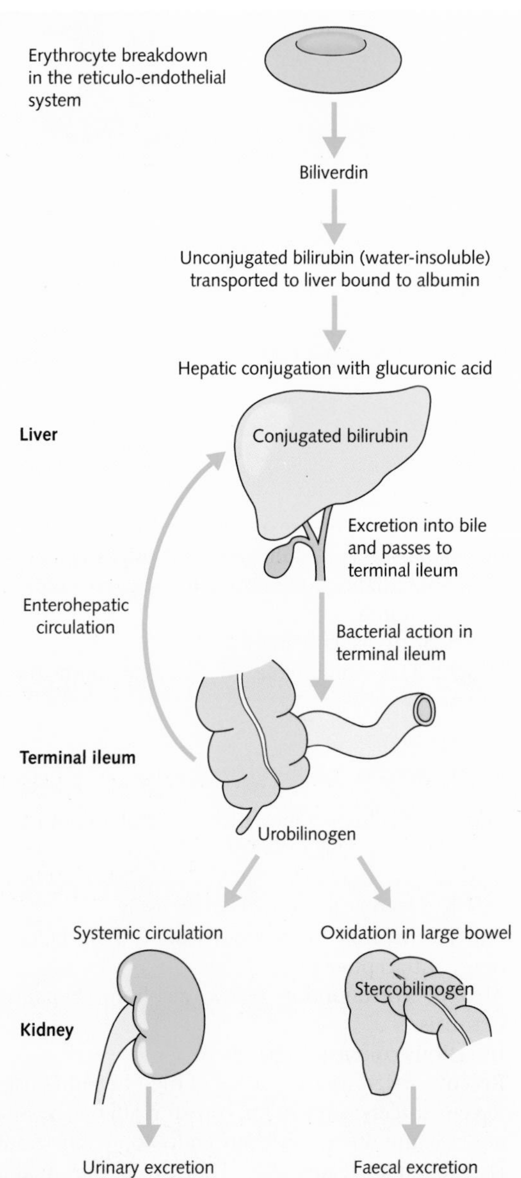

Fig. 13.1 Normal bilirubin metabolism.

clinical examination on any patient that presents with jaundice. Beyond this, there are three important groups of abnormalities that should specifically be looked for in the jaundiced patient:

- How severe is the jaundice? Is there any evidence of encephalopathy?
- Is this an acute or chronic problem? Are there any signs of chronic liver disease?
- Are there any signs of specific disorders? This approach is summarized in Fig. 13.3.

Is there evidence of encephalopathy?

Encephalopathy is defined as disordered brain function. The following factors suggest the presence of encephalopathy:

- Drowsiness: this will eventually progress through stupor to coma.
- Slurred speech.
- Asterixis: flapping tremor of outstretched hands.
- Seizures.
- Constructional apraxia: test by asking the patient to copy a five-pointed star.
- Hepatic fetor: mercaptans pass directly into the lungs due to portal hypertension causing a characteristic odour.

Hepatic encephalopathy can arise as a result of fulminating acute liver failure or when chronic disease decompensates. Precipitating factors, grading and management are described in Ch. 32.

Are there any signs of chronic liver disease?

There are few clinical signs specific to acute liver disease. However, the following signs may commonly be found when liver pathology is long-standing:

- Palmar erythema.
- Leuconychia and oedema: hypoalbuminaemia.
- Clubbing.

Fig. 13.2 The differential diagnosis of jaundice.

Prehepatic (see Ch. 37)	*Hepatic (see Ch. 32)*		*Posthepatic (see Ch. 32)*	
	Acute hepatocellular damage	**Chronic hepatocellular damage**	**Extrahepatic obstruction**	**Intrahepatic obstruction**
Haemolysis	Viral infection (e.g. hepatitis A, B, C, E; EBV; CMV)	Inherited defects (e.g. primary haemochromatosis, Wilson's disease, alpha-1-antitrypsin deficiency)	Gallstones	Primary biliary cirrhosis

Fig. 13.2 The differential diagnosis of jaundice – cont'd.

Prehepatic (see Ch. 37)	Hepatic (see Ch. 32)		Posthepatic (see Ch. 32)	
	Acute hepatocellular damage	**Chronic hepatocellular damage**	**Extrahepatic obstruction**	**Intrahepatic obstruction**
Inherited metabolic defects (e.g. Gilbert's syndrome)	Non-viral infection *(e.g. Leptospira icterohaemorrhagiae)*	Alcohol and other drugs (e.g. methotrexate)	Carcinoma: bile duct, head of pancreas, ampulla of Vater	Alcohol
	Drugs (e.g. paracetamol overdose, alcohol)	Chronic infection (e.g. hepatitis B, C)	Sclerosing cholangitis	Viral hepatitis
	Pregnancy	Cryptogenic	Benign stricture (e.g. post ERCP)	Drugs (e.g. OCP)
		Autoimmune hepatitis Metastatic carcinoma Vascular congestion (e.g. Budd–Chiari, right heart failure)	Pancreatitis Biliary atresia	Pregnancy

CMV, cytomegalovirus; EBV, Epstein–Barr virus; ERCP, endoscopic retrograde cholangiopancreatography; OCP, oral contraceptive pill.

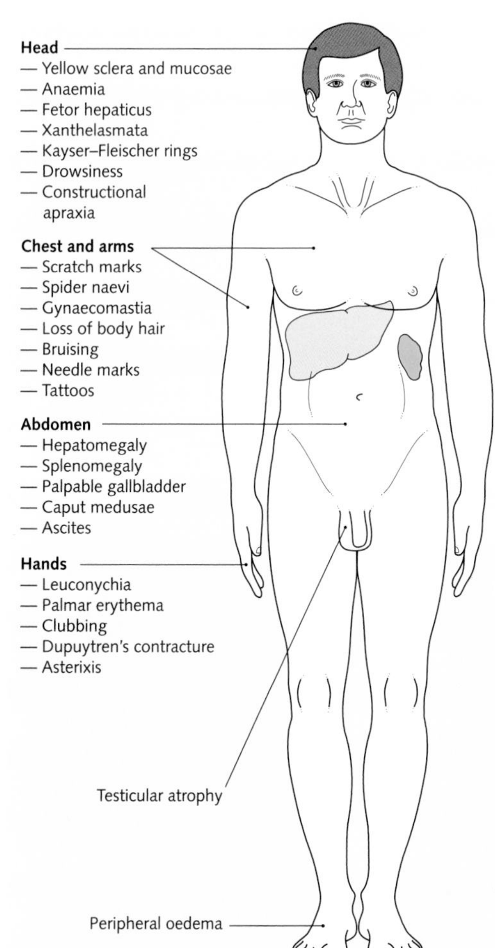

Fig. 13.3 Examining the patient with jaundice.

- Dupuytren's contractures: particularly in alcoholic cirrhosis.
- Spider naevi: more than five in the distribution of the superior vena cava.
- Scratch marks: cholestasis.
- Gynaecomastia, loss of body hair and testicular atrophy: elevated oestrogen.
- Bruising: disordered coagulation.
- Hepatomegaly: not in well-established cirrhosis.
- Splenomegaly, ascites and caput medusae: portal hypertension.

Are there any signs of specific diseases?

- Xanthelasmata: primary biliary cirrhosis.
- Kayser–Fleischer rings: Wilson's disease.
- Slate-grey pigmentation: haemochromatosis.
- Hard, irregular hepatomegaly: malignant metastases.
- Palpable gallbladder: carcinoma of head of pancreas (Courvoisier's law).
- Parotid gland enlargement: alcohol.
- Needle marks or tattoos: hepatitis B, C.

INVESTIGATING THE PATIENT WITH JAUNDICE

The investigation of jaundiced patients falls into two stages. First, the type of jaundice must be determined (prehepatic, hepatic, posthepatic); then, more detailed tests should be performed to determine the specific aetiology. Fig. 13.4 summarizes this approach.

Fig. 13.4 Investigation of the patient with jaundice. CT, computed tomography; ERCP, endoscopic retrograde cholangiopancreatography; EUS, endoscopic ultrasound; MRCP magnetic resonance cholangiopancreatography; PTC, percutaneous transhepatic cholangiography. CT and MRCP are usually performed before ERCP or PTC

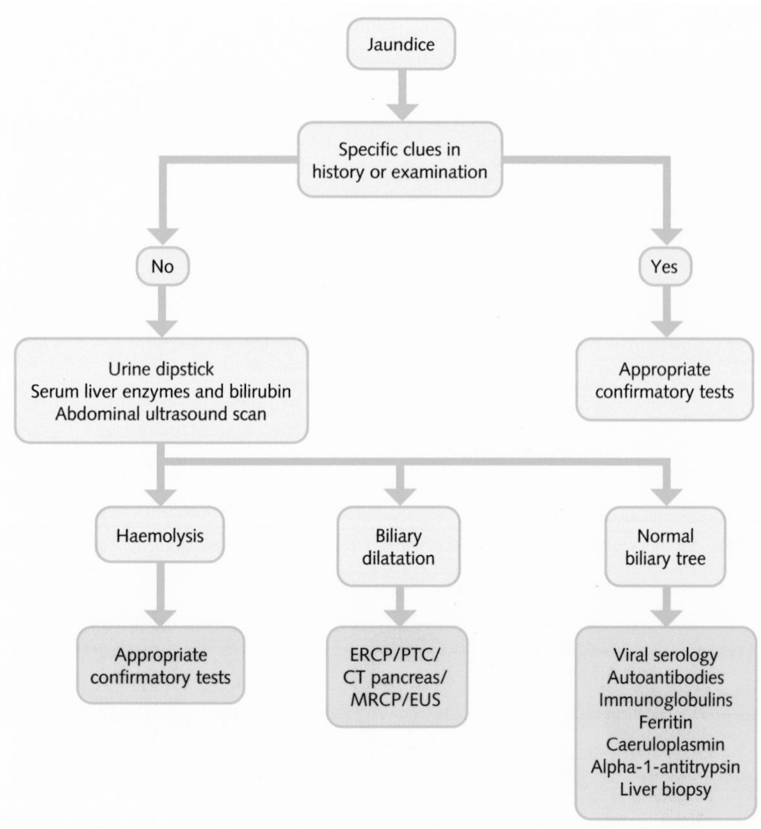

Establish the type of jaundice

Quantification of conjugated bilirubin, along with measurement of serum liver enzymes (alanine aminotransferase, aspartate aminotransferase, alkaline phosphatase, gamma-glutamyltransferase and bilirubin) will give a reasonable indication as to the type of abnormality present (Fig. 13.5). Abdominal ultrasound scan is then essential to exclude biliary obstruction.

The measurement of serum albumin (in the absence of inflammation) and prothrombin time (reflects clotting factor synthesis) help to provide an estimate of hepatic synthetic function.

Tests to determine specific aetiology

The following tests should be used as guided by the above initial investigations.

Haemolysis screen

The haemolysis screen is detailed in Ch. 29.

Fig. 13.5 Biochemical abnormalities in different types of jaundice.

Specimen	Test	Haemolysis	Hepatocellular	Cholestasis
Urine	Urobilinogen Conjugated bilirubin	Raised Absent	Normal or raised Present	Decreased or absent Raised
Faeces	Stercobilinogen	Raised	Normal or decreased	Decreased or absent
Blood	Bilirubin Liver enzymes	Unconjugated Normal	Unconjugated and conjugated AST, ALT	Conjugated Alkaline phosphatase, GGT

ALT, alanine aminotransferase; AST, aspartate aminotransferase; GGT, gamma-glutamyltransferase.

Hepatocellular screen

- Viral serology: hepatitis A, B and C; Epstein–Barr virus (EBV), cytomegalovirus (CMV).
- Autoantibody screen: antimitochondrial antibodies, antismooth muscle antibodies, antinuclear antibodies.
- Ferritin: haemochromatosis, transferrin saturation.
- Serum caeruloplasmin and urinary copper excretion: Wilson's disease.
- Alpha-1-antitrypsin.
- Liver biopsy: definitive diagnostic test for intrinsic liver disease.
- Fasting lipid profile: triglycerides for steatosis.

Cholestasis screen

- CT scan: good images of the pancreas, which is often poorly visualized on an ultrasound scan.
- Magnetic resonance cholangiopancreatography (MRCP) and endoscopic ultrasound: modern techniques for obtaining accurate images of the pancreas and biliary tree.
- ERCP and percutaneous transhepatic cholangiography (PTC): detailed information regarding the biliary tree; also used to perform therapeutic manoeuvres such as bile duct clearance or stent insertion.

HINTS AND TIPS

Liver dysfunction affects the synthesis of clotting factors and therefore the prothrombin time must be checked and corrected before an invasive procedure, e.g. liver biopsy.

Abdominal pain

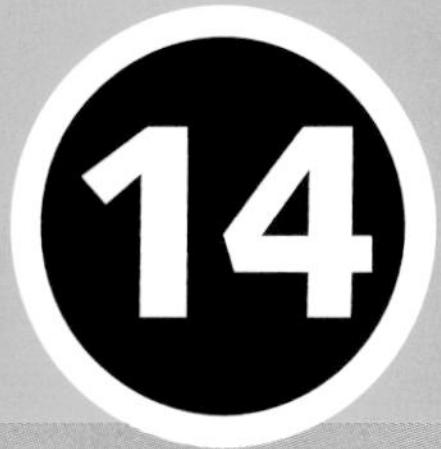

Objectives

The key learning points for this chapter:

- Understand the causes of pain in different regions of the abdomen.
- Assess the patient with abdominal pain.
- Understand the role of investigations in the patient with abdominal pain.

INTRODUCTION

Abdominal pain is a common presenting complaint. Considering the anatomical structures at the site of the pain will often provide clues to its cause.

DIFFERENTIAL DIAGNOSIS OF ABDOMINAL PAIN

The differential diagnosis for abdominal pain is multiple and ranges from benign pathology such as mesenteric adenitis to life-threatening pathology such as a ruptured abdominal aortic aneurysm. Fig. 14.1 summarizes the common causes of abdominal pain.

HISTORY IN THE PATIENT WITH ABDOMINAL PAIN

When a patient presents with abdominal pain, the first priority is to determine whether he or she has an 'acute abdomen' requiring urgent admission to hospital. The history should focus on the pain itself (using the SOCRATES approach) and then associated symptoms.

The presenting complaint

The onset, course, nature and site of the pain must be accurately assessed.

Sudden onset of sustained severe pain is often due to perforation or rupture of a viscus, such as the bowel, spleen or abdominal aorta.

Colicky pain is a griping pain that comes and goes. It is due to muscular spasm in a viscus wall, such as the bowel, ureters and gallbladder. The muscles contract in an attempt to overcome obstruction caused by a stone, tumour, foreign body, stricture, strangulated hernia or intussusception.

Gradual onset with sustained pain can be seen in inflammatory conditions, such as ulcerative colitis or Crohn's disease, infection, including abscess formation or gastroenteritis, and malignancy.

The site and radiation of pain may help to determine the organ involved (as above). Pancreatic and aortic pain may radiate to the back (these are retroperitoneal structures), ureteric pain often radiates from 'loin to groin', and diaphragmatic irritation caused by subphrenic pathology such as an abscess causes referred shoulder tip pain.

Exacerbating and relieving factors may be helpful. Pain from peritoneal irritation is made much worse by movement and relieved by keeping still, whereas patients with colic often curl into a ball and may roll around.

Associated symptoms

The history should now assess other symptoms that may suggest the cause of pain or the consequence of the disease.

Vomiting is common. Haematemesis is seen in upper gastrointestinal bleeding from ulcers or varices, projectile vomiting is seen in pyloric stenosis, and feculent vomiting results from severe large bowel obstruction. Ask the patient specifically about the content of the vomit (bilious, feculent)

Rigors suggest sepsis (e.g. abscess, cholangitis or urinary tract infection). Rigors are particularly common with Gram-negative septicaemia.

Change in bowel habit may be an important symptom. Absolute constipation (no faeces or wind passed rectally) indicates complete bowel obstruction, whereas gastroenteritis or diverticulitis often cause diarrhoea. Constipation alternating with diarrhoea is a feature of colonic malignancy but is also seen in irritable bowel syndrome.

Rectal bleeding may indicate malignancy, inflammatory bowel disease, diverticulitis, dysentery and

Fig. 14.1 Differential diagnosis of abdominal pain.

Site of pain	Causes
Epigastric	Lower oesophageal: oesophagitis, malignancy, perforation Stomach: peptic ulcer, gastritis Pancreas: pancreatitis, malignancy See Ch. 32
Right hypochondrium	Biliary tree: biliary colic, cholecystitis, cholangitis Liver: hepatitis, malignancy, abscess, right ventricular failure Subphrenic space: abscess See Chs 30 & 32
Left hypochondrium	Spleen: traumatic rupture, infarction (sickle cell disease) Pancreas: pancreatitis, malignancy Subphrenic space: abscess See Ch. 32
Central abdomen	Pancreas: pancreatitis, malignancy Small/large bowel: obstruction, perforation, intussusception, ischaemia, Crohn's disease, lymphoma, IBS, adhesions, early appendicitis Lymph nodes: mesenteric adenitis, lymphoma Abdominal aorta: ruptured aortic aneurysm See Ch. 32
Right iliac fossa	Terminal ileum: Crohn's disease, infection (e.g. tuberculosis), Meckel's diverticulum Appendix: appendicitis, tumour (including carcinoid) Caecum/ascending colon: diverticulitis, paracolic abscess, ulcerative colitis, malignancy Ovary/fallopian tubes: malignancy, ectopic pregnancy, pelvic inflammatory disease, cyst (bleeding or torsion) See *Crash Course: Obstetrics and Gynaecology* and Ch. 33
Left iliac fossa	Sigmoid/descending colon: diverticulitis, paracolic abscess, ulcerative colitis, malignancy Ovary/fallopian tube: malignancy, ectopic pregnancy, pelvic inflammatory disease, cyst (bleeding or torsion) See *Crash Course: Obstetrics and Gynaecology* and Ch. 33
Loin	Kidneys: malignancy, pyelonephritis, polycystic disease Ureters: colic due to stone or clot See Ch. 33
Suprapubic	Bladder: UTI, acute urinary retention
Other causes of abdominal pain	Uterus/adnexae: pelvic inflammatory disease, endometriosis (see *Crash Course: Obstetrics and Gynaecology* and Ch. 33) Anxiety (see *Crash Course: Psychiatry*) Myocardial infarction (especially inferior causing epigastric discomfort) (see Ch. 30) Lower lobe pneumonia (causing hypochondrial or loin pain) (see Ch. 31) Vasculitis (especially HSP and PAN) (see Ch. 36) Diabetic ketoacidosis (see Ch. 35) Addison's disease (see Ch. 35) Sickle cell crisis (see Ch. 37) *Very rarely*: lead poisoning, porphyria, familial Mediterranean fever

HSP, Henoch–Schönlein purpura; IBS, irritable bowel syndrome; PAN, polyarteritis nodosa; UTI, urinary tract infection.

angiodysplasia. Dark red bleeding is a feature of bowel infarction.

Dysuria, haematuria and urinary frequency indicate urinary infection. Renal stones are occasionally passed per urethra.

Vaginal discharge will often be present in pelvic inflammatory disease.

Other important points

The remainder of the history is often relevant and must be obtained (e.g. past surgical history, ?adhesions), past medical history (e.g. under follow-up for abdominal aortic aneurysm), details of any similar previous episodes (e.g. recurrent urinary tract infections), family history (e.g. porphyria) and drug history (e.g. opiates causing constipation).

HINTS AND TIPS

It can sometimes be helpful to ask the patient to grade the severity of their pain on a scale of 0–10.

EXAMINING THE PATIENT WITH ABDOMINAL PAIN

The first question that must be asked is 'Is the patient acutely ill?' Signs of shock and peritonism should be looked for. The examination should then focus on specific signs. Fig. 14.2 summarizes the examination approach.

Is the patient acutely unwell?

Pulse and blood pressure

Tachycardia and hypotension indicate shock. Other signs include delayed capillary refill (beware in sepsis, where the peripheries are may be warm because of vasodilation) and reduced urine output. Consider sepsis (particularly Gram-negative), severe bleeding (ruptured abdominal aortic aneurysm, splenic rupture), significant fluid loss (vomiting, diarrhoea, third spacing in bowel obstruction and pancreatitis) and, rarely, acute Addisonian crisis.

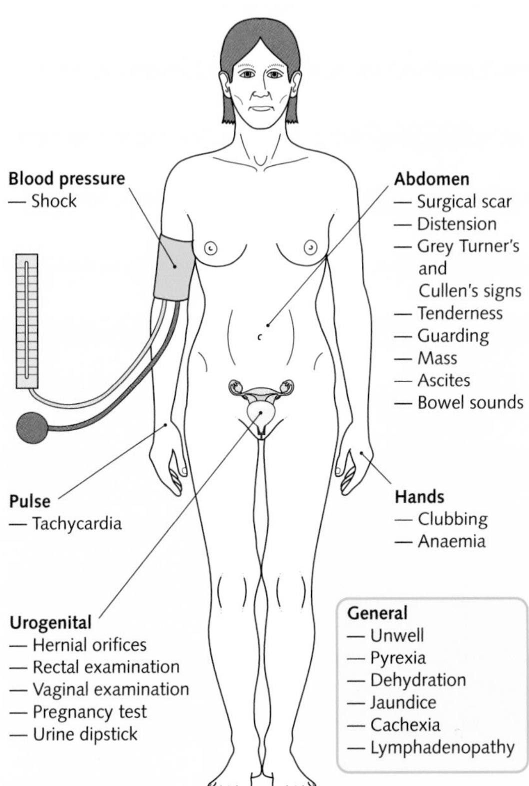

Fig. 14.2 Examining the patient with abdominal pain.

Peritonism

Peritonism is defined as inflammation of the peritoneum. This can be localized or general. The patient often lies still, as movement exacerbates the pain. Look for rebound tenderness and guarding (involuntary spasm of the abdominal wall on palpation). When the peritonism becomes generalized, the abdomen will be rigid and bowel signs will be scanty and high pitched or absent because of paralysis of peristalsis. Causes of peritonism are summarized in Fig. 14.3.

What is the underlying cause?

- Pyrexia: high temperature indicates infection; low-grade pyrexia can be found in malignancy, bowel infarction, inflammatory bowel disease and pancreatitis.
- Jaundice: hepatitis, gallstones or pancreatitis (causing periampullary oedema).
- Dehydration: rapid fluid loss.
- Cachexia: suggests a chronic pathology, particularly malignancy.
- Clubbing: inflammatory bowel disease, small bowel lymphoma or chronic liver disease.
- Lymphadenopathy: lymphoma; or may be due to metastases (remember Virchow's node).
- Cullen's sign (periumbilical or central bruising) and Grey Turner's sign (bruising in the flanks): severe haemorrhagic pancreatitis, rarely leaking abdominal aortic aneurysm. Both are due to retroperitoneal bleeding
- Recent surgical scar: may indicate a source of peritoneal sepsis, such as an anastomotic leak.

Fig. 14.3 Causes of peritonism.

Cause	Examples
Infection	Spread from paracolic/subphrenic abscess following surgery or paracentesis Bowel perforation
Chemical irritation	Bile Faeces Gastric acid Pancreatic enzymes
Transmural inflammation	Crohn's disease Salpingitis

- Older surgical scar: may indicate presence of adhesions.
- Abdominal distension: if marked, indicates bowel obstruction and is accompanied by a resonant percussion note. Occasionally, visible peristalsis may be present. The abdomen may also be distended in generalized peritonitis.
- Tenderness: it is important to consider what structures lie at the site of tenderness. As discussed, rebound tenderness and guarding indicate peritonism.
- Carnett's sign: this is positive when muscles of the anterior abdominal wall are tensed and the pain gets worse; it suggests the abdominal wall, not the abdominal cavity, is the origin of the pain.
- Mass: this can be neoplastic or inflammatory as in Crohn's disease.
- Ascites: malignancy, peritoneal sepsis, pancreatitis, portal hypertension.
- Bowel sounds: high-pitched (tinkling) suggests obstruction; absence indicates an ileus (paralysis of bowel) from whatever cause.
- Hernial orifices (inguinal and femoral): these must be examined, particularly if obstruction is suspected.
- Pelvic and rectal examination: pelvic inflammation, cervical excitation, ectopic pregnancy, rectal mass or bleeding, stool consistency.
- Urine dipstick: should be used to determine the presence of white blood cells (infection), red blood cells (stone, tumour or infection), glucose and ketones.
- Cardiorespiratory examination: consider myocardial infarction and basal pneumonia.

HINTS AND TIPS

Murphy's sign: deep inspiration is arrested by discomfort with two fingers in the right upper quadrant in cholecystitis, examination in the left upper quadrant does not halt inspiration.

Rovsing's sign: a sudden release of pressure in the left iliac fossa causes pain in the right iliac fossa in appendicitis.

INVESTIGATING THE PATIENT WITH ABDOMINAL PAIN

All patients admitted to hospital with abdominal pain should have a full blood count and serum biochemistry performed. The use of radiology and other tests will depend on a focused differential diagnosis. The diagnostic pathway is outlined in Fig. 14.4.

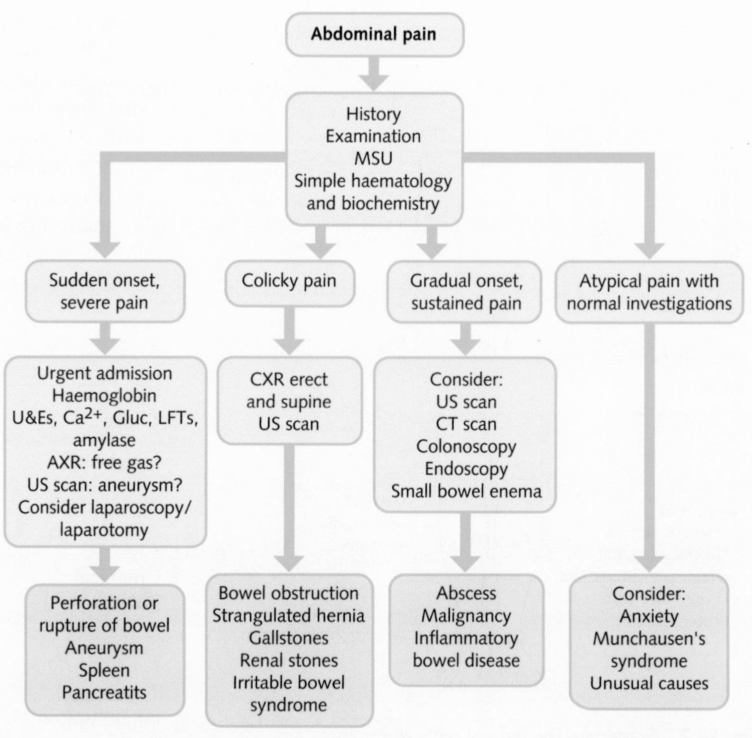

Fig. 14.4 Diagnosis in the patient with abdominal pain. AXR, abdominal X-ray; CT, computed tomography; CXR, chest X-ray; Gluc, glucose; LFTs, liver function tests; MSU, midstream urine; U&Es, urea and electrolytes; US, ultrasound.

Simple tests

- Blood glucose: hypoglycaemia will result from liver failure or Addison's disease; hyperglycaemia will be present in ketoacidosis and may complicate acute pancreatitis.
- Urine dipstick: positive for nitrites and leucocytes indicates UTI; ketone positive may indicate dehydration, anorexia or diabetic ketoacidosis.
- Pregnancy test: any female of childbearing age presenting with abdominal pain *must* have a pregnancy test.

Blood tests

- Full blood count: leucocytosis is seen in infection and occasionally inflammation and malignancy. Anaemia may be due to acute blood loss or chronic pathology such as malignancy.
- Serum amylase: very high in acute pancreatitis but may also be raised in perforated peptic ulcer, diabetic ketoacidosis, cholecystitis, ectopic pregnancy, abdominal trauma and myocardial infarction.
- Urea and electrolytes: dehydration, renal failure as a consequence of obstructive uropathy or shock.
- Serum calcium: hypercalcaemia may cause renal stones and pancreatitis; hypocalcaemia may be a consequence of pancreatitis.
- Liver function tests: abnormal in acute hepatitis, biliary disease and shock.

Imaging

- Abdominal X-ray: erect and supine films should be performed if the following are suspected: perforation (gas under the diaphragm representing free gas); obstruction (dilated loops of bowel with fluid level); pancreatitis (sentinel loop due to ileus in overlying loop of small bowel); infarction ('thumb printing' representing mucosal oedema); renal stone (90% of such stones are radio-opaque).
- Erect chest X-ray: check for free gas under the diaphragm – a sign of viscal perforation.
- Abdominal ultrasound scan: dilatation of biliary tree and ureters; intra-abdominal mass; ascites; abscess.
- CT: useful in diagnosis of abdominal aortic aneurysm, perforation of a viscus. CT pneumocolon allow for detailed imaging of the colon.

Further investigations

- Urine sample: microscopy, culture and sensitivity of midstream urine: to exclude infection.
- ECG to rule out myocardial infarction.
- Stool sample: microscopy, culture and sensitivity. Toxin testing for *C. difficile*.
- Diagnostic laparoscopy: occasionally the above investigations do not yield a diagnosis and the abdominal pain persists. Diagnostic laparoscopic surgery can be helpful in making a diagnosis, but is more commonly useful in ruling out particular pathology.

Urinary symptoms

Objectives

The key learning points for this chapter:

- The causes of urinary symptoms and their underlying physiological basis.
- How to assess a patient with urinary symptoms.
- How to investigate a patient with urinary symptoms.

INTRODUCTION

The volume of water in the circulation is under constant physiological control. Water is normally reabsorbed from the loop of Henle as it passes through the hyperosmolar renal medulla, and is also reabsorbed from the collecting ducts under the control of antidiuretic hormone (ADH), also called arginine vasopressin (AVP) (Fig. 15.1). ADH is synthesized by the hypothalamus and released from the posterior pituitary in response to a rise in serum osmolality or fall in plasma volume. Conversely, a fall in osmolality or rise in plasma volume leads to a decrease in ADH secretion.

Polyuria is defined as the passage of excessive volumes of urine. Urine output depends on fluid intake and loss via other routes (e.g., respiration, sweat, faeces), and typically ranges from 1 to 3.5 L/day. Polydipsia is defined as excessive thirst, often manifested as the ingestion of excessive volumes of fluid, and is usually a consequence of polyuria.

Frequency is the frequent passage of small volumes of urine, and dysuria is pain on passing urine. Symptoms of bladder outflow obstruction, such as those caused by an enlarged prostate gland, include hesitancy (difficulty initiating micturition), terminal dribbling and poor stream. Nocturia, the passage of urine at night, may be associated with frequency or polyuria. Urinary incontinence is common and broadly divided into stress or urge incontinence.

Oliguria and anuria, the passage of small volumes or no urine, respectively, may be due to renal impairment (see Ch. 33) or urinary tract obstruction.

DIFFERENTIAL DIAGNOSIS OF URINARY SYMPTOMS

HINTS AND TIPS

There are many causes of polyuria but those seen most commonly in clinical practice are hyperglycaemia and hypercalcaemia.

The differential diagnosis of polyuria/polydipsia is summarized in Fig. 15.2.

Frequency is commonly due to bladder irritation, which is often due to infection but can also be caused by chemical irritation, tumours or calculi in the bladder. In men, frequency is often caused by prostatic hypertrophy, when it may be accompanied by poor stream, hesitancy and dribbling. Any of the conditions leading to frequency may also cause nocturia.

Dysuria is most commonly due to infection, but can also be caused by chemical irritation. When accompanied by frequency it may indicate cystitis, and in men may also be caused by prostatitis.

Stress incontinence is common in women and often due to weakened pelvic floor muscles due to physical changes following pregnancy and childbirth. Urge incontinence is associated with detrusor instability and inappropriate contraction, which may be a consequence of local factors such as infection or inflammation, or due to damage to the nerve supply. Innervation is mainly from the autonomic nervous system, although there is voluntary control of the external urinary sphincter, and higher control of urination in the micturition centre of the pons.

HISTORY IN THE PATIENT WITH URINARY SYMPTOMS

For many urinary symptoms there will be a simple explanation, for instance infection or prostatic hypertrophy. The history should focus on the following points:

- Frequency: is there coexistent fever, dysuria or cloudy urine (pyuria) which may indicate infection? If so, is there a history of recurrent infection that might indicate a predisposition (e.g. diabetes, urinary stasis, immunosuppression)? In men, are there associated symptoms of prostatic hypertrophy, and if so, are there any associated features of prostate

Fig. 15.1 Water and electrolyte balance in the loop of Henle. ADH, antidiuretic hormone.

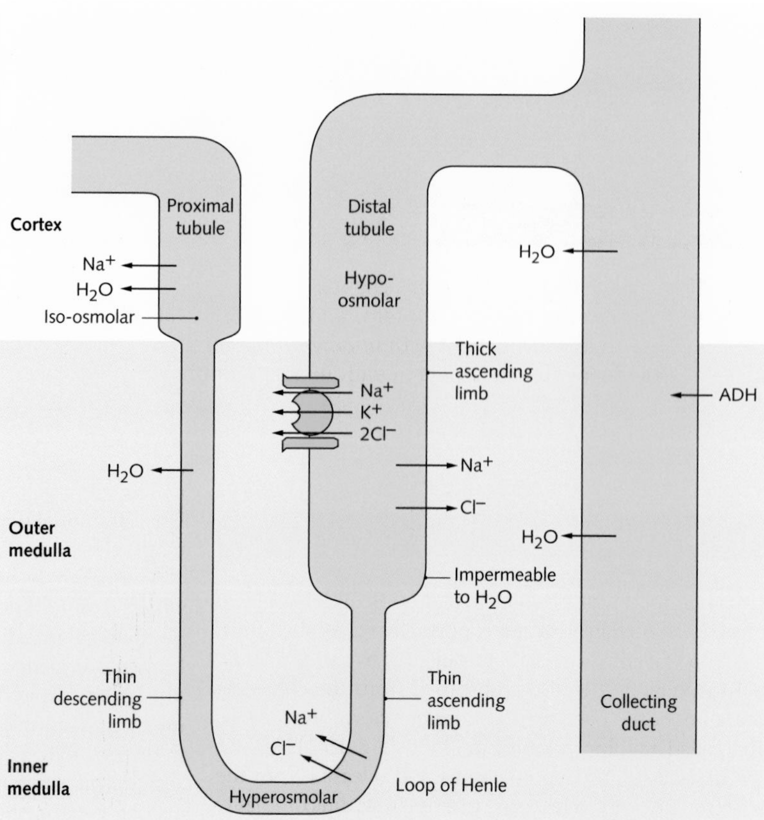

Fig. 15.2 Differential diagnosis of polyuria.

Causes	Examples/notes
Cranial DI (insufficient ADH secretion)	Idiopathic (often familial and commonest form) Post pituitary surgery/irradiation Post head trauma Malignancy (e.g. craniopharyngioma, pinealoma, glioma, metastases) Infections (e.g. meningitis) Infiltrations (e.g. sarcoid and histiocytosis X) Drugs (e.g. alcohol)
Nephrogenic DI (inability of kidney to respond to ADH)	Congenital (primary renal tubular defect) Electrolyte imbalance (hypokalaemia and hypercalcaemia) Lithium toxicity Long-standing pyelonephritis or hydronephrosis
Chronic renal failure	Can result in depressed renal concentrating ability and therefore higher urine volume to excrete a given solute load
Acute renal failure	Diuretic phase of ATN Following relief of obstructive uropathy Early stages of analgesic nephropathy
Osmotic diuresis	Glucose (diabetes mellitus) Calcium (hypercalcaemia)
ANP release	Arrhythmia (e.g. after SVT)
Psychogenic polydipsia	Relatively common psychiatric disturbance characterized by excessive water intake (if prolonged can cause temporary 'renal medullary washout' with reduction of kidney's concentrating ability)

ADH, antidiuretic hormone; ANP, atrial natriuretic peptide; ATN, acute tubular necrosis; DI, diabetes insipidus; SVT, supraventricular tachycardia.

malignancy (e.g. weight loss, bony pain, symptoms of hypercalcaemia)?

- Does the patient have loin pain, or a past history of renal calculi?
- Is there associated haematuria? In the presence of other lower urinary tract symptoms this could be due to infection, calculus or bladder tumour.
- If incontinence is present, be careful to determine the circumstances in which it occurs and the effect it is having on the patient's everyday activities.
- The patient's current medication may provide clues as to the cause.

Polyuria and polydipsia may pose a more difficult diagnostic challenge, and after general questions the enquiry should focus on the following:

- Differentiate between polyuria (an increase in the volume of urine production) and frequency (the frequent passage of small amounts of urine).
- Weight loss: may be associated with diabetes or malignancy: brain metastases can cause pituitary dysfunction; bone metastases may cause hypercalcaemia; myeloma may cause hypercalcaemia and renal failure (due to hypercalcaemia or light chain deposition).
- Headache: primary or secondary brain tumours can cause diabetes insipidus.
- Family history: this is relevant in diabetes mellitus and both forms of diabetes insipidus (cranial and nephrogenic).
- Previous medical history: in particular, consider previous neurosurgery or radiotherapy, head injuries and meningitis.
- Drug history: analgesic abuse may cause renal papillary necrosis; lithium may cause nephrogenic diabetes insipidus; vitamin D or milk-alkali syndrome may lead to hypercalcaemia; nephrotoxic drugs.
- Recurrent infections: may be due to diabetes mellitus.
- Features of hypercalcaemia (see Ch. 35), hypokalaemia (see Ch. 33), chronic renal failure (see Ch. 33) and its common causes – hypertension, diabetes mellitus, polycystic kidneys, urinary tract obstruction, chronic pyelonephritis, glomerulonephritis.
- Brief psychiatric history: especially if thirst is predominant. These patients may drink surreptitiously, resist investigation, have other neurotic symptoms and lack nocturnal symptoms.

EXAMINING THE PATIENT WITH URINARY SYMPTOMS

The examination approach in the patient with urinary symptoms is summarized in Fig. 15.3.

General appearance

- Wasting/cachexia (malignancy and diabetes mellitus) and hydration status.
- Skin manifestations: diabetes mellitus and malignancy (see Ch. 36).
- Nails: brown arcs in chronic renal failure; clubbing – associated with bronchogenic carcinoma, which may produce excess adrenocorticotrophic hormone (and therefore hypokalaemia and nephrogenic diabetes insipidus) or parathyroid hormone (and therefore hypercalcaemia), or may metastasize to brain.
- Anaemia: malignancy or chronic renal failure.
- Lymphadenopathy: malignancy or infiltrative disorder.
- Optic signs: fundal changes of hypertension or diabetes.

Cardiovascular system

Check the heart rhythm (atrial natriuretic peptide production) and the blood pressure for hypertensive nephropathy.

Abdominal examination

Palpate for the kidneys carefully as they may be enlarged in polycystic kidney disease or hydronephrosis. A large bladder may indicate urinary tract obstruction. The liver and spleen may be enlarged in malignancy and infiltrative disorders. An enlarged or craggy prostate can often be palpated on rectal examination.

Neurological examination

The neurological examination should assess the following:

- Peripheral neuropathy (caused by diabetes or infiltrative disorders).
- Hypotonia and areflexia with hypokalaemia.
- Wasting in malignancy.
- Visual fields (classically bitemporal hemianopia with pituitary pathology) and papilloedema (raised intracranial pressure).
- In idiopathic urge incontinence, is there evidence of any underlying neurological abnormality?

INVESTIGATING THE PATIENT WITH URINARY SYMPTOMS

The following investigations should be carried out.

Urine tests

- Simple urinalysis will give an estimate of the specific gravity (a measure of the weight of dissolved particles

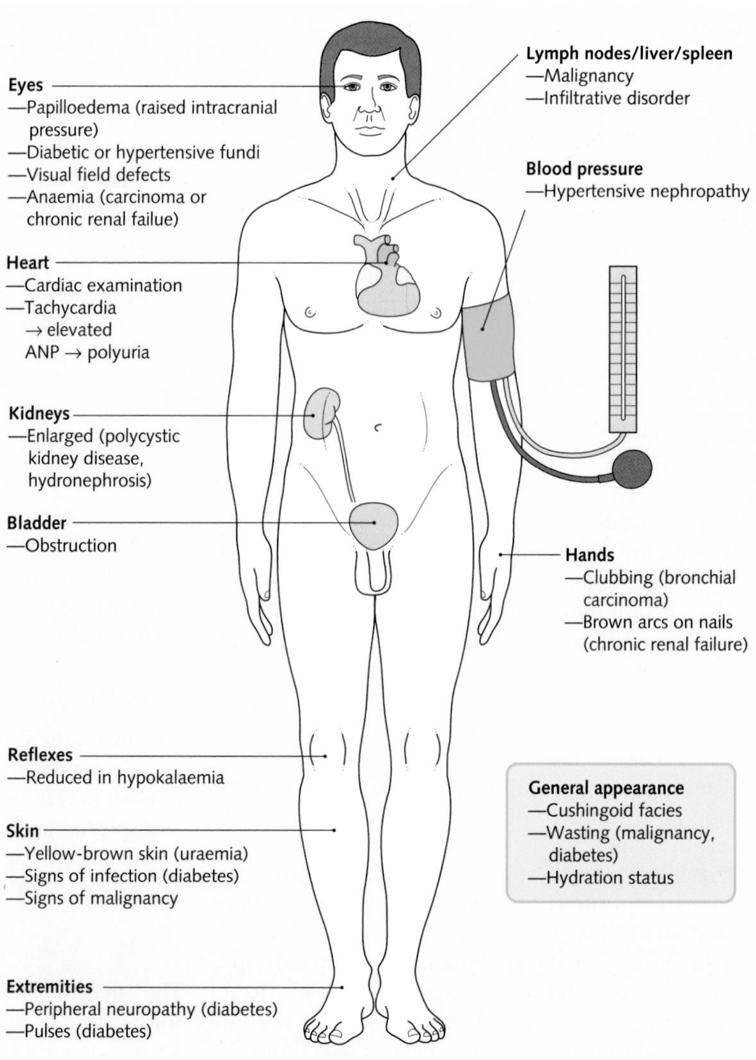

Fig. 15.3 Examining the patient with polyuria or polydipsia. ANP, atrial natriuretic peptide.

in the urine) and will also detect protein, blood, glucose and ketones, as well as leucocytes and nitrites, the presence of which may indicate infection.

- Laboratory urine analysis can measure urine osmolality, which is usually closely related to specific gravity unless there is a small number of large particles, e.g. myeloma. It can also measure the sodium and potassium content.
- Urine microscopy may reveal the presence of blood cells, bacteria or casts, and culture may reveal a pathogenic organism.

Blood tests

- Biochemistry: renal failure (see Ch. 33), hypercalcaemia (see Ch. 35), hypokalaemia (see Ch. 33) and hyperglycaemia (see Ch. 35).
- Full blood count: anaemia with chronic renal failure or malignancy (e.g. leukaemia, myeloma). Evidence of infection.

Imaging

- Chest X-ray: if any suspicion of sarcoidosis, primary or secondary malignancy.
- Renal tract ultrasound can detect abnormal kidney size, cysts and masses, congenital defects of the renal tract, hydronephrosis/hydroureter.
- CT of kidneys/ureters/bladder (CT KUB) if there is suspicion of renal tract calculi.
- CT or MRI of brain to investigate intracranial pathology (e.g. if considering a space-occupying lesion).

Further tests

- Renal concentration tests in polyuria: if either a hypothalamic or pituitary cause or renal tubular dysfunction is suspected. It is mandatory to exclude other potential causes for polyuria, as renal concentration tests may be dangerous. The patient is asked to drink nothing from 16:00 h the day before attending the outpatient department. If the urine osmolality the next morning is not above 800 mmol/kg, inpatient tests are required (Figs 15.4 and 15.5).
- Urodynamic tests: these commonly measure the pre- and post-void bladder volume and flow rate to assess bladder emptying.
- Nuclear renography: radioisotope uptake scans (e.g. DMSA, DTPA, MAG3 scans) can provide detailed information about asymmetric kidney function and can evaluate kidney scarring.

Fig. 15.4 Procedure for testing patients with polyuria and polydipsia.

Weigh the patient
Deprive of all fluids the night before the tests
The next morning, weigh the patient every 2 h (a decrease in weight by >3% indicates dehydration, so stop the test)
Collect urine and blood for osmolality
If the urine osmolality fails to reach 800 mmol/kg give IM DDAVP (DDAVP (desmopressin) is synthetic vasopressin, which acts in the same way as ADH)
Collect blood and urine for osmolality

ADH, antidiuretic hormone; DDAVP, desmopressin, IM, intramuscular.

Fig. 15.5 Interpretation of patient test results.

	Fluid deprivation		*After IM DDAVP*	
	Plasma osmolality	**Urine osmolality**	**Plasma osmolality**	**Urine osmolality**
Pituitary DI	↑	→	↑	↑
Psychogenic polydipsia	↑	↑*	↑	↑
Nephrogenic DI	↑	→	↑	→

DI, diabetes insipidus; IM, intramuscular.
**Urine is concentrated, but less than in normal response; ↑, increase in osmolality; →, no significant change in osmolality.*

Haematuria and proteinuria

Objectives

The key learning points for this chapter:

- Know the definition and causes of haematuria and proteinuria.
- Assess a patient with haematuria or proteinuria.
- Understand the investigations to determine the cause of haematuria and proteinuria.

INTRODUCTION

Haematuria and proteinuria are common presentations of renal disease, although both may also be due to systemic conditions. They are often incidental findings on urine dipstick testing, although macroscopic haematuria is not an uncommon presenting complaint. Microscopically, haematuria is abnormal if there are more than 2 red blood cells per mm^3 of unspun urine; proteinuria is defined as more than 150 mg of protein per 24-h collection of urine. Remember that red-coloured urine may also be due to haemoglobinuria, myoglobinuria, porphyria, drugs (e.g. rifampicin) or even the ingestion of beetroot.

DIFFERENTIAL DIAGNOSIS OF HAEMATURIA AND PROTEINURIA

Haematuria

This is best classified by the site of pathology.

Systemic conditions

- Clotting disorders and anticoagulants.
- Thrombocytopenia.
- Sickle cell disease.
- Endocarditis.
- Vasculitides.

Kidneys

- Glomerular disease (e.g. immunoglobulin A nephropathy, one of the multiple glomerulonephritides, infective endocarditis).
- Infections (e.g. pyelonephritis, tuberculosis).
- Tumours (e.g. renal cell carcinoma, angioma, adenoma, papilloma).
- Cystic disease (e.g. polycystic kidney disease, medullary sponge kidney).
- Interstitial nephritis: drugs (>75% cases) (e.g. penicillins, sulphonamides and non-steroidal anti-inflammatory drugs).
- Trauma (e.g. both spontaneous and after renal biopsy).
- Papillary necrosis.

Ureters

- Calculi.
- Tumours: transitional cell carcinoma, papilloma.
- Trauma.

Bladder

- Cystitis: infection, chemical-induced cystitis, post-radiation cystitis.
- Tumours: transitional cell carcinoma, papilloma.
- Trauma.
- Calculi.
- Infections: tuberculosis and schistosomiasis.

Prostate

- Prostatic carcinoma.
- Tuberculosis.
- Infection: prostatitis.

Urethra

- Calculi.
- Trauma.
- Tumours.
- Foreign bodies (e.g. urinary catheters).

Other sites

Haematuria may result from lesions in adjacent organs (by fistula formation or inflammation) such as:

- Colonic diverticulitis.
- Inflammatory bowel disease.

- Acute appendicitis in a pelvic appendix.
- Acute salpingitis and pelvic inflammatory disease.
- Carcinoma of the colon or genital tract.

Proteinuria

Small amounts of proteinuria can occur in non-renal disease such as urinary tract infection and with vaginal mucus; however, significant proteinuria >1 g/day usually indicates primary renal pathology (Fig. 16.1).

Benign proteinuria

- Functional proteinuria: pyrexia, strenuous exercise, congestive cardiac failure, acute illnesses, pregnancy.
- Orthostatic proteinuria: common in males aged under 30 years; proteinuria when upright but normal when supine.

Pathological proteinuria

This can result from all glomerular disease as the basement membrane is damaged, resulting in increased permeability across it. Differential diagnoses include:

- Diabetes mellitus.
- Glomerulonephritis.
- Other causes of nephrotic syndrome (Fig. 16.2).

In addition to the above, tubular proteinuria, due to tubular or interstitial damage, may occur. Proteinuria results from failure of the tubules to reabsorb some of the plasma proteins that have been filtered by the normal glomerulus. The loss of protein is usually mild and may result from the following:

- Congenital disorders: Fanconi's syndrome, cystinosis, renal tubular acidosis.
- Heavy metal poisoning: lead, cadmium, Wilson's disease.
- Acute tubular necrosis.
- Chronic nephritis and pyelonephritis.
- Renal transplantation.

Fig. 16.1 Levels of proteinuria.

	g/day
Normal	0.02
Microalbuminuria	0.03–0.3
Detectable with urinary dipstick	>0.2
Significant	>1.0
Nephrotic range	>3.0
Heavy	>5.0

Fig. 16.2 Causes of nephrotic syndrome.

Cause	Examples
Renal disease	**Glomerular disorders:** • primary • secondary to cause Reflux nephropathy
Systemic disease	**Amyloidosis** **Systemic lupus erythematosus** Henoch–Schönlein purpura
Metabolic disease	**Diabetes mellitus**
Infection	HIV Infective endocarditis Malaria Hepatitis B
Malignancy	Lymphoma Myeloma
Drugs	Gold Penicillamine Heroin Heavy metals
Familial disorders	Alport's syndrome Finnish-type nephrotic syndrome Sickle cell disease
Allergy	Bee stings Pollen

Common causes are given in bold.

Overflow proteinuria

This is when abnormal amounts of low-molecular-weight protein (filtered at the glomerulus) are neither reabsorbed nor catabolized completely by the renal tubular cells. There is no underlying renal pathology, simply increased protein filtration. The following may be responsible:

- Acute pancreatitis: amylase.
- Multiple myeloma: Bence Jones protein.
- Haemolytic anaemia and march haemoglobinuria: haemoglobin.
- Rhabdomyolysis: myoglobin (e.g. after a crush injury).

HISTORY IN THE PATIENT WITH HAEMATURIA AND PROTEINURIA

HINTS AND TIPS

If haematuria is present in a young woman, it is important to ask about the menstrual cycle and whether she was menstruating when the haematuria was noticed.

The differential diagnosis is vital when taking a focused history in a patient presenting with haematuria or proteinuria.

Presenting complaint

- Ask about the appearance of the urine. Is there frank blood (malignancy), the frothy urine of heavy proteinuria or foreign matter (e.g. vesicocolic fistula)?
- Ask about the urine volume: oliguria may indicate renal failure; polyuria could be a sign of systemic disease (e.g. diabetes or interstitial renal disease and loss of tubular concentrating ability).
- Ask about associated urinary symptoms, such as frequency (urinary tract infection, bladder calculus, prostatism), hesitancy, strangury (the desire to pass something that will not pass, e.g. a calculus) and dysuria (painful micturition reflecting urethral or bladder inflammation).
- When does it occur in the urinary stream? Is the haematuria worse with exercise? This suggests tumour or calculus.
- Ask about loin pain. This suggests pyelonephritis or renal calculi.
- Ask about colicky pain. This suggests a ureteric calculus.
- Is there a history of trauma?
- Does the patient have a vaginal or penile discharge?
- Is the proteinuria only present after vigorous exercise?
- Is the proteinuria absent in early morning specimens (orthostatic proteinuria)?

Associated features

- Is there any evidence of systemic or chronic illness (e.g. arthralgia or rash with vasculitis/connective tissue disease or retinopathy with diabetes mellitus)?
- Ask specifically about diabetes mellitus, hypertension, previous calculi and recurrent urine infections.
- Has there been a history of acute illness, especially fever (e.g. with urinary tract infection or poststreptococcal glomerulonephritis)?
- Are there generalized features of carcinoma (e.g. anorexia and weight loss)?
- Ask about past and current medications (e.g. analgesics (nephropathy) or anticoagulants).
- Is there a history of significant foreign travel (e.g. schistosomiasis or tuberculosis)?
- Is there a family history? Are there clotting disorders – does the patient bruise easily? Is there a history of renal problems (e.g. polycystic kidney disease, sickle cell disease)?
- Are there symptoms of fluid overload or hypoalbuminaemia (e.g. shortness of breath, orthopnoea, ankle swelling)?
- Ask about heavy metal exposure.
- Are there any risk factors for human immunodeficiency virus (HIV) or hepatitis?
- Ensure the patient is not pregnant. While usually benign, never forget pre-eclampsia.
- Do not forget to keep the causes of nephrotic syndrome in mind (see Fig. 16.2).

HINTS AND TIPS

Ask whether the patient has noticed the first appearance of blood when they pass urine. Patients may not volunteer this information because they do not think it is important.

- If the urine is bloodstained at the start of micturition, and clear later on, the site of pathology is likely to be the urethra or prostate.
- If the urine is more bloodstained towards the end of micturition, the site of pathology is likely to be the bladder.
- If the urine is evenly bloodstained throughout micturition, the site of pathology is likely to be the kidney or ureter.

EXAMINING THE PATIENT WITH HAEMATURIA AND PROTEINURIA

The examination approach is summarized in Fig. 16.3.

INVESTIGATING THE PATIENT WITH HAEMATURIA AND PROTEINURIA

An algorithm for the investigation of the patient with haematuria and proteinuria is given in Fig. 16.4. Renal biopsy may provide the best information but is invasive and not without risk (1% of patients have significant bleeding, 1 per 500 need blood transfusion and 1 per 2000 need emergency nephrectomy or die from percutaneous renal biopsy). It is therefore customary to start with urine, blood and radiological tests.

Urine

The following urinary tests should be performed.

Initial tests

- Gross appearance: frank haematuria should always make the doctor consider malignancy.

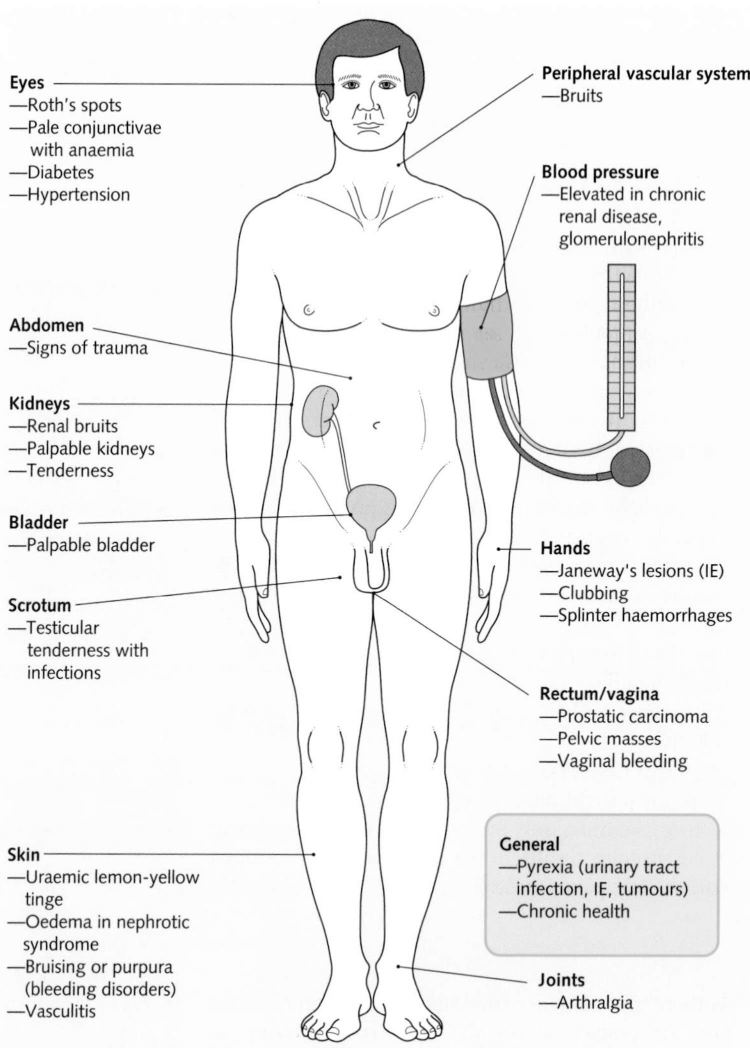

Fig. 16.3 Examining the patient with haematuria and proteinuria. IE, infective endocarditis.

- Urinary dipstick: provides initial information about presence or absence and degree of protein and haematuria. Many sticks also test for nitrites/leucocytes/ketones/pH and glucose.
- Microscopy: red blood cells (dysmorphic or normal), white blood cells, casts (red cell casts imply glomerulonephritis), organisms and crystals.
- Culture: infection.
- Early morning urine: acid-fast bacilli if tuberculosis is suspected.
- Cytology: malignancy.

24-h collection of urine

The precise level of proteinuria is important as an indicator of both the severity and the likely rate of progression of renal disease. It is usually done on a 24-h sample of urine. The glomerular filtration rate (GFR) can be assessed from creatinine measurements in blood and urine. Patients often comply poorly with this test and the results may be erroneous. Many nephrologists and laboratories now use an estimated value (e.g. via the Cockcroft–Gault equation) to monitor the GFR. This estimated value, or eGFR, can be obtained from plasma creatinine levels without the need for urine measurements.

Protein-to-creatinine ratio

This is performed on a single spot urine sample (preferably morning). It correlates well with accurate 24-h urinary protein collection values and is predictive of decline in GFR in diabetic and non-diabetic proteinuric renal failure.

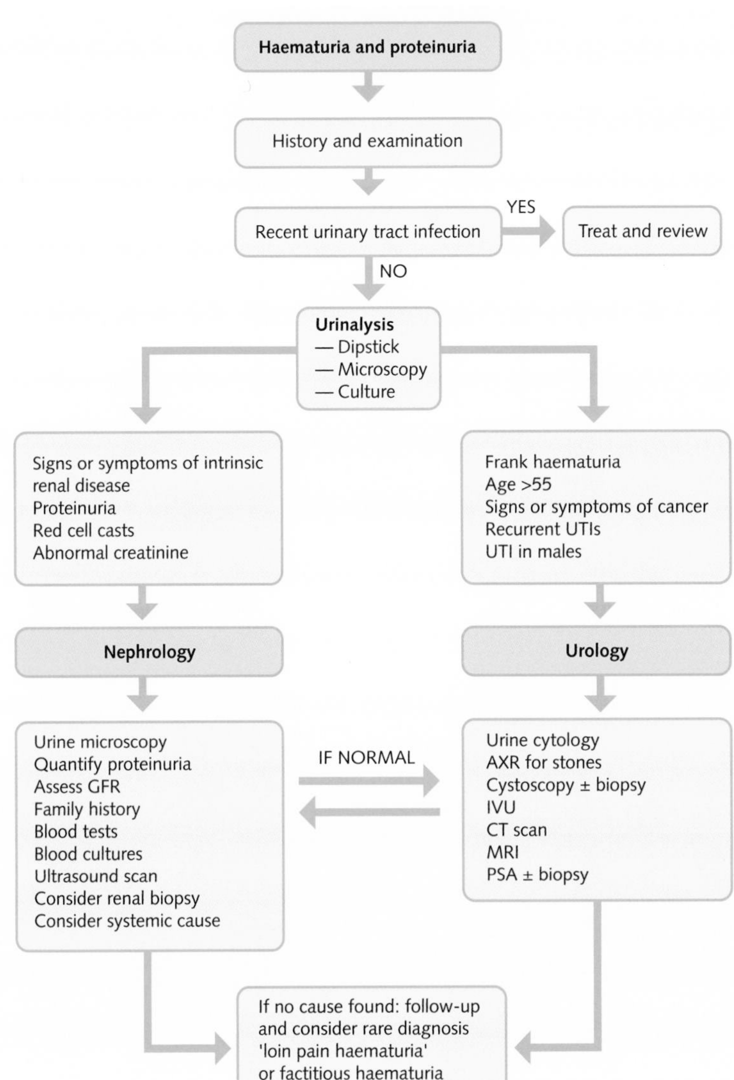

Fig. 16.4 Algorithm for investigation of haematuria and proteinuria. AXR, abdominal X-ray; CT, computed tomography; GFR, glomerular filtration rate; IVU, intravenous urogram; MRI, magnetic resonance imaging; PSA, prostate specific antigen; UTI, urinary tract infection.

It is easier to collect and process and has been widely adopted by diabetologists.

Differential protein clearance

Differential protein clearance (selectivity) is occasionally performed in patients with nephrotic syndrome. Patients with selective proteinuria (low-molecular-weight proteins are cleared more rapidly than large proteins) are more likely to respond to steroid therapy.

Blood tests

The following blood tests should be performed:

- Full blood count: leucocytosis with infections, anaemia with chronic renal failure.
- Erythrocyte sedimentation rate and C-reactive protein (e.g. vasculitis).
- Clotting studies: bleeding diathesis.
- Blood glucose: diabetes mellitus.
- Urea, electrolytes, creatinine and eGFR: renal function.
- Creatine kinase: myoglobinuria.
- Uric acid: gout.
- Blood cultures: infective endocarditis.
- Specialized investigations according to clinical suspicion (e.g. serum complement, antistreptococcal titres and anti-GBM antibodies).
- Protein electrophoresis and urinary Bence Jones protein (myeloma).
- HIV and hepatitis serology: potential causes of nephrotic syndrome.

Imaging

Imaging is of most use in urological practice where structural lesions are suspected. Renal tract ultrasound scanning is useful in nephrological practice to assess size and cortical structure of the kidney and visualize the ureters and bladder to guide further imaging. This may include:

- KUB X-ray (kidney/ureter/bladder): renal outline and stones. 90% of renal calculi are opaque; urate and xanthine stones may be radiolucent.
- Abdominal computed tomography (CT) scan: to visualize the kidneys, adjacent organs and other abdominal masses. CT KUB is now the gold standard for the diagnosis of renal calculi (99% sensitive).
- Abdominal magnetic resonance imaging (MRI) is superior to CT for some solid lesions and for staging of renal cell carcinoma. It is also useful for patients who cannot be administered contrast media because of significant renal impairment.
- Dimercaptosuccinic acid (DMSA) scanning: radionuclide scan that assesses renal function. Particularly useful in diagnosing pyelonephritis.

Other investigations

- Cystoscopy: bladder lesions.
- Ureteroscopy: ureter lesions.

HINTS AND TIPS

When thinking of causes of haematuria, think of the site of pathology along the renal tract. At each site, tumours, calculi, infection and inflammation are possible.

HINTS AND TIPS

Frank haematuria in the elderly needs urological investigation for malignancy first.

Hypertension 17

Objectives

The key learning points for this chapter:

- Understand the definition and differential diagnosis of hypertension.
- Have a logical approach to assessing the patient with hypertension, based on blood pressure levels and overall cardiovascular disease risk.
- Investigate patients presenting with hypertension.

INTRODUCTION

Hypertension is one of the most important modifiable risk factors for cardiovascular disease such as stroke, myocardial infarction and renal disease. The blood pressure (BP) above which someone is 'hypertensive' and requires treatment varies between different countries. However, most clinicians and published British guidelines would initiate drug treatment when the BP is persistently elevated to ≥160/100 mmHg (stage 2 hypertension) and consider it when the BP is ≥140/90 mmHg (stage 1 hypertension). These are arbitrary cut-off points that are influenced by age, the presence of end-organ damage or established cardiovascular disease, and other cardiovascular risk factors for example diabetes mellitus. Approximately 95% of all hypertensive patients have 'essential' or 'primary' hypertension and have no underlying disease. Secondary hypertension can be the result of a range of different pathological processes: for example, renal artery stenosis.

DIFFERENTIAL DIAGNOSIS OF HYPERTENSION

Essential hypertension

Essential hypertension comprises 95% of cases. There is no demonstrable cause, although lifestyle may play a part (e.g. obesity, alcohol, lack of exercise, high salt diet), and is a diagnosis of exclusion.

Secondary hypertension

Secondary hypertension comprises 5% of cases. Factors leading to secondary hypertension are:

- Renal parenchymal disease (e.g. chronic pyelonephritis, glomerulonephritis, polycystic disease, tumour).
- Renal artery disease (e.g. atherosclerosis, fibromuscular dysplasia, vasculitis).
- Obstructive uropathy (e.g. hydronephrosis due to a stone or tumour).
- Congenital (e.g. coarctation of the aorta).
- Drugs (e.g. combined oral contraceptive pill, non-steroidal anti-inflammatory drugs).
- Endocrine (e.g. phaeochromocytoma, hyperaldosteronism, Cushing's syndrome, acromegaly, hypothyroidism, hyperparathyroidism).
- Raised intracranial pressure. Usually coupled with bradycardia, the 'Cushing reflex' (rarely seen as a cause for hypertension in the outpatient setting).
- Obstructive sleep apnoea.

HINTS AND TIPS

95% of patients with hypertension have no identifiable underlying cause.

HISTORY IN THE PATIENT WITH HYPERTENSION

Hypertension is usually asymptomatic and is often found by screening. Ideally, all people should have their blood pressure measured every 5 years as a minimum. The history in a patient with high BP should be approached in three parts.

First, how long has the patient had hypertension and what treatments have been given so far? Second, how severe is the hypertension and has it resulted in complications? Finally, are there any risk factors suggesting that an underlying cause may be present?

Presentation and history of hypertension

Important questions to address are as follows:

- How was the hypertension discovered? For example, at a routine assessment or with malignant (accelerated) hypertension? Liaison with the patient's general practitioner or other health care professionals may be needed for a full history.
- For how long has the blood pressure been monitored? Unless the BP is very high or the patient is at high risk of cardiovascular disease, the diagnosis should not be made until the blood pressure has been persistently elevated for at least 3 months.
- What treatments, if any, has the patient been given so far? If blood pressure control is poor despite taking correct doses of three antihypertensive agents, the patient is said to have 'resistant hypertension'.

How severe is the hypertension and are there complications?

Mild hypertension is asymptomatic. However, when hypertension is severe or chronic, it can be associated with complications resulting from end-organ damage. The following symptoms may occur:

- Headaches.
- Dyspnoea.
- Symptoms of cardiac failure.
- Angina pectoris or myocardial infarction.
- Transient ischaemic attacks or stroke.
- Visual disturbance.
- Hypertensive emergency: hypertensive encephalopathy. This requires immediate HDU/ITU management with IV labetalol or calcium channel blockers, ACE inhibitor or even, although rarely, sodium nitroprusside.

Is the history suggestive of an underlying cause?

Ask about the following:

- Lifestyle history, paying particular attention to smoking (atherosclerosis).
- Precise drug history (e.g. oestrogen-containing contraceptive or non-steroidal anti-inflammatory drugs).
- Previous medical history (e.g. recurrent pyelonephritis, nephrectomy).
- Family history may suggest an underlying disease (e.g. adult polycystic kidney disease).
- Symptoms of phaeochromocytoma are rare but include episodic pallor, headache, tremor, palpitations and nausea.

EXAMINING THE PATIENT WITH HYPERTENSION

Patients with uncomplicated mild essential hypertension will have no associated clinical signs. However, when a patient is found to be hypertensive, one should search for evidence of complications or an underlying cause (Fig. 17.1).

Evidence of an underlying cause

- Palpable kidneys: polycystic disease, renal tumour.
- Peripheral vascular disease and xanthelasmata: renal artery stenosis.
- Renal bruits are rarely heard. Other vascular bruits are equally valid indicators of atherosclerosis: renovascular disease.
- Radiofemoral delay: coarctation of the aorta.
- Neurofibromatosis: renal artery stenosis.
- Cushing's disease, acromegaly.

Evidence of complications

- Atrial fibrillation.
- Displaced, thrusting apex beat indicating left ventricular hypertrophy.
- Cardiac failure.
- Hypertensive retinopathy.
- Previous stroke.

INVESTIGATING THE PATIENT WITH HYPERTENSION

An algorithm for the investigation of the patient with hypertension is given in Fig. 17.2. At presentation all hypertensive patients should have the following tests:

- Urine dipstick for blood and protein: parenchymal disease, urinary tract infection, stone.
- Urea and electrolytes: may indicate renal impairment or suggest a cause (e.g. Conn's syndrome).
- Blood glucose and lipid profile: screen for modifiable cardiovascular risk factors.
- Electrocardiogram: significant hypertension may result in left ventricular hypertrophy.

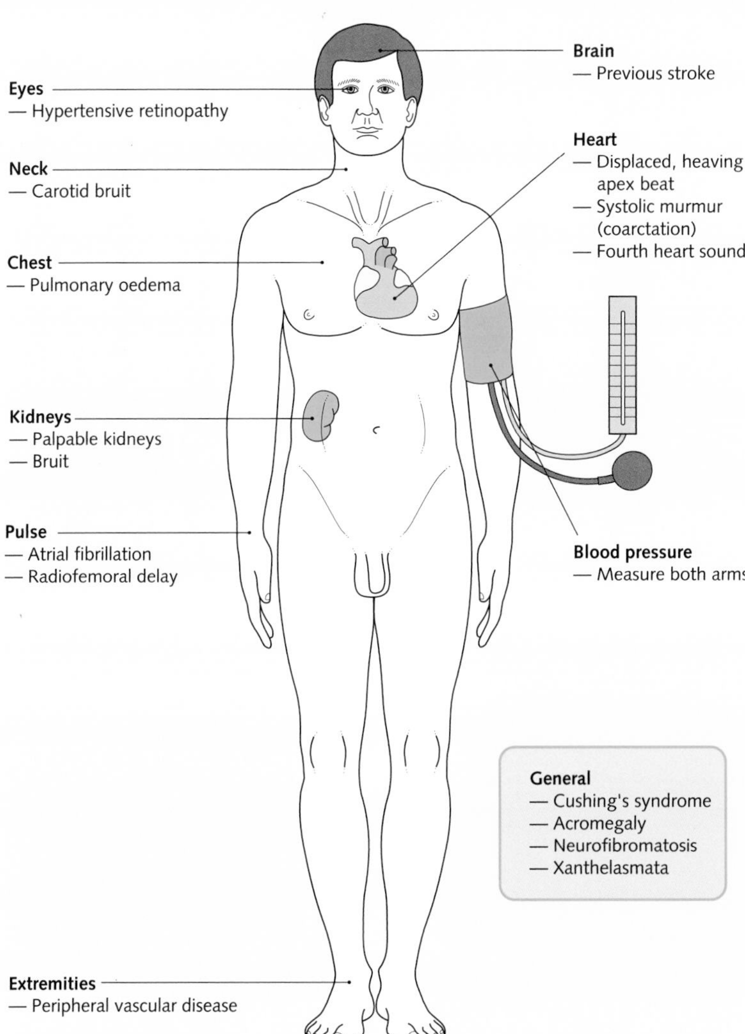

Fig. 17.1 Examining the patient with hypertension.

- Global cardiovascular event risk assessment using a published risk assessment chart.

The blood pressure should be measured reproducibly (i.e. with the correct cuff size, the patient seated, relaxed and the cuff at the level of the heart). Diastolic pressure is recorded when the audible pulse disappears (Korotkoff V). If an automated monitor is being used, it should be one that is validated for the purpose by organizations such as the British Hypertension Society, or the American Heart Association.

Fig. 17.3 shows those patients who should then be investigated further, using the following tests:

- 24-h ambulatory blood pressure measurement (e.g. when blood pressure is abnormally variable, resistant to drug treatment or to exclude 'white coat hypertension').
- 24-h urinary catecholamine and metanephrine excretion: phaeochromocytoma.
- Radiological investigations: renovascular disease, renal parenchymal disease, obstructive uropathy. This

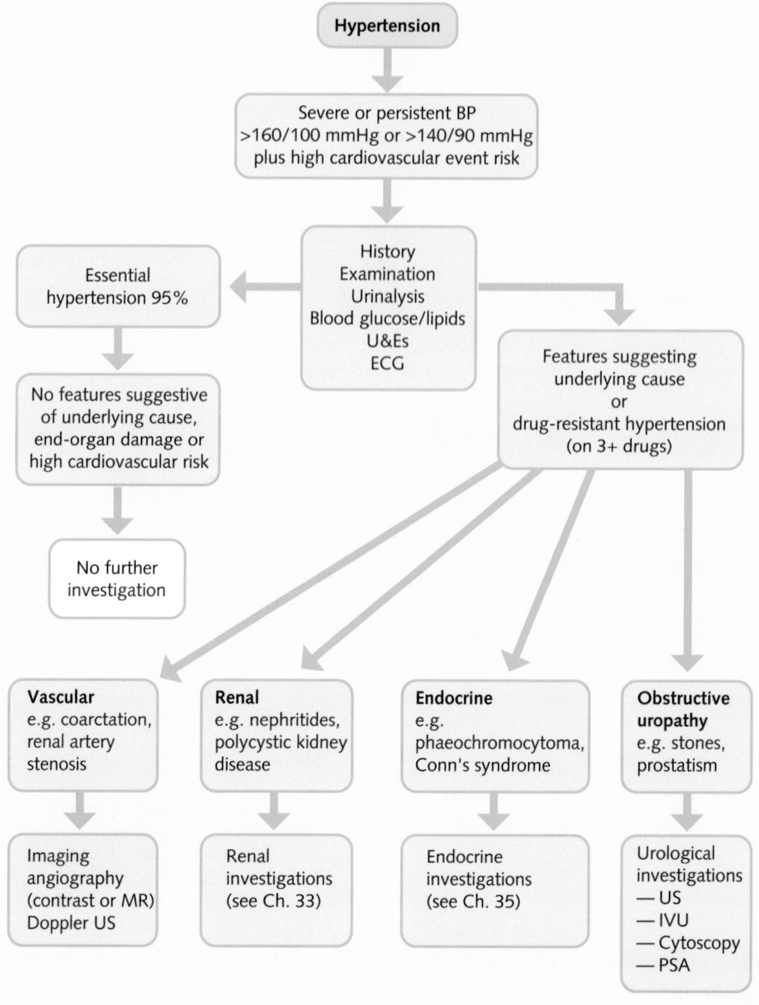

Fig. 17.2 Algorithm for the investigation of the patient with hypertension. ECG, electrocardiogram; IVU, intravenous urogram; MR, magnetic resonance; PSA, prostate specific antigen; U&Es, urea and electrolytes; US, ultrasound scan.

Fig. 17.3 Indications for detailed investigation of hypertension.

Recent onset or worsening of hypertension
Malignant (accelerated) hypertension
Uncontrolled hypertension despite three antihypertensive drugs (beware of and check for non-adherence to medication)
Abdominal bruit
Proteinuria, haematuria, or abnormal renal function
Hypokalaemia not otherwise explained, e.g. by diuretic therapy
Renal failure caused by angiotensin-converting enzyme (ACE) inhibitors
Young age (<30 years)
Severe generalized atherosclerosis
Unexplained ('flash') pulmonary oedema

may include abdominal ultrasound scanning or nuclear medical investigation.

- Renal angiography for renal artery disease; this is a definitive test and should be performed if clinically indicated. Magnetic resonance angiography is now the first-line screening test for suspected renal artery stenosis.

MANAGEMENT OF THE HYPERTENSIVE PATIENT

In August 2011, NICE published a guideline for the management of hypertension in adults. Fig. 17.4 summarizes their recommendations.

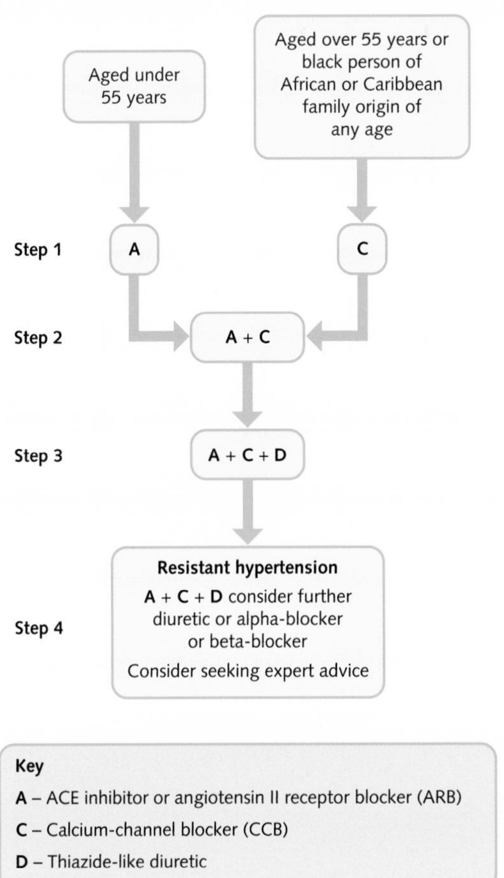

Fig. 17.4 Summary of NICE guideline (August 2011) for the management of adult hypertension.

HINTS AND TIPS

All hypertensive patients should have urine dipstick, urea and electrolytes, cardiovascular risk stratification and an electrocardiogram. Only a few need any further tests.

Headache and facial pain

Objectives

The key learning points for this chapter:

- The causes of headache and facial pain.
- The systematic approach to assessing a patient presenting with headache or facial pain.
- The sequence of investigations to determine the cause of the headache or facial pain.

INTRODUCTION

Headache is one of the most common presenting symptoms. There are often few clinical signs and the history is the main diagnostic tool. Many different pathological processes can result in headache and facial pain. The International Headache Society classification divides headache into primary headache (where the headache is itself the disease), secondary headache (where the headache is due to other disease, e.g. infection) and a third subset which includes facial pain and cranial neuralgias. The more common headaches of all three subsets are considered together here according to the pattern of headache; this list is not exhaustive.

DIFFERENTIAL DIAGNOSIS OF HEADACHE AND FACIAL PAIN

The differential diagnosis of headache and facial pain is summarized in Fig. 18.1.

HISTORY IN THE PATIENT WITH HEADACHE AND FACIAL PAIN

This is the key to diagnosis and the onset, nature and subsequent pattern of pain will usually provide a good shortlist of likely causes. The presence of additional symptoms and risk factors may add further weight to this list.

Solitary acute episode

This pattern is seen in vascular events, infection and trauma. (Note that it may also be the first presentation of the other causes of headache.)

Subarachnoid haemorrhage presents with a sudden onset of severe pain 'as if someone had hit them on the head'. It is often most severe occipitally, and usually reaches maximal severity at onset or within seconds. Nausea, vomiting, neck stiffness and photophobia result from meningeal irritation, but they are not discriminating features. Altered conscious level, seizures and focal neurological deficits may also occur depending on the site and size of the haemorrhage.

Seizures, focal neurological symptoms and symptoms of raised intracranial pressure (see below) can also result from cerebral venous sinus thrombosis. Causal factors include inherited disorders of coagulation, pregnancy, oral contraceptive pill use, dehydration, extension of local infection (e.g. of paranasal sinuses or middle ear) and severe intercurrent illness. Dissection of a carotid or vertebral artery can also cause a sudden onset of pain associated with focal neurology.

Patients with infective meningitis present with a short history of headache, symptoms of infection (malaise, fever and rigors), symptoms of meningeal irritation (vomiting, photophobia, neck pain and stiffness) and may have a rash and altered mental state. However, tuberculous and carcinomatous meningitis, as well as other causes of 'aseptic' meningitis, have a more subacute presentation that can be easily missed. Encephalitis, acute inflammation of the brain, may present with headache and fever. Altered mental state is common and occurs early in the course of the illness.

Cerebral abscess causes headaches, seizures, symptoms of infection and of raised intracranial pressure as the lesion enlarges. The infection may have spread from a local or distant primary focus, such as lung infection (bronchiectasis, abscess), endocarditis, middle ear infection or paranasal sinusitis.

Acute angle-closure glaucoma can cause a severe headache associated with blurred vision, eye pain, cloudiness of the cornea, conjunctival injection and a dilated pupil. There may be nausea and vomiting. It should be considered in hypermetropic, middle-aged or elderly patients. It may occur intermittently with repeated acute attacks.

Fig. 18.1 Differential diagnosis of headache and facial pain (see Ch. 34).

Pattern	Causes
Solitary acute episode	Infection: meningitis, encephalitis, abscess Vascular event: intracranial haemorrhage (especially subarachnoid), venous sinus thrombosis, occasionally infarction (especially if arterial dissection occurred) Trauma First migraine or benign thunderclap headache
Progressive headache	Raised intracranial pressure (including idiopathic intracranial hypertension) Giant cell arteritis
Episodic headache/ facial pain	Migraine Cluster headache and other trigeminal autonomic cephalalgias Trigeminal neuralgia Coital cephalalgia
Chronic headache/ facial pain	Tension headache/analgesic rebound headache Postherpetic neuralgia Post head injury Paget's disease of the skull
Other causes of facial pain	Dental problems Temporomandibular joint Ears/nose/sinuses Cervical spine Eye – especially acute or intermittent angle closure glaucoma Myocardial ischaemia (rarely)

Progressive headache

A headache that comes on gradually over days or weeks and increases in severity is often a feature of a 'space-occupying lesion' (such as tumour or abscess), idiopathic intracranial hypertension (previously 'benign' intracranial hypertension), chronic subdural haematoma or hydrocephalus (which may be due to blockage of CSF flow secondary to other pathology). In all of these the headache results from raised intracranial pressure and has the characteristic features shown in Fig. 18.2. Temporal arteritis also presents gradually, but the nature of the headache is very different.

Cerebral tumours can be primary or secondary, and the patient may have a history of malignancy elsewhere. The most common tumours to metastasize to the brain are those of the bronchus, breast, and melanoma, as well as thyroid, gastrointestinal and renal tumours. In addition to headache, the patient may also develop seizures and focal neurological deficits related to the site of the lesion.

Fig. 18.2 Symptoms of raised intracranial pressure.

Headache worse on coughing, sneezing, stooping down
Headache worse in the morning
Visual disturbance due to papilloedema
Nausea and vomiting
Diplopia (false localizing 6th cranial nerve palsy)

Idiopathic intracranial hypertension is most common in young women. Headache, nausea and visual disturbance are the presenting symptoms. There is an association with obesity, certain drugs and empty sella syndrome. If left untreated, the patient may become blind as a result of infarction of the optic nerve, hence why the condition is no longer termed 'benign'.

Chronic subdural haematoma may follow seemingly minor trauma several weeks previously, and the headache may be associated with cognitive impairment.

Hydrocephalus can be due to either blockage of CSF flow ('non-communicating', e.g. haemorrhage, cysts, malformations) or failure of CSF reabsorption ('communicating', e.g. following meningitis or subarachnoid haemorrhage).

Temporal arteritis predominantly affects older people, and mean age at onset is over 70 years old. The patient presents with a superficial headache overlying the temporal arteries; there is often scalp tenderness which may be exacerbated by brushing or combing the hair. Jaw claudication, and occasionally tongue claudication, may arise as a consequence of inflammation of the branches of the external carotid artery. Visual loss may be temporary (amaurosis fugax) or permanent if the ciliary or central retinal arteries are affected. Weight loss, anorexia, fever and proximal muscle stiffness (but not tenderness) may also occur.

HINTS AND TIPS

Consider temporal arteritis in any patient over 50 years old with a headache.

Recurrent episodic headache and facial pain

Migraine and cluster headaches present with episodes of pain (often severe) interspersed with long symptom-free periods. Paroxysms of pain are also a feature of trigeminal neuralgia and other cranial neuralgias.

Although, classically, migraine is preceded by aura, migraine without aura is more common. Premonitory symptoms precede both types, occur hours to days before the migraine, and include fatigue, nausea and sensitivity to light and noise. Aura, if present, directly precedes the headache, lasts 5–60 min, and most commonly consists of visual features (positive, e.g. flickering lights, spots or lines, or negative, e.g. visual loss), sensory symptoms (paraesthesiae or numbness) or dysphasia. Occasionally, aura may include focal neurological signs including motor weakness; the features must be fully reversible to be defined as aura. The migraine headache is typically unilateral (though may become generalized), pulsating and associated with nausea, photophobia, phonophobia and an aversion to physical activity. The attack resolves spontaneously after 4–72 h and is often followed by sleep. Sometimes the aura can occur without the subsequent headache.

Migraine is more common in women. Provoking factors include menstruation, fatigue, cheese, red wine and the oral contraceptive pill.

Cluster headache is a severe unilateral pain centred around one eye. The pain lasts for 15–180 min if untreated and occurs daily (up to 8 times per day) for several weeks, often waking the patient from sleep. There may be ipsilateral nasal congestion or rhinorrhoea, and the eye can become watery and red; miosis and ptosis can also develop, and occasionally will become permanent. Symptom-free periods of many months occur between attacks. It is more common in men and may be precipitated by alcohol. Cluster headache is the commonest of a group of headaches called the trigeminal autonomic cephalalgias, which share headache and parasympathetic activation as their cardinal features.

Trigeminal neuralgia is characterized by paroxysms of lancinating pain in the distribution of the 5th cranial nerve. It is often stimulated by touching 'trigger zones' on the face such as the lips, or by eating or drinking, but can occur spontaneously. The pain lasts for up to 2 min and does not occur during sleep. Spontaneous remissions can last several months.

Chronic headache and facial pain

Persistent pain is a feature of postherpetic neuralgia, post-traumatic headache, Paget's disease of the skull and tension headache.

Following shingles of the trigeminal nerve (usually the ophthalmic division), a persistent burning pain known as postherpetic neuralgia may develop. Facial scarring is usually apparent and the pain may disturb sleep. It is uncommon in the young.

Tension-type headache is the commonest cause of headache presenting to doctors. The feeling is often described as 'a tight band around the head', is most often constant and bilateral, and tends to be worse towards the end of the day or at times of particular stress.

Following head injury, which may not necessarily be severe, a few patients develop persistent headache, similar to a tension headache. It is associated with poor memory and concentration, dizziness, irritability and symptoms of depression.

With any frequent or chronic headache, medication-overuse headache may be superimposed; it can occur with practically any of the medications commonly used for headache. Criteria for diagnosis are outlined by the International Headache Society classification.

EXAMINING THE PATIENT WITH HEADACHE AND FACIAL PAIN

The diagnosis is often clear from the history. On examination look for evidence of the pathological processes, such as raised intracranial pressure and meningism. Focal neurological deficits, if present, help to determine the site of the lesion. Fig. 18.3 summarizes the examination approach.

Signs of raised intracranial pressure

- Papilloedema: commonly, the only sign.
- False localizing sign (ipsilateral then bilateral 6th cranial nerve palsy).
- Altered level of consciousness, bradycardia with hypertension (the Cushing reflex – a late sign), which can progress to decerebrate posturing and death.

Signs of meningism

- Irritability: with a preference for a quiet, darkened room.
- Neck stiffness and photophobia.
- Positive Kernig's sign: spasm and pain in hamstrings on knee extension.
- Positive Brudzinski's sign: neck flexion causes hip and knee flexion.
- Delirium, fever and petechial rash: may be present in infectious meningitis.

If subarachnoid haemorrhage is suspected, look for subhyaloid (retinal) haemorrhage, bruit of an arteriovenous malformation and a 3rd cranial nerve palsy caused by direct pressure from a posterior communicating artery aneurysm.

Signs of temporal arteritis

- Temporal artery tenderness.
- Loss of temporal artery pulsation – there may be overlying erythema.
- Optic atrophy (seen as optic disc pallor).
- Low-grade pyrexia.

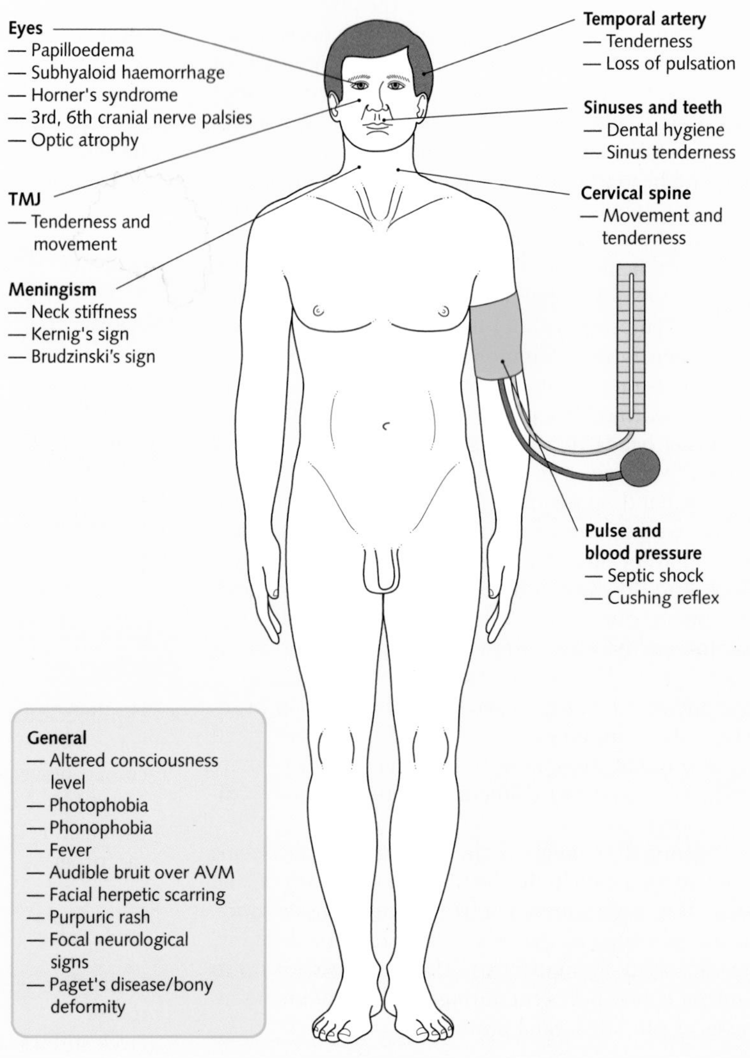

Fig. 18.3 Examining the patient with headache and facial pain. AVM, arteriovenous malformation; TMJ, temporomandibular joint.

Focal neurological deficit

Focal neurological signs will help to determine the site of the lesion (see Chs 24 and 26) and may be found in addition to other signs, such as meningism or raised intracranial pressure.

INVESTIGATING THE PATIENT WITH HEADACHE AND FACIAL PAIN

An algorithm for the investigation of the patient with headache and facial pain is given in Fig. 18.4. Investigations include the following.

Blood tests

- Full blood count: normochromic normocytic anaemia suggests chronic pathology (e.g. temporal arteritis, tuberculous meningitis); leucocytosis will be seen in infection.
- Erythrocyte sedimentation rate: high in temporal arteritis but may also be raised in infection and malignancy.
- Clotting studies may be important in the context of intracerebral bleeding.

Imaging

- CT or MRI scans of the head: presence of blood, space-occupying lesion (tumour, abscess) or hydrocephalus.

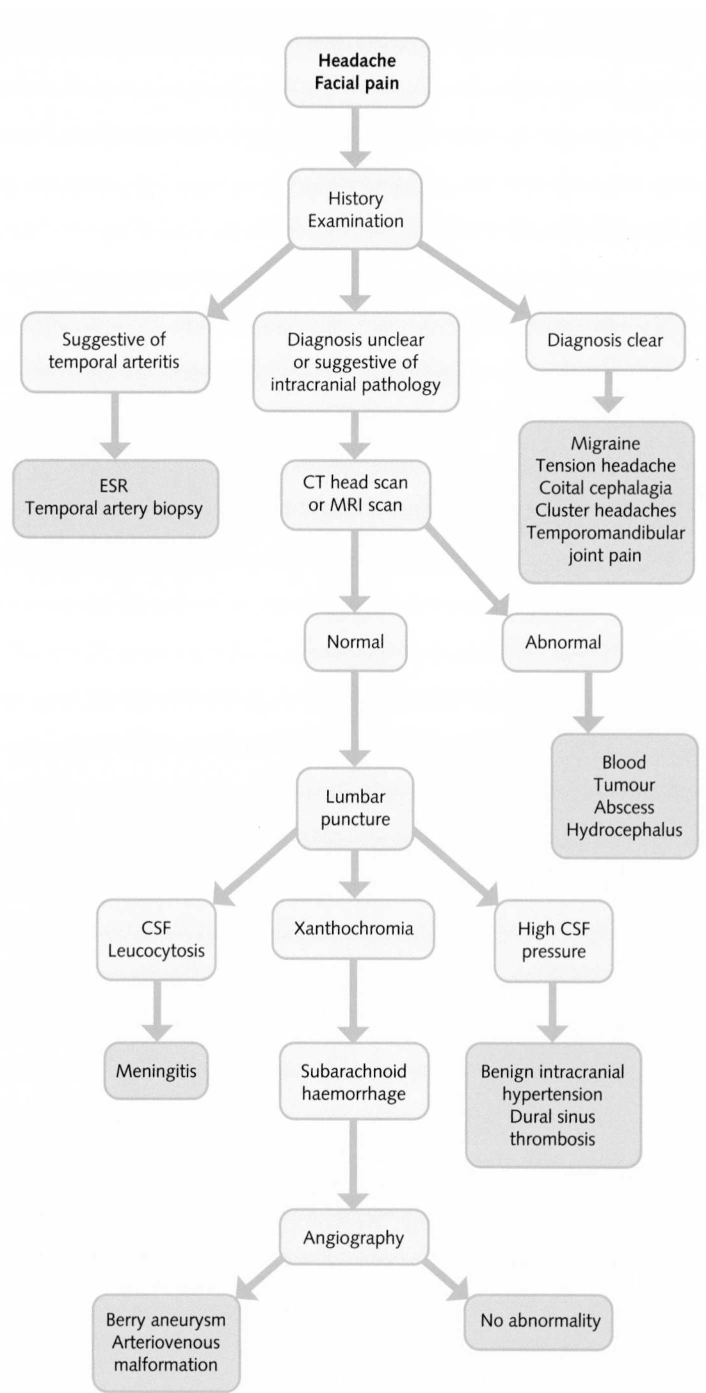

Fig. 18.4 Algorithm for the investigation of the patient with headache and facial pain. CSF, cerebrospinal fluid; CT, computed tomography; ESR, erythrocyte sedimentation rate; MRI, magnetic resonance imaging.

Contrast enhancement may help determine the nature of a lesion.

Further tests

- Temporal artery biopsy: temporal arteritis. This is a definitive test but, as there is often patchy vascular involvement ('skip lesions'), a negative result does not exclude the diagnosis.
- Lumbar puncture: this should never be performed when raised intracranial pressure is a possibility, as it may cause cerebellar tonsil herniation ('coning'). Cerebrospinal fluid (CSF) examination is invaluable in the diagnosis of meningitis. CSF should be sent to the laboratory for assessment of glucose and protein, microscopy, culture and cytology (see Ch. 26). CSF sampling and spectrophotometry may also diagnose a small number of subarachnoid haemorrhages not detected on CT.
- CT angiography, MR angiography or digital subtraction angiography (DSA): to identify the precise cause (e.g. berry aneurysm or arteriovenous malformation) in subarachnoid haemorrhage.
- Visual fields: these should be serially measured in patients with idiopathic intracranial hypertension, which carries a serious risk of optic nerve infarction.
- Electroencephalography: herpes simplex encephalitis shows characteristic features.
- Intraocular tonometry: pressure will be raised in glaucoma.

HINTS AND TIPS

When meningitis is suspected clinically, treat with antibiotics (after blood cultures if in hospital) and then complete investigations. Patients can die awaiting confirmation of the diagnosis.

Joint disease 19

Objectives

The key learning points for this chapter:

- Understand the differential diagnosis of joint disease.
- Have a logical approach to assessing the patient with painful joints.
- Direct investigations to establish the cause of the joint disease.

DIFFERENTIAL DIAGNOSIS OF JOINT DISEASE

Possible causes of joint disease are many, although in practice the common conditions include the following:

- Rheumatoid arthritis (RA).
- Osteoarthritis (OA).
- Gout.
- Seronegative arthritides: ankylosing spondylitis, Reiter's syndrome and psoriatic arthritis.
- Septic arthritis.
- Trauma.

HINTS AND TIPS

The causes of a single hot, red joint is a favourite question. They are as follows:

- Septic arthritis – until proven otherwise.
- Trauma.
- Gout.
- Pseudogout.
- Haemarthrosis.
- Rheumatoid arthritis.

Arthritis and arthralgia may also be a feature of systemic disease, including connective tissue diseases, especially systemic lupus erythematosus (SLE).

Less common causes include the following:

- Enteropathic arthropathies (e.g. inflammatory bowel disease).
- Behçet's syndrome.
- Leukaemia and lymphoma.
- Metastases: bronchial, breast, thyroid, kidney and prostate carcinomas.
- Hypertrophic pulmonary osteoarthropathy: bronchial carcinoma.
- Endocrine causes: acromegaly, myxoedema and hyperparathyroidism.
- Metabolic diseases: Wilson's disease, haemochromatosis, chondrocalcinosis, ochronosis, pyrophosphate arthropathy.
- Others: familial Mediterranean fever, sarcoidosis, amyloidosis, sickle cell disease, Wegener's granulomatosis.

A systematic approach to the differential diagnosis of joint disease is illustrated in Fig. 19.1.

HISTORY IN THE PATIENT WITH JOINT DISEASE

The different types of joint disease have many features in common, and examination will provide further additional important clues to the aetiology. Ask about the following.

Presenting complaint

- Onset: rapid or slowly progressive.
- Persistent or relapsing.
- Early morning stiffness and effect of rest and exercise: classically inflammatory arthritis (e.g. RA is worse first thing in the morning and relieved by exercise). Degenerative arthritis (e.g. OA is worse at the end of the day and relieved by rest, although there is considerable overlap).
- Pain: the site, character and exacerbating and relieving factors should be elucidated. Arthralgia is joint pain, whereas arthritis indicates an inflammatory process (i.e. swelling, heat and erythema).
- Weakness: with or without wasting of muscles.

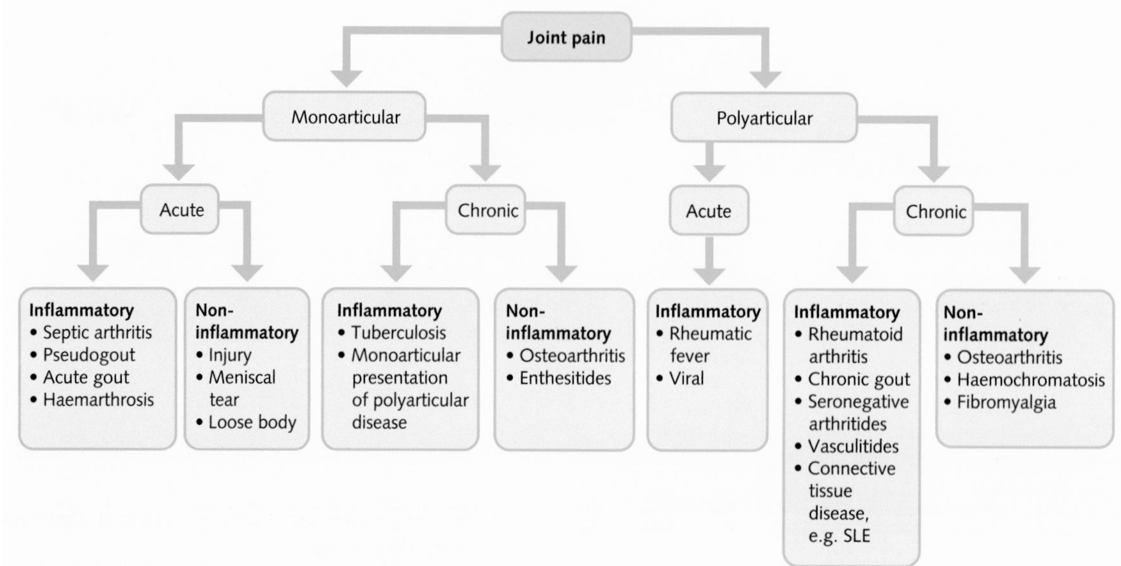

Fig. 19.1 Differential diagnosis algorithm for joint disease.

- Swelling and deformity.
- In patients with chronic arthritis, it is important to explore the extent of loss of function. How limited are the activities of daily living? This often correlates poorly with the disease activity.
- Distribution of the affected joints (see below): symmetrical or asymmetrical, mono- or polyarthritis.
- Patient's age: RA classically affects women aged 25–55 years, and OA usually occurs in the over 40s age group.
- Any history of trauma.

Associated features

- Recent infection (e.g. viral illness and reactive arthritis or septic arthritis).
- Drug therapy: gout may be precipitated by thiazides and loop diuretics, allopurinol, pyrazinamide.
- Systemic features associated with different arthropathies: inflammation of the eye (RA and seronegative arthropathies), shortness of breath (fibrosis in RA and ankylosing spondylitis), paraesthesiae (entrapment neuropathies), gastrointestinal symptoms (enteropathic arthropathies).

HINTS AND TIPS

Chronic arthritis and the associated reduction in function can lead to feelings of helplessness and depression. Assessment of these features is an important part of the history in patients with arthritis.

HINTS AND TIPS

Causes of joint pain can be remembered by the mnemonic SOFTER TISSUE: Sepsis, Osteoarthritis, Fractures, Tendon/muscle, Epiphyseal, Referred, Tumour, Ischaemia, Seropositive arthritides, Seronegative arthritides, Urate, Extra-articular rheumatism (e.g. polymyalgia).

EXAMINING THE PATIENT WITH JOINT DISEASE

Rheumatoid arthritis

RA is a systemic connective tissue disorder, the joints being one of many body parts affected. Look for the following (see Fig. 36.1):

- Symmetrical deforming arthropathy.
- Swelling of the proximal interphalangeal (PIP) and metacarpophalangeal (MCP) joints.
- Wasting of the small muscles of the hand.
- Nodules on the elbows and extensor tendons.
- Ulnar deviation of the fingers: subluxation and dislocation at the MCP joints.
- Swan-neck deformity: hyperextension of the PIP joints and flexion of the MCP and terminal interphalangeal (TIP) joints.
- Boutonnière deformity: flexion of the PIP joints and extension of the TIP and MCP joints.

- 'Z-shaped' thumb.
- Trigger finger.
- Iatrogenic Cushing's disease: steroids used in treatment.
- Involvement of other joints.
- Cervical spine disease: subluxation very important.
- Anaemia.
- Arteritic lesions: nail-fold infarcts, chronic leg ulceration and purpuric rash.

You must also carry out a general examination. In particular, look for the following:

- Eye signs: keratoconjunctivitis sicca, keratitis, episcleritis, scleromalacia perforans, cataracts due to steroids.
- Dry mucous membranes: Sjögren's syndrome.
- Chest signs: pleural effusion, fibrosing alveolitis.
- Neurological signs: peripheral neuropathy, mononeuritis multiplex, entrapment neuropathy.
- Vasculitic leg ulceration.
- Felty's syndrome: splenomegaly, neutropenia.
- Cardiac signs: pericarditis, myocarditis, conduction defects and valvular incompetence.
- Secondary amyloidosis.
- Other autoimmune disorders.

HINTS AND TIPS

Five causes of anaemia in rheumatoid arthritis:
- Normochromic normocytic anaemia of chronic disease.
- Microcytic anaemia from chronic blood loss secondary to drug treatment.
- Bone marrow suppression from treatment (e.g. gold or penicillamine).
- Megaloblastic anaemia from impaired folate release or pernicious anaemia.
- Felty's syndrome.

HINTS AND TIPS

Be aware that when introducing yourself to the patient with rheumatoid arthritis shaking hands may be painful.

Osteoarthritis

In the hands in OA look for the following:

- Heberden's nodes: swelling of the TIP joints.
- Bouchard's nodes: swelling of the PIP joints.
- Subluxation of the first metacarpal: square hand appearance.
- Crepitus of affected joints.
- Wasting and weakness of the muscle groups involved around the joint.
- Positive Trendelenburg's sign: this is a downward tilting of the pelvis on the opposite side to the stance leg when the patient stands on the affected leg – a sign of weak hip abduction.
- Joint effusions.
- Intermittent locking of the joints due to loose bodies.
- Loss of function.

Gout

Acute gout presents with severe pain, swelling and erythema of the affected joint. Traditionally this is the first metatarsophalangeal joint (podagra when the great toe is affected).

Chronic tophaceous gout follows from recurrent attacks. Look for the following:

- Asymmetrical swelling of the small joints of the hands and feet.
- Tophi: look especially on the helix of the ear and tendon sheaths.
- Causes of secondary hyperuricaemia (e.g. diuretic use or tumour lysis syndrome).

Seronegative arthritides

Psoriatic arthritis

Look for the following:

- Asymmetrical arthropathy.
- Usually involvement of the TIP joints.
- Pitting of the fingernails and onycholysis.
- Thickened nails.
- Psoriatic plaques: look particularly at the elbows, extensor aspects of limbs, scalp, behind the ears, and the navel.
- Other forms of psoriatic arthropathy: arthritis mutilans, an RA-like picture, asymmetrical mono- or oligoarthropathy, ankylosing spondylitis.

Ankylosing spondylitis

Ask the patient to sit or stand up. Look for the following:

- Loss of lumbar lordosis and a fixed kyphosis and hyperextension of the neck.
- A stooped, 'question mark' posture.
- Rigid spine.
- Reduced chest expansion.
- Prominent abdomen.

Also examine for complications and extra-articular manifestations:

- Eyes: iritis.
- Cardiovascular system: aortitis (listen for aortic regurgitation and conduction defects).
- Chest: apical fibrosis.

- Neurological: atlantoaxial dislocation leading to paraplegia or sciatica.
- Secondary amyloidosis: feel for organomegaly (pretty uncommon!)

Reactive arthritis

This is a triad of urethritis, conjunctivitis and seronegative arthritides. It follows non-specific urethritis or occasionally dysentery. Look for the following:

- Large joint mono- or oligoarthritis.
- Iritis.
- Keratoderma blennorrhagica (hyperkeratotic brown, aseptic abscesses on the soles and palms).
- Mouth ulcers.
- Circinate balanitis.
- Enthesopathy (plantar fasciitis or Achilles tendinitis).
- Aortic regurgitation.

Septic arthritis

This must be recognized and treated promptly because of potential destruction of the joint and widespread infection. It usually presents as a monoarthritis but can involve multiple joints. The affected joint is swollen, painful, hot and red. The patient will keep the joint still and even minimal passive movement will cause significant pain.

INVESTIGATING THE PATIENT WITH JOINT DISEASE

History and examination of the patient presenting with joint disease will often guide appropriate investigations. Below is a list of investigations that can aid in diagnosis.

Blood tests

- Full blood count: anaemia; raised white cell count in infection and occasionally in RA, leucopenia and thrombocytopenia in SLE, neutropenia in Felty's syndrome.
- Erythrocyte sedimentation rate and C-reactive protein: non-specific but raised in the presence of inflammation (therefore often high in RA but less so in OA).
- Rheumatoid factor: positive in about 75% of patients with RA. It may also be positive in SLE, mixed connective tissue diseases, scleroderma and Sjögren's syndrome.
- Antinuclear antibodies: positive in 30% of patients with RA and in 80% of patients with SLE.
- Anti-double-stranded DNA antibodies: high titres in SLE.
- Other autoantibodies according to clinical suspicion (e.g. anti-RoSSA and anti-LaSSB antibodies in Sjögren's syndrome, and anti-Scl70 antibodies in scleroderma).
- Viral serology: if a viral cause for the arthropathy is suspected (e.g. rubella, mumps, infectious mononucleosis, Coxsackie virus and hepatitis B virus).
- Urea and electrolytes: associated renal involvement.
- Liver function tests: liver involvement or drug treatment.
- Creatine kinase: myositis.
- Serum urate: usually high in gout but beware of false positives and false negatives.

Joint aspiration

- Note that this should be done prior to starting antibiotics if septic arthritis is suspected, but if there is no expertise available antibiotics should be started.
- Appearance: purulence indicates infection, frank blood indicates haemarthrosis or traumatic tap.
- Microscopy and culture for bacteria, polarized light microscopy for crystals: monosodium urate indicates gout, calcium pyrophosphate indicates pseudogout.
- White cell count: high in inflammatory arthropathies.
- Culture: gonococci, tubercle bacillus or fungi when indicated.

HINTS AND TIPS

In pseudogout, crystals are positively birefringent in plane-polarized light. Remember this by the 'P's. In gout, the crystals are negatively birefringent.

Imaging

- Plain X-ray for RA: soft tissue thickening, juxta-articular osteoporosis, loss of joint space, bony erosions, subluxation.
- Plain X-ray for OA: loss of joint space, subchondral sclerosis and cysts, marginal osteophytes.
- Plain X-ray for gout: soft tissue swelling and punched-out lesions in juxta-articular bone.
- Plain X-ray for ankylosing spondylitis: 'bamboo spine' (squaring of the vertebrae and obliteration of sacroiliac joints); also found in reactive arthritis and inflammatory bowel disease.

- A chest X-ray should be performed to look for associated diseases or complications of RA:
  - pleural effusion
  - diffuse pulmonary fibrosis
  - rheumatoid nodules or cavities
  - obliterative bronchiolitis
  - rheumatoid pneumoconiosis: Caplan's syndrome.
- Magnetic resonance imaging is now widely used to provide images of soft tissue injury including ligaments, muscle and intervertebral discs.
- Computed tomography is very good for assessing bones and joints. Reconstruction of the images using improved software gives three-dimensional pictures of the anatomy of an injury.

Further investigations

- Arthroscopy allows direct visualization inside the joint space, and can be used for biopsy and the removal of foreign bodies.

HINTS AND TIPS

Ask the patient how the joint disease affects their daily activities. Your concerns are not always the same as those of your patient, but the eventual management plan should be patient-centred.

Back pain 20

Objectives

The key learning points for this chapter:

- The differential diagnosis of back pain.
- How to differentiate non-specific back pain from other causes.
- How to assess a patient with back pain.
- A logical approach to the investigation of back pain.

INTRODUCTION

Back pain is a common problem, affecting up to two-thirds of adults at some point, and as such is a common presenting complaint placing a considerable burden on health services. The majority of cases are benign, non-specific and will resolve within a few weeks; up to 85% of patients will not receive a precise diagnosis. However, there are many significant causes and detecting those that need further investigation and treatment is an important skill.

Patients with back pain frequently develop chronic pain, and the effective management of this problem is often a challenge.

DIFFERENTIAL DIAGNOSIS OF BACK PAIN

Back pain is usually due to a mechanical or structural cause; this may have a neuropathic element to it such as in the case of spinal stenosis or nerve root pain secondary to a prolapsed disc. The pathology may be due to an underlying predisposition, e.g. crush fracture secondary to osteoporosis.

Non-mechanical back pain is less common but important to detect, and includes pain due to inflammatory conditions, infection and cancer.

Back pain may also be referred from other viscera. The causes of back pain are summarized in Fig. 20.1.

HISTORY IN THE PATIENT WITH BACK PAIN

Presenting complaint

Characteristics of the pain

- Site (e.g. level of spine, central or paraspinal) and radiation.
- Character (e.g. shooting in nerve root pain) and severity (is it affecting their daily activity?)
- Time course including speed of onset, progression, variation over the day (e.g. worse in the morning with inflammatory arthritis). Is the pain present at night?
- Aggravating and relieving features (e.g. pain due to disc prolapse may be worsened on leaning forward; pain due to neoplasia is often unremitting).

Associated features

- Weakness and sensory loss: can this be localized to a single myotome/dermatome (e.g. disc prolapse) or is it more generalized (e.g. cauda equina syndrome)?
- Incontinence (cauda equina syndrome).
- Stiffness (inflammatory disease).
- Fever (infection, lymphoma).
- Weight loss (inflammatory disease, neoplasia, chronic infection).
- Involvement of other joints (inflammatory arthritis).
- Pseudoclaudication: leg pain on walking, similar to ischaemic claudication (spinal stenosis).
- Features of anaemia (e.g. myeloma, colorectal cancer), change in bowel habit (colorectal cancer), new cough (lung cancer) or urinary symptoms (prostate cancer).
- Clues suggesting referred pain.
- Depression, anxiety, psychosocial factors (see Fig. 20.2 – yellow flags).

Other important points

- Age (see Fig. 20.3 – red flags).
- Trauma: may be seemingly innocuous.
- Past medical history: immune compromise, chronic infection, cancer.
- Response to previous or current medication. Immunosuppressive therapy.
- Family history: inflammatory arthritis.

Fig. 20.1 Differential diagnosis of back pain.

Mechanical back pain (possibly causing neurogenic pain)	Unknown cause/ non-specific pain	Lumbar strain/sprain
	Degenerative disease	Facet joint arthritis
	Disc prolapse	
	Spinal fracture	Pathological fracture (e.g. due to neoplasia or osteoporosis) Traumatic fracture
	Spinal stenosis	
	Spondylolysis and spondylolisthesis	
Non-mechanical pain	Neoplastic infiltration	Myeloma Metastatic carcinoma Direct invasion of retroperitoneal tumours Lymphoma/leukaemia Spinal cord tumours
	Infection	Osteomyelitis Discitis Abscess
	Inflammatory conditions	Ankylosing spondylitis Reactive arthritis Enteropathic arthritis Sacroiliitis
	Paget's disease	
Referred pain from visceral disease	Pelvic	Prostatitis Endometriosis Pelvic inflammatory disease
	Renal	Calculi Neoplasia Pyelonephritis
	Gastrointestinal	Pancreatitis Ulcer disease
	Aortic aneurysm	
Other	Fibromyalgia	

Fig. 20.2 Yellow flags: factors associated with development of chronic pain.

Physical/pain related	Obesity, older age, increased severity of pain, disability, neurological involvement, previous episode of pain
Psychological	Anxiety, depression, emotional distress, somatization
Social	Lack of education
Behavioural	Smoking, poor coping skills, avoidance of activity due to fear of pain, prior inactivity
Occupational	Highly physical employment, dissatisfaction with job, lack of employer flexibility on type of work done
Other	Involvement in litigation

Fig. 20.3 Red flags suggesting significant underlying disease in back pain.

Age >50 or <20 years old	Neoplasia more common in the older population; inflammatory disease in the young
Morning stiffness	Inflammatory disease
Nocturnal pain, constant pain	Malignancy
History of trauma	Vertebral fractures
Systemic symptoms such as fever, weight loss	Inflammatory, infectious or neoplastic disease
Immunosuppression	Infectious disease
Prolonged steroid use	Predisposes to osteoporosis and crush fractures
Neurological symptoms including sphincter disturbance	Nerve root disease, cauda equina syndrome, spinal cord compression

- Social history: smoking (lung cancer), alcohol (trauma, osteoporosis), occupation (sprain/strain), sport (trauma).

HINTS AND TIPS

Remember that with inflammatory causes the pain is worse first thing in the morning, associated with stiffness, and improves after 30–60 min as the patient moves around. Conversely, mechanical back pain is often worse with movement and better at rest.

EXAMINING THE PATIENT WITH BACK PAIN

Examination should start with the affected area of the spine and subsequently be directed by the history. If concerning features are present, a detailed systemic examination should be performed to look for an underlying disease process causing the back pain, and for any neurological sequelae.

Spinal examination

- Look: obvious abnormalities are postural abnormality, kyphosis, scoliosis, trauma, masses.
- Feel: assess spine and paraspinal region for tenderness, inflammation. Evaluate any masses fully.
- Move: is there a reduced range of movement or pain on movement?
- Special tests: straight leg raise.

Other systems/evidence of underlying disease

- Other joints: inflammatory arthritis.
- Neurological exam: if there is any hint of neurological involvement this needs to be detailed, assessing motor and sensory function fully.
- Rectal exam: assess anal tone (cauda equina syndrome) and palpate the prostate for masses.
- Respiratory: fibrosis (ankylosing spondylitis), cancer.
- Eyes: uveitis (inflammatory arthritis).
- Abdomen: masses (cancer, aortic aneurysm), tenderness (referred pain).

INVESTIGATING THE PATIENT WITH BACK PAIN

Investigations should be requested according to clinical suspicion, and only if there are features of the history or examination suggesting a significant underlying cause, or if the pain does not resolve within a few weeks. Over-investigation should be avoided; most patients do not require investigation for back pain.

Blood tests

- Full blood count: anaemia in malignancy, chronic disease. Raised white cell count in infection.
- CRP/ESR: non-specific markers of inflammation but may be useful in detecting inflammatory arthritis. Will also often be raised in infection and malignancy.
- Renal function, liver function, calcium, parathyroid hormone, vitamin D, myeloma screen: may be useful depending on suspected underlying pathology.

Imaging

- Plain X-rays of spine and pelvis: these are useful for detecting fractures (traumatic and compression fractures), disc space narrowing, degenerative change, spondylolisthesis, and changes of inflammatory disease (e.g. sacroiliitis, squaring of the vertebrae).
- Cross-sectional imaging: MRI or CT is occasionally required urgently if there is a suspicion of spinal cord compression or cauda equina syndrome. In other circumstances they provide detailed information on spinal pathology. MRI is preferred for soft tissue lesions (metastases, abscesses, herniated discs) and can provide useful information regarding infectious processes (discitis, osteomyelitis). CT provides better images of bone and is useful when further delineation of fractures is required, for spondylolisthesis, and when MRI is contraindicated.

Skin lesions and rash

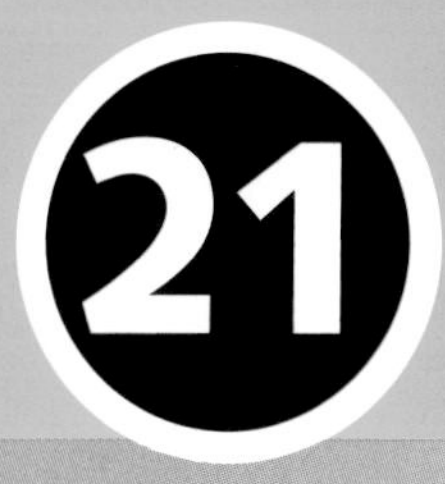

Objectives

The key learning points for this chapter:

- The differential diagnosis and description of lesions affecting the skin.
- How to assess a patient presenting with skin disease.
- The investigations needed to identify the cause of the skin disease.

Dermatology is potentially a large subject for the student and junior doctor. Skin disease may be primary or the manifestation of a systemic condition. Students should become familiar with the descriptive terminology used and learn how to manage the most common conditions. For exams a picture book is essential for revision. Many conditions are covered further in Ch. 36.

DIFFERENTIAL DIAGNOSIS BY APPEARANCE

Pigmented lesions

- Freckles (ephelides): flat, brown spots arising on sun-exposed areas.
- Lentigo: similar to freckles but often larger, and not affected by sunlight, although they may develop due to sun exposure.
- Seborrhoeic keratosis: benign, beige/brown plaques, 3–20 mm in diameter, with a velvety or warty surface.
- Melanocytic naevus (mole): there are many subtypes, including the blue naevus (small, slightly elevated blue-black lesions) and dysplastic naevus (usually a larger naevus, >5 mm, with an irregular, blurred border and mixed pigmentation and texture).
- Melanoma: flat or raised pigmented lesion with possibly a recent change in appearance. It has varying colours and typically irregular borders.
- Melasma: well-demarcated patches of increased pigmentation with an irregular border, usually on the face and predominantly in women.

Scaly lesions

- Psoriasis: silvery, scaled, well-demarcated plaques on skin, usually over the extensor surfaces. It can also be pustular or guttate (widespread small lesions) and involve the nails.
- Atopic dermatitis/eczema: dry, pruritic skin on the face, neck, wrists and hands, and in the flexures of the elbows and knees, common in children but possible at any age. Over time the excoriated areas may become lichenified.
- Seborrhoeic dermatitis: greasy plaques with yellowish scale affecting the face, scalp, armpits, groin and trunk.
- Xerosis: dry skin.
- Lichen simplex chronicus: chronic rubbing or scratching in response to itch, causing pigmented, lichenified skin lesions with exaggerated markings.
- Tinea corporis: fungal infection causing ring-shaped lesions with a scaly border and central healing, or scaly inflamed patches with a distinct border.
- Pityriasis versicolor (also tinea versicolor): scaly, discoloured macules or patches, which may be slightly elevated. They may be pale or hyperpigmented and are usually on the chest or back.
- Secondary syphilis: pigmented papules with slight scale.
- Pityriasis rosea: oval, pink/red, scaly lesions following the skin tension lines of the trunk. It is commonly preceded by a herald patch.
- Discoid lupus erythematosus: well-defined red patches, usually on the face. There is scaling, follicular plugging, atrophy and telangiectasia of involved areas. The patches may thicken and often leave scars.
- Exfoliative dermatitis: widespread skin erythema (erythroderma) with scaling or peeling.
- Actinic (solar) keratoses: small, pink lesions that are rough, crusted and scaly in texture. They are due to sun damage and are considered to be premalignant.
- Bowen's disease (intraepidermal squamous cell carcinoma): small, well-demarcated, slightly raised, pink-to-red, scaly plaques.
- Extramammary Paget's disease: a rare form of adenocarcinoma, this resembles chronic eczema and may involve apocrine areas such as the genitals.

- Intertrigo: rash in body/skin folds due to excess moisture and often infection, causing fissuring, erythema and superficial denudation.

HINTS AND TIPS

Dermatitis and eczema are interchangeable terms (though 'eczema' is commonly used to refer to the atopic form). There are several types, and different types may exist simultaneously.

Vesicular lesions

- Herpes simplex: recurrent, small, grouped vesicles on an erythematous base, especially around the oral and genital areas.
- Herpes zoster ('shingles'): vesicular lesions in a dermatomal distribution, usually preceded by pain and general malaise.
- Pompholyx (dyshidrotic eczema): small, intensely pruritic vesicles or bullae on the palms, soles and sides of fingers.
- Dermatophytid reaction: an allergic reaction to fungal infection causing pruritic, grouped, vesicular lesions in a variable distribution, distant to the site of primary infection.
- Dermatitis herpetiformis: pruritic papulovesicular lesions mainly on the elbows, knees, buttocks, shoulders and scalp. It is associated with gluten-sensitive enteropathy.
- Miliaria (heat rash): superficial, aggregated, small vesicles, papules or pustules on covered areas of the skin.
- Scabies: pruritic vesicles and pustules especially between the fingers.

Weepy or encrusted lesions

- Impetigo: vesiculopustular lesions with thick, golden-crusted exudate, associated with group A streptococci or *Staphylococcus aureus*. Bullous impetigo, with clear blisters, is associated with *S. aureus*.
- Acute allergic contact dermatitis: erythema and oedema, with pruritus, often followed by vesicles and bullae in an area of contact with a suspected agent. They may later weep, crust and become infected.
- Atopic, nummular or vesicular dermatitis may ooze and become crusted.

Pustular lesions

- Acne vulgaris: the most common skin condition, characterized by open and closed comedones and frequently accompanied by cysts, papules and pustules. It varies from mild, purely comedonal to pustular inflammatory acne. Scarring is common.
- Acne rosacea: papules, pustules and erythema over the forehead, cheeks and nose, with telangiectasia and a tendency to flush easily. Hyperplasia of the soft tissue of the nose (rhinophyma) may occur.
- Folliculitis: pustules in the hair follicles.

Figurate erythema

These are lesions that look like rings or arcs.

- Urticaria: eruptions of evanescent (short-lasting) wheals or hives.
- Erythema multiforme: erythematous lesions in a symmetrical distribution initially over the extensor surfaces of the limbs, spreading to the trunk. Palms, soles and mucous membranes may be involved. Lesions start as macules which evolve to become papular, urticarial, bullous or purpuric. Target lesions with clear centres and concentric erythematous rings may develop.
- Erythema migrans: an enlarging red patch or ring around an initial papule. The centre may clear or become indurated, vesicular or necrotic. It is a feature of Lyme disease.
- Erysipeloid: discrete red/purple lesions, most often on a finger or the back of the hand, which gradually enlarge. Caused by *Erysipelothrix insidiosa*, it is often seen in fishermen and meat handlers.

Bullous lesions

- Bullous impetigo (see Weepy or encrusted lesions).
- Pemphigus: relapsing crops of flaccid bullae appearing on normal skin, which rupture easily leaving erosions and ulcerations. Mucous membrane (especially oral) involvement is usually the first sign. There may be superficial exfoliation after slight pressure (Nikolsky's sign).
- Bullous pemphigoid: tense blisters, typically in flexural areas. They may be preceded by urticarial or eczematous lesions.
- Porphyria cutanea tarda: blistering on exposed areas.
- Erythema multiforme: see above.

Papular and nodular lesions

- Hyperkeratotic: warts, corns, seborrhoeic keratoses.
- Purple: lichen planus (see Ch. 36); Kaposi's sarcoma – malignant skin lesions with dark plaques or nodules on cutaneous or mucosal surfaces, common in people with human immunodeficiency virus infection.
- Flesh-coloured and umbilicated: molluscum contagiosum – a viral infection causing single or multiple, rounded, dome-shaped, waxy papules,

2–5 mm in diameter, which are umbilicated and contain a caseous plug; keratoacanthoma – a rapidly growing, usually benign skin tumour with a crater topped with keratin debris.
- Pearly: basal cell carcinoma – most commonly nodular with a central erosion and rolled edges, though can be superficial, waxy or pigmented; intradermal naevi.
- Small, red, and inflammatory: acne, miliaria, candidiasis, intertrigo, scabies, folliculitis.
- Erythema nodosum: painful red nodules without ulceration on the anterior aspects of the legs; they may regress over weeks to resemble contusions.
- Furuncles (boils): painful inflammatory swellings of a hair follicle forming an abscess, usually caused by *S. aureus*.
- Epidermoid cyst.

Photodermatoses

Painful erythema, oedema and vesiculation on sun-exposed surfaces, usually the face, neck, hands and upper chest. Causes include drugs (e.g. amiodarone, phenothiazines, sulphonamides and related drugs), polymorphic light eruption and systemic lupus erythematosus (SLE).

Maculopapular lesions

- Morbilliform drug eruptions, most commonly due to antibiotics and anti-epileptics.
- Exanthemata due to viral (e.g. measles) or bacterial infection (e.g. scarlet fever).
- Secondary syphilis.

HINTS AND TIPS

Drug eruptions may mimic any inflammatory skin condition. They usually start abruptly and are a widespread, symmetrical, erythematous eruption. Constitutional symptoms such as malaise, arthralgia, headache and fever may be present.

Erosive lesions

- Any vesicular or blistering lesion can leave behind an erosion, for instance impetigo, vesicular dermatitis or pemphigus.
- Erosive lichen planus: affects the mucous membranes.

Ulcerated lesions

- Decubitus ulcers: bed sores or pressure sores.
- Skin cancers.
- Parasitic infections, e.g. leishmaniasis.
- Syphilis: primary chancre.
- Venous or arterial insufficiency.
- Neuropathic ulcers: particularly in diabetes.

Petechial and purpuric lesions

- Thrombocytopenia: primary or secondary.
- Coagulation disorders, e.g. disseminated intravascular coagulation.
- Vascular disorders, e.g. vasculitis.

Miscellanous lesions

- Candidiasis: superficial, denuded, red areas with or without satellite vesicopustules. There are whitish, curd-like concretions on the oral and vaginal mucous membranes.
- Cellulitis: a hot, red, diffuse, spreading infection of the skin.
- Erysipelas: oedematous, spreading, circumscribed, hot, erythematous area, with or without vesicle or bulla formation, frequently involving the face.
- Stevens–Johnson syndrome and toxic epidermal necrolysis: usually caused by a reaction to medication. There is a rapidly spreading erythematous rash which may merge to form large areas of skin detachment. Mucosal involvement is common and mortality is high.
- Staphylococcal scalded skin syndrome: widespread erythematous blistering skin lesions due to release of staphylococcal toxins.

HISTORY IN THE PATIENT WITH SKIN RASHES

The following long list of factors should be assessed when taking a history in the patient with skin rashes:

- Rash: onset, duration.
- Aggravating factors: physical or chemical agents; cold (cold urticaria or cryoglobulinaemia); heat (worsens seborrhoeic conditions and superficial skin conditions).
- Precipitants: stress may lead to alopecia or eczema.
- Site of origin: contact dermatitis and pityriasis rosea (herald patch).
- Rate of progression or alteration of lesions.
- Timing of change in skin lesions, particularly for moles.
- Associated hair and nail abnormalities.
- Possible infective agents: foreign travel (tropical infections), pets (papular urticaria or animal scabies), farm animals (orf (poxvirus), ringworm), close contacts.

- Chemical exposure: at home or work, acting as antigens or direct irritants. Ask about soap and laundry detergent.
- Foods: nuts and shellfish.
- Light exposure: herpes simplex, SLE and vitiligo.
- Occupation.
- Current medication, including over-the-counter drugs; steroids may make the rash better (as in dermatitis) or worse (as in acne). Have any drugs been recently started or altered?
- General health and past medical history.
- Family history: important in eczema, psoriasis, inherited skin disorders.
- Patient's explanation for rash.

Systemic symptoms should be assessed, and may take the following forms:

- Itching (Fig. 21.1): atopy or urticaria, scabies, eczema, dermatitis herpetiformis, lichen planus, flexural psoriasis.
- Pain: inflammatory conditions, skin tumours.

Finally, the mode of spread is significant and may take the form of an annular appearance (e.g. erythema annulare, erythema multiforme and fungal infections) or irregular spread (e.g. pyoderma gangrenosum or malignancy).

HINTS AND TIPS

Fixed drug eruptions occur at the same site each time a patient takes a medication. With repeated exposure, the number of involved sites may increase.

Fig. 21.1 Possible causes of generalized and localized itching.

Generalized itching	Localized itching
Uraemia Cholestasis Lymphoma Iron-deficiency anaemia Hypo- and hyperthyroidism Pregnancy Carcinoma Allergies, e.g. atopic eczema Morphine ingestion Diabetes mellitus Multiple sclerosis Syphilis Intestinal parasites	Scabies and other mite infestations Contact eczema Dermatitis herpetiformis (associated with coeliac disease) Urticaria ('nettle rash') Lichen planus Prickly heat Winter itch Aquagenic pruritus Old age Pruritus ani Pruritus vulvae

COMMUNICATION

Skin diseases affecting exposed areas such as the face can have a devastating effect on patients that is often disproportionate to the severity of the disease. Careful questioning of the patient's concerns and appropriate reassurance that the condition can be treated are important aspects of managing dermatological problems.

EXAMINING THE PATIENT WITH A SKIN RASH

Always examine the entire skin, but maintain the dignity of the patient, and look in the mouth (e.g. with lichen planus, herpes simplex and zoster, and infective exanthemata). Rashes may change with time and become characteristic or diagnostic of common dermatoses, such as the infectious exanthemata. Look at the distribution of lesions:

- If widespread and symmetrical, suspect systemic disease.
- If only areas exposed to the sun are involved, suspect light sensitivity.
- A dermatomal distribution suggests herpes zoster.
- Dermatitis involving the hands, face, axillae, ears and eyelids suggests contact dermatitis.
- Dermatitis involving the axillae, groins, scalp, the central chest and back, eyebrows, ears and beard suggests seborrhoeic dermatitis.
- Dermatitis involving the popliteal and cubital fossae and the face suggests atopic dermatitis.

Describe the lesions. Terms and characteristics of dermatological lesions are given in Fig. 21.2. Certain features may be especially helpful, for instance:

- Bizarrely shaped lesions suggest that the cause is an external agent (e.g. caustic liquid or a self-induced injury – 'dermatitis artefacta').
- Fungal infections are characterized by slow growth, a smooth outline, an active edge with a healing centre and asymmetry.
- Non-blanching lesions quickly narrow the differential diagnosis.

COMMUNICATION

When referring a patient with skin lesions ensure you have fully examined the patient and are confident you can describe the lesions accurately.

Fig. 21.2 Terms and characteristics of dermatological lesions.

Term	Characteristics
Alopecia	Hair loss
Atrophy	Loss of skin thickness
Blister or bulla	Vesicle >1 cm diameter
Crust	Dried exudate on skin surface
Cyst	Epithelium-lined cavity containing fluid or semi-solid material
Erythema	Area of reddened skin that blanches with pressure
Fissure	Linear crack in epidermis
Indurated	Hard and thickened
Köbner's phenomenon	Skin lesions occurring at sites of external injury
Lichenification	Thickened skin with exaggerated skin markings
Macule	Circumscribed change in the skin colour ≤1 cm diameter. It is not elevated above the surface
Nodule	Solid elevated skin lesion >1 cm diameter
Papule	Solid raised palpable area ≤1 cm diameter
Patch	Macule >1 cm across
Petechiae	Pinpoint haemorrhages
Plaque	Palpable plateau-like elevation of skin
Purpura	Area of reddened skin caused by extravasation of blood that does not blanch with pressure
Pustule	Circumscribed, pus-filled lesion
Scale	Flake of hard skin
Scar	Connective tissue replacement following loss of dermal tissue
Ulcer	Irregularly shaped break in surface continuity of epithelium
Vesicle	Fluid-filled lesion <1 cm diameter
Wheal	Raised, palpable lesion with pale centre

INVESTIGATING THE PATIENT WITH SKIN RASHES

HINTS AND TIPS

In the patient presenting with subcutaneous nodules, think of the following:

- Rheumatoid nodules.
- Rheumatic fever.
- Polyarteritis.
- Xanthelasmata.
- Tuberous sclerosis.
- Neurofibromatosis.
- Sarcoidosis.

The history and examination may be enough to determine the diagnosis. If the patient is not unwell it may be possible to examine for skin changes over time, thereby allowing the development of characteristic lesions. The following investigations should be considered:

- Blood tests: full blood count, urea and electrolytes, bacterial and viral titres with immunological tests for tropical diseases if appropriate, and blood cultures.
- Skin scrapings and nail clippings: fungi.
- Examination of the skin under UV light (e.g. fungal/bacterial infections, tuberous sclerosis, porphyria).
- Examination of brushings of household pets: mites.
- Culture of fluid-containing lesions.
- Skin biopsy.
- Investigations for suspected systemic diseases or malignancy suggested by the history, examination or initial investigations.

Loss of consciousness

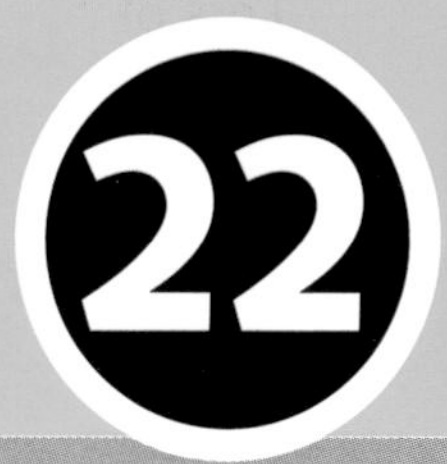

Objectives

The key learning points for this chapter:

- The differential diagnosis of an episode of loss of consciousness.
- The systematic approach to assessing a patient presenting with loss of consciousness.
- How to investigate patients and identify the underlying cause.

INTRODUCTION

Loss of consciousness may be transient ('blackouts') or ongoing (coma). Many patients are admitted to hospital with 'collapse?cause'. This term is rarely helpful as patients use the word 'collapse' to describe a variety of situations, and it is essential to determine whether or not the patient has actually lost consciousness. In addition, the collapse may be mistakenly labelled as a transient ischaemic attack (TIA) when there is little supporting evidence of posterior circulation ischaemia, and other diagnoses are more likely.

COMMUNICATION

Many patients use the terms dizziness, light-headedness, fall, faint, loss of consciousness and collapse interchangeably. Careful questioning is needed to establish whether the patient had a true syncopal episode, as this is key to making the correct diagnosis.

DIFFERENTIAL DIAGNOSIS OF LOSS OF CONSCIOUSNESS

Blackouts

Many patients describe transient episodes of blacking out, which are often recurrent. Some of these patients have syncope: a transient loss of consciousness and postural tone due to a reduction in cerebral perfusion with spontaneous recovery. The causes of blackouts are summarized in Fig. 22.1.

Coma

In coma, the patient remains unconscious and is unrousable. The causes of coma are summarized in Fig. 22.2.

HISTORY IN THE PATIENT WITH LOSS OF CONSCIOUSNESS

COMMUNICATION

Always try to obtain a collateral history from a witness, even if the patient has regained consciousness.

When a patient presents unconscious, relatives or the general practitioner should be contacted to gain information regarding previous medical history, prodromal illness, known alcohol or drug abuse, and whether the events leading to the coma were witnessed by anyone.

In syncope, the history should focus on the following details.

Before the event

- Find out what the patient was doing at the time.
- Ask about any symptoms occurring prior to the event.
- Syncope due to postural hypotension often occurs after standing up suddenly.
- Prior to an epileptic seizure, there is often an aura.
- In arrhythmia, the patient can be aware of palpitations, chest pain or dyspnoea before blacking out.
- Episodes of bradycardia may cause collapse without any warning (Stokes–Adams attacks).
- Exertional syncope is seen in aortic stenosis and hypertrophic cardiomyopathy (HCM).
- Occasionally, syncope can occur following cough, micturition, swallowing or straining during defecation.
- Syncope on head-turning may suggest carotid sinus hypersensitivity or rotational vertebrobasilar insufficiency. Very rarely, subclavian steal may cause syncope during exercise of an arm.

Fig. 22.1 Differential diagnosis of blackouts.

Causes	Subgroups	Examples and notes
Syncope (see Chs 30 & 34)	Orthostatic (postural) syncope	Old age, drugs (antihypertensives and others), autonomic neuropathy
	Neurocardiogenic (vasovagal) syncope	Characterized by inappropriate vagal outflow in response to stimulus (e.g. prolonged standing, fear, pain)
	Carotid sinus syndrome	Syncope on minor stimulation of the carotid sinus (e.g. head turning, shaving)
	Situational syncope	Cough, micturition, defecation
	Cardiogenic syncope	Arrhythmia (Stokes–Adams attack) or structural heart disease (e.g. AS, HCM)
	TIA/vertebrobasilar insufficiency	Transient ischaemia in posterior circulation causing LOC (i.e. needs to affect RAS in the brainstem; as this is diffuse, TIAs rarely cause LOC alone – other brainstem structures are affected), subclavian steal
Epilepsy (see Ch. 34)	Complex partial seizure	Focal epileptic activity with altered consciousness (e.g. temporal lobe epilepsy)
	Generalized seizure	Generalized epileptic activity
	Pseudoseizure	Behaviour mimicking a seizure but no epileptic activity in brain
Hypoglycaemia (see Ch. 35)	Fasting	See list in Ch. 35
	Postprandial	Dumping syndrome

AS, aortic stenosis; HCM, hypertrophic cardiomyopathy; LOC, loss of consciousness; TIA, transient ischaemic attack; RAS, reticular activating system.

Fig. 22.2 Differential diagnosis of coma.

Causes	Examples
Neurological (see Ch. 34)	Trauma – especially closed head injury
	Cerebrovascular event – intracranial haemorrhage or infarction
	Epilepsy (postictal or non-convulsive status epilepticus)
	Meningitis, encephalitis, overwhelming septicaemia
	Space-occupying lesion
Metabolic	Hypo- or hyperglycaemia
	Myxoedema or Addisonian crisis (see Ch. 35)
	Hypothermia (see Ch. 35)
	Hypoxia or CO_2 narcosis (see Ch. 31)
	Severe electrolyte disturbance (see Ch. 35)
	Uraemic encephalopathy
	Hepatic encephalopathy (see Ch. 32)
	Drugs and toxins (see Ch. 39)

The attack itself

- What happened during the episode itself? This is where the history of a witness is vitally important.
- Prolonged seizure activity associated with tongue biting, particularly the side of the tongue, are suggestive of epilepsy. Any cause of cerebral hypoxia may result in brief anoxic seizures, which may be more prolonged if the patient is upright. Urinary incontinence can be a feature of both syncope and epilepsy.
- In Stokes–Adams attacks, the patient typically becomes very pale, with flushing on recovery. The length of time that the patient remained unconscious should be recorded.
- If available, the pulse rate during the episode can help (e.g. bradycardia or absent pulse in Stokes–Adams attack). If the attack occurs in hospital the blood pressure and blood glucose should be recorded during the episode.

Following the event

- How quickly did the patient recover? Syncope is generally followed by rapid recovery. However, in epilepsy there is usually postictal sleepiness or disorientation.

- Focal neurological impairment after recovery of consciousness may suggest TIA (though TIA only rarely presents with blackout) or Todd's paresis following a seizure (see Ch. 34).
- It is also very important to ask whether the patient hurt themselves during the episode. If there is significant injury, consider cardiac syncope (lack of warning) or seizure.

Risk factors

- Is there a previous history of similar episodes or of epilepsy, cardiac disease, cerebrovascular disease or obstructive airways disease?
- Does the patient have cardiovascular risk factors or a relevant family history (e.g. HCM)?
- Is the patient on insulin or a healthcare worker with access to insulin?
- Is there a history of drug abuse or depression?
- Has there been any previous head trauma?

EXAMINING THE PATIENT WITH LOSS OF CONSCIOUSNESS

Fig. 22.3 summarizes the examination approach. The emphasis of the examination differs between the sick comatose patient and one with recurrent blackouts. These approaches are outlined below.

Coma patient

- Always start with ABCDE: Airway, Breathing, Circulation, Disability (i.e. Glasgow coma scale – see Fig. 22.4), Exposure.
- Urgent observations: pulse, blood pressure, respiratory rate, oxygen saturation, capillary glucose and arterial blood gas.
- Survey for injuries: especially closed head injury and evidence of skull fracture such as blood or cerebrospinal fluid in ears, or Battle's sign (bruising over the mastoid process).

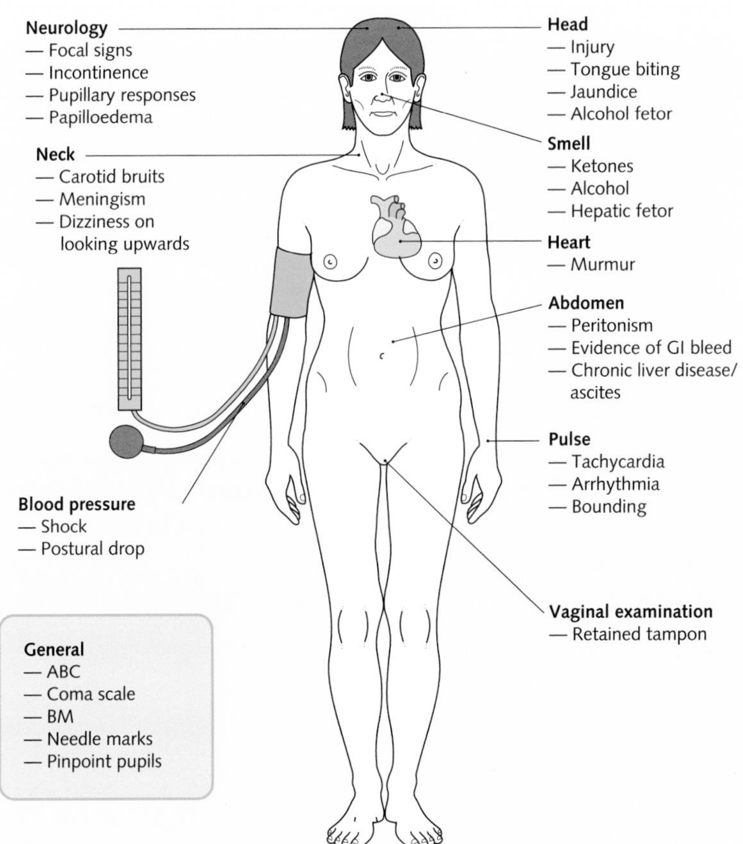

Fig. 22.3 Examining the patient with loss of consciousness. ABC, the Airway–Breathing–Circulation first-aid mnemonic; BM, stick test for blood sugar; GI, gastrointestinal.

Fig. 22.4 The Glasgow coma scale.

Category	Response	Score
Best verbal response	Orientated Confused conversation Inappropriate speech Incomprehensible sounds No speech	5 4 3 2 1
Best motor response (i.e. best response of any limb)	Obeys commands Localizes to pain Withdraws to pain Flexes to pain (decorticate) Extends to pain (decerebrate) No response	6 5 4 3 2 1
Eye opening	Spontaneous To speech To pain No eye opening	4 3 2 1

The Glasgow coma scale is used in assessing loss of consciousness in a patient.

- Check for evidence of liver disease, diabetes mellitus, IV drug use (e.g. signs of chronic liver disease or injection sites). Consider hepatic encephalopathy, diabetic coma, opiate or other overdose.
- Is there a characteristic smell: alcohol, ketones, hepatic fetor?
- Look for signs of meningism (meningitis or subarachnoid haemorrhage) and rash (meningococcal meningitis classically gives petechial or purpuric rash).
- Examine pupils and eye movement (see Fig. 22.5).
- Cardiovascular examination: arrhythmia (including atrial fibrillation which predisposes to stroke), murmurs or other evidence of bacterial endocarditis.
- Respiratory: focal consolidation, evidence of COPD and carbon dioxide retention.
- Abdomen: gastrointestinal haemorrhage, ascites (which may be infected), organomegaly, peritonism.
- Neurological examination: focal neurology suggests intracranial cause.

HINTS AND TIPS

Remember to look for items hinting as to the cause of loss of consciousness, i.e. medic alert bracelets, neck tags or wallet cards.

Patient with blackouts

- Lying and standing blood pressure.
- Thorough cardiovascular and neurological examination.
- Remember to examine fully for any injuries sustained.

Fig. 22.5 Examination of the eyes in the coma patient.

Test	Findings	Interpretation
Visual fields (by visual threat – normal response is to blink)	Hemianopia	Suggests contralateral hemisphere lesion
Pupil reactions	Normal direct and consensual	Intact midbrain
	Midposition, unreactive to light, irregular	Midbrain lesion
	Unilateral, fixed, dilated	Third nerve compression (e.g. due to tentorial herniation)
	Small, reactive	Pontine lesion, opiate overdose
	Horner's syndrome	Ipsilateral lateral medullary or hypothalamic lesion
Doll's head manoeuvre to test vestibulo-ocular reflex (*perform only if cervical spine normal*)	Normal if pupils fixed on same point in space when head moved quickly	Brainstem from 3rd to 7th nerve nucleus intact
Fundoscopy	Papilloedema	Raised intracranial pressure (occasionally CO_2 narcosis)
	Subhyaloid haemorrhage	Subarachnoid haemorrhage
	Hypertensive retinopathy	? Hypertensive encephalopathy

INVESTIGATING THE PATIENT WITH LOSS OF CONSCIOUSNESS

HINTS AND TIPS

A blood glucose test should be performed urgently in all unconscious patients to exclude hypoglycaemia.

Investigation will be guided by findings in the history and clinical examination. The following investigations are useful in the different clinical scenarios:

- Full blood count: anaemia in severe haemorrhage or haemolysis (malaria); leukocytosis in sepsis.
- Urea and electrolytes: hypo- or hypernatraemia.
- Calcium: hypocalcaemia.
- Glucose: hypoglycaemia/hyperglycaemia.
- Creatine kinase: rhabdomyolysis (if lying unconscious for a prolonged period).
- Liver function tests (biochemistry and synthetic function): liver failure.
- Thyroid function tests: hypothyroidism (myxoedema coma).
- Electrocardiogram: arrhythmia, left ventricular hypertrophy in aortic stenosis and HCM.
- Arterial blood gases: hypercapnia, hypoxia, acid–base status. The ABG may also give you a quick potassium and glucose reading.
- Chest X-ray: pulmonary disease, aspiration pneumonia.
- Septic screen: cultures of blood, urine, ascitic fluid.
- Drug screen of urine and blood.
- Computed tomography head scan: intracranial pathology.
- Carotid Dopplers: carotid artery stenosis.
- 24-h or 7-day ECG monitoring for arrhythmia.
- Echocardiogram: heart rhythm, source of emboli, aortic stenosis, HCM.
- Lumbar puncture: meningitis, subarachnoid haemorrhage.
- Tilt-table testing: patients are moved from a recumbent to an upright position with monitoring of their pulse, blood pressure, electrocardiogram and symptoms. Those with orthostatic (postural) hypotension show an early drop in blood pressure (within 2–3 min) whereas those with vasovagal syndrome show a delayed response (up to 45 min) in which the blood pressure alone may drop (vasodepressor response), bradycardia may occur, causing hypotension (cardioinhibitory response), or a mixture of the two. In some centres, carotid sinus massage is performed in combination with tilt-table testing to increase its sensitivity at diagnosing carotid sinus hypersensitivity (which may also manifest with a vasodepressor response, cardioinhibitory response or a mixture of the two).
- Electroencephalogram (EEG): epilepsy (including non-convulsive status epilepticus), viral encephalitis.

HINTS AND TIPS

Carotid Dopplers should only be requested for clinical syndromes suggesting unilateral anterior cerebral circulation infarction where carotid intervention would be considered.

Confusional states

Objectives

The key learning points for this chapter:

- The definition and causes of confusional states.
- How to assess a confused patient.
- How to approach the investigation of confusional states.

INTRODUCTION

Confusion can be acute, subacute, or chronic, and may be reversible or progressive. It is often divided into delirium (acute or subacute onset of fluctuating disturbance of consciousness with change in cognition) or dementia (progressive disease of the brain causing impairment of higher cortical function without impairment of consciousness). Any cause of delirium can precipitate an acute exacerbation of dementia – 'acute on chronic confusion'. Confusional states are very common, particularly in the elderly, and are often worsened by admission to hospital.

COMMUNICATION

When a patient presents with confusion it is essential to talk to family members or carers. Try to establish whether the problem is long-standing and getting worse or is a new presentation.

DIFFERENTIAL DIAGNOSIS OF CONFUSIONAL STATE

Delirium

There are many causes of delirium in the elderly patient; the most common are summarized in Fig. 23.1.

Dementia

The causes of dementia are summarized in Fig. 23.2.

HINTS AND TIPS

It is important to remember that depression can sometimes mimic dementia ('pseudodementia'). Other psychiatric illnesses causing psychosis and severe anxiety may present in a very similar manner to acute confusional states with an organic cause.

HISTORY IN THE CONFUSED PATIENT

The first step is to establish whether the patient is newly confused or if there is a history of dementia, and if so whether the confusion is worse than normal. A good account from relatives, carers or close friends is almost always the only way of getting a true picture of the pattern of disease. The previous hospital notes can be an invaluable source of information, and a thorough social history is essential to put the patient's problems in context. The history should then focus on possible underlying causes.

Pattern of confusion

HINTS AND TIPS

Severe symptoms of 'delirium tremens' due to alcohol withdrawal may occur 24–48 h after the patient's last drink, and long after their admission to hospital.

Delirium develops over hours or days. It is characterized by clouding of consciousness that fluctuates in severity,

Fig. 23.1 Differential diagnosis of delirium.

Causes	Examples
Infection	Any – commonly urinary tract, pneumonia, cellulitis, meningitis, encephalitis
Drug intoxication	Opiates, anxiolytics, steroids, tricyclics, anticonvulsants, drugs of abuse (see Ch. 39)
Drug withdrawal	Alcohol, benzodiazepines
Metabolic	Liver, kidney, cardiorespiratory failure (hypoxia and hypercapnia), hyper- or hyponatraemia, hypoglycaemia, hypercalcaemia
Endocrine	Thyroid disorders, electrolyte and glucose abnormalities may be caused by Addison's disease, diabetes and parathyroid disorders
Vitamin deficiency	Wernicke-Korsakoff syndrome (thiamine deficiency) (see *Crash Course: Psychiatry*)
Cerebral pathology	Abscess, tumour, haemorrhage, infarction, trauma, epilepsy/postictal, encephalitis (both infectious and autoimmune) (see Ch. 34)
Pain	Any cause
New surroundings	Hospital ward, possibly without hearing (hearing aid?) or vision (spectacles?)

Fig. 23.2 Differential diagnosis of dementia (see *Crash Course: Psychiatry*).

Categories	Causes
Common causes	Alzheimer's disease, vascular dementia, Lewy body dementia, frontotemporal dementias
Rarer causes	Chronic alcohol abuse, Huntington's chorea, Creutzfeldt–Jakob disease, Parkinson's disease, Pick's disease, HIV, subacute sclerosing panencephalitis, progressive multifocal leukoencephalopathy, pellagra (niacin deficiency)
Treatable causes (which **must** therefore be excluded)	B_{12}/folate deficiency, hypothyroidism, thiamine deficiency, subdural haematoma, normal pressure hydrocephalus, neurosyphilis, resectable tumour, depression (pseudodementia)

often worse at night with lucid periods in the day. It can be accompanied by poor recent memory, disorientation and hallucinations. As a result, the patient may be agitated, uncooperative and sometimes paranoid, though behaviour may also be underactive.

Dementia usually has a gradual onset over months or years. It is characterized by a global deterioration in higher cerebral function with no change in level of consciousness, tends to be progressive and is often exacerbated when the patient is removed from familiar surroundings, such as by admission to hospital. Vascular dementia may present as 'multi-infarct' dementia, progressing in a stepwise fashion, or slowly and gradually in a manner indistinguishable from Alzheimer's disease.

A more rapid onset is seen in Creutzfeldt–Jakob disease (CJD), hydrocephalus and depression. The depressed patient often complains of memory loss (unlike patients with early dementia, who may not be aware of the problem), makes poor effort at testing and may have a personal or family history of depression.

Possible underlying causes

The following should be assessed, as they may reveal an underlying cause:

- Age: dementia becomes increasingly common after the age of 60 years. A thorough search for a treatable underlying cause should be made, particularly in younger patients.
- Symptoms of focal infection (see Ch. 8).
- Symptoms of raised intracranial pressure (see Ch. 18).
- Risk factors for, or known, vascular disease (see Ch. 30).
- Dietary history: vitamin deficiency.
- Alcohol intake: while chronic alcohol abuse can cause dementia in its own right, it may also be associated with thiamine deficiency (Wernicke–Korsakoff syndrome) as well as folate and B_{12} deficiency, both of which may increase the risk of dementia.
- Previous head injury or evidence of falls: subdural haematoma.
- Other neurological symptoms: cerebrovascular disease, multiple sclerosis, cerebral tumour/abscess, inflammatory or autoimmune neurological disease.
- Symptoms of endocrine disease, particularly hypo- or hyperthyroidism.
- Previous medical history of any disease may be relevant: long-standing renal disease (uraemia), liver disease (encephalopathy), malignancy (cerebral metastases, hypercalcaemia or paraneoplastic syndromes, e.g. encephalitis), diabetes (insulin overdose), endocrine disease (thyroid disorders, Addison's disease).
- Drug history: particular attention should be given to sedatives, anticonvulsants and steroids. Has the patient ever used illegal drugs?

- Family history: Wilson's disease (autosomal recessive); Huntington's chorea (autosomal dominant); depression.
- Brief psychiatric history: notably for features of depression.
- Sexual history may provide information regarding the possibility of HIV, hepatitis or syphilis.

EXAMINING THE CONFUSED PATIENT

Since the causes of confusion are so varied, a thorough clinical examination is mandatory. This approach is summarized in Fig. 23.3. Particular attention should be given to the following:

- Consciousness: the level of consciousness should be recorded using the Glasgow coma scale (see Fig. 22.4).
- Blood pressure: hypotension may be due to sepsis or cardiac failure. Hypertension is a risk factor for cerebrovascular events and can also be a response to raised intracranial pressure.
- Cyanosis: hypoxia is a common cause of confusion in patients in hospital. The oxygen saturation should be measured.

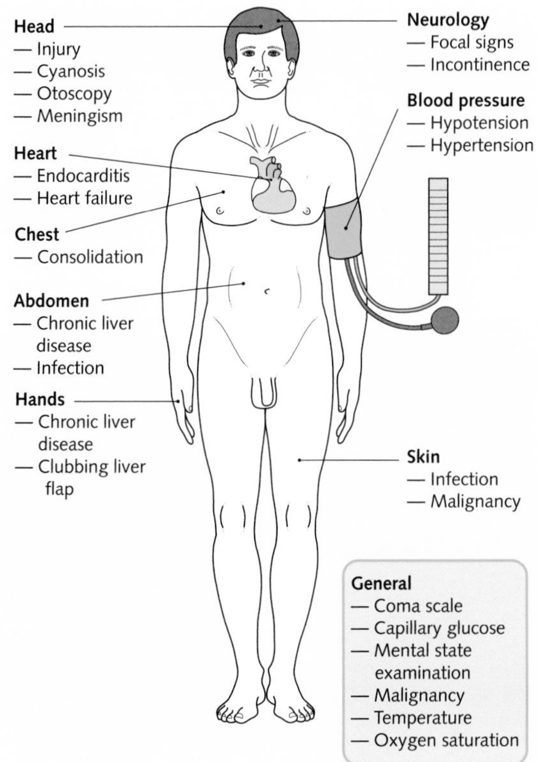

Fig. 23.3 Examining the confused patient.

- Capillary glucose: hypoglycaemia or hyperglycaemia (DKA and HONK syndrome).
- Evidence of head injury: subdural haematoma.
- Signs of infection: measure temperature, look for neck stiffness, consolidation in the chest, signs of endocarditis, abdominal tenderness, otitis media on otoscopy, pressure areas and skin for evidence of cellulitis (see Ch. 8).
- Mental state: The 10-point abbreviated mental test score (see Fig. 23.4) is useful for confirming confusion and may be used serially to monitor progress. The 30-point MMSE (mini-mental state examination) is mandatory if querying a new diagnosis of dementia, to document cognitive function and provide a baseline for future assessment. In many cases more comprehensive assessment is required in due course, for instance with the Addenbrooke's cognitive examination.
- Focal neurological deficit and the pattern of signs may give important clues as to the diagnosis (see Chs 24 and 26): fundoscopy should be performed looking for papilloedema (raised intracranial pressure), optic atrophy (demyelination) or subhyaloid haemorrhages (subarachnoid haemorrhage). Parkinsonism may be present in Parkinson's disease and Parkinson plus syndromes. Myoclonus, extrapyramidal signs and aphasia are features of CJD.
- Signs of chronic liver disease, particularly a liver flap (asterixis): hepatic encephalopathy commonly causes confusion. Chronic liver disease may also indicate chronic alcohol abuse or rare disorders such as Wilson's disease.
- Malignancy: examine thoroughly – breasts, digital rectal examination for prostate and bowel pathology,

Fig. 23.4 The abbreviated mental test score.

1	Age
2	Date of birth
3	Time (to nearest hour)
4	Year
5	Address for recall at end of test – to be repeated by patient to ensure it has been heard correctly: 42 West Street
6	Name of this place
7	Recognition of two people (e.g. nurse and doctor)
8	Year of First World War (or similar)
9	Name of monarch
10	Count backwards from 20 to 1

One point is awarded for each correct answer. A score of less than 7/10 strongly suggests confusion.

lymph nodes and skin for dermatological malignancy and cutaneous manifestations of malignancy.

- Signs of endocrine disorders, particularly thyroid disease and Addison's disease (see Ch. 35).

COMMUNICATION

It is often difficult to examine confused patients and signs can be missed. Having a family member or nurse present may help to calm and position the patient.

INVESTIGATING THE CONFUSED PATIENT

There is much overlap in the investigation of delirium and dementia despite the difference in urgency. The following tests should be considered.

Initial tests

Routine observations, including oxygen saturation, capillary glucose, urinalysis and ECG, can all be performed quickly and may give an almost immediate clue as to the underlying cause.

Blood tests

- Full blood count: reactive blood picture in malignancy, infection or inflammation; anaemia with raised mean corpuscular volume in vitamin B_{12} or folate deficiency.
- Erythrocyte sedimentation rate: raised in malignancy, infection, inflammation.
- Urea and electrolytes: hypo- or hypernatraemia and renal failure.
- Liver function tests: abnormal in liver disease. Gamma-glutamyltransferase may indicate recent excess alcohol consumption.
- Thyroid function tests: thyroid stimulating hormone (TSH) usually raised in hypothyroidism and low in hyperthyroidism.
- Serum calcium: hyper- or hypocalcaemia.
- Serum glucose: hypoglycaemia.
- Arterial blood gases for hypoxia.
- Blood cultures if considering infection.
- Vitamin B_{12} and folate levels: deficiency. Red blood cell folate is a more reliable indicator of long-term deficiency than serum folate.
- Syphilis serology: tertiary syphilis may cause dementia.

Radiology

A chest X-ray may show pneumonia, cardiac failure or malignancy. Computed tomography scanning or magnetic resonance imaging of the head should be considered to look for tumour, infarction, haematoma, hydrocephalus and abscess.

Further tests

Consider the following when clinically indicated:

- Urine: toxicology screen, culture for urinary infection.
- Red cell transketolase for thiamine deficiency.
- Electroencephalogram: typical temporal lobe seizure foci of herpes simplex encephalitis.
- Lumbar puncture and cerebrospinal fluid examination: protein, glucose, microscopy, culture and oligoclonal bands.
- Autoimmune screen including autoimmune encephalitis antibodies.
- Ammonia – often raised in liver disease. Also caused by defects in metabolism (see Ch. 34).
- Serum copper and caeruloplasmin (reduced) and 24-h urinary copper excretion (increased): Wilson's disease.
- *Borrelia* serology for Lyme's disease.
- Thick and thin blood films: malaria.
- HIV serology.

Stroke and transient ischaemic attack

24

Objectives

The key learning points for this chapter:

- The definitions and differential diagnosis of stroke and transient ischaemic attack (TIA).
- A logical approach to assessing the patient with a stroke or TIA.
- The investigation of patients presenting with acute neurological deficits.

INTRODUCTION

A stroke is a neurological deficit due to vascular disturbance that develops over minutes (sometimes hours) and persists for at least 24 h. Identical deficits lasting less than 24 h are termed transient ischaemic attacks (TIAs). Stroke is often also called 'cerebrovascular accident' (CVA) or 'cerebrovascular event' (CVE), but the term 'stroke' should be used to avoid confusion. Cerebral infarction (mainly embolism or thrombosis) accounts for 80% of strokes; 20% are caused by intracerebral haemorrhage. Fig. 24.1 outlines the principal types and causes.

DIFFERENTIAL DIAGNOSIS OF STROKE

The diagnosis is often clear from the history and examination but the following pathologies can also produce a clinical picture that is identical to stroke and should be considered in atypical presentations:

- Subdural haematoma: particularly in the elderly and in alcohol misuse.
- Space-occupying lesions: e.g. tumour (primary or secondary) or cerebral abscess (consider if patient has bronchiectasis or heart murmur suggesting endocarditis).
- Epilepsy: postictal (Todd's) paresis following seizure (generalized or partial).
- Hemiplegic migraine: typical features of migraine also present, resolving within 24 h.
- Toxic/metabolic cause: hypo- and hyperglycaemia, hyponatraemia, drug overdose.
- Demyelination: e.g. multiple sclerosis.

HISTORY IN THE STROKE PATIENT

The history should focus on three distinct areas. First, does the history fit with the diagnosis of stroke? Second, where is the anatomical site of the lesion? Finally, are any risk factors present?

The pattern of onset

The key feature in stroke is that the symptoms develop rapidly over a few minutes, or less commonly hours, but once the deficit is complete it remains stable and usually improves. If there has been gradual neurological deterioration, consider one of the differential diagnoses or hydrocephalus secondary to the stroke (oedema or blood preventing free drainage of cerebrospinal fluid). Improvement can be complete but there is often some residual deficit.

The site of the lesion

Any intracranial artery can be involved in stroke. The symptoms and signs will reflect which artery and therefore which part of the brain has been involved. This is summarized in Fig. 24.2.

Underlying risk factors

Fig. 24.3 shows the main risk factors for stroke; many are common to all vascular disease (see Ch. 30).

HINTS AND TIPS

If the patient has atrial fibrillation calculate their risk of further stroke using a risk-scoring system such as the CHADS2 score (see Ch. 34) to allow a reasoned decision regarding anticoagulation.

EXAMINING THE STROKE PATIENT

Clinical examination gives information regarding four important areas in the stroke patient.

Fig. 24.1 Types of stroke.

Type	Aetiology
Haemorrhagic	Hypertension Aneurysm (particularly Charcot–Bouchard microaneurysms; also berry and mycotic aneurysms) Arteriovenous malformation (AVM) Tumours Bleeding tendency (thrombocytopenia, coagulopathy, anticoagulants) Drugs (amphetamines, ecstasy, cocaine) Haemorrhagic transformation of infarction
Ischaemic (thrombotic, hypotensive, occlusive)	Hypertension Intracranial arterial atheroma Vasculitis (e.g. temporal arteritis, SLE, PAN, neurosyphilis) Prolonged hypotension (e.g. cardiac arrest) Thrombophilia (hyperviscosity, antiphospholipid syndrome) Drugs (amphetamines, ecstasy, cocaine) Arterial dissection (cervical or vertebral)
Ischaemic (embolic)	Carotid or vertebral atheroma Cardiac: • atrial fibrillation with left atrial thrombosis • endocarditis • ventricular thrombus, e.g. due to MI or ventricular aneurysm • atrial myxoma Paradoxical: • venous thrombus can reach the cerebral circulation via an atrial septal defect

MI, myocardial infarction; PAN, polyarteritis nodosa; SLE, systemic lupus erythematosus.

- What are the neurological abnormalities and do they fit with the diagnosis of stroke?
- Is there any evidence of an underlying cause?
- Have any complications arisen as a result of the stroke?
- What acute treatment is needed?

Fig. 24.4 summarizes this examination approach.

Has the patient had a stroke?

A thorough neurological examination should be performed, including a Glasgow coma score (GCS). Does the pattern of neurological deficit fit with disruption of the cerebral vascular supply (see Fig. 24.2)? Remember that the GCS is imperfect in stroke as dysphasia and aphasia reduce the verbal score. Pay particular attention to the pattern of upper motor neurone weakness, hemianopia, dysphasia and sensory/visual inattention. This enables you to place the patient in the Bamford classification, which has important prognostic implications (Fig. 24.5).

COMMUNICATION

Taking a history from a patient with a stroke can be challenging. The patient may have a receptive or expressive dysphasia and could have visual impairment from a homonymous hemianopia. It is important to position yourself where the patient can see you to maximize communication with the patient. A collateral history may be required.

Determining the likely site of the lesion helps to focus the search for an underlying cause (e.g. carotid bruits in an anterior or middle cerebral artery stroke).

Is there any evidence of an underlying cause?

There are many causes and risk factors for stroke. However, pay particular attention to the following:

- Carotid bruits: carotid atheroma.
- Murmurs: endocarditis, valvular disease, atrial septal defect.
- Pulse: atrial fibrillation.
- Blood pressure: hypertension can be the cause or result of stroke; prolonged hypotension can also cause stroke.
- Diminished peripheral pulses and femoral bruits: peripheral vascular disease.
- Xanthelasmata, xanthomata: underlying hyperlipidaemia
- Temporal artery tenderness: giant cell arteritis.
- Tar-stained fingers from smoking.

Have any complications developed?

Complications are very common following stroke, both acutely and during recovery, and are related to the extent of cerebral damage and the degree of neurological deficit. The more common problems, and protective measures, are outlined in Fig. 24.6.

What acute intervention is needed?

There is strong evidence that the acute management of stroke influences outcome. At present this involves the use of antiplatelet agents, good fluid balance, glycaemic

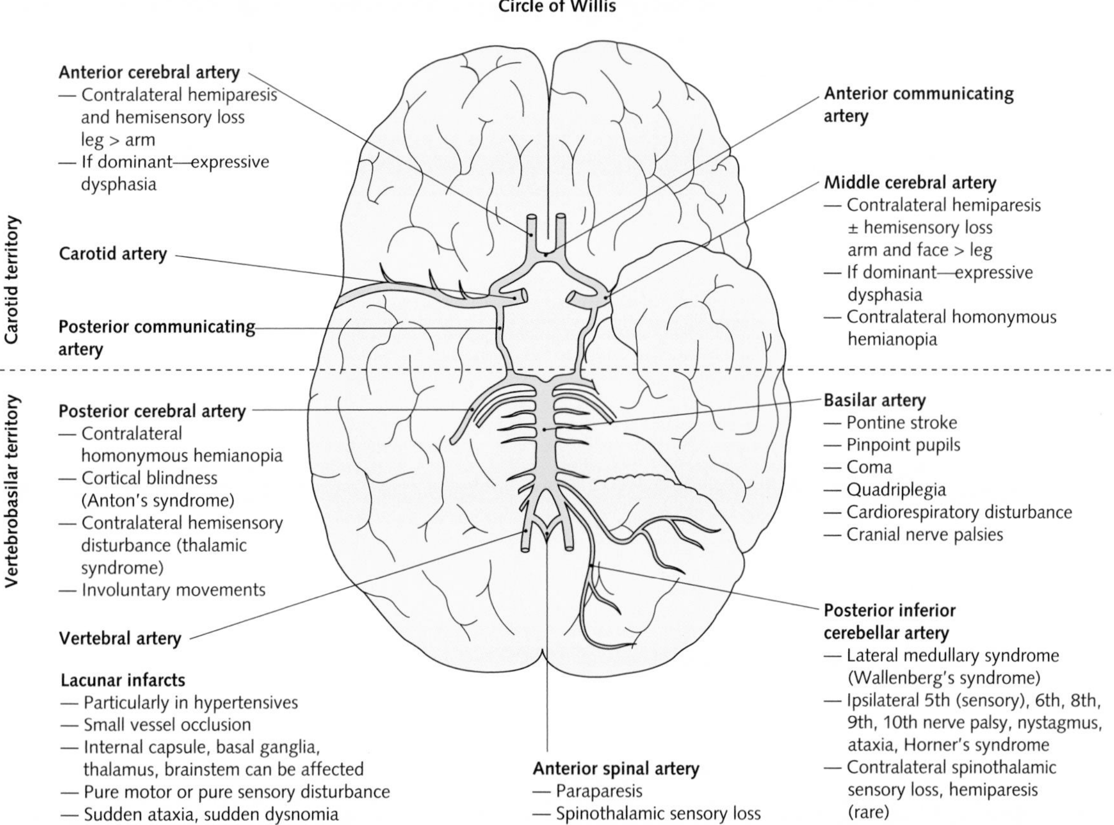

Fig. 24.2 Symptoms and signs associated with different strokes. Note that haemorrhagic strokes have symptoms and signs determined by the site of the bleed. Patients may also develop headache, loss of consciousness and vomiting as a result of raised intracranial pressure.

Fig. 24.3 Risk factors for stroke.

Previous stroke or transient ischaemic attack
Poorly controlled hypertension
Atrial fibrillation
Established vascular disease (carotid bruit, coronary artery disease, peripheral vascular disease)
Diabetes mellitus
Hypercholesterolaemia
Thrombophilia
Family history
Smoking
Oral contraceptive pill
Obesity
Alcohol excess

control, normothermia and correction of hypoxia. Acute thrombolysis is widely used in the UK; trials indicate that there is a benefit in patients who present up to 4.5 h after the onset of symptoms, despite the increased risk of haemorrhage, but the cut-off time of 3 h is more widely used. It is performed following exclusion of intracerebral haemorrhage by computed tomography (CT) scanning or magnetic resonance imaging (MRI) and done in centres with expertise and experience in the treatment. Exclusion criteria are numerous and among others include mild or rapidly improving neurological deficits, severely uncontrolled hypertension, recent surgery and current anticoagulant therapy. The NIHSS score must be calculated prior to administration of thrombolysis; this score takes into account features of the patient's syndrome to assess severity and whether thrombolysis is warranted.

INVESTIGATING THE STROKE PATIENT

The diagnosis of stroke remains a clinical one. The purpose of acute investigations is to look for treatable causes and offer the best supportive care. In the acute stroke patient the following investigations should be considered.

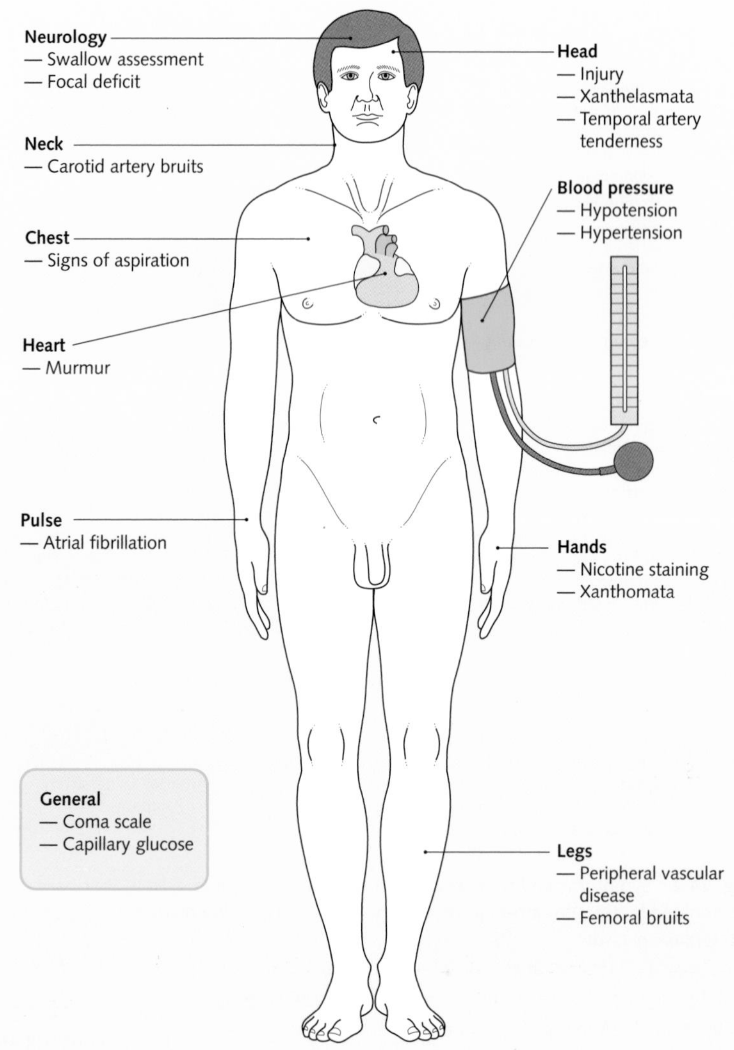

Fig. 24.4 Examining the stroke patient.

HINTS AND TIPS

Calculation of the risk of further vascular events following a TIA using a risk scoring system such as the ABCD2 score (see Ch. 34) may be helpful in guiding clinical decisions.

Simple early tests

- Capillary glucose: to rule out hypoglycaemia.
- Routine bedside observations: blood pressure, pulse and oxygen saturations will give a quick indication of the development of complications.
- ECG: this may show atrial fibrillation, or potentially (and much more rarely) ventricular aneurysm following recent myocardial infarction.

Blood tests

- Full blood count: polycythaemia may cause a stroke; a reactive picture may indicate inflammation (e.g. temporal arteritis).
- Erythrocyte sedimentation rate/C-reactive protein: elevated in inflammation, vasculitis, infection and malignancy.
- Urea and electrolytes: renal impairment may either be due to, or the cause of, hypertension. It may also result from reduced oral intake or concurrent sepsis.
- Blood glucose: diabetes is associated with increased risk of stroke. Hypoglycaemia may present with stroke-like symptoms or signs, and prolonged severe hypoglycaemia may result in permanent brain injury.
- Fasting lipids: hypercholesterolaemia is an important, treatable, risk factor for stroke.

Fig. 24.5 The Bamford classification of stroke.

Category	Percentage of overall strokes	Clinical findings	*Percentage at 1 year*	
			Deceased	Living independently
TACS (total anterior circulation stroke)	20	All three of: (i) Weakness of two or more of face, arm and leg (ii) Homonymous hemianopia (iii) Disturbance of higher cerebral function, e.g. dysphasia, dyspraxia, inattention If the patient is drowsy then (ii) and (iii) are assumed	60	5
PACS (partial anterior circulation stroke)	35	Any of the following: (i) Two of the components of TACS (ii) Higher cortical function deficit alone (iii) Limited sensory or motor deficit	15	55
LACS (lacunar stroke)	20	i) Pure motor or sensory stroke affecting {2/3} of face/arm close space and insert/leg. ii) Sensorimotor stroke affecting ≥{2/3} face/arm/leg iii) Ataxic hemiparesis iv) Dysarthria – clumsy hand syndrome **No** disturbance of higher function	10	60
POCS (posterior circulation stroke)	25	i) Brainstem and/or cerebellar deficits ii) Isolated homonymous hemianopia	20	60

- Clotting: to assess level of anticoagulation if the patient is receiving warfarin or to investigate suspected coagulopathy.

Imaging

- CT brain scan: this is indicated within 24 h of admission in all stroke cases, although it is increasingly performed within just a few hours of presentation. In some situations it is required urgently; these are outlined in Fig. 24.7. Most patients with TIA will also need acute imaging of the brain.
- MRI brain scan: this is indicated if posterior circulation stroke is suspected, and is recommended following TIA due to its increased sensitivity for small lesions.
- Chest X-ray: this is not routinely required, but should be performed if the clinical scenario indicates.

Further investigations

Depending on the patient and the clinical scenario, further tests may be required. The following further investigations should be considered, especially in young patients with no obvious risk factors:

- Blood cultures: infective endocarditis.
- Carotid imaging (ultrasound or CT/MR angiography): if anterior circulation stroke and carotid intervention would be considered.
- Echocardiogram: cardiac source of embolus – vegetations or thrombus. The echo can be contrast enhanced ('bubble echo') to look for septal defects, e.g. patent foramen ovale (PFO).
- Autoantibodies: may provide evidence of vasculitis (antinuclear antibodies, antineutrophil cytoplasmic antibodies), antiphospholipid syndrome (anticardiolipin antibodies) or cerebral lupus (anti-double-stranded DNA).
- Thrombophilia screen.
- Cerebral angiography/venography or radiological equivalent: this may be performed if there are additional signs or symptoms suggesting an unusual cause of infarction or haemorrhage, such as venous sinus thrombosis, arterial dissection or subarachnoid haemorrhage.
- 24-h electrocardiogram monitoring: paroxysmal atrial fibrillation.
- Syphilis serology: neurosyphilis.

Fig. 24.6 Complications of stroke and measures to prevent them.

Complications	Prophylactic measures
Acute	
Cerebral oedema ('malignant MCA syndrome')	Particularly in haemorrhagic stroke and usually non-preventable (avoid overenthusiastic rehydration). Surgical decompression is becoming more commonly performed
Aspiration pneumonia	Patient should be kept nil by mouth until they can swallow safely
Seizures	None. Can be treated with anti-epileptics. They may also occur later in the illness course as the brain remodels
Subacute and long term	
Pressure sores	Careful nursing with regular turning on air mattress
Contractures and spasticity	Regular skilled physiotherapy
Malnutrition	Feeding via nasogastric tube or, later, gastrostomy
Depression	Provision of adequate social and practical support
Deep vein thrombosis	Physiotherapy, antiembolism stockings Heparin not used routinely

Fig. 24.7 Indications for urgent CT brain scan.

It is required prior to thrombolysis
The patient is taking anticoagulants or has a known bleeding tendency
There is uncertainty as to the diagnosis (e.g. subdural or subarachnoid haemorrhage)
There was severe headache at the onset of symptoms
There are progressive or fluctuating neurological signs
There is a reduced conscious level (GCS <13)
There are symptoms or signs of raised intracranial pressure (e.g. papilloedema)

Lymphadenopathy and splenomegaly

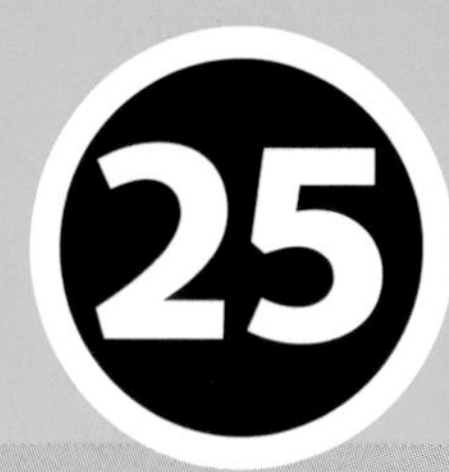

Objectives

The key learning points for this chapter:

- The differential diagnosis of lymphadenopathy and splenomegaly.
- How to systematically assess a patient presenting with lymphadenopathy or splenomegaly.
- The sequence of investigations necessary to establish the underlying cause.

INTRODUCTION

Splenomegaly is often a focus of short case or objective structured clinical examinations because many of its causes are chronic. Lymphadenopathy is a common presentation to healthcare services; it may be localized or generalized.

DIFFERENTIAL DIAGNOSIS OF LYMPHADENOPATHY AND SPLENOMEGALY

Localized lymphadenopathy

Consider which structures have lymphatic drainage to the nodes affected and examine these carefully for the following:

- Local infection: bacterial, viral, TB.
- Metastases: local malignancy (e.g. the breast in axillary lymphadenopathy).
- Lymphoma: Hodgkin's disease or non-Hodgkin's lymphoma.

Generalized lymphadenopathy

- Infection: particularly viral (Epstein–Barr virus (EBV), cytomegalovirus (CMV), HIV, rubella), but also bacterial (tuberculosis (TB), syphilis, brucellosis) and protozoal (toxoplasmosis).
- Lymphoproliferative: Hodgkin's disease or non-Hodgkin's lymphoma, chronic lymphocytic leukaemia, acute lymphoblastic leukaemia, acute myeloblastic leukaemia.
- Connective tissue disorders: systemic lupus erythematosus, rheumatoid arthritis, Kawasaki disease.
- Infiltration: sarcoidosis.
- Drugs: phenytoin occasionally causes lymphadenopathy with significant constitutional symptoms ('pseudolymphoma'). Other causes include allopurinol and isoniazid.
- Other: lipid storage diseases, rare haematological causes.

Splenomegaly

Traditionally splenomegaly is divided into three groups, massive, moderate and mild splenomegaly. However, it is often difficult to distinguish accurately (see Ch. 2).

Massive splenomegaly

- Myeloproliferative disease: chronic myeloid leukaemia, myelofibrosis (also called agnogenic myeloid metaplasia), and, less commonly, polycythaemia vera.
- Malaria: rare in developed countries.
- Kala-azar (visceral leishmaniasis): rare in developed countries.
- Gaucher's disease (lipid storage disorder).
- Lymphoproliferative disorders (see Ch. 37).
- Thalassaemia major.

Mild and moderate splenomegaly

The above plus:

- Portal hypertension, commonly with liver cirrhosis of any cause.
- Acute leukaemias.
- Infection: infectious mononucleosis, infectious hepatitis, infective endocarditis, TB, brucellosis, schistosomiasis.
- Haemolytic anaemias (see Ch. 37).
- Connective tissue disease: systemic lupus erythematosus (SLE), rheumatoid arthritis (Felty's syndrome).
- Infiltration: amyloid, sarcoid, metastasis of solid malignancy.

- Myeloproliferative disorders: essential thrombocythaemia.
- Megaloblastic anaemias (see Ch. 37).
- Immune thrombocytopenic purpura (ITP) may occasionally cause mild splenomegaly.

HISTORY IN THE PATIENT WITH LYMPHADENOPATHY OR SPLENOMEGALY

It is often not possible to make a diagnosis on the basis of the history in these patients. However, important clues in the history can help to focus the clinical examination and further investigations.

Localized lymphadenopathy

Pain and rate of node enlargement

Lymphadenopathy associated with infection is often painful and develops quickly. When due to lymphoma or other malignancy, it is commonly painless and enlarges more slowly. Therefore, the acutely painful lymph node, while more distressing to the patient, may be of comfort to the examining doctor!

Sometimes the lymphadenopathy will not be noticed until it is large enough to cause disfigurement or rubs against clothes.

Symptoms in local structures

Has the patient noticed pain, erythema or a mass in any of the structures draining into the affected node, e.g. cellulitis in inguinal lymphadenopathy or a breast mass in axillary lymphadenopathy? Neurological signs may be present due to a nodal mass pressing on a nerve or plexus distant from the deficit.

Systemic symptoms

In lymphoma the patient may experience pruritus or 'B symptoms' (fever, drenching night sweats, weight loss). 'B symptoms' indicate more extensive disease and a worse prognosis (see Ch. 37).

COMMUNICATION

In patients with suspected Hodgkin's lymphoma, ask about alcohol use. Although rare, alcohol can produce dramatic pain in the lymphadenopathy associated with Hodgkin's disease and the patient may have given up drinking because of it.

Generalized lymphadenopathy

Infection and underlying malignancy – be it lymphoma or metastatic – are the two top diagnoses here and questions are asked with this in mind. A full systemic enquiry is essential in these patients as most of the causes of generalized lymphadenopathy can affect multiple systems, and a suggestion of distant primary malignancy may only become clear with thorough questioning. Special attention should be paid to the following:

- Malaise, anorexia and general debility: common but non-specific.
- 'B symptoms': haematological malignancy.
- Skin rash: rubella, SLE and sarcoidosis.
- Arthralgia and arthropathy: SLE, rheumatoid arthritis and (rarely) syphilis (arthritis in secondary syphilis or Charcot joints in advanced tertiary syphilis).
- Infectious contacts: rubella, TB and EBV.
- Risk factors for HIV infection (see Ch. 38).
- Travel, sexual and occupational history.
- Contact with animals (zoonoses).
- Drug history: phenytoin.

Splenomegaly

Previous medical history

Enquire carefully about any pre-existing illness (as listed above) or previous conditions that might cause or be related to splenomegaly, e.g. chronic liver disease resulting in portal hypertension; connective tissue disease; previous malignancy; damaged cardiac valves (rheumatic fever or prosthetic valve) that might underlie subacute infective endocarditis.

Recent travel abroad or infectious contacts

Consider infectious mononucleosis, TB, schistosomiasis, kala-azar and malaria.

Systemic symptoms

Systemic symptoms suggestive of an underlying cause include arthralgia, rash, anorexia and 'B symptoms' (as above).

Symptoms of haematological disturbance

In bone marrow failure, splenomegaly may occur as a result of extramedullary haematopoiesis; in splenomegaly from other causes, the enlarged spleen may itself cause deficiencies in any of the three cell lines ('hypersplenism'). There may be malaise, breathlessness and lethargy if anaemia is present; recurrent infection may occur with leukopenia; and mucosal and petechial bleeding may indicate thrombocytopenia.

EXAMINING THE PATIENT WITH LYMPHADENOPATHY OR SPLENOMEGALY

When lymphadenopathy or splenomegaly is present, a full clinical examination of the lymphatic system should be made. The examination should then focus on possible underlying causes. Fig. 25.1 summarizes this examination approach.

Assessment of involved nodes and splenomegaly

First, the extent, sites, size, consistency, tenderness and fixation of enlarged lymph nodes should be documented. Normal reactive nodes are generally less than 1 cm in diameter, feel soft, are not fixed and can be tender. Lymphomatous nodes are often larger and feel rubbery but are not fixed. Lymph nodes infiltrated by carcinoma feel hard and may be fixed to surrounding tissue. Cervical, occipital, supraclavicular, axillary and inguinal areas should be palpated carefully. Small (shotty) inguinal nodes may be palpable in slim, healthy individuals.

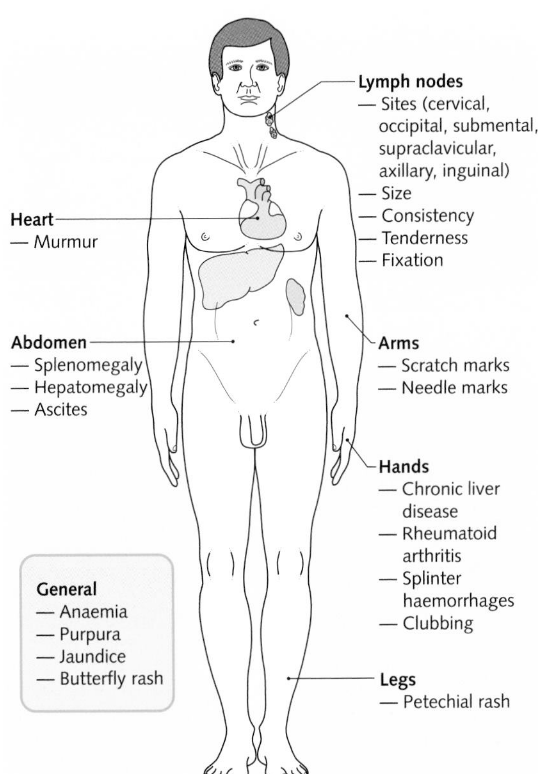

Fig. 25.1 Examining the patient with lymphadenopathy and/or splenomegaly.

Fig. 25.2 Characteristic clinical features that distinguish between the spleen and left kidney.

Spleen	Left kidney
No palpable upper border	Palpable upper border
Not bimanually palpable (not ballottable)	Bimanually palpable (ballottable)
Notch on medial border	No notch
Moves inferomedially on inspiration	Moves inferiorly on inspiration
Dull to percussion	Resonant to percussion (overlying bowel)

If splenomegaly is present, the size from the left costal margin must be recorded.

It is important to distinguish the left kidney from the spleen when palpating a mass in the left hypochondrium and the differences between the two are commonly asked for in examinations (see Fig. 25.2). The presence or absence of hepatomegaly is important in clinical practice, and hepatosplenomegaly is a common scenario in exams.

Assessing for evidence of an underlying cause

Anaemia and petechial bleeding/purpura may be present as described above. Jaundice may result from liver disease or haemolysis. Cachexia should warn of underlying malignancy.

Fig. 25.3 summarizes clinical findings that may point to particular diagnoses. Evidence of chronic liver disease, rheumatoid arthritis and SLE should also be looked for as described in Chs 13 and 19. Needle marks of drug misuse may indicate previous exposure to HIV and hepatitis B or C, and be a portal of entry for bacteria in infective endocarditis.

Localized lymphadenopathy

Examine those structures with lymphatic drainage to the affected nodes. Erythema, increased temperature and tenderness suggest infection, while a hard, non-tender mass may indicate malignancy. When there is isolated cervical lymphadenopathy, a formal ear, nose and throat examination should also be performed since oropharyngeal malignancies commonly metastasize to these nodes.

Splenomegaly and generalized lymphadenopathy

Where there is both splenomegaly and generalized lymphadenopathy consider lymphoproliferative disorders, infection, connective tissue disease and sarcoidosis. A full and thorough examination should be performed.

Fig. 25.3 Additional clinical features of some conditions presenting with splenomegaly.

Disease	Clinical features
Portal hypertension	Caput medusae, venous hum, ascites
Infectious mononucleosis	Palatal petechiae, severe pharyngitis, fever, lymphadenopathy, jaundice, tender hepatomegaly, rash (often after penicillins)
Bacterial endocarditis	Clubbing, splinter haemorrhages, Osler's nodes, Janeway lesions, Roth's spots (see Ch. 2), changing murmurs, haematuria, pyrexia
AA and AL amyloid	Cardiac failure and arrhythmia, hepatomegaly, macroglossia, renal failure
Sarcoidosis	Bilateral hilar lymphadenopathy, erythema nodosum, lupus pernio, uveitis, hypercalcaemia

HINTS AND TIPS

Remember, massive splenomegaly crosses the patient's midline into the right iliac fossa, so palpation for the spleen needs to start there.

INVESTIGATING THE PATIENT WITH LYMPHADENOPATHY OR SPLENOMEGALY

Haematology

- A full blood count may show anaemia, leukopenia, lymphopenia, thrombocytopenia or a combination of these. In lympho- or myeloproliferative disease it may show an excess of any of the three cell lines.
- A blood film can provide diagnostic information (Fig. 25.4).
- Erythrocyte sedimentation rate/plasma viscosity will be elevated in infection, malignancy and inflammation.

Biochemistry

- LFTs: infective hepatitis of any cause, including CMV and EBV, will cause abnormal transaminase levels; elevation of alkaline phosphatase and gamma-glutamyltranspeptidase will occur when the porta hepatis is obstructed by enlarged lymph nodes; unconjugated hyperbilirubinaemia will be present in haemolysis.

Fig. 25.4 Blood film abnormalities in conditions presenting with lymphadenopathy or splenomegaly.

Disease	Blood film
Acute leukaemia	Circulating blasts (Auer rods in AML)
Chronic lymphocytic leukaemia	Lymphocytosis, smear cells
Chronic myeloid leukaemia	Leukocytosis due to spectrum of myeloid cells
Myelofibrosis	Tear drop poikilocytes, leukoerythroblastic blood film
Lymphoma	Often normal (occasionally mild eosinophilia in Hodgkin's disease)
Haemolysis	Reticulocytosis (polychromasia), spherocytosis, erythroblasts, red cell fragments (schistocytes)
EBV, infectious hepatitis, toxoplasmosis	Atypical lymphocytes
Malaria (thick and thin films)	Parasitaemia, thrombocytopenia, haemolysis

Many of these disorders may also be associated with a normocytic anaemia. A leukoerythroblastic film will be seen wherever there is heavy bone marrow involvement or severe illness. Autoimmune haemolytic anaemia may also arise in lymphoma and chronic lymphocytic leukaemia. AML, acute myeloid leukaemia; EBV, Epstein–Barr virus.

- C-reactive protein will be elevated in infection, malignancy and inflammation.
- Lactate dehydrogenase: a useful prognostic marker in lymphoma, and is often raised in haemolysis.
- Serum calcium: may be raised in malignancy, sarcoidosis and sometimes lymphoma.
- Serum uric acid: raised when there is rapid cell turnover, as in malignancy (especially haematological).
- Beta-2 microglobulin: this may give prognostic information in lymphoma.

Immunology

- Autoimmune profile: useful in the diagnosis of many autoimmune diseases, particularly connective tissue disease (see Ch. 36).

Microbiology

- Monospot test: EBV.
- Serology: EBV, CMV, HIV, rubella, viral hepatitis, toxoplasmosis. Further serology (e.g. brucellosis, leishmaniasis) as per clinical suspicion.

- Blood cultures: repeated if infective endocarditis is suspected.
- Sputum culture: TB.

Imaging

- Chest X-ray: bilateral hilar lymphadenopathy (caused by lymphoma, sarcoidosis and TB).
- Abdominal ultrasound scan: will confirm the presence of splenomegaly. It is poor at imaging the retroperitoneal lymph node chains.
- CT scan of the chest, abdomen and pelvis: gives clear staging information in malignancy and particularly lymphoma, where retroperitoneal lymphadenopathy may often be missed by ultrasound scan.

Further investigations

- Lymph node excision biopsy: this allows thorough assessment of lymph node infiltration and architecture, often providing a definitive diagnosis of lymphadenopathy and its classification. Fine needle aspiration (FNA) is often inadequate.
- Bone marrow examination: this includes aspiration, trephine and cytogenetic analysis. It is indicated if the blood count or film suggest haematological abnormalities and it is useful in the diagnosis of leukaemias, myeloproliferative disorders, immune thrombocytopenias and pancytopenia. Occasionally, it is helpful in storage diseases, lymphoma and carcinoma, where there is marrow infiltration.
- If TB is suspected, induced sputum samples can be obtained; if these are negative, bronchoscopy and bronchoalveolar lavage fluid samples may be required.
- Very rarely, a splenic biopsy is required to diagnose the cause of splenomegaly.

HINTS AND TIPS

To enhance chances of palpating the spleen, lie the patient on their right side and fix the lower ribs with the left hand whilst palpating with the right hand in inspiration.

Sensory and motor neurological deficits

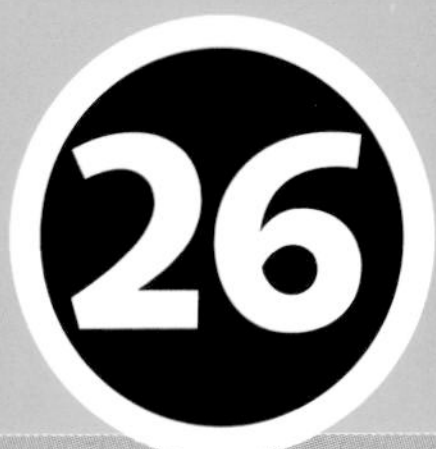

Objectives

The key learning points for this chapter:

- A basic understanding of neuroanatomy.
- How to use this as a guide to understanding the causes of sensory and motor neurological deficits.
- How to assess patients with neurological deficits and identify how these impact on their function.
- How to investigate patients presenting with neurological deficits.

INTRODUCTION

Muscle weakness or abnormal sensation can result from disease occurring anywhere along the pathway from the skin or muscle to the spinal cord and brain. The pathological processes are outlined below.

DIFFERENTIAL DIAGNOSIS OF SENSORY AND/OR MOTOR NEUROLOGICAL DEFICITS

The differential diagnosis is approached logically according to the likely anatomical site (the level of the lesion) and the possible causes at that location (Fig. 26.1).

HISTORY IN THE PATIENT WITH SENSORY AND/OR MOTOR NEUROLOGICAL DEFICITS

It is often a daunting prospect to be faced with a patient with neurological symptoms or signs. However, despite the vast number of potential underlying pathologies, a lesion at a particular point in the pathway between brain and muscle or skin will always produce the same clinical signs regardless of the cause. There are five important aspects to consider in the history.

Pattern of deficit

Fig. 26.2 summarizes characteristic symptoms and signs that arise as a consequence of a lesion at a particular neurological level. If the neurological abnormalities do not fit with a single localized lesion, consider MS, motor neurone disease, paraneoplastic neuropathy, multi-system disorders (e.g. sarcoidosis or vasculitis) or, lastly, a functional disorder.

Onset

This is extremely important. Sudden onset usually indicates a vascular problem such as infarction or haemorrhage. Lesions such as those due to trauma (e.g. enlarging haematoma), multiple sclerosis (MS), infection (e.g. abscess), acute prolapsed disc and myelitis can also develop rapidly, e.g. over hours. An insidious onset, over weeks to months, is more typical of cervical spondylosis, motor neurone disease, neoplasm or myopathy.

Precipitants

Trauma may result in muscular and neurological deficits. Acute myasthenia can be precipitated by intercurrent illness (particularly infection) or drugs (aminoglycosides or penicillamine). The incidence of MS relapses may increase postpartum and during systemic infections, and symptoms may be exacerbated by exertion, hot weather, or by a hot bath.

Progression

Many lesions cause gradually progressive, unremitting disease, including tumours, motor neurone disease, hereditary ataxias, syringomyelia and degenerative brain diseases. Intermittent deficits can be due to transient ischaemic attacks, epilepsy, migraine and myasthenia gravis. MS is characterized by the development of lesions which are dissociated in time and site. Symptoms and signs due to trauma or vascular events may slowly improve with time or remain static following the initial event.

Evidence of cause

The following factors provide evidence of cause:

- Family history: e.g. hereditary ataxias, phenylketonuria, neurofibromatosis.

Fig. 26.1 Differential diagnosis of sensory and/or motor neurological deficits.

Site of lesion	Examples
Muscle (see Chs 34–36)	*Congenital*
	Dystrophy: Duchenne, Becker, limb girdle, facioscapulohumeral
	Myotonia: myotonic dystrophy, myotonia congenita (Thomsen's disease)
	Acquired
	Drugs: steroids, cholesterol-lowering drugs (statins and fibrates), penicillamine
	Endocrine: Cushing's syndrome, thyrotoxicosis, hypothyroidism and hyperparathyroidism
	Infection: viral (influenza, HIV), parasitic (toxoplasmosis, trichinosis) and bacterial (*Borrelia*, *Clostridium perfringens*)
	Inflammation and autoimmune: polymyositis, dermatomyositis and sarcoidosis
	Metabolic: periodic paralyses, glycogen storage diseases and mitochondrial myopathy
	Toxin: alcohol
	Tumour: sarcoma and paraneoplastic syndromes
Neuromuscular junction (see Ch. 34)	Myasthenia gravis
	Lambert-Eaton myaesthenic syndrome (LEMS)
	Clostridium botulinum infection (botulism)
Peripheral nerves (see Chs 34–38)	Mononeuropathy (only one nerve involved)
	Entrapment: carpal tunnel syndrome (median nerve), and meralgia paraesthetica (lateral cutaneous nerve of thigh)
	Stretching: ulnar nerve neuropathy with increased carrying angle
	Trauma
	Compression: e.g. by tumour, as in neurofibromatosis, or AVM
	Infarction: e.g. due to vasculitis
	Mononeuritis multiplex/multifocal neuropathy (two or more nerves involved)
	Connective tissue disease: PAN, SLE, RA
	Infection: leprosy, herpes zoster, HIV, Lyme disease
	Inflammation: sarcoidosis
	Metabolic: DM
	Infiltration: amyloidosis
	Tumour: infiltration, paraneoplastic syndrome, neurofibromatosis
	Polyneuropathy (with symmetrical deficit most marked distally)
	Congenital
	Charcot–Marie–Tooth disease (hereditary sensorimotor neuropathy)
	Refsum's disease
	Friedreich's ataxia (spinal cord pathology usually coexists)
	Acquired
	Connective tissue disease: PAN, SLE, RA
	Drugs: nitrofurantoin, metronidazole, vinca alkaloids, platinum-containing drugs, isoniazid

Fig. 26.1 Differential diagnosis of sensory and/or motor neurological deficits – cont'd.

Site of lesion	Examples
	Inflammation: AIDP (Guillain–Barré), CIDP, multifocal motor neuropathy
	Metabolic: DM, renal failure (uraemic neuropathy), porphyria
	Toxins: alcohol, lead, mercury and arsenic
	Tumour: paraneoplastic syndrome and paraproteinaemias
	Infiltration: amyloidosis
	Vitamin deficiency: thiamine (B_1), niacin (B_6), B_{12}, folate
Brachial or lumbar plexus	Compression: cervical rib, thoracic outlet syndrome
	Idiopathic: neuralgic amyotrophy
	Metabolic: DM
	Trauma: birth injury (Erb's and Klumpke's palsies) and, classically, motorbike accidents
	Tumour: malignant infiltration (e.g. Pancoast tumour)
Spinal nerve root	Infection (e.g. pyogenic meningitis, syphilis, CMV)
	Prolapsed intervertebral disc and spondylosis
	Spinal stenosis
	Tumour
	Vertebral fracture dislocation
Anterior horn cell (see Ch. 34)	Motor neurone disease
	Spinal muscular atrophy
	Poliomyelitis
Spinal cord (see Ch. 34)	Degeneration: osteoarthritis (osteophytes may cause spinal stenosis or foraminal stenosis)
	Infection: abscess, HIV, TB (Pott's disease)
	Inflammation: MS, sarcoidosis, RA (atlanto-axial subluxation)
	Metabolic: Paget's disease causing spinal stenosis or compression
	Trauma: direct; prolapsed intervertebral disc; radiotherapy
	Tumour: metastases, neurofibroma, meningioma, glioma, ependymoma
	Vascular: anterior spinal artery occlusion, aortic dissection, aortic aneurysm (emboli), AVM, vasculitis
	Vitamin deficiency: subacute combined degeneration of the cord (vitamin B_{12})
	Others: syringomyelia, spina bifida, motor neurone disease
Cerebellum (see Ch. 34)	*Congenital*
	Friedreich's ataxia and spinocerebellar ataxias
	Ataxia telangiectasia
	Acquired
	Endocrine: hypothyroidism
	Infection: abscess, meningoencephalitis, post-infectious encephalitis
	Inflammation: MS
	Toxins: alcohol, lead, anticonvulsants

Continued

Fig. 26.1 Differential diagnosis of sensory and/or motor neurological deficits – cont'd.

Site of lesion	Examples
	Trauma: 'punch-drunk' syndrome
	Tumour: metastases, acoustic neuroma, haemangioblastoma (von Hippel–Lindau disease), paraneoplastic degeneration
	Vascular: infarction, haematoma, AVM
Cerebral hemispheres (see Ch. 34)	Degenerative disease
	Hydrocephalus: primary or secondary
	Infection: abscess, meningitis, encephalitis; HIV (e.g. AIDS dementia complex), malaria, rabies, tuberculosis, syphilis
	Inflammation: sarcoidosis, SLE, MS
	Metabolic: phenylketonuria, Wilson's disease (basal ganglia), other inborn errors of metabolism
	Toxic: alcohol
	Trauma: haematoma, diffuse axonal injury
	Tumour: primary or secondary
	Vascular: infarction, haemorrhage, AVM, aneurysm
	Vitamin deficiency: thiamine (B_1), niacin (B_6), B_{12}

AIDP, acute inflammatory demyelination polyneuropathy; AVM, arteriovenous malformation; CIDP, chronic inflammatory demyelinating polyneuropathy; CMV, cytomegalovirus; DM, diabetes mellitus; HIV, human immunodeficiency virus; MS, multiple sclerosis; PAN, polyarteritis nodosa; RA, rheumatoid arthritis; SLE, systemic lupus erythematosus; TB, tuberculosis.

- Drug history: e.g. phenytoin (cerebellar signs), vinca alkaloids and platinum-containing drugs (peripheral neuropathy), penicillamine (myasthenia).
- Dietary history: intake of vitamins B_1, B_6, B_{12} and folate.
- Alcohol history.
- Pre-existing illness: e.g. diabetes, hypertension (cerebrovascular disease), rheumatoid arthritis, tuberculosis or malignancy.
- History of trauma.
- Associated features: e.g. swinging pyrexia and rigors (abscess), vasculitic symptoms (connective tissue disease), anorexia and weight loss (malignancy), symptoms of hypo- or hyperthyroidism.
- Travel history (exposure to infections, e.g. Lyme disease) and risk factors for HIV.

EXAMINING THE PATIENT WITH SENSORY AND/OR MOTOR NEUROLOGICAL DEFICITS

When assessing a patient in clinic or hospital, a full neurological examination should be performed (see Ch. 2). However, in medical school examinations you will usually only be expected to assess a specific part of the system, such as the eyes, face, legs, arms or gait. The most common neurological short cases are peripheral neuropathy (usually due to diabetes mellitus), Parkinson's disease, stroke and multiple sclerosis, but be prepared for anything!

It is important to remember that, in sensory problems, subjective sensation is usually more sensitive than physical examination, which should be used to elicit the pattern and delineate and clarify the problem.

The clinical examination should aim to answer three questions. First, where is the anatomical site of the lesion or lesions? Second, is there anything to suggest the underlying pathological process? Finally, what disability does the patient have as a consequence of their neurological deficit?

The anatomical site of the lesion

From the moment you meet the patient, observe them carefully. How does the patient shake your hand? Can they lift their arm up? Can they let go of your hand (myotonia)? Watch how they undress or get on to the bed. A severe deficit will often become apparent before you start the examination. Examine the area of interest very carefully.

Fig. 26.2 Symptoms and signs associated with different anatomical lesions.

Site of anatomical lesion	Symptoms	Specific signs	Muscle	Reflexes	Sensation
Brachial or lumbar plexus	Muscle weakness Sensory disturbance		Wasting Fasciculation Reduced tone Reduced power in distribution of affected nerves	Reduced or absent	Deficit in distribution of affected nerves
Anterior spinal root	Muscle weakness		Wasting Fasciculation Reduced tone Reduced power in distribution of affected root	Reduced or absent	Normal
Posterior spinal root	Pain in skin and muscle supplied by that root		Normal	Reduced or absent	Deficit in distribution of affected root
Anterior horn cell	Muscle weakness		Wasting Fasciculation Reduced tone Reduced power in distribution of affected nerve	Reduced or absent	Normal
Spinal cord	Pain at site of lesion worse on coughing, sneezing, at night Urinary/bowel disturbance Leg weakness Sensory disturbance		At level of lesion: wasting, fasciculation Reduced tone Reduced power Below lesion: spasticity Increased tone Reduced power	At level of lesion: reduced or absent Below lesion: increased, upgoing plantars	Below lesion: ipsilateral posterior column loss (proprioception, vibration sense) contralateral spinothalamic loss (pain and temperature)
Cerebellum	Unsteadiness Tremor Altered speech Falls Poor coordination	Broad-based gait Falling to side of lesion Intention tremor Past-pointing dysdiadochokinesis Nystagmus Staccato speech	Reduced tone Normal power	Pendular	Normal
Cerebral hemispheres	Determined by site of lesion (see Ch. 21) Weakness Seizures Altered speech Disturbed higher functions	Postural drift Dysphasia Dysarthria Visual disturbance	Increased tone 'Clasp-knife' rigidity Wasting only if disuse Reduced power in pyramidal distribution (flexors stronger than extensors in arms, extensors stronger than flexors in legs)	Brisk Plantars upgoing	Deficit determined by site of lesion

Continued

Fig. 26.2 Symptoms and signs associated with different anatomical lesions – cont'd.

Site of anatomical lesion	Symptoms	Specific signs	Muscle	Reflexes	Sensation
Muscle	Weakness (particularly climbing stairs, getting out of chair) Pain (inflammation)	Myotonia in myotonia dystrophica Calf pseudohypertrophy and Gowers' sign in Duchenne muscular dystrophy	Wasting (usually proximal) Tone normal or reduced Power reduced	Usually normal; reduced or absent in severe muscle disease only Plantars downgoing	Normal
Neuromuscular junction	Diplopia Dysphagia Altered voice Proximal muscle weakness	Fatiguable weakness with repetition in myasthenia gravis Increasing strength with repetition in LEMS	Wasting only if severe Tone normal Power alters with repetition	Normal	Normal
Peripheral nerve	Muscle weakness Sensory disturbance May be purely sensory, purely motor or mixed	Mononeuropathy and mononeuritis multiplex – signs in distribution of affected nerves Polyneuropathy – signs symmetrical and distal (glove and stocking)	Wasting Fasciculation Reduced tone Reduced power	Reduced or absent	Deficit of all modalities (glove and stocking distribution)

Fig. 26.2 should help you identify where the anatomical lesion is likely to be on the basis of the neurological signs present.

The underlying cause

Once the site of the lesion is identified, think of the differential diagnosis as outlined at the beginning of this chapter. Are there any clues around the patient? Look for diabetic drinks (for peripheral neuropathy or amyotrophy).

If the patient is young, looks well and is sitting in a wheelchair, consider MS as the most likely diagnosis. An elderly patient with a hemiparesis is most likely to have had a stroke – is there a blood pressure chart? Is the patient in atrial fibrillation?

Look at the patient's face for myotonic facies (myotonic dystrophy), Cushing's syndrome (proximal myopathy) or hypothyroidism (myopathy or cerebellar dysfunction). Does the patient have neurofibromatosis (spinal cord or peripheral nerve lesions) or connective tissue disease such as rheumatoid arthritis (entrapment mononeuropathy, mononeuritis multiplex or peripheral neuropathy)?

The resultant disability

COMMUNICATION

Often the most important thing for the patient is what the lesion prevents them from doing. Assess and distinguish impairment, disability and handicap, and address the problems accordingly.

It is important to distinguish three related concepts: impairment refers to a problem of body function or structure (e.g. right arm weakness following stroke); disability refers to a particular activity (e.g. cannot write); and handicap refers to social function (e.g. cannot work).

Think what tasks the affected part of the body normally performs and ask the patient to show you how they manage, such as doing up buttons (for peripheral neuropathy), brushing hair or standing up from a chair (for proximal myopathy). Watching the patient walk is an important part of the examination and can give useful information (Fig. 26.3).

Fig. 26.3 Abnormalities of gait.

Lesion	Gait
Hemiplegia	Foot is plantar flexed; leg is stiff and dragged through a semicircle
Spastic paraplegia	Legs stiff; walk in 'scissor fashion', like 'walking through mud'
Proximal myopathy	Waddling gait; trunk moves to swing legs forward; difficulty in climbing stairs or standing out of a chair
Parkinsonism	Stooped posture, hesitation in starting, shuffling, festinant (accelerating), difficulty turning, poor arm swing and may freeze
Cerebellar dysfunction	Broad-based, ataxic with a tendency to fall to the side of the lesion; unable to perform tandem gait (heel to toe).
Dorsal column disease	Stamping; wide-based with patient looking at the ground as unable to sense where foot is; clumsy and slaps feet to ground
Foot drop	Stepping; legs lifted high off the ground as no dorsiflexion of the foot
Musculoskeletal disease	Limping; patient avoids weight bearing on affected side because of pain

INVESTIGATING THE PATIENT WITH SENSORY AND/OR MOTOR NEUROLOGICAL DEFICITS

The pathway of investigation is very much determined by the history and clinical examination findings. The following tests may be useful but each patient will require only those relevant to their presentation.

Blood tests

- Full blood count and erythrocyte sedimentation rate: reactive picture in inflammation, infection and neoplasm, and raised MCV in vitamin B_{12} deficiency and alcohol abuse.
- Urea and electrolytes: raised urea and creatinine in renal failure, potassium high or low in periodic paralyses.
- Serum calcium: raised in hyperparathyroidism, sarcoidosis, malignancy.
- Serum glucose: raised in DM.
- Liver function tests: raised gamma-GT in alcohol abuse, raised alkaline phosphatase in Paget's disease and deranged transaminases in metastases, infection and Wilson's disease.
- Thyroid function tests: hyper- or hypothyroidism.
- Creatine kinase: markedly raised in muscle inflammation and muscular dystrophies.
- Autoantibodies: in systemic disease, e.g. rheumatoid arthritis, systemic lupus erythematosus and polyarteritis nodosa, and in many specific neurological diseases – see Fig. 26.4.
- Serology: human immunodeficiency virus (HIV), herpes and syphilis where appropriate.
- Immunoglobulins: paraproteinaemias.

Fig. 26.4 Autoantibodies in specific neurological disease.

Autoantibody target	Associated disease
Ganglioside M1 (GM1)	Multifocal motor neuropathy
Ganglioside Q1b (GQ1b)	Miller Fisher syndrome
Voltage-gated calcium channel (VGCC)	LEMS
Voltage-gated potassium channel (VGKC)	Autoimmune encephalitis
NMDA receptor	Autoimmune encephalitis
Acetylcholine receptor (AChR) and muscle specific kinase (MUSK)	Myasthenia gravis
Aquaporin-4 (AQP4)	Neuromyelitis optica
Anti-Hu, Ri, Yo	Paraneoplastic neurological syndromes
GAD	Stiff person syndrome

Cerebrospinal fluid analysis

- A lumbar puncture is often required and many different tests can be performed on the CSF. These are outlined in Fig. 26.5.

Imaging

- Plain radiographs may demonstrate degenerative and destructive bone lesions and fractures.
- Magnetic resonance imaging (MRI) of the brain and spine is extremely useful in diagnosing and localizing central lesions. It provides greater anatomical detail than CT and contrast can be given to show blood vessels or areas of blood–brain barrier breakdown.
- Computed tomography (CT) scanning remains useful in the acute setting, e.g. for detecting

Fig. 26.5 CSF analysis and interpretation.

Test	Interpretation
Microscopy	Direct visualization of microorganisms or malignant cells
Culture and sensitivity	Infection
PCR	Detection of viral RNA or DNA
Low glucose (<{2/3} blood glucose)	Bacterial/TB/fungal/carcinomatous meningitis
Very high protein (>2 g/L)	GBS, Froin's syndrome*, TB/fungal meningitis, Behçet's syndrome
High protein (0.4–2 g/L)	Bacterial meningitis, viral encephalitis, cerebral abscess, cerebral malignancy
Oligoclonal bands	Multiple sclerosis, SLE, neurosyphilis, neurosarcoidosis, Behçet's syndrome, SSPE
Neutrophils	Bacterial meningitis
Lymphocytes	Partially treated bacterial meningitis, viral encephalitis/meningitis, TB meningitis, CNS vasculitis, Behçet's syndrome, HIV-associated, lymphoma/leukaemia, SLE
Xanthochromia (yellow CSF due to haemoglobin breakdown); usually by spectrophotometry	Subarachnoid haemorrhage (xanthochromia from 12 h after event)

**Froin's syndrome – raised CSF protein and xanthochromia but normal cell count, seen below a block in spinal cord compression.*
CNS, central nervous system; GBS, Guillain–Barré syndrome; HIV, human immunodeficiency virus; SLE, systemic lupus erythematosus; SSPE, subacute sclerosing panencephalitis; TB, tuberculosis.

haemorrhage, and also provides accurate imaging of bony structures.

- Myelography can be useful in demonstrating compressive cord lesions but this technique has been largely superseded by CT scans and MRI.

Further tests

- Electromyogram (EMG): useful in primary muscle disease (typical changes in myotonia and myasthenia); it also shows denervation but not its cause.
- Nerve conduction studies demonstrate peripheral neuropathies and the site and type of individual nerve lesions.
- Evoked potentials: visual evoked potentials (VEP) demonstrate previous retrobulbar neuritis in MS. Auditory and somatosensory evoked potentials may also be performed to look for lesions in these pathways.
- Biopsy: consider if the diagnosis is in doubt despite history, examination and non-invasive procedures. Muscle, nerve and brain biopsies can be performed to give a definitive histological diagnosis.

Vertigo and dizziness

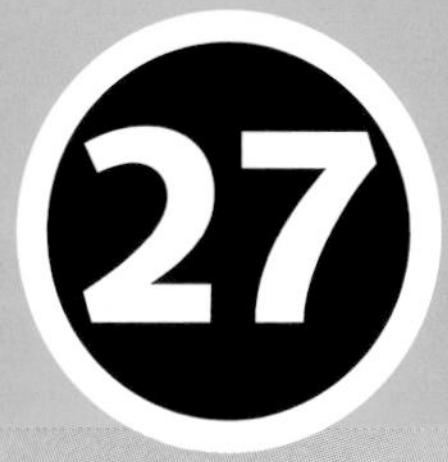

Objectives

The key learning points for this chapter:

- The importance of distinguishing true vertigo from dizziness or unsteadiness.
- The causes of vertigo resulting from pathology at various points of the neurological pathway, from the inner ear to the brainstem.
- How to assess the patient with vertigo.
- How to approach the investigation of patients with vertigo.

INTRODUCTION

True vertigo is the illusion of movement, usually rotation but also swaying or tilting, of a patient or their surroundings. This is often accompanied by nausea, vomiting and postural instability. It results from disease either in the labyrinth (the most common cause), the 8th cranial nerve or its connections in the brainstem, including the cerebellum.

Dizziness or unsteadiness without vertigo can result from a variety of unrelated disorders; these are discussed in more detail in their appropriate chapters. It is important to bear in mind that occasionally patients with vestibular dysfunction will not complain of vertigo, and that patients with presyncope occasionally complain of a mild spinning sensation.

COMMUNICATION

When a patient presents with 'vertigo' or 'dizziness' it is vital to establish whether true vertigo is present or not, as these symptoms result from different pathologies.

DIFFERENTIAL DIAGNOSIS IN THE PATIENT WITH VERTIGO OR DIZZINESS

Vertigo

The differential diagnosis in the patient with vertigo includes labyrinth disorders, 8th cranial nerve disease or brainstem lesions and is summarized in Fig. 27.1. Rarely, vertigo can be a feature of temporal lobe pathology (e.g. temporal lobe epilepsy).

Dizziness

The differential diagnosis of dizziness is summarized in Fig. 27.2.

HISTORY IN THE PATIENT WITH VERTIGO

The diagnosis in patients with vertigo is largely made on the history. It is important to elicit the time course of the vertigo and the likely site of the lesion by asking about other auditory and neurological symptoms. Typical features of specific diseases are shown in Fig. 27.3.

Onset and pattern of vertigo

The following should be established:

- Onset: peripheral lesions generally cause acute severe symptoms; central lesions tend to cause a gradual onset with less severe vertigo, unless caused by ischaemia.
- Duration and recurrence: is it a single episode (e.g. ischaemia or migrainous) or recurring (e.g. benign positional vertigo)? Are the attacks brief (seconds to minutes) or prolonged (hours to days)?
- Aggravating features: is there a relation to specific positions or movements? Is it worse on coughing/sneezing?

Aural symptoms

The presence of aural symptoms suggests that the lesion is peripheral, involving the labyrinth or 8th cranial nerve:

- Deafness (fluctuating or progressive).
- Tinnitus.
- Ear discharge or pain.
- A sensation of ear 'fullness' (Ménière's disease).

Fig. 27.1 Differential diagnosis of vertigo (see Ch. 34).

Location of lesion	Examples
Labyrinth	Middle ear disease (e.g. otitis media)
	Ménière's disease
	Benign positional vertigo
	Labyrinthitis
	Traumatic vertigo
	Perilymphatic fistula
8th cranial nerve	Vestibular neuronitis
	Acoustic neuroma
	Ramsay Hunt syndrome: herpes zoster of the geniculate ganglion
	Ototoxic drugs: aminoglycosides such as gentamicin
	Petrous temporal bone pathology (e.g. Paget's disease)
Brainstem/ cerebellum	Vertebrobasilar ischaemia: TIA, posterior circulation stroke (including lateral medullary syndrome), rotational ischaemia Multiple sclerosis: demyelination
	Migraine
	Encephalitis
	Tumour
	Alcohol abuse
	Episodic ataxia (inherited autosomal dominant disorders)
	Syringobulbia

Neurological symptoms

The following symptoms suggest central pathology or acoustic neuroma:

- Other cranial nerve involvement: facial weakness, facial numbness, diplopia, dysarthria, dysphagia.
- Seizures.
- Weakness, altered sensation, limb ataxia.

History suggestive of an underlying cause

- Recent viral illness may suggest vestibular neuronitis.
- Head injury may cause vertigo via a range of mechanisms such as labyrinth concussion or benign positional vertigo.
- Previous otological surgery.

Fig. 27.2 Differential diagnosis of dizziness without true vertigo.

Causes	Further information
Low cardiac output	See Ch. 27
Non-specific dizziness – often due to psychiatric disorder, e.g. anxiety	See *Crash Course: Psychiatry*
Anaemia	See Ch. 37
Hypoglycaemia	See Ch. 35
Postural hypotension	See Ch. 30
Visual disturbance	See *Crash Course: Neurology*
Cerebrovascular disease	See Ch. 34
Pyrexia	See Ch. 38

- Drug history (e.g. aminoglycosides).
- Recent flying or diving (e.g. barotrauma – perilymphatic fistula).
- Associated headache with photophobia or phonophobia suggests migrainous vertigo.
- Past medical history: risk factors for vascular disease (ischaemia), multiple sclerosis, migraine.
- Family history of vertigo: inherited episodic ataxia (channelopathies).

EXAMINING THE PATIENT WITH VERTIGO

The clinical examination is often normal. The following specific abnormalities should be looked for carefully:

- Nystagmus: observe the direction of slow and fast phases, and whether they change direction or amplitude with direction of gaze. Are there features of a peripheral or central cause (see Ch. 2)?
- Hallpike's manoeuvre: the patient's neck is extended and head turned to one side; they are then asked to lie down quickly with their head over the end of the bed. In benign positional vertigo there will be a latent period of a few seconds followed by horizontal and torsional nystagmus.
- Head thrust test: the patient is asked to fix their vision on a target; their head is then quickly turned through 15° horizontally. It is positive if the eyes are moved away from the point of fixation and quickly corrected, and suggests a peripheral lesion.
- Focal neurological signs: if present, these suggest a central lesion, acoustic neuroma or Ramsay Hunt syndrome. Pay particular attention to assessment of the 8th cranial nerve, gait and cerebellar signs.

Fig. 27.3 Characteristic features of conditions causing vertigo.

Disease	Cause	Length of vertigo	Aural symptoms	Neurological symptoms	Natural history
Ménière's disease	Excess endolymphatic fluid (hydrops)	20 min–24 h Often preceded by sensation of fullness in the ear	Fluctuating but progressive sensorineural deafness Tinnitus	None	Episodic, unilateral at first becomes bilateral in 25–45% Frequency diminishes with duration
Vestibular neuronitis	Possibly viral	Days to weeks Explosive onset	None	None	Spontaneously resolves in weeks
Benign positional vertigo	Debris within the semicircular canals Can follow head injury and vestibular neuronitis	Less than a minute Precipitated by changes in head position	None	None	Episodic attacks Spontaneous resolution over weeks to months, but may recur after a symptom-free period.
Perilymphatic fistula	Rupture of round window membrane Often due to barotrauma Can be spontaneous	Frequent, short-lasting episodes, persisting for months to years	Deafness and tinnitus	None	Often resolves with bed rest Can be surgically repaired
Vertebrobasilar insufficiency	Compression of vertebral arteries by osteophytic cervical vertebrae	Seconds Precipitated by neck extension or rotation	None	Dysarthria Diplopia Visual loss Syncope	Episodic attacks
Acoustic neuroma	Schwannoma of vestibular nerve	Gradual onset Progressive	Unilateral deafness and tinnitus	5th and 7th cranial nerve palsies Ipsilateral cerebellar signs	Symptoms progress until surgical removal
Central lesions	Tumour Demyelination Vascular Migraine	Dependent on underlying pathology	Often spared	Usually present and dependent on site of lesion	Tumour/ demyelination: symptoms progress until underlying cause treated

- Eyes: papilloedema (tumour with raised intracranial pressure), optic atrophy (demyelination) and ophthalmoplegia (cranial nerve defect, demyelination).
- Ears: otoscopy may reveal otitis media or a herpetic rash. Herpetic lesions may also be found on careful examination of the surrounding skin.
- Lying and standing blood pressures: postural hypotension.
- Neck movements: are they limited or do they provoke the symptoms? Rarely, cervical spondylosis can cause 'rotational vertebrobasilar ischaemia' on head-turning.

Fig. 27.4 summarizes the examination approach.

HINTS AND TIPS

Remember: benign positional vertigo is diagnosed with *Hallpike's* manoeuvre and treated with *Epley's* manoeuvre.

INVESTIGATING THE PATIENT WITH VERTIGO

- Simple tests including routine observations, blood glucose and ECG should be considered to look for

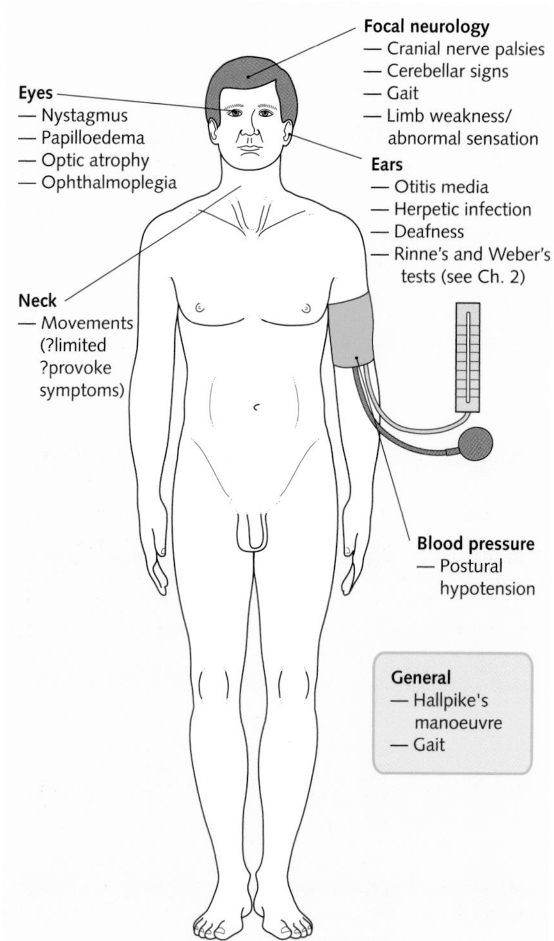

Fig. 27.4 Examining the patient with vertigo.

Fig. 27.5 Indications for brain imaging in acute vertigo.

New-onset headache (raises possibility of haemorrhage)
Intact head impulse tests (increased likelihood of central lesion)
Other cranial nerve symptoms/signs suggesting central cause
Nystagmus with features of a central lesion
Acute deafness (raises possibility of labyrinthine stroke)

N.B. The presence of significant cardiovascular risk factors should increase the suspicion of a vascular event.

a cause. Similarly, routine blood tests may reveal infection or evidence of other underlying disease.

- Imaging: MRI should be performed if a central lesion or acoustic neuroma is suspected. If posterior circulation infarction is suspected, this may need to be performed urgently. See Fig. 27.5 for other indications.
- Audiometry: this will help distinguish between conductive and sensorineural deafness.
- Caloric tests: normally, running cold and then warm water into the external auditory meatus causes nystagmus with the fast phase away and towards, respectively; where there is pathology in the ipsilateral labyrinth, 8th cranial nerve or brainstem this normal response will be reduced or absent.
- Electronystagmography: a more accurate assessment of the presence and type of nystagmus.

Excessive bruising and bleeding

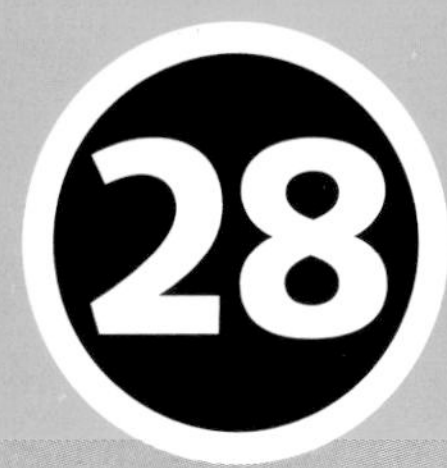

Objectives

The key learning points for this chapter:

- The differential diagnosis of bruising and bleeding.
- The approach to assessing a patient presenting with bruising or bleeding.
- How to focus investigations to identify the precise cause of the bruising or bleeding.

INTRODUCTION

Excessive bruising and bleeding (prolonged, spontaneous or following an insignificant injury) arise when there is abnormal haemostasis; this may occur due to abnormalities of the coagulation pathway, abnormalities of platelet number or function or abnormalities of the blood vessel (e.g. fragility of the vessel wall). This chapter is intended to help with stable patients who have a documented increased tendency to bleed and is not about resuscitating the shocked patient.

DIFFERENTIAL DIAGNOSIS OF BRUISING AND BLEEDING

Platelet abnormalities

Platelets may be reduced in number or function.

Thrombocytopenia

- Reduced production: bone marrow failure, drugs (commonly cytotoxics, quinine and co-trimoxazole), post chemotherapy or post radiotherapy, viral infections (including HIV), hereditary syndromes.
- Increased consumption: immune thrombocytopenic purpura (ITP), disseminated intravascular coagulation (DIC), thrombotic thrombocytopenic purpura (TTP), haemolytic uraemic syndrome (HUS), systemic lupus erythematosus (SLE), HIV-associated and hyper-splenism.
- Abnormal distribution: splenic pooling in splenomegaly.
- Dilutional: massive transfusion.
- Factitious: isolated thrombocytopenia may be related to aggregation caused by EDTA used in full blood count bottles.

Heparin is the most common drug-related cause of thrombocytopenia in hospitalized patients. There are two types; the most common is a relatively benign, non-immune form due to a direct effect on platelet activation. It usually resolves and does not need withdrawal or future withholding of heparin. The less frequent, immune mediated form has the potentially serious sequelae of arterial and venous thrombosis.

HINTS AND TIPS

Remember, heparin-induced thrombocytopenia is a procoagulant state.

Platelet dysfunction

- Hereditary: Glanzmann's thrombasthenia (deficiency of glycoprotein IIb/IIIa receptor on platelet surface).
- Acquired: aspirin, heparin, thienopyridines (e.g. clopidogrel), dipyridamole, uraemia.
- Myeloproliferative disease and paraproteinaemia.

Coagulation abnormalities

Coagulopathies may be due to vitamin K deficiency, factor deficiency (which can be specific or combined, inherited or acquired) or acquired clotting factor inhibitors.

Vitamin K deficiency

Factors II, VII, IX and X are dependent on vitamin K.
Deficiency may be caused by:

- Malabsorption: bowel pathology such as coeliac disease or biliary obstruction (vitamin K is fat-soluble).
- Antagonist drugs: coumarins (warfarin).

Factor deficiency

- Hereditary: haemophilia A (factor VIII), haemophilia B (factor IX), von Willebrand's disease (von Willebrand factor).
- Acquired: liver disease (decreased production of clotting factors as synthetic function fails), DIC (massive consumption of clotting factors resulting in deficiency).

Acquired factor inhibitors

These are most commonly directed against factor VIII:

- Postpartum.
- Autoimmune disease: SLE and rheumatoid arthritis.
- Malignancy.

Vessel wall abnormalities

Vessel wall abnormalities may be inherited or acquired.

Hereditary

- Hereditary haemorrhagic telangiectasia (Osler–Weber–Rendu disease).
- Connective tissue disease: pseudoxanthoma elasticum, Ehlers–Danlos syndrome.

Acquired

- Trauma.
- Physiological: senile purpura.
- Drugs: corticosteroids.
- Infections: meningococcal septicaemia (damage due to endotoxin and inflammation).
- Vitamin deficiency: scurvy (vitamin C).
- Endocrine: Cushing's syndrome.

HISTORY IN THE PATIENT WITH BRUISING AND BLEEDING

The history should focus on three areas. First, what is the pattern and extent of the bleeding and bruising? Second, are there any clues as to the possible underlying cause? Finally, have complications occurred?

What is the pattern and extent of bleeding and bruising?

As a general rule:

- Platelet abnormalities (deficiency or dysfunction) cause skin or mucosal purpura and haemorrhage, with prolonged bleeding following trauma or often minor surgery. Most cases of von Willebrand's disease also follow this pattern.
- Vessel wall abnormalities cause petechiae and ecchymoses due to bleeding from small vessels, usually in the skin but also in mucous membranes.
- Coagulopathies cause haemarthroses, muscle haematomas, postoperative or traumatic bleeding and palpable ecchymoses, and if inherited start early in life.

COMMUNICATION

Abnormal bruising or bleeding can be a very alarming initial presentation. It is important to ask the patient about specific concerns they may have, for example that the condition might signal leukaemia or other malignancy. For patients with hereditary haemophilia bruising and bleeding are common symptoms and they often know more about their condition than the non-specialist doctor. Each patient should be counselled according to their individual needs.

What is the underlying cause?

- Bleeding and bruising: first, determine whether it is within the spectrum of 'normal' and related to recent trauma, or possibly due to an underlying haemostatic abnormality.
- Age: senile purpura seen mostly on the upper limbs.
- Liver disease: intrinsic liver disease (coagulopathy) or biliary obstruction (may cause reduced platelet function and vitamin K deficiency).
- Drug history: aspirin, clopidogrel, heparin, warfarin, steroids, previous chemotherapy.
- Family history (e.g. haemophilia, hereditary haemorrhagic telangiectasia).
- Symptoms of underlying bone marrow failure (e.g. recurrent infection, symptoms of anaemia).
- Hyperextensibility of the skin or joints: Ehlers–Danlos syndrome, pseudoxanthoma elasticum.
- Poor diet: scurvy (ecchymoses predominantly on the lower limbs).
- Known acquired immune deficiency syndrome or risk factors for HIV infection.

HINTS AND TIPS

Von Willebrand factor is necessary for platelet adhesion and prevents factor VIII from degradation; vWf deficiency may therefore cause bleeding consistent with both platelet abnormalities and coagulopathy.

Have complications occurred?

- Evaluate the severity of the bleeding: was it life-threatening or a minor irritant?

- Symptoms of anaemia (see Ch. 29).
- Muscle pain or mass.
- Joint pain or deformity.

EXAMINING THE PATIENT WITH BRUISING AND BLEEDING

The examination should be approached in a similar manner to the history. Fig. 28.1 summarizes the examination approach.

What is the pattern and extent of bruising and bleeding?

The sites and types of lesions should be documented (see above). 'Petechiae' usually denotes small, pinpoint bleeding into skin or mucosa; 'purpura' denotes small bruises; and 'ecchymosis' refers to anything larger than 1–2 cm.

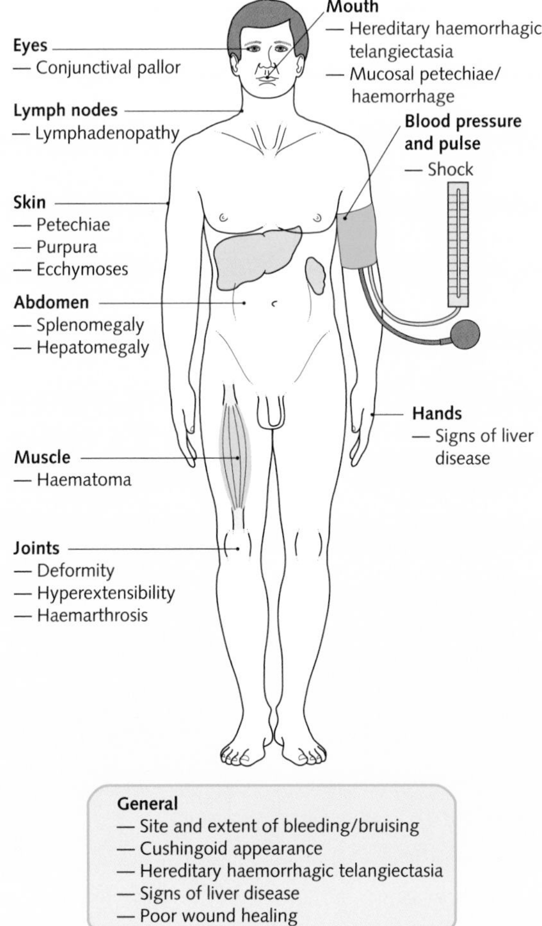

Fig. 28.1 Examining the patient with bruising and bleeding.

Are there signs suggestive of a specific underlying cause?

- Signs of liver disease (see Ch. 13) or immune deficiency.
- Splenomegaly (of any cause): platelet sequestration.
- Cushingoid appearance and fragile skin: steroid therapy, endocrinopathy.
- Hereditary haemorrhagic telangiectasia: characteristic petechiae on the tongue and lips.
- Scurvy: corkscrew hairs with hyperkeratosis of the follicles, perifollicular haemorrhages, gum hypertrophy, poor wound healing.
- Ehlers–Danlos syndrome: hyperextensible skin and joints, 'fish-mouth' wounds due to slow healing, and pseudotumours under scars and over bony prominences.
- Pseudoxanthoma elasticum: loose skin in neck, axillae, antecubital fossae and groins, 'chicken skin', blue sclera, angioid streaks in the retina, hyperextensible joints.

How severe has the bleeding been and are there complications?

Look for evidence of anaemia, which may be due to chronic bleeding or an acute haemorrhage (see Ch. 29). Finally, look for joint deformities (haemarthrosis) or a muscle mass (haematoma).

INVESTIGATING THE PATIENT WITH BRUISING AND BLEEDING

When an abnormality of haemostasis is suspected, a platelet count and simple coagulation assays should be performed; more specific tests to diagnose the underlying cause can then be considered. Fig. 28.2 summarizes the normal coagulation pathway.

An algorithm for investigating the patient with bruising and bleeding is given in Fig. 28.3; the common tests are summarized in Fig. 28.4.

Full blood count and blood film

- Platelet count: if thrombocytopenia is present, request a blood film to exclude an artefactual result due to platelet clumping and to look for a primary haematological cause. A bone marrow aspirate should be performed (see below).
- Other indices: haemoglobin level may give an indication of severity of bleeding, and an abnormal

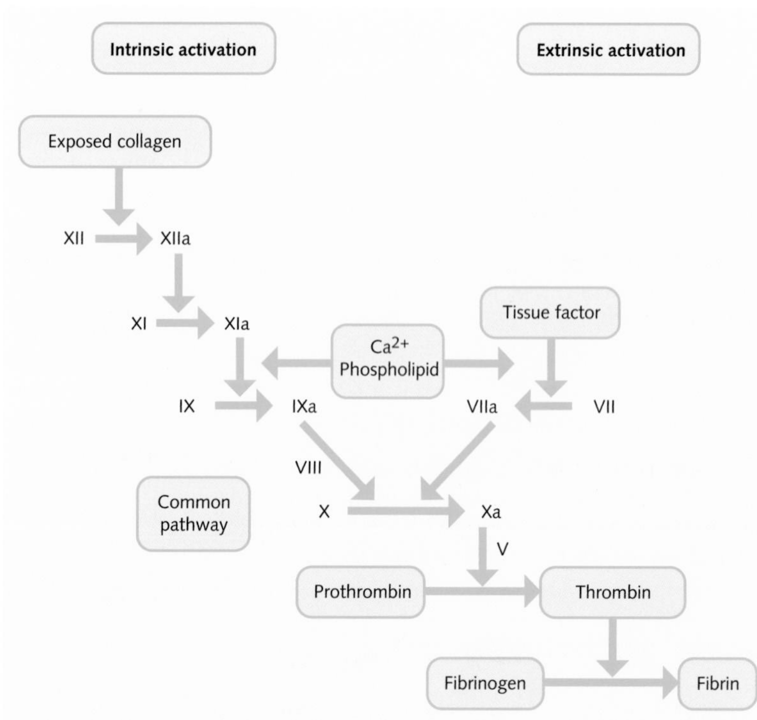

Fig. 28.2 The normal coagulation pathway. INR (international normalized ratio) measures extrinsic pathway, APTT (activated partial thromboplastin time) measures intrinsic pathway.

white cell count may indicate underlying bone marrow disease or infection. The mean cell volume may inform whether the bleeding is chronic or acute.

Coagulation studies

- Prothrombin time: this measures the extrinsic system (tissue factor and VII) and common pathway (X, V, prothrombin and fibrinogen). It is prolonged in liver disease and warfarin therapy, and is generally expressed as international normalized ratio (INR).
- Activated partial thromboplastin time: this measures the intrinsic system (XII, XI, IX and VIII) and common pathway (X, V, prothrombin and fibrinogen). It is prolonged in unfractionated heparin therapy (not newer low-molecular-weight heparins), factor deficiency such as factor VIII (haemophilia A) and factor IX (haemophilia B, Christmas disease), acquired factor inhibition and the presence of a lupus anticoagulant.
- Thrombin time: this measures the activity of thrombin and fibrinogen in the common pathway. It is prolonged in fibrinogen deficiency (disseminated intravascular coagulation) or dysfunction. Prolonged thrombin time may also result from heparin therapy (inhibition of thrombin activity).
- Mixing studies: if the above tests are prolonged, the sample can be mixed 1:1 with normal serum and reassessed; correction of the test implies a deficiency, whereas continued prolongation implies the presence of an inhibitor. Further tests, e.g. the dilute Russell viper venom test, can be employed to look for inhibitors, e.g. a lupus anticoagulant.

Platelet function studies

- Platelet function assay (PFA-100 analyser): this is performed using a laboratory analyser that measures platelet adhesion and aggregation with greater sensitivity and specificity than bleeding time. It is useful in the diagnosis of von Willebrand's disease and other inherited disorders of platelet function, and can discriminate between aspirin/NSAID-induced dysfunction and other causes. It returns a parameter called 'closure time'.
- Bleeding time: this is now rarely performed.

Fibrinogen, fibrin degradation products and D-dimers

- Fibrinogen: inherited disorders of fibrinogen are rare and may cause reduced levels or complete lack of fibrinogen. Fibrinogen levels are low in DIC (due to massive consumption) and may be reduced in liver disease (reduced synthesis).

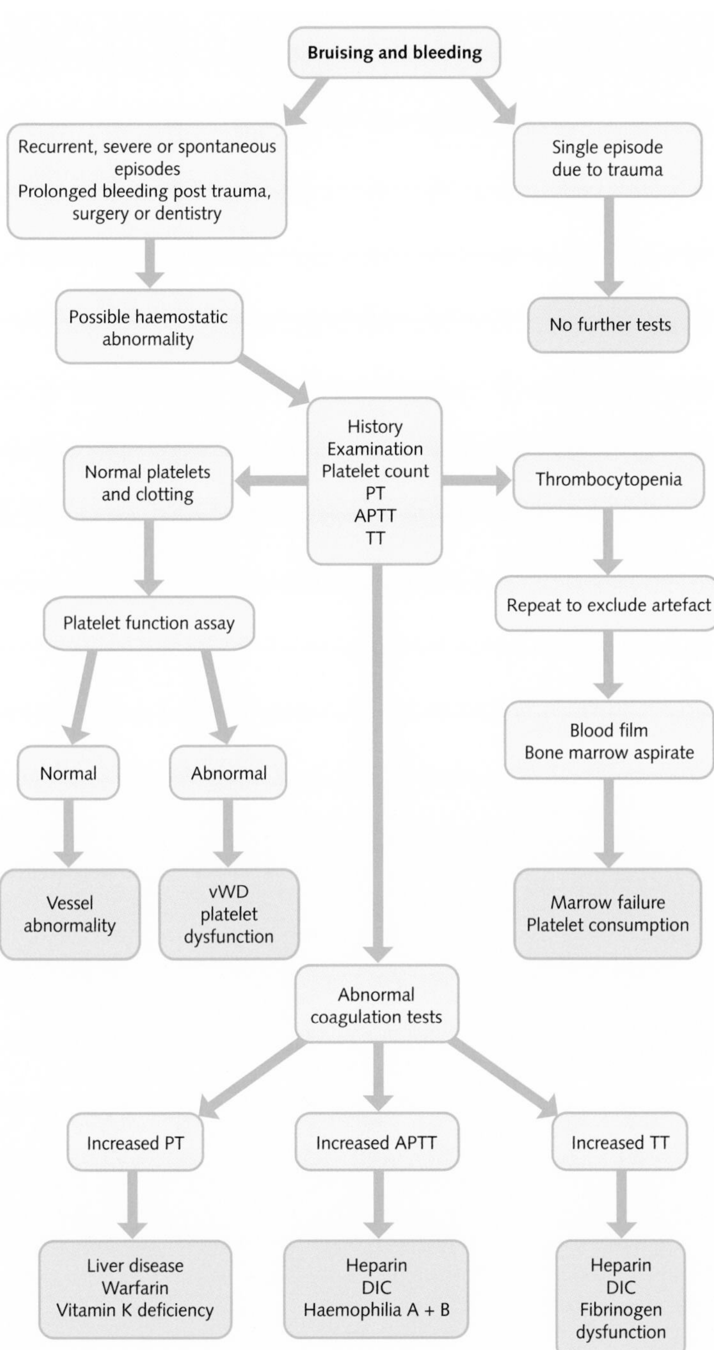

Fig. 28.3 Algorithm for investigating the patient with bruising or bleeding. APTT, activated partial thromboplastin time; DIC, disseminated intravascular coagulation; PT, prothrombin time; TT, thrombin time; vWD, von Willebrand's disease.

- Fibrin degradation products, including D-dimers, will be grossly elevated in DIC and may be raised in other conditions including malignancy, renal disease and the systemic inflammatory response syndrome (SIRS).

Other tests

- Bone marrow aspirate and trephine biopsy: this should be performed in significant thrombocytopenia without clear cause (increased megakaryocytes in consumptive thrombocytopenia, e.g. idiopathic

Fig. 28.4 Summary of the common tests of clotting.

	Platelet dysfunction including aspirin	**Haemophilia**	**Vitamin K deficiency/ warfarin**	**Intrinsic liver disease**	**vWD**	**Heparin**
Platelet count	N	N	N	N	N	N/−
INR	N	N	+	+	N	N/+
APTT	N	+	N/+	N/+	+	+
TT	N	N	N	N/+	N	+
Platelet function	Abnormal	N	N	Possibly abnormal	Abnormal	N

+, Increased; −, decreased; APTT, activated partial thromboplastin time; INR, international normalized ratio; N, normal; TT, thrombin time; vWD, von Willebrand's disease.

thrombocytopenic purpura, or reduced megakaryocytes in bone marrow failure) and if there is any suspicion of underlying bone marrow disease.

- Specific tests for other diseases given in the differential diagnosis list should be performed as indicated from the history, examination and basic laboratory tests.

Bear in mind that normal range results in many tests do not exclude a bleeding disorder. There are increasing numbers of sophisticated tests of platelet function and coagulation that are beyond the scope of this book. Referral to a haematologist specializing in haemostasis is recommended.

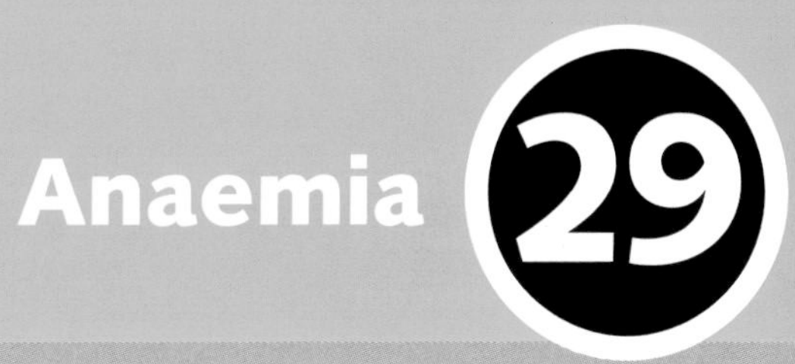

Anaemia

Objectives

The key learning points for this chapter:

- The classification and causes of anaemia.
- How to assess a patient presenting with anaemia.
- The investigations required to determine the likely cause of anaemia.

INTRODUCTION

Anaemia is not a diagnosis but a consequence of an underlying problem. A patient is anaemic when the haemoglobin concentration in the blood is less than 13.5 g/dL in men and 11.5 g/dL in women. Anaemia is common, as up to 10% of women in the UK are iron-deficient as a result of menorrhagia.

DIFFERENTIAL DIAGNOSIS OF ANAEMIA

The mean corpuscular volume (MCV) of the red blood cells gives important clues to the likely underlying cause of the anaemia.

Microcytic red blood cells

Microcytic red blood cells (RBCs) have an MCV of less than 80 femtolitres (fL). Causes include:

- Iron-deficiency anaemia (Fig. 29.1).
- Thalassaemia.
- Anaemia of chronic disease (see Ch. 37).
- Sideroblastic anaemia.
- Lead poisoning.

Normocytic red blood cells

Normocytic RBCs have a MCV of 80–95 fL. Causes include:

- Anaemia of chronic disease (see Ch. 37).
- Haemolysis (Fig. 29.2); may also lead to a mild macrocytosis.
- Acute blood loss.
- Bone marrow hypoplasia.
- Myelodysplastic syndrome.

Macrocytic red blood cells

Macrocytic RBCs have an MCV of more than 95 fL. Causes include:

- Megaloblastic anaemia: folate deficiency (Fig. 29.3), vitamin B_{12} deficiency (Fig. 29.4).
- Normoblastic anaemia: alcohol, liver disease, hypothyroidism, pregnancy, reticulocytosis.

HISTORY IN THE ANAEMIC PATIENT

It is important to establish the severity of any symptoms caused by the anaemia. The history should then focus on whether any complications of anaemia are present and whether there are any clues as to the likely underlying diagnosis.

Symptoms of anaemia

When anaemia develops over a long time, the haemoglobin can be very low before symptoms occur. Anaemia is tolerated less well in the elderly. The following symptoms may be reported:

- Lethargy and fatigue.
- Shortness of breath: most marked on exertion.
- Light-headedness.
- Palpitations.
- Pulsatile tinnitus.

Symptoms of complications

- Symptoms of cardiac failure (see Chs 4 and 5).
- Angina.
- Ischaemic claudication.

Fig. 29.1 Causes of iron-deficiency anaemia.

Mechanism	Examples
Reduced iron intake	Poor diet Malabsorption (e.g. gastrectomy, coeliac disease) Proton pump inhibitors can reduce iron absorption
Increased iron utilization	Infancy, adolescence, pregnancy
Abnormal iron loss	Chronic bleeding from gastrointestinal tract, urinary tract or uterus

Fig. 29.2 Causes of haemolytic anaemia.

	Mechanism	Examples
Inherited	Red blood cell membrane defects	Hereditary spherocytosis Hereditary elliptocytosis
	Enzyme deficiencies	Glucose-6-phosphate dehydrogenase deficiency Pyruvate kinase deficiency
	Abnormal haemoglobin	Thalassaemia Sickle cell disease
Acquired	Immune	ABO incompatibility (blood transfusion) Haemolytic disease of the newborn Autoimmune (warm, IgG): idiopathic, viral infection, lymphoma, CLL, SLE, drugs Autoimmune (cold, IgM): idiopathic, lymphoma, CLL, mycoplasma, Epstein–Barr virus.
	Non-immune	Mechanical heart valves Extensive burns Malaria Microangiopathic (DIC, TTP, pre-eclampsia) Paroxysmal nocturnal haemoglobinuria Liver disease (especially alcoholic), uraemia

CLL, chronic lymphocytic leukaemia; DIC, disseminated intravascular coagulation; SLE, systemic lupus erythematosus; TTP, thrombotic thrombocytopenic purpura.

Fig. 29.3 Causes of folate deficiency.

Mechanism	Examples
Reduced intake	Poor diet, e.g. old age, poverty, alcoholism
Reduced absorption	Coeliac disease, extensive Crohn's disease, tropical sprue, achlorhydria, gastrectomy
Increased utilization	Physiological, e.g. pregnancy, lactation, prematurity Increased cell turnover, e.g. malignancy, chronic inflammation, haemolysis, dialysis
Drugs	Trimethoprim, sulfasalazine, anticonvulsants, methotrexate

Folic acid is present in most fruit and vegetables, especially citrus fruits and green, leafy vegetables.

Fig. 29.4 Causes of vitamin B_{12} deficiency.

Mechanism	Examples
Reduced intake	Vegans
Reduced absorption	Stomach pathology, e.g. gastrectomy, pernicious anaemia Small intestinal disease, e.g. Crohn's, ileal resection, ileal TB or UC
Increased utilization	Blind loop syndrome (bacterial overgrowth – folate often normal or raised), fish tapeworm (*Diphyllobothrium latum*)
Abnormal metabolism	Transcobalamin II deficiency (autosomal recessive), abnormal IF
Drugs	Nitrous oxide, metformin

Vitamin B_{12} is presents in all foods of animal origin.
IF, intrinsic factor; TB, tuberculosis; UC, ulcerative colitis.

Evidence to suggest underlying cause

- Specific symptoms: menorrhagia, change in bowel habit, dyspepsia, weight loss, change in stool or urine colour.
- Pre-existing illness: chronic inflammatory disease (e.g. rheumatoid arthritis), previous abdominal surgery, chronic renal failure.
- Family history: haemolytic anaemia.
- Drug history: non-steroidal anti-inflammatory drugs, steroids, anticoagulants (iron deficiency), anticonvulsants (folate deficiency).

- Diet: vegans (vitamin B_{12} deficiency), alcoholics (folate deficiency).
- Pica (craving for specific and often bizarre foods): iron deficiency.
- Pregnancy: folate deficiency.

HINTS AND TIPS

Remember that the rate of drop in haemoglobin is as important as the level; if blood loss is chronic, very low levels can be tolerated with only mild symptoms occurring. If acute, a fall of just 2 g/dL can cause significant symptoms.

EXAMINING THE ANAEMIC PATIENT

Signs of anaemia and its complications

Fig. 29.5 summarizes the examination approach. The following signs of anaemia should be noted:

- Pallor: mucous membranes (mouth and conjunctivae), nails, skin creases.
- Hyperdynamic circulation: tachycardia, collapsing pulse (due to increased stroke volume causing wide pulse pressure), systolic flow murmur.
- Cardiac failure.

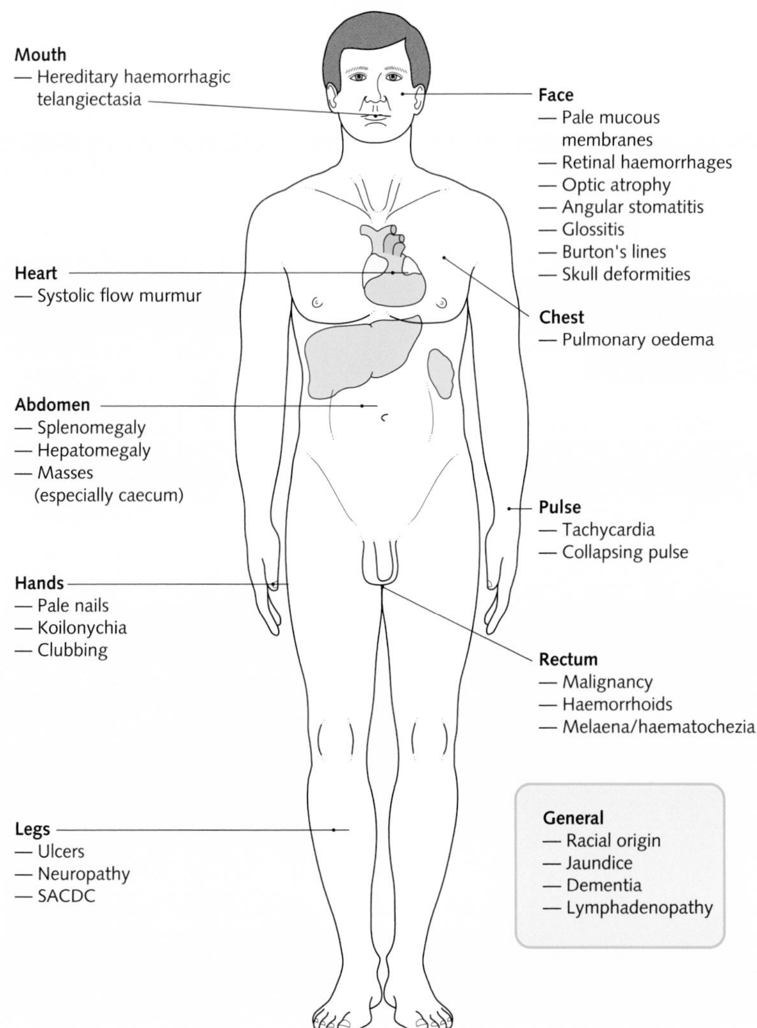

Fig. 29.5 Examining the anaemic patient. SACDC, subacute combined degeneration of the cord.

Evidence of underlying disease

A full general examination should always be performed, including breast examination and rectal examination in iron deficiency. Specific abnormalities include the following:

- Glossitis: megaloblastic anaemia, iron deficiency.
- Angular stomatitis and koilonychia: iron deficiency, folic acid and vitamin B_{12} deficiency.
- Jaundice: haemolysis, megaloblastic anaemia (mild).
- Splenomegaly: haemolysis, megaloblastic anaemia, marrow infiltration and hypoplasia (see Ch. 25).
- Leg ulcers: rheumatoid arthritis, sickle cell disease.
- Bone deformities: thalassaemia.
- Peripheral neuropathy, optic atrophy, subacute combined degeneration of the cord and dementia are all neurological sequelae of vitamin B_{12} deficiency.
- Blue line on the gums (Burton's lines), peripheral motor neuropathy and encephalopathy are seen in lead poisoning.
- Haemosiderin deposition in the skin may be evidence of multiple transfusions.

Note the racial origin of the patient as thalassaemia is more common in people from the Mediterranean to south-east Asia, while sickle cell anaemia is more common among people of Black African origin.

> **COMMUNICATION**
>
> Iron-deficiency anaemia may be a sinister finding in older adults and always needs an explanation. A careful dietary and medical history should be taken to try and identify an underlying cause.

INVESTIGATING THE ANAEMIC PATIENT

General blood tests

Full blood count

- Haemoglobin: severity of anaemia.
- Mean corpuscular volume (80–95 fL): underlying pathologies.
- White cell count (4.0–11.0 × 10^9/L): if low, consider bone marrow failure; if high, consider infection, inflammation or malignancy.
- Platelet count (150–400 × 10^9/L): if low, consider bone marrow failure; if high, consider infection, inflammation or malignancy.
- Red cell distribution width (RDW): this is a measure of the spread of the MCV. In a mixed population of microcytic and macrocytic red cells (anisocytosis), the overall MCV may still be normal, but the RDW will be raised.

Erythrocyte sedimentation rate (ESR) and plasma viscosity (PV)

The ESR and PV will be raised in infection, inflammation or malignancy.

Reticulocyte count

Reticulocytes are immature erythrocytes that normally constitute only 0.5–2.0% of circulating RBCs. The reticulocyte count and percentage rises if RBC production and release increases in response to peripheral loss or breakdown. This occurs following haemorrhage, in acute or chronic haemolysis, or during vitamin B_{12}, folate or iron replacement therapy for anaemia caused by deficiency.

Blood film

The blood film is mandatory and can provide diagnostic information, as shown in Fig. 29.6.

Haematinics

A request can often be made to a haematology lab to perform 'haematinics' and this usually includes ferritin (the iron storage protein and best non-invasive estimate of iron stores), folate and vitamin B_{12}. All these tests should be performed as deficiencies often coexist. Levels cannot be reliably interpreted following blood transfusion.

Other tests

- Tissue transglutaminase to look for malabsorption due to coeliac disease.
- Thyroid function tests.

Specific blood tests

> **HINTS AND TIPS**
>
> Ferritin is an acute phase protein, so falsely elevated or normal results may occur with inflammation.

An algorithm is presented in Fig. 29.7 to outline the diagnosis of anaemia.

Iron deficiency

See Fig. 29.8 for a summary of iron studies in different conditions.

Fig. 29.6 Abnormalities on the blood film in anaemia.

Abnormality	Changes on blood film
Iron deficiency	Hypochromic, microcytic RBCs, target cells, pencil cells, poikilocytosis (variation in RBC shape), anisocytosis (variation in RBC size), often thrombocytosis
Vitamin B_{12}/ folate deficiency	Oval-shaped macrocytosis, neutrophil nuclei hypersegmented (more than six lobes), poikilocytosis; white blood cell and platelet count may be low
Haemolysis	Reticulocytosis, microspherocytes, erythroblasts Many spherocytes in hereditary spherocytosis Elliptocytes in hereditary elliptocytosis
Thalassaemia	Hypochromic, microcytic RBCs, basophilic stippling, target cells, reticulocytosis
Sickle cell disease	Sickle cells, target cells Features of hyposplenism in adults (Howell–Jolly bodies, Pappenheimer bodies, target cells)
Anaemia of chronic disease	Normochromic, normocytic RBCs Neutrophilia and thrombocytosis may be present
Liver disease	Macrocytic RBCs, target cells Features of iron deficiency and folate deficiency may also be present

RBC, red blood cell.

- Serum ferritin: low in iron deficiency but raised in iron overload, haemochromatosis and anaemia of chronic disease (occasionally).
- Serum iron: low, though this is less sensitive than other measures.
- Total iron-binding capacity: increased.
- Transferrin saturation (serum iron/total iron-binding capacity): $<15\%$.

Vitamin B_{12} deficiency

- Serum vitamin B_{12}: low.
- Bilirubin and lactate dehydrogenase (LDH): may be mildly raised due to intramedullary destruction of abnormal RBCs.
- Gastric parietal cell antibodies: positive in 80% of patients with pernicious anaemia.
- Intrinsic factor antibodies: positive in approximately 50% of patients with pernicious anaemia.
- Schilling test (now rarely performed): the patient is given a loading dose of 1000 mg vitamin B_{12} intramuscularly followed by a small oral dose of radioactive vitamin B_{12}, and absorption is estimated by measuring the vitamin B_{12} excreted in the urine. Intrinsic factor is then given if malabsorption is present; in pernicious anaemia this will correct the malabsorption, but it will persist despite the use of intrinsic factor in intestinal disease.

HINTS AND TIPS

Vitamin B_{12} deficiency can cause a profound pancytopenia in addition to anaemia.

Folate deficiency

- RBC or serum folate: low.
- Bilirubin and LDH: mildly raised – intramedullary destruction of abnormal RBCs.
- Further tests for intestinal malabsorption may be necessary (see below).

Haemolysis

- Serum bilirubin: raised and unconjugated.
- Serum haptoglobins: reduced or absent.
- LDH: raised.
- Stercobilinogen (faecal) and urobilinogen (urinary): raised.
- Reticulocyte count: raised.
- Haemoglobin electrophoresis: abnormal in thalassaemia and sickle cell disease.
- Direct antigen test (Coombs' test): positive in immune-mediated haemolytic anaemias (autoimmune, drug-induced or alloimmune haemolytic disease of the newborn).
- Osmotic fragility: increased if spherocytes are present.
- Enzyme assays: available in specialist centres only for glucose-6-phosphate dehydrogenase and pyruvate kinase deficiencies.
- Ham's (acid haemolysis) test: positive in paroxysmal nocturnal haemoglobinuria. Ham's test is an examination favourite but increasingly rare in clinical practice.

Anaemia of chronic disease

- Ferritin: often high (ferritin is an acute phase protein).
- Serum iron: low.
- Total iron-binding capacity: low.
- Serum vitamin B_{12}: normal.
- RBC/serum folate: normal.

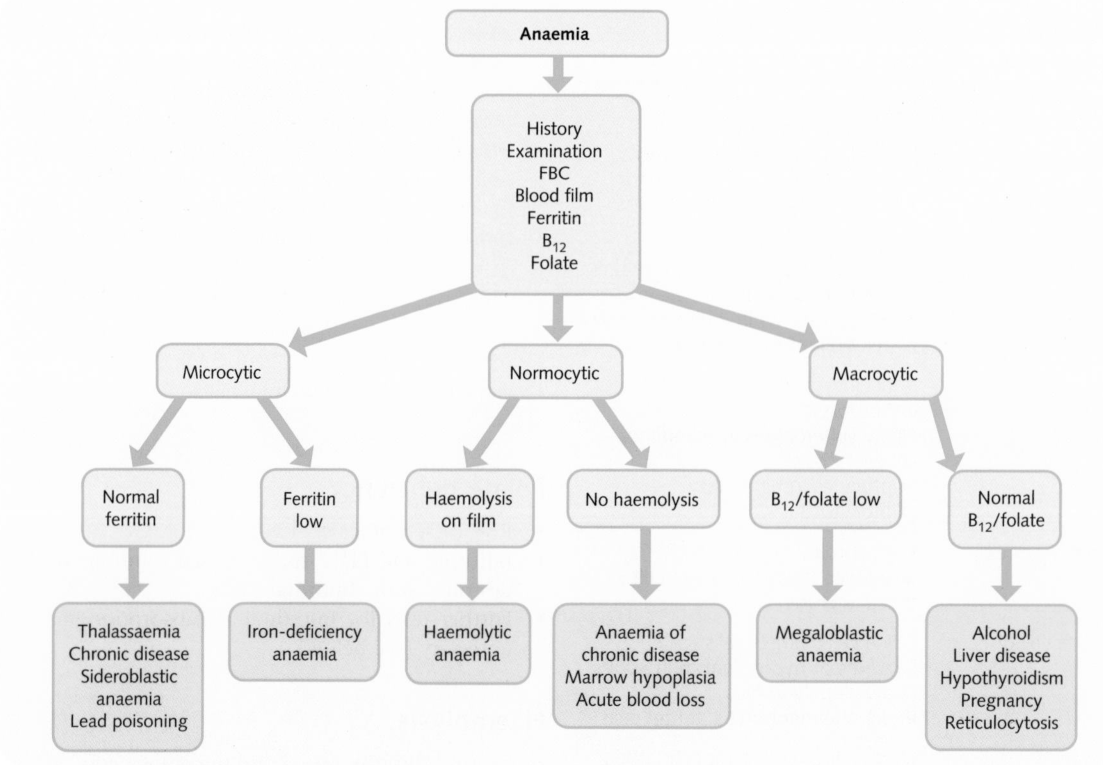

Fig. 29.7 Algorithm for the diagnosis of anaemia. FBC, full blood count.

Fig. 29.8 Interpretation of iron storage results.

	Ferritin	Serum iron	Percentage of transferrin saturation	Total iron-binding capacity
Iron-deficiency anaemia	↓	↓	↓	↑
Anaemia of chronic disease	→ or ↑	↓	↓	↓
Thalassaemia	→ or ↑	→ or ↑	→ or ↑	→
Sideroblastic anaemia	↑	↑	↑	→
Haemochromatosis	↑	↑	↑	↓

→, Normal; ↓, reduced; ↑, increased.

The clinical scenario should direct other investigations. Consider erythrocyte sedimentation rate, C-reactive protein, autoantibody screen, sepsis screen and search for occult malignancy.

HINTS AND TIPS

Mixed deficiency can cause a normocytic anaemia: in these cases remember to check the RDW and request a blood film.

Further tests

There may be a clear cause, for instance menorrhagia or pregnancy in iron deficiency, meaning that further tests are not necessary. However, further investigation is often required.

Bone marrow

- Not necessary when the diagnosis is obvious (e.g. iron deficiency).

- Bone marrow aspirate gives information regarding the development and proportion of different cell lines, infiltration by abnormal cells (e.g. blast cells or metastatic carcinoma) and the presence of iron stores. Samples can be used for cytogenetics.
- Bone marrow trephine biopsy provides structural information regarding bone marrow architecture, overall cellularity and accurate assessment of infiltration.

Gastrointestinal investigations

- Upper gastrointestinal endoscopy and colonoscopy should always be considered in iron deficiency. Coeliac disease is a common cause of iron deficiency and duodenal biopsy often shows characteristic changes.
- If no cause of iron deficiency is found, consider capsule endoscopy to look for angiodysplasia. If bleeding is acute, a mesenteric angiogram may be helpful.
- Tests looking for causes of malabsorption may be necessary, such as contrast studies (barium or water-soluble contrast), colonoscopy and terminal ileal biopsy, enteroscopy and jejunal biopsy. Capsule endoscopy may be useful.

Cardiovascular system

Objectives

The key learning points for this chapter:

- Know the most important risk factors for ischaemic heart disease.
- Describe differences between the management of ST-segment elevation myocardial infarction (STEMI) and non-ST-segment elevation myocardial infarction (NSTEMI).
- Know the drugs used for a patient with stable angina in an outpatient clinic.
- Describe the ECG characteristics of arrhythmias.
- Describe the action of drugs that improve survival in systolic heart failure.
- Understand how drugs are combined in the treatment of hypertension.
- Describe the clinical findings of common heart valve lesions.
- Describe the usual presentations of infective endocarditis.

ISCHAEMIC HEART DISEASE

Introduction

Ischaemic heart disease (IHD) is the result of an imbalance between myocardial oxygen supply and demand. The term covers a group of clinical syndromes, including chronic angina pectoris and the acute coronary syndromes (ACS), which include 'unstable angina', non-ST-segment elevation myocardial infarction (NSTEMI) and ST-segment elevation myocardial infarction (STEMI). The commonest underlying pathology is atherosclerosis of the coronary arteries. More rarely, IHD can result from coronary artery spasm, emboli, coronary ostial stenosis, aortic stenosis, hypertrophic obstructive cardiomyopathy, arrhythmias causing decreased coronary perfusion pressures, and anaemia. Cardiac ischaemia in the presence of normal coronary arteries is termed cardiac syndrome X. It is thought to be due to abnormalities of small coronary vessels resulting in a reduction of coronary flow reserve and is therefore also referred to as microvascular angina.

The prevalence of IHD shows gross geographical variation, reflecting both genetic and lifestyle factors. In the UK it is estimated 6.5% of men and 4% of women suffer with IHD. Prevalence is highly age dependent; less than 0.5% of the population under the age of 40 has IHD, yet greater than 25% of those over 75 suffer with IHD.

Risk factors for ischaemic heart disease

A number of predictors have been found to be associated with an increased likelihood of developing IHD and are called risk factors (Fig. 30.1).

The complete list of possible risk factors for IHD is extremely long and includes environmental factors as well as personal characteristics. Not all these factors will ultimately be shown to be truly causal. For example, obesity may act as a risk factor because it is associated with raised serum cholesterol, hypertension and decreased glucose tolerance. Typically, risk factors are divided into modifiable and non-modifiable.

Non-modifiable risk factors

Age

As discussed in the introduction the prevalence of IHD rises steeply with increasing age. This may be due to the cumulative effects of raised serum cholesterol, hypertension, cigarette smoking and other factors over time.

Sex

The rate in young men is about six times higher than in women of the same age, although this difference diminishes with increasing age. Premenopausal women are thought to be protected by their hormonal status, and this protection diminishes progressively during and after the menopause such that the ratio of IHD in men and women aged 70 years is equal.

Family history

The effect of family history appears to be independent of other major risk factors if first-degree relatives below the age of 50 years are affected. Although high levels of serum total cholesterol may cluster in families, only a very small proportion of these are associated with the genetic condition 'familial hypercholesterolaemia'.

Fig. 30.1 Major risk factors for coronary artery disease.

Type	Risk factors
Non-modifiable	Age Male sex Positive family history Race
Modifiable	Cigarette smoking Hyperlipidaemia Hypertension Diabetes mellitus Left ventricular hypertrophy

Race

The prevalence of IHD in British Asians is high compared with their family members remaining in the Indian subcontinent. The explanation is only partly accounted for by low HDL cholesterol and a higher prevalence of DM and glucose intolerance.

Modifiable risk factors

Smoking

The risk of developing coronary artery disease is directly proportional to the number of cigarettes smoked. The rate of IHD in current smokers is about three times that of those who have never smoked. Giving up smoking leads to an initial rapid decrease in the risk of developing IHD, followed by a more gradual decline in risk; the risk of IHD is almost the same as a non-smoker after approximately 10 years.

HINTS AND TIPS

The description of symptoms in ischaemic heart disease is very variable. Patients often use words such as heaviness, tightness or restriction rather than pain.

Blood lipid profile

The risk of IHD increases as serum total cholesterol and low-density lipoprotein (LDL) cholesterol increases. High-density lipoprotein (HDL) cholesterol is 'protective' for IHD, and the risk of IHD decreases as HDL increases. Triglycerides are also positively related to IHD risk, although, when the relationship of IHD to other blood lipids is taken into account, the independent contribution of triglycerides to IHD may be small.

Hypertension

Both systolic and diastolic hypertension are associated with the risk of developing IHD, as well as hypertensive heart disease, stroke and renal failure. Treatment of hypertension with drugs reduces the incidence of cardiac events, particularly in the elderly.

Diabetes mellitus

In countries where IHD is prevalent, diabetes mellitus (DM) is associated with an approximately threefold increase in the risk of a major IHD event.

Weight

Overweight individuals have twice the risk of a major IHD event. This is probably mediated through increased blood pressure levels, total cholesterol, insulin resistance and with decreased HDL and physical activity.

Obstructive sleep apnoea

Although associated with obesity and hypertension, obstructive sleep apnoea appears to have an independent association with cardiovascular and cerebrovascular disease.

Novel risk factors

In recent years, newer risk factors have been suggested; these include elevated C-reactive protein (CRP) and hyperfibrinogenaemia plus hyperhomocysteinaemia. Whether these are truly independent risk factors or markers of underlying inflammation should become clear from further studies.

Psychosocial factors

Although stress and other strong emotional responses can precipitate major IHD events in individuals with severe atherosclerosis, it remains to be shown whether stress plays a role in the pathogenesis of coronary artery disease in the absence of other standard risk factors.

Combining risk factors is a more accurate way of predicting those at risk from IHD than relying on any one individual risk factor. Many models and scoring systems have been devised incorporating the different risk factors so that those at high risk may be targeted for preventative treatment. The commonly used cardiovascular risk prediction charts can be found at the back of the *British National Formulary*. They are an aid to decision making but should not replace clinical judgement. In addition, this should be accompanied by population-based measures to reduce the risk of IHD.

Pathophysiology

Atherosclerosis is a slowly progressive focal proliferation of connective tissue within the arterial intima that begins as early as the second decade of life. It is linked to high lipid levels. LDL is the main atherogenic lipid, although the principal constituent of atherosclerotic plaques is collagen synthesized by smooth muscle cells.

The initial process consists of endothelial dysfunction in association with a high circulating cholesterol, inflammation and shear forces. Macrophages enter the arterial wall between endothelial cells, taking up lipids and forming 'foam cells'. The accumulation of lipid-laden macrophages in the subendothelial zone leads to the formation of fatty streaks. Toxic products released from the macrophages lead to the adhesion of platelets and result in smooth muscle cell proliferation and thrombus formation. This then becomes organized, leading to the development of an atherosclerotic plaque surrounded by a fibrotic cap. Progressive enlargement of these lesions leads to segmental narrowing of the lumen, which, when sufficient to be flow-limiting on exercise, causes stable exertion-associated angina.

Atherosclerotic plaques are liable to rupture, resulting in sudden thrombosis, which is responsible for acute coronary syndromes. Factors associated with plaque disruption and consequent thrombosis include a large lipid core, a high monocyte density and low smooth muscle cell density.

The association of high levels of CRP and other inflammatory markers with IHD has led many to suggest that atherosclerosis may be an inflammatory process. Various pathogens have been advanced, including *Helicobacter pylori* and *Chlamydia pneumoniae*, although this remains speculative.

Clinical features

Ischaemic heart disease clinically presents in broadly two categories: chronic 'stable' angina and acute coronary syndromes (ACS). Stable angina is due to a 'predictable' mismatch between oxygen supply and demand of cardiac myocytes – cardiac ischaemia. This is brought on by exertion and relieved by rest. Symptoms are central chest pain, heaviness or discomfort commonly radiating to the jaw or arm and may be associated with shortness of breath, sweating, nausea or faintness (see Ch. 4). ACS presents with the same symptoms but, unlike stable angina, occurs suddenly and is often a result of athrosclerotic plaque rupture.

Investigations

Although stable angina and ACS present with similar symptoms they are investigated differently. ACS is a medical emergency and requires urgent inpatient diagnosis which guides management (see later). Stable angina is commonly managed in primary care with diagnostic investigations arranged as an outpatient.

Assessment of risk factors

The risk factors for IHD have been summarized above. All modifiable risk factors should be addressed as part of investigating patients with suspected IHD. Baseline blood pressure measurement, lipid profile and glucose levels should be performed. If the patient is a smoker, smoking cessation advice should be provided.

Electrocardiogram

A normal ECG does not exclude a diagnosis of stable angina or ACS. During attacks, there may be ST-segment depression or symmetrical T wave inversion. T wave inversion in leads V_1–V_3 often indicates left anterior descending coronary artery stenosis. The ECG may show signs of an old myocardial infarction (MI) or left ventricular hypertrophy. Comparison with an old ECG is very useful (and therefore doing a routine ECG for anyone attending A&E over the age of 60 is a good idea).

Exercise electrocardiogram

In IHD the exercise ECG is an indicator of exercise performance and is an independent indicator of prognosis. It is contraindicated in ACS, severe aortic stenosis, severe pulmonary hypertension and significant rhythm disturbances. The test is usually regarded as positive if there is more than 1 mm of downsloping ST-segment depression after the J point (the junction of the ST segment and the T wave). If the pre-test probability of angina is high, the number of false positives is low. Causes of false-positive tests include hyperventilation, digoxin, hypokalaemia, hypertension, valvular heart disease, left ventricular hypertrophy and pre-excitation syndromes. The test should be terminated if there is more than 3 mm of ST depression, a fall in blood pressure, ventricular tachycardia, pallor, indicating peripheral circulatory collapse or if the end point is reached.

Echocardiography

This can be used to assess ventricular function and localize areas of ventricular wall involvement. In patients with angina but no evidence of infarction, the echocardiogram may be normal. With diffuse ischaemic changes, left ventricular function may be globally impaired. Exercise or pharmacological stress echocardiography may be used to detect areas of 'hibernating' myocardium. These are areas that show reduced function with exercise, due to decreased blood flow secondary to decreased coronary flow reserve, but which show improved function at rest. They indicate areas that may improve with revascularization procedures.

CT coronary angiography

Recent advances in computed tomography technology have allowed for non-invasive assessment of the coronary arteries. CT scans can be used in stratifying IHD risk through a 'calcium score' – a proven indicator for atherosclerosis, or as a non-invasive method for assessing coronary artery patency.

Nuclear imaging

This technique may be used to assess myocardial structure and function. A radioactive isotope (e.g. thallium, technetium (MIBI or MUGA scan)) is injected during exercise and an image is taken soon after. The isotope is taken up by healthy myocardium whereas areas of infarction show up as 'cold spots'. If exercise is not feasible, pharmacological stress can be induced with agents such as adenosine. Repeat images are taken at rest to obtain a redistribution image. The disappearance of the cold spot implies ischaemia provoked by exertion and reversed by rest; a fixed cold spot indicates infarction. It is a useful technique when the exercise test is equivocal or contraindicated, or to indicate the clinical significance of angiographically equivocal stenoses.

Coronary angiography

This is a technique for visualizing the coronary arteries radiographically, measuring intracardiac pressures, blood oxygen saturation in different cardiac chambers and cardiac output. The test is usually used to determine the exact coronary anatomy and to decide on further management (i.e. medical therapy, coronary angioplasty or coronary artery bypass surgery). In stable angina, it is usually reserved for patients with:

- Angina resistant to optimal medical treatment.
- Strongly positive exercise tests indicating a poor prognosis.
- Evidence of reversible ischaemia on stress testing with reduced left ventricular function.
- After confirmed troponin-positive acute coronary events, especially if pain continues.

More rarely, coronary angiography is used as a diagnostic test when other non-invasive tests have not been helpful and symptoms persist.

The mortality from the procedure is approximately 1 in 1000. Complications include:

- Haemorrhage and haematoma at the site of arterial puncture.
- Emboli into arteries resulting in coronary or peripheral ischaemia.
- Stroke.
- Arrhythmias.
- Coronary artery dissection.

Treatment of ischaemic heart disease

Chronic stable angina provides considerable morbidity for patients and a high workload for health services. Similar to all chronic disease, the optimal management comprises patient education, lifestyle change and medication. Non-coronary causes for angina should be sought and treated (e.g. valvular heart disease and anaemia). NICE guidelines are now available for the management of stable angina (July 2011), unstable angina and NSTEMI (March 2010) and chest pain of recent onset (March 2010). Guidance on STEMI is due to be published in July 2013.

General measures

Risk factors should be sought and addressed. Weight loss, smoking cessation, exercise within the capacity of the patient and healthy diet should all be encouraged. Exercise may improve the collateral circulation in the heart in the same way as in peripheral vascular disease. Factors precipitating angina (e.g. cold weather or extremes of emotion) should be avoided. All patients should be provided with a sublingual nitrate, either spray or tablet, for relief of acute attacks or prophylactic use before exercise.

Pharmacological management

Antiplatelet drugs

All patients should be prescribed aspirin 75 mg daily as this lowers the incidence of subsequent MI and death. There is a risk of gastrointestinal bleeding so patients should be given advice to take the aspirin with food and made aware of warning signs such as melaena; if a history of previous bleeding is present, a proton pump inhibitor can be added. If aspirin is contraindicated, then clopidogrel, an inhibitor of platelet aggregation, is an alternative. Furthermore, clopidogrel has recently come off licence and its use is likely to increase in the coming years, potentially instead of aspirin, to treat pathologies where atherosclerosis is the underlying disease process.

Beta-blockers

Beta-blockers improve oxygen supply and demand balance by lowering heart rate and blood pressure, decreasing end systolic stress and contractility and prolonging diastole, permitting more coronary flow. Beta-blockers are the first-line drug in preventing symptoms and meta-analyses have shown they improve mortality.

Typical beta-blockers include atenolol, bisoprolol and metoprolol. Relative contraindications include asthma and peripheral vascular disease with skin ulceration. They are contraindicated in second- and third-degree heart block.

Nitrates

Nitrates cause peripheral vasodilatation, especially in the veins. This reduces venous return and ventricular preload is decreased. Reduction in the distension of the heart wall decreases oxygen demand, resulting in relief of angina. Nitrates work by conversion to nitric oxide, which results in an increase in intracellular cyclic guanosine monophosphate (cGMP) in smooth muscle. This stimulates calcium-binding processes and the free calcium available to trigger muscle contraction is reduced.

Short-acting nitrates are the mainstay of relief of acute angina and, when combined with rest, they relieve the pain in minutes. If it continues, then this should be a warning sign to patients. Longer-acting nitrates are more stable and can be effective for several hours. Isosorbide dinitrate (ISDN) is rapidly metabolized by the liver to mononitrate, which is the main active metabolite. Isosorbide mononitrate (ISMN) may avoid the variable absorption and unpredictable first-pass metabolism of the dinitrate.

Adverse effects are normally due to arterial dilatation and include headaches, flushing, hypotension and rarely fainting. Patients may become tolerant to nitrates, reducing their effectiveness. Nitrate 'holidays' are the traditional way of minimizing the problem, although newer once-daily preparations reduce this effect.

Calcium channel blockers

Calcium antagonists inhibit the influx of calcium into the myocyte during the action potential and relax peripheral vascular smooth muscle. They reduce angina by a combination of reduced afterload and hence myocardial oxygen demand plus reduced heart rate and increased coronary vasodilation. They are especially useful if there is a degree of coronary artery spasm. Dihydropyridines such as nifedipine can cause reflex tachycardia secondary to peripheral vasodilatation and therefore may be combined with a beta-blocker. Diltiazem has slight negative inotropic and chronotropic effects, and the patient should be monitored if on beta-blockers for the development of bradycardias. Verapamil is the drug of choice for supraventricular tachycardias if beta-blockers are contraindicated (verapamil and beta-blockers must never be coprescribed). All calcium channel blocking drugs are negatively inotropic to some degree and, although amlodipine has demonstrated its safety in heart failure, extreme care should be taken with prescribing any of them to patients with impaired left ventricular function.

Side effects include headache, flushing, dizziness, constipation and gravitational oedema.

Potassium channel activators

Nicorandil has arterial and venous vasodilating properties and is useful in patients refractory to treatment with other antianginal agents.

ACE inhibitors

Patients with stable angina and proven left ventricular dysfunction should be on an ACE inhibitor unless contraindicated. The benefit of ACE inhibitors in stable angina with normal ventricular function is controversial and several large RCTs have been contradictive.

Lipid-lowering drugs

Statins (HMG-CoA reductase inhibitors) are the mainstay of lipid-lowering therapy. The current maxim is 'the lower the better'. Statins may also help to stabilize atherosclerotic plaques and reduce the frequency of acute cardiac events. Most patients with IHD should be on a statin even if their cholesterol is within the normal range.

Angioplasty and stenting

After plaque visualization at angiography, coronary artery stenoses can be dilated using a balloon to improve perfusion. The best results in terms of patency and flow are achieved with stent insertion. This is a very safe procedure and is now preferred to surgery in most cases. Use of clopidogrel and glycoprotein IIb/IIIa receptor antagonists has further reduced stent re-stenosis. Drug-eluting stents (e.g. with sirolimus) may further enhance this, although trials are still ongoing. Patients need only stay in hospital overnight and they return to activity quickly compared to surgery.

Surgical management

Coronary artery bypass graft (CABG) surgery should be considered in patients who have angina despite optimal medical therapy and are not suitable for, or have failed, angioplasty. It has a low mortality in otherwise well patients (2%). Bypass using one or both of the internal mammary arteries is preferred to the traditional vein graft. They result in better patency, flow and graft survival. Certain patient groups are better served by surgery rather than stents (Fig. 30.2). Postoperatively, the number and dose of antianginal drugs can be reduced.

Fig. 30.2 Patient factors associated with reduction in mortality with coronary artery bypass surgery.

Left main stem stenosis
Triple-vessel coronary artery disease
Two-vessel disease with proximal LAD disease
Benefit is greater in those with left ventricular impairment

LAD, left anterior descending coronary artery.

ACUTE CORONARY SYNDROMES

The terminology used to classify acute cardiac ischaemic events has changed in the last few years. Subendocardial and non-Q-wave myocardial infarctions (MI) are now termed non-ST-segment elevation MI (NSTEMI). Acute MI with ST-segment elevation is hence an STEMI. This reflects the fact that the key to appropriate treatment is the presence or absence of ST-segment elevation because there are good evidence-based guidelines for their different management. When combined with unstable angina, all three are the 'acute coronary syndromes' (ACS). ACS is common (incidence 15/1000): of these roughly one-third will present with an NSTEMI; one-third with an STEMI; and one-third with unstable angina. Prognostic scoring systems have been validated and will be discussed later in this section.

ST-SEGMENT ELEVATION MYOCARDIAL INFARCTION (STEMI)

Myocardial infarction affects 5 in 1000 of the general population per year in the UK and is the most common cause of mortality in the Western world. Ninety percent of transmural MIs are caused by an occlusive intracoronary thrombus overlying an ulcerated or fissured stenotic plaque. Underlying most cases there is a dynamic interaction between severe coronary atherosclerosis, an acute atheromatous plaque change, superimposed thrombosis, platelet activation and vasospasm. The microscopic changes of acute MI follow a predictable sequence (Fig. 30.3).

The overall fatality from acute MI has improved markedly in the last 20 years with better medical care, the development of coronary care units and the recognition of the importance of opening the occluded artery to reperfuse the damaged myocardium and limit infarct size.

Presentation and symptoms

Patients commonly present with acute-onset central chest pain (see Ch. 4), although occasionally ACS may be 'silent'. Associated features include nausea, vomiting, sweatiness, palpitations, dyspnoea, syncope and/or pulmonary oedema. The pain may radiate into the jaw, one or both arms or may even be epigastric. The patient will often be distressed.

Fig. 30.3 Changes induced by acute myocardial infarction.

Time after onset of symptoms	Macroscopic changes	Microscopic changes
Up to 18 h	None	None
24–48 h	Pale oedematous muscle	Oedema, acute inflammatory cell infiltration, necrosis of myocytes
3–4 days	Yellow rubbery centre with haemorrhagic border	Obvious necrosis and inflammation, early granulation tissue
3–6 weeks	Silvery scar becoming rough and white	Dense fibrosis

Diagnosis

The diagnosis of MI is based on the presence of at least two out of three of the following features: (1) A typical or suggestive cardiac history (See Ch 4), (2) specific ECG changes, (3) Cardiac enzyme changes. These are criteria set be by the World Health Organisation (WHO).

Electrocardiogram

The earliest ECG changes or 'hyperacute' changes consist of tall, pointed T waves followed by elevation of the ST segment. This is followed by T wave inversion, the R wave voltage decreases and Q waves develop. After weeks or months, the T wave may become upright again but the Q waves remain (Fig. 30.4).

The site of the infarction may also be deduced from the affected leads on the ECG:

- Inferior MI: involves leads II, III and aVF.
- Anterior MI: affects the precordial leads.
- Anteroseptal MI: affects leads V_1–V_3.
- Lateral MI: affects leads I and aVL, and V_4–V_6.
- Posterior MI: there is a dominant R wave in leads V_1–V_3 with ST-segment depression and upright T waves.

There may also be 'reciprocal' ECG changes with ST-segment depression in leads opposite to the site of infarction.

Diagnostic criteria for STEMI are as follows:

- ST-segment elevation >2 mm in 2 or more chest leads.
- ST-segment elevation >1 mm in 2 or more limb leads.
- Posterior MI (see above).
- New-onset LBBB.

Cardiac enzymes

Cardiac enzymes are intracellular enzymes which leak out of infarcted myocardium into the bloodstream (Fig. 30.5):

- Elevated troponin I or T concentrations in the blood are highly reliable markers of myocardial damage.

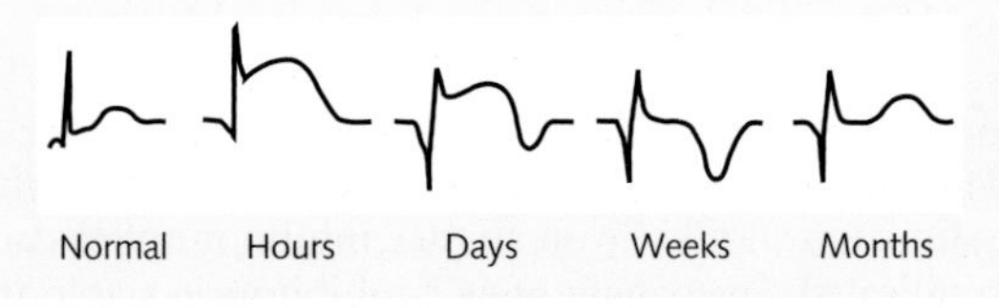

Fig. 30.4 Progressive electrocardiogram changes in myocardial infarction.

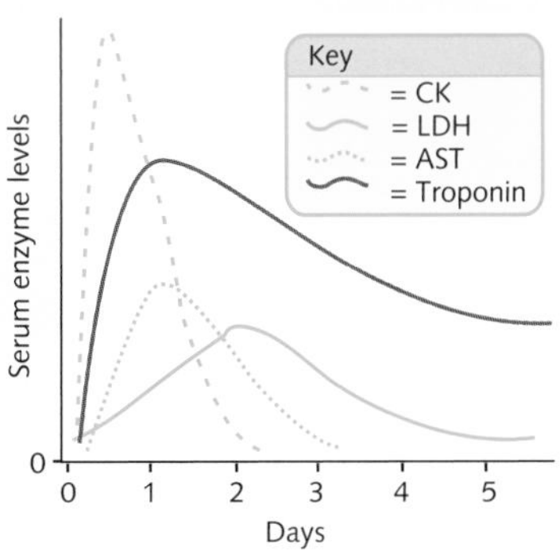

Fig. 30.5 The pattern of serum markers after acute myocardial infarction. AST, aspartate aminotransferase; CK, creatine kinase; LDH, lactate dehydrogenase.

They are not 'enzymes' but proteins involved in myocyte contraction. They are most reliable 8–12 h post event and remain elevated for several weeks.

- Creatine kinase (CK) peaks within 24 h. It is a cardiac enzyme that is also produced by skeletal muscle and brain. In cases of doubt, the myocardium-bound isoenzyme fraction of CK (CK-MB) can be requested, which is specific for heart muscle damage. The site of the infarct is related to the serum level of enzyme. CK is therefore still used to assess reinfarction in patients whose troponin is elevated from a previous MI.
- Aspartate aminotransferase and lactate dehydrogenase were formerly used to assess MI as they remain elevated for several days after CK has settled. Their use is now largely obsolete.

Further tests

- A full blood count (FBC): anaemia.
- Urea and electrolytes (U&Es): renal and electrolyte abnormalities.
- Chest X-ray (CXR): aortic dissection, signs of heart failure and to assess cardiac size.
- Blood glucose.

Management

Emergency care

The main aims are to prevent or treat cardiac arrest and to relieve pain – the patient should ideally be managed on a coronary care unit with continuous cardiac monitoring. The ABC principles should be followed in the emergency setting. Oxygen, sublingual nitrates, intravenous nitrate and opiates such as diamorphine are given for pain relief. Diamorphine relieves pain, but also alleviates sympathetic activation associated with the pain, which causes vasoconstriction and increases the work of the heart. Antiemetics should be administered with opiates. Aspirin (300 mg) should be given as soon as possible and is often done by the paramedic crew. Anxiety is a natural response to the pain and to the circumstances surrounding a heart attack. Reassurance of patients and those closely associated with them is therefore of great importance.

Primary percutaneous coronary intervention

Immediate primary angioplasty and stenting leads to better immediate and long-term outcomes in acute STEMI than thrombolysis. Patients with an STEMI should therefore be treated immediately with primary percutaneous coronary intervention (PCI). If the admitting hospital does not have 24-h PCI facilities, urgent transfer should be arranged. Patients undergoing primary percutaneous coronary intervention should be treated with a glycoprotein IIb/IIIa receptor antagonist.

Thrombolytic treatment

UK guidelines now state that if primary percutaneous coronary intervention cannot be provided within 90 min of diagnosis, patients with an ST-segment elevation acute coronary syndrome should receive immediate thrombolytic therapy.

Contraindications to thrombolytic therapy are given in Fig. 30.6. Major bleeding complications are seen in approximately 1–3% of patients.

The two main thrombolytics are streptokinase and alteplase, a recombinant tissue plasminogen activator (tPA). Streptokinase induces an antibody response, which reduces the effectiveness of a repeat dose and increases the risk of an anaphylactic reaction. It should therefore not be readministered in the period between 5 days and a minimum of 2 years following initial treatment. Streptokinase is now rarely used.

Fig. 30.6 Contraindications to thrombolytic therapy.

Contraindications	Stroke Major surgery, trauma or head injury within 3 weeks Gastrointestinal bleed Known bleeding disorder Suspected dissecting aneurysm Cerebral neoplasm
Relative contraindications	Transient ischaemic attack in the preceding 6 months Warfarin therapy Pregnancy Non-compressible punctures Traumatic resuscitation Refractory hypertension (SBP >200 mmHg) Recent retinal laser treatment

SBP, systolic blood pressure.

Other therapy in the acute phase

Antiplatelet agents

Aspirin therapy 300 mg should be prescribed early. This leads to a 30% reduction in deaths or 24 lives saved in 1000 treated. If aspirin sensitivity is present then clopidogrel should be used.

Beta-blockers

In the absence of hypotension or bradycardia, administration of beta-blockers in the acute phase, preferable intravenously, potentially limits infarct size, reducing the risk of fatal arrhythmias. There is a 15% reduction in mortality at 1 week. It is particularly appropriate when the patient has a tachycardia (in the absence of heart failure), relative hypertension or pain unresponsive to opioids. If the intravenous formulation is not available, start oral therapy.

Angiotensin-converting-enzyme inhibitors

All patients should be commenced on ACE inhibitors if tolerated as they produce survival benefit. ACE inhibitors are of most value in patients with clinical symptoms or signs of heart failure, or impaired left ventricular function echocardiographically. Opinions differ as to the best time to initiate treatment – whether acutely or after a few days. The benefits appear to be a class effect, and doses should be titrated to the target dose.

Statins

Statins should be started on admission, regardless of cholesterol levels, as they may improve outcomes by anti-inflammatory plaque-stabilizing effects.

Heparin

Patients with an ST-segment elevation acute coronary syndrome who do not receive reperfusion therapy should be treated immediately with low-molecular-weight heparin.

Control of glucose

Patients with a STEMI and diabetes mellitus or marked hyperglycaemia (>11.0 mmol/L) should have immediate intensive blood glucose control, commonly through an insulin sliding scale regime. This should be continued for at least 24 h.

NON-ST-SEGMENT ELEVATION MYOCARDIAL INFARCTION (NSTEMI) AND UNSTABLE ANGINA

Symptoms

The patient may have characteristic central ischaemic chest pain (see Ch. 4) or more non-specific symptoms. Patients with chronic stable angina may note that their pain is no longer relieved fully by glyceryl trinitrate (GTN), that it is increasing in intensity or that it is occurring at rest. These are all symptoms requiring urgent assessment.

> **HINTS AND TIPS**
>
> Don't forget that ACS can present with atypical pain such as epigastric pain or scapular pain. Diabetic patients may not experience any pain, a 'silent' MI, due to peripheral neuropathy.

Diagnosis

The diagnosis of NSTEMI and unstable angina is based on the presence of two out of three from a typical history, ischaemic ECG changes (but not meeting STEMI criteria), positive cardiac enzyme test.

History

The history and clinical features are the same as those for STEMI.

ECG

The ECG may show ST-segment depression, T wave flattening, biphasic changes or inversion. The deeper the changes, the more worrying they are. The initial ECG may be normal and serial ones are needed, preferably when pain occurs, to demonstrate the dynamic ischaemia.

> **HINTS AND TIPS**
>
> Old ECGs are invaluable in assessing patients with chest pain, allowing for comparison.

Cardiac enzymes

The measurement of troponin I or T concentration at 8–12 h after the onset of pain is crucial. As well as being a highly specific marker of myocardial damage, it has shown prognostic value, although interpretation may be more difficult with renal impairment. Therefore, patients with non-evolving ECGs who are pain-free and with a negative troponin result can safely be discharged and have an exercise test and cardiovascular risk stratification as outpatients. Patients with positive troponin NSTEMI events are at high risk for further events (30% chance of STEMI at 1 month) and should be evaluated for revascularization procedures as inpatients.

Risk scoring

All patients that present with ACS should have risk stratification using clinical scores. This allows clinicians to identify those patients who are most likely to benefit

Fig. 30.7 Components of GRACE score.

Age
Heart rate
Systolic blood pressure
Creatinine
Congestive heart failure
Cardiac arrest on admission
ST-segment elevation on ECG
Elevated cardiac enzymes

from early therapeutic intervention. Various scoring systems exist, but NICE now recommends the use of the Global Registry of Acute Cardiac Events (GRACE) score (Fig. 30.7). The GRACE score is validated as a prognostic tool to predict in hospital death and MI and mortality and MI at 6 months. As such, those patients that have a high-risk benefit from early intervention such as PCI or CABG.

Management

Emergency care

The initial emergency management of NSTEMI and unstable angina is identical to that of STEMI: aspirin 300 mg, morphine and nitrates. The role of oxygen is controversial and newer guidelines do not comment on this. The safest approach is to give oxygen, aiming for saturations between 94 and 98%. In the case of a cardiac arrest secondary to ACS, high-flow oxygen must given.

Pharmacological management

Antiplatelet agents

Aspirin

Aspirin (300 mg) should be given straight away and is often administered by paramedics. It should be continued daily at 75 mg.

Clopidogrel

Clopidogrel has been demonstrated to significantly improve outcomes in combination with aspirin in patients with NSTEMI. It should also be used if aspirin is contraindicated. The first dose is 300 mg and subsequently 75 mg daily. This should be continued for 3 months.

Glycoprotein IIb/IIIa receptor antagonists

These are potent antiplatelet agents that block the binding of fibrinogen to the IIb/IIIa receptor on the platelet surface. They are started if the pain continues or ECG changes progress. They may settle the acute events on their own but are usually part of a strategy including cardiac catheterization. The most common agents are tirofiban or eptifibatide. They have a significant risk of causing bleeding, which should be assessed.

Heparin and heparin-like agents

In the presence of ischaemic ECG changes or elevation of cardiac enzymes, patients with an acute coronary syndrome should be treated immediately with low-molecular-weight heparin or fondaparinux. Heparin should be given for at least 3–5 days and until pain-free for 24 h. It is usually given as twice-daily enoxaparin.

Beta-blockers

Unless contraindicated (e.g. asthma, overt heart failure or known marked left ventricular dysfunction), beta-blockers should be started. They have immediate anti-anginal effects and reduce the progression to acute STEMI, reduce arrhythmias and improve survival. Examples include metoprolol, atenolol and carvedilol.

Rate-limiting calcium channel antagonists

For example diltiazam. This is an antianginal drug that has negatively chronotropic effects. If beta-blockers are contraindicated, then it is an alternative agent.

Statins

Statin therapy should be started immediately as per management of STEMI.

ACE inhibitors

Angiotensin-converting-enzyme (ACE) inhibition should start early in patients with NSTEMI. It is reasonable to start at a low dose and wait 12 h until the acute event has settled, as hypotension is a risk.

Over 90% of patients with NSTEMI will become pain-free and respond well to the above treatments. If pain continues, complications such as cardiogenic shock ensue and/or the ECG changes progress, then additional therapy is needed and the patient should be transferred to a centre with interventional cardiology support.

Role of percutaneous coronary intervention

The big differential between NSTEMI and STEMI is the role of PCI – it is not indicated in patients without STEMI or new left bundle branch block (LBBB) because it has no demonstrated benefit. However, angiography and angioplasty is recommended in ongoing NSTEMI or those at moderate or high risk of mortality or future MI within the first 96 h of admission (as calculated by GRACE score).

Subsequent inpatient management of patients with ACS

General

Patients should be on bed rest for the first 24 h. If uncomplicated, the patient can then sit out of bed, use a commode and undertake self-care and self-feeding. Ambulation can be started the next day and exercise is gradually built up to climbing stairs within a few days.

In patients with proven NSTEMI the mortality at 1 year is up to 20%. All patients should have their cardiovascular risks assessed and modified. Long-term antiplatelet medications, statins, beta-blockers and ACE inhibitors should be prescribed unless contraindicated. The need for angioplasty or bypass surgery should be considered with stress testing or angiography.

Thromboprophylaxis

Deep vein thrombosis and pulmonary embolism may be prevented by subcutaneous heparin when in bed. If they do occur, the patient should be treated initially with heparin, followed by oral anticoagulation. Patients are usually started on a low-molecular-weight heparin after admission to the coronary care unit.

Further investigations and risk stratification

Post-MI patients should undergo echocardiography to assess valve and systolic function. Most patients can safely undergo a limited exercise test after being pain-free for 5–7 days. If normal, they can be followed up in clinic with no further testing. Increased risk of further events and death include:

- Continuing angina.
- Heart failure.
- Positive exercise or pharmacological stress test.

These patients should then have angiography prior to discharge.

Complications of myocardial infarction

A summary of the complications that may occur as a result of MI is given in Fig. 30.8.

Cardiac failure and cardiogenic shock

Left ventricular failure during the acute phase of MI is associated with a poor prognosis. Repeated examination of the heart and lungs for signs of incipient heart failure should be performed in all patients (Fig. 30.9).

Echocardiography can be helpful in the assessment of ventricular function, mitral regurgitation and ventricular septal defects.

The management of heart failure is described later in this chapter. Cardiogenic shock is defined as an inability to perfuse end organs, resulting in tissue hypoxia secondary to pump failure.

Other causes of shock should be excluded such as hypovolaemia, vasovagal reactions, drugs or arrhythmias. Ventricular and valvular function should be evaluated by echocardiography. Inotropic agents are of value: dobutamine (5–20 μg/kg/min) is first line. Correction of acidosis is important for myocardial function,

Fig. 30.8 Complications of myocardial infarction.

Complication	Interval	Mechanism
Sudden death	Usually within hours	Often ventricular fibrillation
Arrhythmias	First few days	–
Persistent pain	12 h to a few days	Progressive myocardial necrosis (extension of MI)
Angina	Immediate or delayed (weeks)	Ischaemia of non-infarcted muscle
Cardiac failure	Variable	Ventricular dysfunction following muscle necrosis; arrhythmias
Mitral incompetence	First few days	Papillary muscle dysfunction, necrosis or rupture
Pericarditis	2–4 days	Transmural infarct with inflammation of the pericardium
Cardiac rupture and ventricular septal defects	3–5 days	Weakening of wall following muscle necrosis and acute inflammation
Mural thrombus	One week or more	Abnormal endothelial surface following infarction
Ventricular aneurysm	4 weeks or more	Stretching of newly formed collagenous scar tissue
Dressler's syndrome	Weeks to months	Autoimmune
Pulmonary emboli	1 week or more	Deep venous thrombosis in lower limbs
Late ventricular arrhythmias	–	–

Fig. 30.9 Killip classification for assessment of heart failure.

Class	Features
1	No crepitations or third heart sound
2	Crepitations over less than 50% of lung fields or third heart sound
3	Crepitations over 50% of the lung fields
4	Shock

although improving cardiac output itself improves lactic acidosis, which is the usual cause.

Emergency angiography and angioplasty or surgery should be considered.

Cardiac rupture

Free wall rupture, if acute, is usually fatal within minutes. If subacute, there is haemodynamic deterioration with hypotension and signs of cardiac tamponade. Immediate surgery is needed.

Ventricular septal defect (VSD) occurs in 1% of all infarctions, appearing early after MI. Without surgery, the mortality is 50% within the first week and 90% within the first year. It should be suspected if there is clinical deterioration and a loud pansystolic murmur at the left sternal edge. Treatment is by surgical closure of the defect and bypass grafts as necessary.

Mitral regurgitation

The incidence of moderately severe or severe mitral regurgitation is approximately 4% and the mortality without surgery is high at approximately 20%. Valve replacement is the procedure of choice in papillary muscle dysfunction and rupture.

Arrhythmias and conduction disturbances

These are extremely common in the early period following MI. Often, the arrhythmias are not hazardous in themselves but are a manifestation of a serious underlying disorder such as continuing ischaemia, vagal overactivity or electrolyte disturbance that requires attention, particularly potassium and magnesium. Arrhythmias can also occur following reperfusion. The management of arrhythmias is covered in detail in this chapter.

Ventricular arrhythmias

Ventricular arrhythmias may present as ventricular ectopics, ventricular tachycardia (VT), or ventricular fibrillation (VF).

Ventricular ectopics are almost universal on the first day and require no treatment if the patient is asymptomatic.

Short episodes of VT may be well tolerated and require no treatment. More prolonged episodes may cause hypotension and heart failure. Amiodarone or lidocaine are the drugs of choice. Direct current (DC) cardioversion may be required if haemodynamically significant VT persists.

Ventricular fibrillation is associated with approximately 5% of MI. It is not compatible with life. If VF occurs, immediate defibrillation should be performed as part of the Advanced Life Support protocol.

When arrhythmias occur late in the course of MI, they are liable to recur and are associated with a high risk of death. If it is probable that the arrhythmia is induced by ischaemia, revascularization should be considered. If this is unlikely, antiarrhythmic agents (e.g. beta-blockers and amiodarone) and electrophysiologically guided treatment may be given. In some cases, an implantable defibrillator is indicated.

Supraventricular arrhythmias

Atrial fibrillation (AF) complicates 15–20% of MIs and is often associated with severe left ventricular damage and heart failure; it is usually self-limiting. If the heart rate is fast, bisoprolol or digoxin are effective in slowing the rate but amiodarone is more efficacious in terminating the arrhythmia.

Other supraventricular arrhythmias are rare but are also usually self-limiting. They may respond to carotid sinus massage. Beta-blockers may be effective and DC shock should be employed if the arrhythmia is poorly tolerated.

Sinus bradycardia and heart block

Sinus bradycardia is common early on, especially in inferior MI, and responds to atropine in boluses titrated against response, although large doses of atropine should be avoided.

Atrioventricular (AV) block is common in inferior MI as the right coronary artery supplies the AV node and may respond to atropine, although patients may go on to need a permanent pacemaker. However, it may take up to 14 days before normal conduction is restored.

Heart block with anterior MI is ominous because it indicates a large infarct. The development of LBBB or bifascicular block may presage complete heart block and is an indication for temporary pacemaker insertion. If complete heart block does occur and persists, a permanent pacemaker will be needed.

Pericarditis

This can occur within the first few days, causing pain that is sharp in nature and varies with posture and respiration. The diagnosis can be confirmed by a pericardial rub. If troublesome, it may be treated with high-dose aspirin, non-steroidal anti-inflammatory drugs (NSAIDs) or steroids. Dressler's syndrome is fever, leucocytosis, pericarditis and serositis occurring up to 3 months after

MI because of an autoimmune response to the damaged myocardium. Treatment is as for pericarditis.

Rehabilitation

Rehabilitation is aimed at restoring the patient to as full a life as possible and must take into account physical, physiological and socioeconomic factors. The process should start as soon as possible after hospital admission and should be continued in the succeeding weeks and months. Depression and denial are common. Lifestyle advice should be individualized and include advice on diet, exercise and smoking cessation.

Secondary prevention

Smoking

Observational studies show that those who stop smoking have a mortality in the succeeding years of less than half that of those who continue to smoke. It is potentially the most effective of all the secondary prevention measures. All smokers should be counselled to stop smoking. Nicotine replacement therapy may be of value.

Hypertension

The blood pressure should be controlled to below 130/85 mmHg.

Fasting glucose, lipids and diet

Assessment for diabetes before discharge is essential as it indicates a worse prognosis. Immediately after MI, lipid levels are unreliable and all patients should be on statin therapy. Fasting lipid levels should be part of routine follow-up in clinic over subsequent years.

All patients should be discharged on the 'big four' drugs (listed below) unless contraindicated, because all show benefit in secondary prevention.

Weight reduction should be encouraged if overweight by a combination of diet and exercise.

Antiplatelet treatment

Aspirin 75 mg daily reduces the risk of reinfarction and death by 25%. There is no clear benefit of oral anticoagulation over antiplatelet therapy, although it may be considered for patients with left ventricular aneurysm, atrial fibrillation or echocardiographically proven left ventricular thrombus.

Beta-blockers

Beta-blockers reduce the risk of mortality and reinfarction by 20–25%. Approximately 25% of patients have relative contraindications to beta-blockers because of uncontrolled heart failure, respiratory disease or other conditions. Calcium channel blockers such as diltiazem and verapamil may be used if beta-blockers are contraindicated.

Angiotensin-converting-enzyme inhibitors

Provided there are no contraindications, ACE inhibitors are of benefit to all after MI. However, patients at low risk gain only marginal benefit, and these drugs are often reserved for people with clinical or echocardiographic signs of heart failure or anterior MI.

Lipid-lowering agents

There are clear benefits from treatment with statins. The risk of subsequent major coronary heart disease events is lowered. All subgroups of patients appear to benefit from treatment even if initial levels of cholesterol are 'normal'.

ARRHYTHMIAS

Introduction

An arrhythmia is a disturbance of normal sinus cardiac rhythm. Arrhythmias are very common, often intermittent, but may cause cardiac compromise. They are commonly secondary to IHD, particularly after MI. Ventricular ectopic beats are extremely common in the first 24 h following an MI, but any arrhythmia including conduction disturbances may occur. Other causes include drugs (prescribed or illicit), cardiomyopathy, myocarditis, thyroid dysfunction and electrolyte disturbances.

Clinical features

Arrhythmias may present with palpitations (see Ch. 6), dizziness, angina, shortness of breath (see Ch. 5), syncope, cardiac arrest or sudden death; they may also be symptomless. The history should focus on symptoms and possible underlying aetiologies.

HINTS AND TIPS

Ask the patient to tap out the rhythm – it helps in determining whether the rhythm is regular or irregular and gives you some idea of the heart rate.

Investigations

An ECG with a long rhythm strip will allow diagnosis of the arrhythmia if present at the time of the test. Make sure to look for signs of ischaemia when assessing the ECG. For infrequent symptoms, 24-h Holter monitoring (with a diary of events) may record the rhythm disturbance. Other routine investigations should include FBC, U&Es, calcium, magnesium, thyroid function tests (TFTs) and a chest radiograph. An echocardiogram should be considered to look for structural cardiac disease. More prolonged ambulatory monitoring over weeks or months should be considered in difficult problems. Echocardiography may be useful in diagnosing an underlying structural cause such as mitral valve disease or hypertrophic cardiomyopathy.

Finally, electrophysiological studies may reveal an arrhythmogenic focus; radiofrequency ablation can destroy this focus and response to treatment may be assessed, but this is only available in specialized centres.

Supraventricular arrhythmias

Sinus tachycardia

This is defined as a heart rate of >100 bpm originating from the SA node. It can be entirely physiological (e.g. during exercise), but may be pathological. Causes include anaemia, pulmonary embolism, pain, sepsis, thyroid toxicosis, hypovolaemia or heart failure. Treating the underlying cause should resolve the tachycardia. Rarely patients suffer with idiopathic inappropriate sinus tachycardia, which is though to be due to abnormal autonomic tone.

Atrial fibrillation

Aetiology and pathophysiology

This is an irregular, chaotic atrial rhythm at a rate of 300–600 bpm. It is transmitted to the ventricles via the AV node at different intervals leading to an irregular heart rate, dependent on the speed of conduction and refractoriness down the AV node. The incidence rises with age and is over 10% in those over 75 years old. It may be idiopathic, secondary to chronic heart disease or a response to acute illness. Causes include:

- IHD.
- Mitral valve disease.
- Hyperthyroidism.
- Hypertension.
- Cardiomyopathy.
- Excess alcohol consumption.
- Pericarditis.
- Pneumonia.
- Atrial myxoma.
- Endocarditis.
- Infiltrative diseases of the heart (e.g. sarcoidosis).

Clinically, there is an irregularly irregular pulse and the apical rate can be greater than the rate at the radial artery since the pulse volume varies. The first heart sound is of variable intensity.

The ECG shows absent P waves and irregular narrow complex QRS complexes (unless there is associated BBB) (Fig. 30.10).

Complications

The most common complication associated with AF is thromboembolic disease. Poor synchronization of atrial contraction results in the formation of thrombus. The thrombus can embolize anywhere in the systemic circulation, but frequently causes stroke, although ischaemic gut is also encountered. Patients should therefore be anticoagulated to reduce the risk of systemic emboli. Anticoagulation can be achieved with either warfarin or aspirin depending on risk profile (CHADS score). If the patient has contraindications to warfarin, aspirin should be used but it is less effective in preventing strokes. A new oral anticoagulation agent, dabigatran etexilate, is a direct thrombin inhibitor. Current trials are looking promising and NICE are in the process of its technical appraisal. It is likely that it will play a major role in anticoagulation for patients with atrial fibrillation, mechanical heart valves or post orthopaedic operations.

Heart failure can be a result of uncontrolled AF. The management of heart failure is discussed in this chapter.

Management

In long-standing atrial fibrillation there is debate as to whether conversion back to sinus rhythm or simple rate control is best. The ventricular rate can usually be

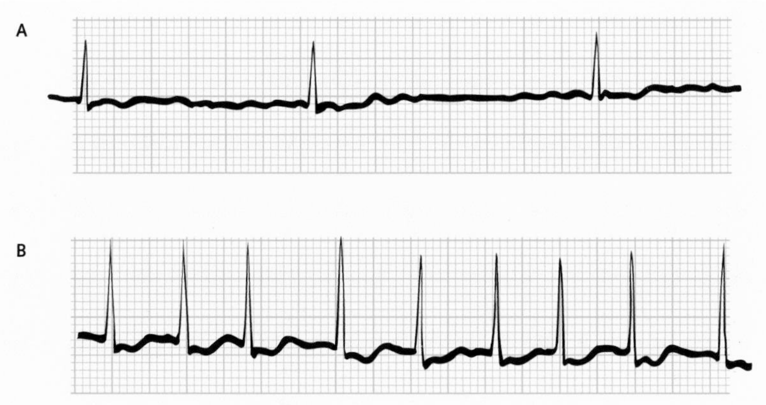

Fig. 30.10 Electrocardiogram of atrial fibrillation with a slow ventricular rate (A) and fast ventricular rate (B).

controlled with a beta-blocker, calcium antagonist or digoxin. Other classes of drug may sometimes be required. If the atrial fibrillation is of recent onset, DC cardioversion or intravenous flecainide to restore sinus rhythm may be attempted. After more than 2 days of atrial fibrillation the patient should be fully anticoagulated for at least 1 month before cardioversion. If this is unsuccessful, the aim is control of the ventricular rate.

Atrial flutter

This is due to a regular circus movement of continuous atrial depolarization. As the AV node cannot conduct that fast, it is usually transmitted with a degree of block (e.g. 2:1, 3:1, etc.).

The causes and treatment are similar to those for atrial fibrillation.

The ECG shows a 'sawtooth' appearance to the baseline at 300 bpm due to flutter or F waves (Fig. 30.11). The ventricular rate is usually divisible into this (e.g. 150 bpm in 2:1 block or 100 bpm in 3:1 block).

> **HINTS AND TIPS**
>
> If the heart rate is 150 bpm, always consider atrial flutter with 2:1 block as the diagnosis.

Paroxysmal supraventricular tachycardias

Paroxysmal SVT is normally due to the presence of a second pathway between the atria and ventricles. An impulse is conducted normally through one AV connection and is then conducted retrogradely up the other, causing a premature atrial contraction. This is then conducted down the first AV connection. On each occasion, the ventricle also depolarizes, giving rise to a fast ventricular rate. The refractory period for an accessory pathway may be shorter than the AV node, leading to ventricular rates exceeding 200 bpm. Broadly speaking, supraventricular tachycardias are divided into AV re-entry (AVRT) and AV nodal non-re-entry tachycardias (AVNRT) rhythms.

AVNRT

This is the commonest cause of a narrow complex tachycardia. By definition the re-entry is through the AV node. The predominant symptom is palpitations. The condition is commonly benign and may require no treatment beyond termination of the tachycardia (see below).

AVRT

This condition is due to a re-entry accessory circuit not involving the AV node. Patients tend to present at a younger age, as these pathways are often congenital and specialist referral is mandatory. AVRT frequently settle with flecainide, but may require accessory pathway ablation to cure the condition. Wolff–Parkinson–White (WPW) syndrome is an example of a congenital AVRT.

Management

Non-pharmacological

Initially, try vagal stimulation, which can be achieved in the following ways:

- Valsalva manoeuvre: ask the patient to blow against resistance (the closed glottis) for approximately 15 s, as if straining at stool. The tachycardia usually terminates in the relaxation (parasympathetic) phase.
- Carotid sinus massage: massage of the carotid artery at the level of the thyroid cartilage.
- Diving reflex: the patient holds his breath while the face is wetted with cold water.
- Eye pressure: this should not now be done as it may cause retinal detachment.

> **HINTS AND TIPS**
>
> Intravenous adenosine can be administered to reveal the underlying rhythm in supraventricular tachycardias by temporarily blocking the AV node.

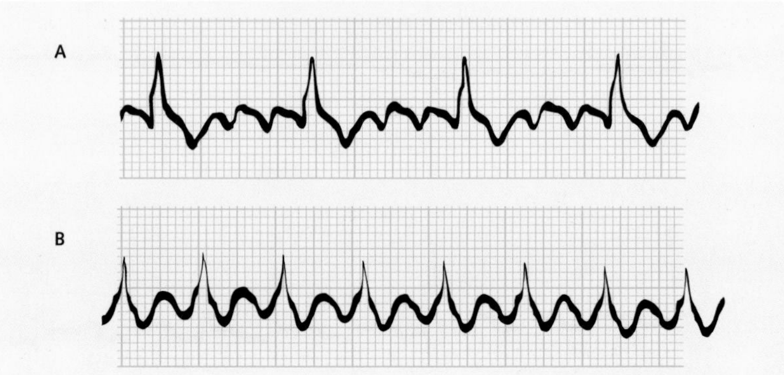

Fig. 30.11 Electrocardiogram of atrial flutter. (A) Atrial flutter with 4:1 block. (B) Atrial flutter with 2:1 block.

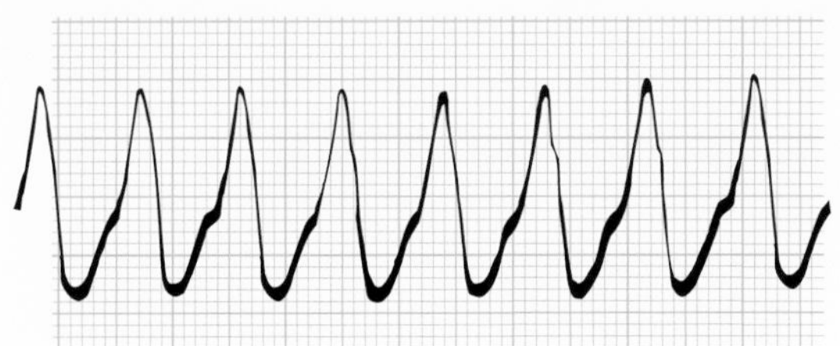

Fig. 30.12 Electrocardiogram of ventricular tachycardia.

Pharmacological

Intravenous adenosine is the treatment of choice in AVNRT. Digoxin or intravenous beta-blockers may also be effective, although care must be taken if there is any evidence of pre-excitation. Intravenous verapamil can be useful for patients without MI or valvular disease. If the arrhythmia is poorly tolerated, synchronized DC shock usually provides rapid relief.

Potassium and magnesium levels should be checked and corrected.

If the patient is already on digoxin, the levels should be checked to exclude toxicity.

Ventricular tachycardia

Diagnosis

VT is defined as three or more consecutive ventricular extrasystoles with a rate greater than 120 bpm (Fig. 30.12).

Management

If there is no pulse, or circulatory collapse, then treat with DC shock as per advanced life support algorithms or synchronized DC cardioversion, respectively. If conscious, the patient will require an anaesthetic. Electrolyte abnormalities should be corrected. If the patient has a stable blood pressure, then response to amiodarone can be assessed in a monitored environment.

Drug treatment is also used for prophylaxis of recurrent attacks. The most common setting is after MI; amiodarone is the preferred therapy for emergency use. Other options include lidocaine or procainamide.

Torsades de pointes ('twisting of the points')

This is a special form of so-called 'polymorphic' VT, which tends to occur in the presence of a long QT interval. It may progress to VF and is often refractory to treatment, which is with intravenous magnesium sulphate. Antiarrhythmics may further prolong the QT interval and worsen the condition. Overdrive pacing may be effective.

Ventricular fibrillation

VF is an emergency and requires immediate Advanced Life Support©, DC shock with cardiopulmonary resuscitation (Fig. 30.13).

HINTS AND TIPS

Patients have different interpretations of the word 'palpitations'. Make sure they are clear with what is meant. They may mean a fast rate or a sensation of a single beat, or an awareness of normal heart rate. Tap out different rates or rhythms for them to get more information.

Bradycardias

Sinus bradycardia

Sinus bradycardia is defined as a resting pulse rate of <60 bpm. For notes on sinus bradycardia see Ch. 6.

Sick sinus syndrome

This is due to dysfunction of the sinus node and can lead to periods of sinus bradycardia with periods of asystole, and tachycardia. Dual-chamber pacemakers are now fitted as standard, although they will only function as an atrial pacemaker if there is no AV conduction defect.

Heart block

This refers to aberrant conduction through the heart and has three forms, termed first-, second- and third-degree block. As the 'degree of block' increases so does the

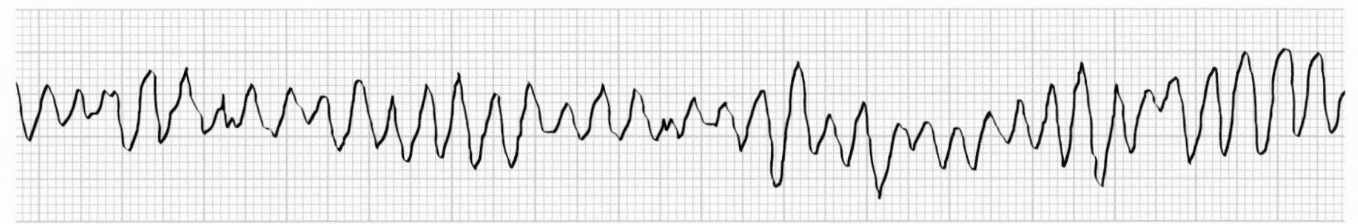

Fig. 30.13 Electrocardiogram of ventricular fibrillation. Coordinated activity of the ventricles ceases. The electrocardiogram shows irregular waves of no defined shape. In this trace there are short periods suggestive of ventricular flutter.

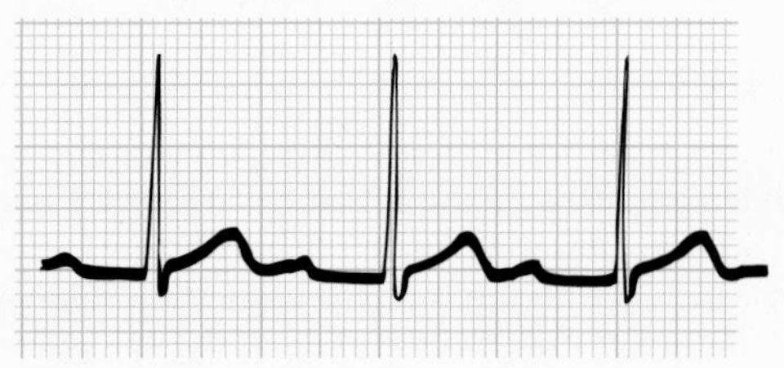

Fig. 30.14 Electrocardiogram of first-degree heart block.

seriousness of the problem (i.e. first-degree block is usually unimportant whilst third-degree block is an emergency).

First-degree heart block

The ECG shows a prolonged PR interval (more than 0.2 s) (Fig. 30.14). All impulses are conducted to the ventricles.

Second-degree heart block

Only some of the atrial impulses are conducted via the AV node. In Wenckebach (Mobitz type I) heart block, there is progressive widening of the PR interval, culminating in non-conduction through the AV node. The cycle then continues (Fig. 30.15). Mobitz type II heart block is intermittent failure of AV conduction (Fig. 30.16). This is the more serious of the two because the block is below the AV node in the His bundle, which may lead to third-degree block. The block occurs in the AV node and hence escape rhythms are more stable in Wenckebach block.

Third-degree (complete) heart block

This is complete dissociation between atrial and ventricular contraction (Fig. 30.17). The ventricular rate assumes a slow 'escape' rhythm with a rate between 30 and 50 bpm. All negatively chronotropic drugs should be stopped. If the patient is symptomatic, atropine can be tried. If this fails, a temporary pacing wire needs to be inserted. Isoprenaline infusion is no longer used routinely. If the patient remains stable or the rhythm problem does not resolve, as they commonly do post MI, then a permanent pacemaker can be fitted as a semi-elective procedure.

HINTS AND TIPS

In complete heart block, work out the atrial rate and the ventricular rate separately by marking them on a piece of paper. They should both be regular but at different rates.

Antiarrhythmic drugs

Traditionally, antiarrhythmics are classified according to their effects on the action potential (Vaughan Williams classification; Fig. 30.18). However, this is now of less clinical relevance than a classification based on the site of action in the heart – supraventricular, ventricular and both. Examples of antiarrhythmic drugs are given below.

Supraventricular arrhythmias only

Adenosine

Adenosine is used for terminating paroxysmal SVT. It is a purine nucleoside, which causes transient AV block. The half-life is 8–10 s but is longer if the patient is taking dipyridamole. It can cause flushing, chest pain and bronchospasm – it is important to warn patients of these prior to giving the drug.

Verapamil

Verapamil is an L-type calcium channel blocker and an alternative to adenosine and should not be used for wide-complex tachycardias unless a supraventricular origin has been established beyond doubt. It should not be used with beta-blockers.

Digoxin

Digoxin is a purified cardiac glycoside (derived from foxgloves) and, although its mechanism is not fully understood, is thought to have its effect through binding to the Na/K ATPase of cardiac myocytes. Its main role is in reducing ventricular rate. It has a mildly positive ionotropic effect. Digoxin toxicity can be dangerous and levels should be monitored.

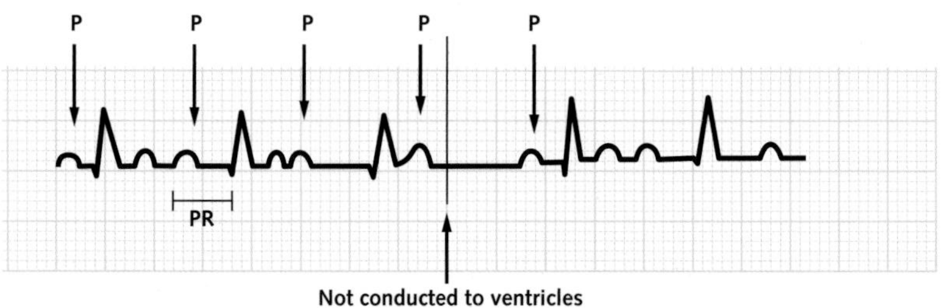

Fig. 30.15 Electrocardiogram of Wenckebach heart block.

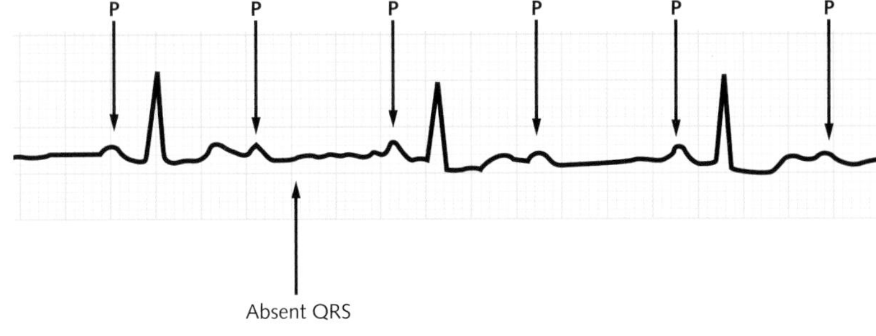

Fig. 30.16 Electrocardiogram of Mobitz type II heart block showing two P waves for each QRS complex (i.e. 2:1 block).

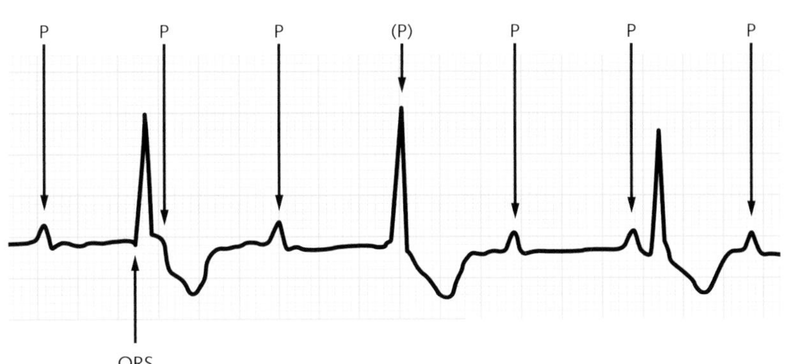

Fig. 30.17 Electrocardiogram of complete heart block. No relationship between atria (P) and ventricles (QRS).

Supraventricular and ventricular arrhythmias

Amiodarone

Amiodarone is effective in both types of arrhythmia with little deleterious effect on haemodynamics. This means it is widely used on coronary care units in acute settings (e.g. post MI). In chronic dysrhythmias, its main indication is in prevention of life-threatening VF/VT. In this, it is less effective than an implanted defibrillator. Otherwise, it should only be used when other drugs are ineffective or contraindicated, and usually under hospital supervision. It can be used orally or intravenously for rapid effect. The half-life is several weeks. It may therefore take some weeks to achieve steady-state plasma concentration.

Fig. 30.18 The Vaughan Williams classification of antiarrhythmic drugs.

Class	Features
Ia,b,c	Membrane sodium channel blockers (e.g. quinidine, lidocaine and flecainide, respectively)
II	Beta-blockers
III	Amiodarone, bretylium, sotalol
IV	Calcium channel blockers (excluding dihydropyridines, e.g. nifedipine)

It is an iodine-containing compound and side effects include hypo- and hyperthyroidism and liver dysfunction. TFTs and liver function tests (LFTs) should therefore be checked at baseline and every 6 months. It may cause pulmonary fibrosis, corneal microdeposits (which are reversible on stopping treatment) and photosensitivity.

Beta-blockers

Beta-blockers act mainly by attenuating the effects of the sympathetic nervous system on automaticity and conductivity within the heart. Sotalol is a beta-blocker that also has class III actions. It is used widely to control paroxysmal atrial fibrillation (PAF).

Flecainide

Flecainide is used acutely to cardiovert patients in new atrial fibrillation, if there is no structural heart disease or heart failure, with good success rates. It is excellent for the control of PAF. In a trial in which it was successfully used to suppress premature ventricular contractions post MI, it was associated with increased mortality compared to placebo – demonstrating the maxim 'treat the patient, not the result'.

Procainamide

Procainamide is used for ventricular arrhythmias and PAF. It can cause a syndrome resembling systemic lupus erythematosus with prolonged use.

Ventricular arrhythmias

Lidocaine

Lidocaine was used commonly for VT after an MI but it can only be given intravenously. It can be used in patients with haemodynamically stable VT to attempt to cardiovert to sinus rhythm. In most situations, amiodarone is now preferred. The dose should be decreased with cardiac or liver failure to avoid convulsions, depression of the central nervous system or depression of the cardiovascular system.

Magnesium

Magnesium sulphate is indicated in broad complex tachycardias in the presence of hypokalaemia (potassium less than 4.0 mmol/L). Magnesium sulphate is also indicated in cardiac arrest for refractory ventricular fibrillation in the presence of suspected hypomagnesaemia or refractory ventricular tachycardia in the presence of suspected hypomagnesaemia.

HEART FAILURE

Heart failure occurs when the heart is unable to maintain sufficient cardiac output to meet the demands placed on it by the body. It is a syndrome as a direct consequence of an underlying pathology such as IHD or cardiomyopathy. The problem is usually one of failure of myocardium, although excess pre- and afterload plus rhythm disturbances and increased demand beyond that of a normal heart's capacity are possible. Failure can be systolic, due to impairment of contraction, diastolic, an impairment of relaxation, or a combination of both. The incidence rises with age and almost 1 million adults in the UK have heart failure. It is classified by its severity (Fig. 30.19). The mortality in severe heart failure is approximately 40% at 1 year.

Fig. 30.19 The New York Heart Association classification of heart failure.

Class	Features
I	No limitation of physical activity
II	Slight limitation of physical activity, breathless climbing two flights of stairs
III	Marked limitation of physical activity, breathless walking 100 m on flat
IV	Inability to carry out any physical activity without discomfort

Aetiology

Heart failure secondary to intrinsic heart disease

Cardiogenic heart failure is due to an abnormality of the heart and can be unmasked when a heart with reduced reserve is unable to cope with the often seemingly minor stresses placed on it. These may manifest at rest or more usually on exertion. Causes include the following:

- IHD (65% of new UK cases per year).
- Hypertension.
- Valvular heart disease.
- Infection: viruses, Chagas' disease.
- Toxins: alcohol, chemotherapy.
- Nutritional deficiency: beriberi.
- Post partum.
- Tachycardia-induced: atrial fibrillation, atrial flutter.
- Genetic: hypertrophic obstructive cardiomyopathy, Duchenne muscular dystrophy.

High-output heart failure

A normal heart is unable to maintain an increased cardiac output in the face of grossly elevated requirements. It is then unable to meet these requirements. Conditions causing this include:

- Thyrotoxicosis.
- Anaemia.
- AV shunts.
- Beriberi.
- Fever.
- Paget's disease.
- Pregnancy.

Such conditions may also cause a previously silent cardiac problem to manifest itself.

Clinical features

Left heart failure

In left ventricular failure inadequate cardiac output leads to elevated left atrial pressures and these combine to give the majority of clinical findings. Symptoms include:

- Exertional dyspnoea (most common).
- Orthopnoea.
- Paroxysmal nocturnal dyspnoea (PND).
- Fatigue.
- Wheeze ('cardiac asthma').
- Cough.
- Haemoptysis (rare).

Signs include:

- Tachypnoea.
- Tachycardia.

- Pulsus alternans (alternating large- and small-volume pulse).
- Peripheral cyanosis and low pulse volume.
- Cardiomegaly.
- Third heart sound ('S3 gallop').
- Functional mitral regurgitation secondary to dilatation of the mitral valve annulus.
- Basal crepitations indicating pulmonary oedema.
- Pleural effusions.

Acute left ventricular failure is a medical emergency and typically presents with severe dyspnoea due to pulmonary oedema. Patients will be sitting up, distressed, pale and sweaty and may even be coughing up pink frothy sputum. Clinical features will include tachycardia, fine crackles and a raised JVP.

Right heart failure

This may occur secondary to chronic lung disease, multiple pulmonary emboli, primary pulmonary hypertension, right heart valve disease, left-to-right shunts or isolated right ventricular cardiomyopathy. It is commonly associated with left ventricular failure, in which case the term congestive cardiac failure is used. Elevated right atrial pressures lead to peripheral fluid retention. Symptoms include:

- Fatigue.
- Nausea.
- Wasting.
- Swollen ankles.
- Abdominal discomfort.
- Anorexia.
- Breathlessness.

Signs include:

- A raised jugular venous pressure (JVP).
- Smooth hepatomegaly.
- Liver tenderness.
- Pitting oedema.
- Ascites.
- Functional tricuspid regurgitation.
- Tachycardia.
- Right ventricular third heart sound.

Congestive cardiac failure

Congestive cardiac failure (CCF) is failure of both the right and the left ventricles. As such the clinical findings are a combination of those listed above. Bilateral pleural effusions tend to be a common feature.

Investigations

The cause for the heart failure must always be sought because heart failure itself is an inadequate diagnosis. After the history and examination, investigations include the following.

Blood tests

- FBC: anaemia.
- U&Es: renal dysfunction or electrolyte abnormalities.
- LFTs: liver congestion.
- Cardiac enzymes/troponin: if acute onset, to exclude acute coronary syndromes.
- Thyroid function tests.

Imaging

- CXR: cardiomegaly, alveolar oedema, 'bat's wings shadowing', prominent upper lobe vessels, Kerley B lines, pleural effusions.
- Echocardiography: remains the gold standard investigation and can assess ventricular and valvular function.

Other investigations

- ECG: IHD, arrhythmias and left ventricular hypertrophy. Finding a normal ECG has a very strong negative predictive value against heart failure.
- Exercise testing: functional severity and prognosis.
- Cardiac catheterization: assess and treat ischaemic/valve lesions or rarely biopsy myocardium with cardiomyopathy.
- Nuclear techniques: ejection fraction, cardiac function and reversible ischaemia.
- Brain (B-type) natriuretic peptide: this a marker of ventricular dysfunction and may help in the assessment of suspected cardiac failure. A low plasma level makes the diagnosis of heart failure unlikely. It can be used to determine the need for echocardiography.

Management of chronic heart failure

General

Hear failure is a complex syndrome of symptoms and should be managed according to recent NICE guidelines (August 2010). The underlying cause of the heart failure should be sought and treated appropriately. Exacerbating factors such as anaemia and hypertension should be treated. Patients should be advised to maintain an optimal weight, avoid excessive salt intake and alcohol consumption and stop smoking.

Drug treatment

These are divided into drugs which improve symptoms of heart failure, namely diuretics and digoxin, and those which are improving prognosis, namely ACE inhibitors, certain beta-blockers and spironolactone. They reduce the risk of MI and increase survival. Treatment is best planned as a stepped care plan in outpatients when stable.

ACE inhibitors

The renin–angiotensin–aldosterone system is activated in heart failure. ACE inhibitors reduce angiotensin-mediated vasoconstriction, reducing afterload, and decrease aldosterone-mediated salt and water retention. This improves the function of the damaged heart. Many studies have been performed using various ACE inhibitors in settings from post acute MI to cardiomyopathy in outpatients. Their effects are class effects, and they have revolutionized systolic heart failure treatment by reducing symptoms, hospitalizations and mortality. They should therefore be started early in any patient with heart failure.

Side effects include cough, first-dose hypotension, hyperkalaemia and worsening renal function, especially in people with bilateral renal artery stenosis. As such, they should be commenced at a low dose and increased gradually with regular electrolyte monitoring. Commonly used drugs include ramipril, enalapril, perindopril and lisinopril.

Beta-blockers

For many years, it was assumed that these were contraindicated in heart failure because the sympathetic nervous system was compensating for the failing heart and blocking this was deleterious. This remains true in the acute setting, where the negatively inotropic and chronotropic effects of beta-blockade can be harmful. However, it is thought that high circulating levels of catecholamines cause progressive myocardial damage. Indeed, the level appears to correlate with prognosis.

Three beta-blockers have shown improved function and survival for patients with moderate to severe heart failure. They are carvedilol, bisoprolol and metoprolol. They can be considered to interfere with the renin–angiotensin–aldosterone axis from the opposite end to ACE inhibitors and spironolactone. These should only be commenced in stable patients by experienced clinicians. The progress should be carefully monitored and the dose increased slowly – 'start low, go slow'.

Spironolactone

Spironolactone is an aldosterone antagonist that was more commonly used in ascites as a diuretic. Aldosterone may act directly as a deleterious growth factor on myocytes in addition to its salt- and water-retaining effects. In a study using low (non-diuretic) doses, it improved morbidity and mortality (RALES trial). Side effects include hyperkalaemia and, because it is usually given with ACE inhibitors, electrolytes need monitoring.

Angiotensin II receptor blockers

Similar to ACE inhibitors, these interfere with the renin–angiotensin–aldosterone system. Their exact place in therapy is less certain. They are usually used in patients who cannot tolerate an ACE inhibitor (e.g. for cough). They can be used in addition to ACE inhibitors as these do not completely suppress angiotensin II production.

Loop diuretics

Loop diuretics, commonly furosemide and bumetanide, are very effective at reducing symptoms in patients with heart failure in both acute and chronic care. They help manage the fluid balance of patients. Side effects include hypovolaemia and renal impairment if diuresis is excessive, electrolyte disturbance and rarely ototoxicity. Renal function should be monitored regularly. They have not demonstrated improvement in survival in any trial.

Thiazide diuretics

These are rarely used alone in cardiac failure. Metolazone is reserved for severe symptomatic heart failure because, when coupled with a loop diuretic, it can produce very profound diuresis.

Digoxin

As well as its effectiveness in rate control of patients with atrial fibrillation, digoxin is a mild positive inotrope because of its effect in increasing intracellular calcium. As such, it may have benefits in cardiac failure even in patients with sinus rhythm. It does not improve survival but may reduce symptoms and hospital admissions. Side effects causing concern include rhythm disturbances, nausea and visual disturbances. Therapeutic drug monitoring allows effective dosing to minimize complications. Digoxin should only be added to patients in sinus rhythm with heart failure not responding to accepted best practice.

Nitrates and hydralazine

These are powerful vasodilating drugs that can improve the symptoms of heart failure and may improve prognosis. Their only use currently is in patients who are unable to take ACE inhibitors. They may be more effective in black patients than standard therapy.

Ionotropic therapy

In chronic heart failure in the UK, there is little role for intravenous therapy with positive inotropic drugs other than as a bridge to transplantation in end-stage disease. Inotropes used include milrinone, a phosphodiesterase inhibitor, and the beta-agonist dobutamine.

Warfarin

Patients with severe heart failure and cardiomyopathy are at risk of thrombus formation and systemic embolization and, accordingly, warfarin should be considered in patients with poor systolic function regardless of atrial fibrillation.

Non-drug therapy

General

Patients should be encouraged to stop smoking. Alcohol intake should be discussed, and those who suffer with alcohol-related cardiomyopathy should be encouraged to abstain completely. Annual vaccinations for influenza and a one-off pneumococcal vaccination should be offered.

Cardiac rehabilitation

Graded supervised group-based exercise programmes and patient education encourage activity and independence. NICE recommends the inclusion of a psychological and educational component in the rehabilitation programme.

Biventricular pacemakers

Patients with intraventricular conduction delay (as shown by a widened QRS complex) have poorly coordinated ventricular contraction, which further reduces ejection fraction. Resynchronizing this using a standard right atrial and right ventricular pacemaker plus a left ventricular pacing wire via the coronary sinus improves cardiac output in some patients. If coupled with first-degree heart block, the effect can be further improved. The long-term benefit is uncertain.

Implantable cardioverter/defibrillator

Patients with cardiomyopathy often have abnormal conduction systems and are at an increased risk of dysrhythmias, in particular VF and tachycardia. One therapy is long-term amiodarone, although its effectiveness is doubted. If the risk is significant, then an implantable defibrillator is the preferred option.

Left ventricular assist devices

Left ventricular assist devices (LVADs) are mechanical circulatory devices that can be used to partially or completely replace the function of the failing heart. Their most common clinical indication is post cardiac surgery where the device allows for cardiac recovery.

Transplantation

Heart transplantation can be performed as a treatment for chronic heart failure. The extent of the surgery and postoperative immunosuppression does mean only a select patient group is suitable for transplantation. Furthermore, the heart is a particularly sensitive organ when it comes to ischaemia and, as a result, the number of organs available are substantially lower than, for example, donor kidneys. The current prognosis for heart transplantation is very good, with 70% of all-comers alive at 5 years.

Management of acute heart failure

This is an emergency characterized by acute breathlessness, orthopnoea, wheezing, anxiety and sweating. There may be pink, frothy sputum and ischaemic chest pain, as well as signs of pulmonary oedema. The first aim is to relieve symptoms and stabilize the patient, the second is to support other organs with adequate perfusion and the third is to find and treat the cause. If severe, the management should begin before investigations are performed:

- Sit the patient upright.
- Give high-concentration oxygen unless there is coexisting chronic hypercapnia due to long-standing respiratory failure.
- Respiratory support with continuous positive airway pressure to improve oxygenation or non-invasive ventilatory support can be used effectively. If failing, involve an anaesthetist early.

Traditional therapy involves:

- Diamorphine (2.5–5 mg IV) slowly with an antiemetic to reduce anxiety and reduce venous capacitance to reduce preload.
- Diuresis with furosemide (40–80 mg IV if renal function normal). Furosemide may work initially by vasodilatation.
- Give IV venodilators (e.g. GTN) if systolic blood pressure is greater than 100 mmHg. This will reduce preload.

Many cardiologists feel that, in acute cardiogenic shock, where the patient is not overloaded with fluid but where it is merely wrongly distributed due to the failing haemodynamics of the heart, first-line therapy should be with a nitrate, sublingual if needed, and that furosemide is of secondary importance.

Treat other conditions that may compromise cardiac function:

- Fast atrial fibrillation: digoxin, orally or intravenously. Other arrhythmias should be treated appropriately. DC cardioversion may be needed.

Further management if the above is inadequate needs to be in a critical care unit (CCU/HDU/ICU):

- Intravenous inotropic agents may be of value if there is hypotension. If pulmonary congestion is dominant, dobutamine is preferred at 5 μg/kg/min, increasing gradually to 20 μg/kg/min if needed. Remember, dobutamine has vasodilating properties and so may not have the effect on blood pressure that is expected. It can be combined with low doses of noradrenaline (norepinephrine).
- If the pulmonary oedema is not improving, then acute haemofiltration can remove fluid rapidly and prevent intubation.

- Intra-aortic balloon counterpulsation in primary cardiac failure may be available (in specialist units only) to support the heart while therapy is planned.

HINTS AND TIPS

Remember LMNOP for the management of acute left ventricular failure: Loop diuretic, Morphine, Nitrates, Oxygen and Position.

HYPERTENSION

Hypertension is defined as a systemic blood pressure persistently above 140/90 mmHg. The prevalence of hypertension differs depending on blood pressure cut-off points, age, sex and race. It increases with age, and is more common in men and Afro-Caribbeans. The risk of morbidity and mortality rises continuously with increasing blood pressure, and marginal risk is greater at higher blood pressures. Similarly, the lower the blood pressure achieved with treatment, the lower the risk of complications of hypertension. However, the benefit of lowering diastolic blood pressure to below 90 mmHg is minimal in uncomplicated hypertension in young or middle-aged patients.

Blood pressure should be taken sitting or lying after 2–3 min rest. The air bladder within the cuff should cover at least 80% of the arm circumference, otherwise, in obese patients, artificially high readings are observed. The dial or mercury column should fall slowly and be read to the nearest 2 mmHg. The diastolic pressure is recorded at the disappearance of sounds (i.e. Korotkoff phase V). Readings should be taken on separate occasions and in both arms before a formal diagnosis of hypertension can be made. If the reading is >140/90 mmHg in clinic, the patient should be offered ambulatory blood pressure monitoring to confirm the diagnosis.

Essential hypertension

In 95% of people, the diagnosis of hypertension is idiopathic ('essential') (i.e. no cause can be found).

Aetiology

Genetic influences on blood pressure regulation have been suggested by family studies. Factors implicated include defects in the renin–angiotensin–aldosterone axis, problems with sodium handling and increased sympathetic nervous system activation. A number of environmental factors are also associated with the development of hypertension. These include obesity, alcohol, dietary sodium intake, dietary potassium and smoking.

Fig. 30.20 Age and hypertension – factors associated with advancing age.

Greater likelihood of hypertension (>50%)
Greater damage when hypertensive
Diastolic threshold for treatment 90 mmHg
As much or more benefit from treatment
No increase in treatment side effects
Elderly should be offered treatment unless suffering other life-shortening illness
Erect pressures should be measured

Age

The prevelance of hypertension increases with age in both men and women. Around 30% of the population aged between 45 and 55 have hypertension. This number increases to approximately 70% in those over 75 years old. Factors relating to hypertension associated with advancing age are summarized in Fig. 30.20.

Obesity

There is a continuous linear relationship between excess body fat and blood pressure levels. Obstructive sleep apnoea is more common in, although not unique to, overweight individuals and appears to be an independent risk factor for hypertension and cardiovascular disease.

Alcohol

Increased alcohol consumption is related to higher blood pressure levels, and the effects are additive to those of obesity.

Dietary sodium

Salt intake has a small effect on population blood pressure levels. Salt restriction may reduce systolic blood pressure by 3–5 mmHg in hypertensives and is most clear-cut in older subjects and those with more severe hypertension.

Dietary potassium

Dietary sodium and potassium intake are generally inversely related. Dietary potassium may have a blood pressure lowering effect.

Smoking

This leads to an acute elevation in blood pressure, which subsides within 15 min of finishing a cigarette. Regular smokers can have slightly lower blood pressures than non-smokers, although the small potential benefit is greatly outweighed by the increased cardiovascular and respiratory risks.

Secondary hypertension

A definite underlying cause for hypertension is more common in younger people, and should be looked for specifically in those aged under 35 years:

- Renal disease: chronic glomerulonephritis, chronic pyelonephritis, renal artery stenosis and polycystic kidney disease. Although it only accounts for 1% of all hypertension, the diagnosis of renal artery stenosis is important as it is the commonest curable cause.
- Endocrine disease: Cushing's and Conn's syndromes, phaeochromocytoma and acromegaly.
- Pregnancy-induced hypertension and pre-eclampsia: associated with oedema and proteinuria.
- Coarctation of the aorta.
- Drugs: oestrogen-containing oral contraceptive pill, NSAIDs, steroids, sympathomimetics in cold cures, carbenoxolone and liquorice.

History

Patients with hypertension are usually asymptomatic. The history should concentrate on environmental predisposing factors, associated cardiovascular risk factors and the symptoms of underlying secondary causes. For example, patients with phaeochromocytoma may have symptoms of panic, headache, sweating, nausea, tremor and pallor. Accelerated hypertension may lead to symptoms secondary to heart failure, renal failure, headaches, nausea and vomiting, visual impairment or fits.

HINTS AND TIPS

In hypertension, explanation to the patient of the needs and expectations of treatment is very important. Patients need to understand that they are taking treatment to reduce future risks and not to improve current health. Work together to achieve a combination of lifestyle changes and drug treatment that achieves control with minimal side effects.

Examination

The clinical approach to the patient with hypertension is summarized in Fig. 30.21 and Ch. 17. Apart from the blood pressure itself, the examination should focus on complications of hypertension or underlying secondary causes. The patient should be examined for left ventricular hypertrophy, coarctation of the aorta (difference in blood pressure in the arms, weak femoral pulses, radiofemoral delay), renal bruits for possible underlying renal artery stenosis, and palpable kidneys, e.g. in polycystic kidney disease. There may be retinopathy, classified by the Keith–Wagener changes (Fig. 30.22).

Fig. 30.21 Clinical evaluation of the patient with hypertension.

Causes of hypertension	Drugs causing hypertension? Paroxysmal features? (phaeochromocytoma) Present, past or family history of renal disease? General appearance? (Cushing's syndrome) Radiofemoral delay? (coarctation) Kidney(s) palpable? (polycystic, hydronephrosis, neoplasm) Abdominal or loin bruit? (renal artery stenosis)
Contributory factors	Overweight? Alcohol intake?
Complications	Cerebrovascular disease Left ventricular hypertrophy or cardiac failure Ischaemic heart disease Fundal haemorrhages and exudates (accelerated phase)
Contraindications to drugs	Gout, diabetes (thiazides) Asthma, heart failure, heart block (beta-blockers) Heart failure, heart block (verapamil)
Cardiovascular risk	Assessment of other cardiovascular risk factors

Look for the five 'C's.

Investigations

In all patients

The minimum tests include urinalysis and serum biochemistry for evidence of renal disease, and ECG for evidence of left ventricular hypertrophy or ischaemia.

Consideration should also be given to the following:

- Chest radiograph: cardiac size and signs of heart failure.

Fig. 30.22 The Keith–Wagener classification of retinopathy.

Grade	Features
I	Arterial narrowing and increased tortuosity
II	Arteriovenous nipping
III	Haemorrhages and soft exudates
IV	Grades I–III and papilloedema

- Fasting lipids and glucose: cardiovascular risk.
- Echocardiography: left ventricular hypertrophy and left ventricular function.
- Fundoscopy: indicates end-organ damage.

In younger patients

Further investigations are warranted in young patients where a secondary cause is more likely, in patients with rapidly rising blood pressure or severe hypertension, in patients with hypertension resistant to treatment, and in patients with deranged U&Es. These investigations include urinary catecholamines for phaeochromocytoma and renal tract ultrasound for structural abnormalities; if renovascular disease is suspected, then contrast or magnetic resonance renal arteriography is indicated.

Further investigations depend on clinical suspicion (e.g. aortography for coarctation of the aorta).

HINTS AND TIPS

Most patients find visiting their doctor stressful and will often have a raised blood pressure – 'white-coat hypertension'. A diagnosis of hypertension can therefore only be made after ambulatory blood pressure monitoring.

Management

NICE published guidelines on the clinical management of primary hypertension in adults in August 2011. For secondary hypertension, treatment of the underlying condition may be indicated (e.g. treatment of an underlying endocrine condition or surgical correction of aortic coarctation).

An algorithm of the decision-making process in patients with hypertension is given in Fig. 17.4. The presence of other risks is crucial to proper therapy. The aim is to reduce blood pressure to below 140/90 mmHg. A target of 130/85 mmHg is indicated in high-risk groups, such as diabetics and patients with nephropathy.

In hypertension, as in many chronic disorders, drugs are best added 'stepwise' until control has been achieved. An attempt can then be made to 'step down' treatment under supervision. Monotherapy controls blood pressure in only 30–50% of patients and most patients therefore need two or more drugs. In uncomplicated mild hypertension, drugs may be substituted rather than added.

As a rule, it is the response to therapy rather than the class of drugs used that is the most important factor. For uncomplicated hypertension in the elderly, combining thiazide diuretics with calcium channel blockers is the recommended first choice. In specific situations, other choices are best (e.g. ACE inhibitors in diabetes, proteinuria or heart failure).

It has been suggested that hypertension can be divided into two groups: the first is renin-dependent hypertension, most common in young white patients. This responds better to ACE inhibitors (A) or angiotensin receptor antagonists. The second group is low-renin hypertension that is poorly responsive to ACE and responds better to calcium antagonists (C) or diuretics (D).

Drug treatment

Thiazide diuretics

Thiazides lower blood pressure mainly by lowering body sodium stores. Initially, blood pressure falls because of a decrease in blood volume, venous return and cardiac output. Gradually, the cardiac output returns to normal but the hypotensive effect remains because the peripheral resistance decreases. Side effects include impaired glucose tolerance and gout. Low doses (bendroflumethiazide 2.5 mg) cause little biochemical disturbance without loss of the antihypertensive effect. Higher doses are never usually needed, nor are potassium supplements. Thiazides are better tolerated in women than in men and are more effective in the elderly.

ACE inhibitors

ACE inhibitors act by inhibiting the renin–angiotensin–aldosterone axis with an increase in vasodilating bradykinin. They are more effective in patients with higher renin levels and so are best in young white patients versus Afro-Caribbean patients. The indications for ACE inhibitors grow yearly as new patient groups to benefit emerge. They are highly effective in heart failure, proteinuric nephropathy and diabetes. As such, they are now often started as monotherapy and are very potent combined with a diuretic or calcium channel blocker.

Side effects include a dry cough, secondary to bradykinin, hyperkalaemia and a usually transient worsening in serum creatinine (or glomerular filtration rate) as intraglomerular pressure falls. Acute renal failure is uncommon without another pathology (e.g. bilateral renal artery stenosis, sepsis or hypovolaemia). Monitoring of electrolytes is essential as the dose is titrated.

Angiotensin II receptor blockers

They block the renin–angiotensin system, producing effects similar to ACE inhibitors. They are effective in conditions in which ACE inhibitors have shown benefit. They are useful for people in whom chronic cough limits therapy with ACE inhibitors because they do not affect bradykinin production. There is some suggestion that they may have a cardiovascular protective effect over and above their blood pressure reduction.

Calcium channel blockers

Calcium antagonists are a heterogeneous group and work in different ways on both the heart and peripheral vasculature. The dihydropyridines (e.g. nifedipine) are good vasodilating drugs that may cause a reflex tachycardia. Diltiazem also has negatively inotropic and chronotropic effects. They are relatively contraindicated in heart failure. They are effective as monotherapy in 50% of patients and amlodipine (which has demonstrated its safety in heart failure) has become the most common antihypertensive worldwide. Side effects include flushing, headache, oedema and constipation. The oedema does not respond to diuretics.

Potassium-sparing diuretics

Potassium-sparing diuretics may be used for the prophylaxis or treatment of diuretic-induced hypokalaemia. They are now also indicated as a 'step 4' medication in treatment-resistant hypertension.

Beta-blockers

Beta-blockers were until relatively recently part of the 'ABCD' approach to managing hypertension. In the recent NICE guidelines they have fallen out of favour and are now only recommended in the management of hypertension in the very young or as a 'step 4' agent in treatment-resistant hypertension. Beta-blockers initially produce a fall in blood pressure by decreasing cardiac output. With continued treatment, the cardiac output returns to normal but the blood pressure remains low because the peripheral resistance is 'reset' at a lower level and renin levels are reduced.

Side effects include negative inotropism, provocation of asthma and heart block. Less serious side effects include cold hands and fatigue.

Alpha adrenergic receptor blockers

Alpha-blockers reduce both arteriolar and venous resistance, and maintain a high cardiac output.

Central acting agents

Methyldopa stimulates alpha-2 receptors in the medulla and reduces sympathetic outflow. In 20% of patients it causes a positive Coombs' test and, rarely, haemolytic anaemia. Drug-induced hepatitis with fever may also occur.

Vasodilators

Minoxidil is a potent vasodilator and decreases peripheral resistance. It may cause a reflex tachycardia, which can be prevented by combination with a beta-blocker. It may also cause fluid retention, which responds to a diuretic, and hirsutism. This is its other therapeutic use for men.

Management of accelerated ('malignant') hypertension

Malignant hypertension or very severe hypertension (diastolic blood pressure >140 mmHg) requires urgent treatment in hospital. Treatment is normally given orally with beta-blockers or calcium antagonists to reduce diastolic blood pressure to 100–110 mmHg within the first 24 h. Over the next few days, further antihypertensives should be given to lower blood pressure further.

Very rapid falls in blood pressure should be avoided because the reduction in cerebral perfusion may lead to cerebral infarction, blindness, worsening renal function and myocardial ischaemia. Intravenous antihypertensive drugs such as nitroprusside, GTN or labetalol are rarely required. Sublingual nifedipine is best avoided because of its unpredictable response.

Management of hypertension in pregnancy

Good blood pressure control in pregnancy is important – oral methyldopa is safe. Beta-blockers are effective and safe in the third trimester; labetalol is used relatively frequently, but may cause intrauterine growth retardation when used earlier in pregnancy. Hydralazine may also be used. Its side effects include drug-induced lupus.

Follow-up

Concordance with treatment is an important issue in a chronic, asymptomatic condition such as hypertension, where treatment is aimed at reduction of later complications; 25–50% of patients default or discontinue treatment, so an effective recall system is needed. When the blood pressure is satisfactorily controlled, it should be checked once a year. More frequent checks are needed during dose titration if the control is borderline, if compliance is a problem or if the treatment regimen is complex. On routine visits, the blood pressure and weight should be measured and the patient should be asked about side effects. The urine should be checked for protein and glucose yearly.

Apart from this, routine re-examination or investigation is unnecessary and should only be performed if there is a special indication (e.g. variable or borderline blood pressure control, or at the onset of new symptoms).

Prognosis

Patients with untreated malignant hypertension have a 90% mortality in 1 year, and treatment is therefore lifesaving. The risk of hypertension in other cases depends on the level of blood pressure, the presence of complications (e.g. cardiac or renal failure) and the presence of other cardiovascular risk factors (e.g. male sex, smoking, diabetes and older age). Those at highest risk gain most benefit from treatment.

VALVULAR HEART DISEASE AND HEART MURMURS

Introduction

Valvular heart disease is any disease that affects any of the four heart valves. It is a common condition that may be congenital or acquired. Clinically most heart valve abnormalities are asymptomatic and only discovered by the presence of a heart murmur on careful auscultation of the precordium. Heart murmurs are due to vibration caused by turbulent blood flow within the heart. The commonest causes in examinations and real clinical practice are left-sided valvular heart disease and tricuspid regurgitation. Non-valvular causes include:

- Innocent 'flow' murmurs, especially in children.
- High cardiac output states, e.g. pregnancy, thyrotoxicosis and fever.
- Congenital heart disease, e.g. atrial septal defect (ASD), ventricular septal defect (VSD), patent ductus arteriosus (PDA) and coarctation of the aorta.

The classification of heart murmurs includes ejection systolic murmurs, pansystolic murmurs, diastolic murmurs and continuous murmurs.

Mitral stenosis

The cause of mitral stenosis is usually rheumatic fever, although only approximately half of all patients give a positive history. It is four times more common than mitral regurgitation in rheumatic fever and is more common in women than in men.

Progressive stenosis of the mitral valve, via thickening of the cusps and fusion of the commissures, results in a pressure gradient between the left atrium and the left ventricle. As the stenosis worsens, ventricular filling becomes impaired, and this is compounded by fibrosis of the subvalvar apparatus leading to left atrial dilatation and hypertrophy, atrial fibrillation and thrombus formation. Pulmonary congestion ensues as left atrial pressure rises, and an increase in pulmonary artery pressure may lead to right heart failure.

Clinical features

Dyspnoea on exertion is an early symptom and may progress to orthopnoea and PND. Breathlessness often worsens considerably with the onset of atrial fibrillation (loss of atrial systole) and is often accompanied by palpitations. Cough and haemoptysis may occur because of bronchitis, pulmonary infarction, pulmonary congestion and bronchial vein rupture. Systemic emboli may occur in patients, particularly in atrial fibrillation. Fatigue and cold extremities are late symptoms, probably secondary to a low cardiac output. Chest pain occurs in a few people and may be due to coronary artery embolism or severe pulmonary hypertension. The patient may have coexistent coronary artery disease. On examination the patient may have a malar flush. The pulse may be low volume and irregular (AF). The apex beat will non-displaced and tapping. On auscultation there will be a loud S1 opening snap followed by a mid-diastolic rumbling murmur, heard best in expiration. A summary of the clinical signs of mitral stenosis are given in Fig. 30.23.

Management

Maintenance of sinus rhythm confers haemodynamic benefit as ventricular filling is improved. Cardioversion should be considered if atrial fibrillation is present and the chamber dimensions are favourable. Anticoagulation is indicated in patients with atrial fibrillation although some would anticoagulate all patients with mitral stenosis. The risk of emboli is greater with a large left atrium or left atrial appendage.

It may be necessary to add in other rate-controlling drugs such as beta-blockers or verapamil.

If symptoms persist, the patient should be considered for mitral valve replacement or valvotomy. If the valve is not calcified and the leaflets are pliable, balloon valvuloplasty may be attempted.

Mitral regurgitation

The incidence of mitral regurgitation is equal in men and women. It is usually secondary to rheumatic fever, floppy prolapsing mitral valve leaflets, papillary muscle dysfunction, rupture after an inferior MI, cardiomyopathy, or ventricular dilatation or dysfunction. Less common causes include congenital malformations, which may be associated with an ostium primum atrial septal defect, infective endocarditis, rupture of the chordae tendineae, cardiomyopathy, rheumatoid arthritis, or left atrial tumour interfering with mitral valve closure.

The circulatory changes depend on the speed of onset and severity of mitral regurgitation. Acute regurgitation may lead to acute pulmonary oedema, whereas chronic regurgitation allows for compensatory left ventricular and atrial dilatation.

Clinical features

Progressive exertional dyspnoea, palpitations and fatigue are common, with symptoms of pulmonary oedema if severe. Atrial fibrillation, systemic emboli and

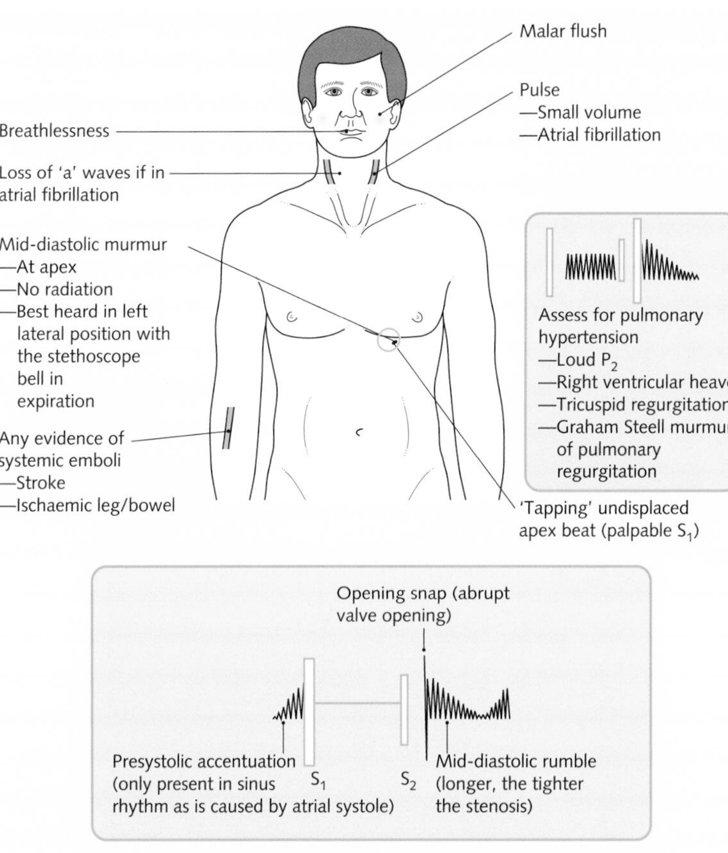

Fig. 30.23 Mitral stenosis.

chest pain are less common than in mitral stenosis. On examination the apex beat may be displaced and hyperdynamic. There will be a pansystolic murmur radiating to the axilla. A summary of the clinical signs of mitral regurgitation are given in Fig. 30.24.

Management

Diuretics are used for pulmonary congestion, and vasodilators are helpful in acute regurgitation. Digoxin and anticoagulants are given to patients in atrial fibrillation.

Mitral valve replacement is indicated if symptoms are severe and uncontrolled by medical treatment, or if pulmonary hypertension develops. Good results are achieved if left ventricular function is preserved, and early referral may allow repair of the valve rather than replacement.

Mitral valve prolapse

This is due to prolapse of the mitral valve leaflets into the left atrium during ventricular systole. Prolapse is common in floppy valves and myocardial disease, and should be distinguished from benign mitral prolapse syndrome. It may affect up to 5% of the population and is three times commoner in women. Mitral valve prolapse is associated with Turner's syndrome, Marfan's syndrome, osteogenesis imperfecta, patent ductus arteriosus and atrial septal defects.

Clinical features

This condition is often asymptomatic and found incidentally. An apical midsystolic click is heard, associated with a late systolic murmur if the valve is regurgitant. It may be associated with palpitations and atypical chest pain, although the latter is more common in people aware of their condition. Systemic emboli and syncope are rare.

The ECG may show inferolateral ST/T segment changes. Arrhythmias may be confirmed by Holter monitoring and the commonest rhythm disturbance is ventricular extrasystoles. Echocardiography is diagnostic.

Management

Treatment is only indicated for complications (e.g. anti-arrhythmic drugs for significant rhythm disturbances, or anticoagulants for emboli).

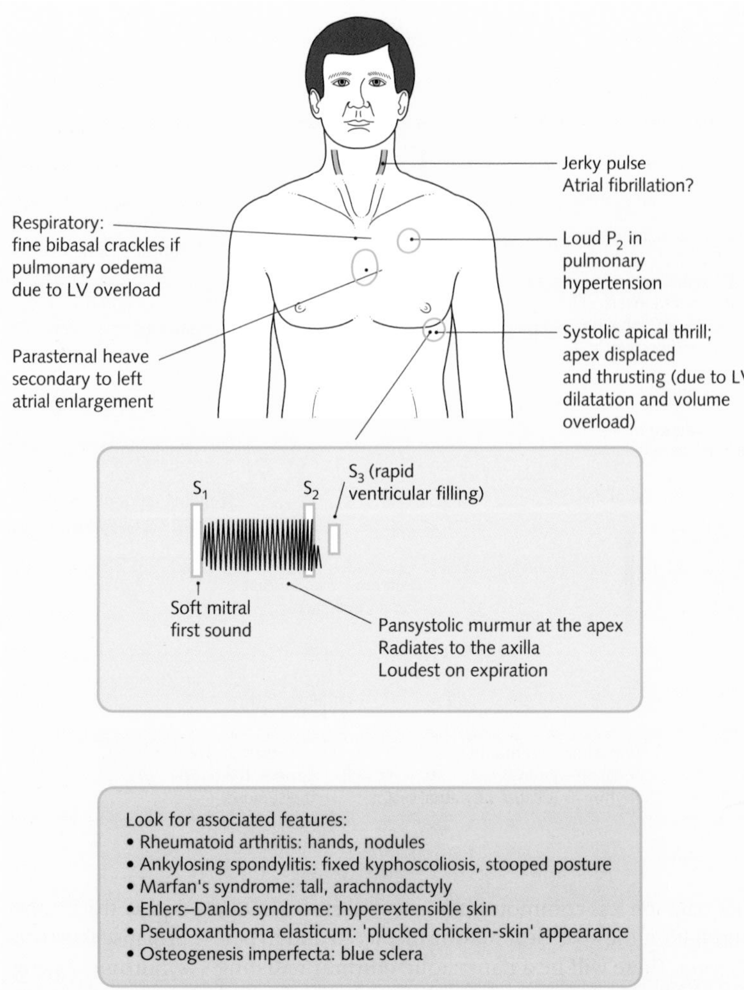

Fig. 30.24 Mitral regurgitation. LV, left ventricle.

Aortic stenosis

The commonest cause of aortic stenosis under the age of 65 is a calcified bicuspid valve, and this is more common in men. In younger patients, the cause may be congenital or due to rheumatic fever. In patients over 65 the commonest cause is senile calcific aortic stenosis, which is commoner in women. Aortic stenosis tends to progress gradually, causing obstruction to the left ventricular outflow with resultant hypertrophy. Ventricular dilatation and heart failure are late complications. Conduction defects may result from calcification extending into the ventricular system.

Clinical features

Initially the patient may be asymptomatic. Classically late symptoms are angina pectoris, exertional dyspnoea and syncope. Sudden death may occur, probably secondary to ventricular dysrhythmias. On examination the patient may have a slow rising pulse with narrow pulse pressures. The apex beat is non-displaced and a left ventricular heave may be palpable. On auscultation there is a ejection systolic murmur radiating to the carotids. Occasionally the stenosis is so severe that minimal flow causes no murmur. A summary of the clinical signs in aortic stenosis are given in Fig. 30.25.

Aortic sclerosis is a distinctly different condition secondary to senile degeneration of the aortic valve. Clinically it does result in an ejection systolic murmur, but this does not radiate to the carotid artery; nor does it cause a change in the character of the pulse.

Management

Valve replacement is indicated for severe stenosis because of the risk of sudden death, or for symptomatic aortic stenosis. Valve replacement surgery can either be open or, more recently, by means of transcatheter

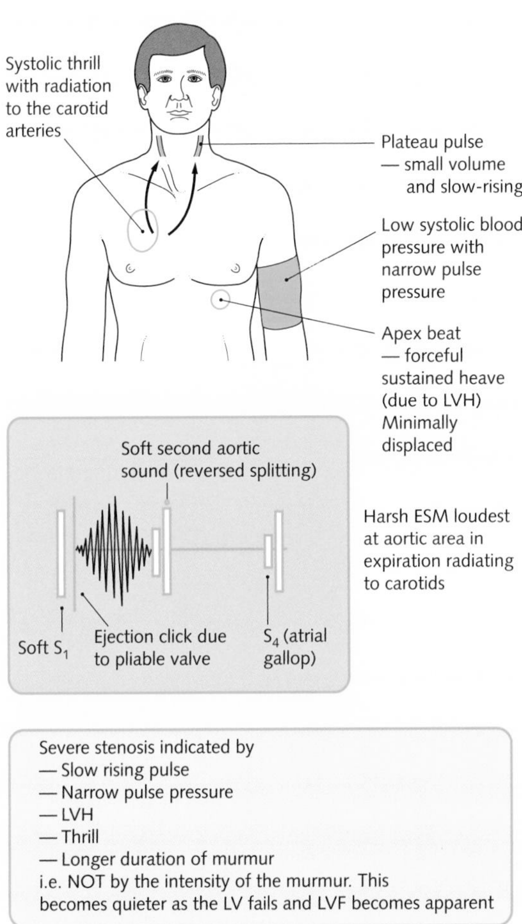

Fig. 30.25 Aortic stenosis. ESM, ejection systolic murmur; LV, left ventricle; LVT, left ventricular failure; LVH, left ventricular hypertrophy.

aortic valve implantation (TAVI). It should be done whilst left ventricular function is preserved. The management of asymptomatic moderate stenosis (i.e. surgery versus medical therapy) is uncertain. Drugs do not alter the progression of the disease, although diuretics and digoxin can be given for heart failure. Many cardiovascular drugs are contraindicated in aortic stenosis; these are predominantly vasodilating medications. The decrease in systemic vascular resistance increases the gradient across the valve, increasing the work the ventricle has to perform.

Aortic regurgitation

The more common causes include cusp malformation (e.g. bicuspid valve) and cusp erosion (e.g. infective endocarditis).

Other causes include:

- Cusp distortion (e.g. senile calcification and rheumatic fever).
- Loss of support (e.g. VSD).
- Aortic wall disease due to inflammation (e.g. syphilis).
- Ankylosing spondylitis.
- Reiter's syndrome.
- Psoriatic arthropathy.
- Aortic wall disease due to dilatation (e.g. hypertension with or without dissection).

Clinical features

The patient is usually asymptomatic until the ventricle fails, giving rise to symptoms of heart failure. Angina rarely occurs. Clinical signs in aortic regurgitation are given in Fig. 30.26. The pulse has a sharp rise and fall ('collapsing' or 'water hammer') with a wide pulse pressure. Other manifestations of this are visible pulsation in the nail bed (Quincke's sign), visible arterial pulsation in the neck (Corrigan's sign), head bobbing (de Musset's sign), 'pistol shot' femoral artery sound (Traube's sign) and a diastolic murmur following distal compression of the artery (Duroziez's sign).

Management

Valve replacement is indicated for symptomatic patients. In the meantime, diuretics and digoxin may be given to control symptoms of heart failure. The prognosis is good while ventricular function is good, but death usually occurs within 2–3 years after the onset of ventricular failure.

Tricuspid regurgitation

This may be functional secondary to right heart failure, commonly as a result of pulmonary hypertension. It may also be rheumatic in association with mitral valve disease, or due to endocarditis in intravenous drug users.

Clinical features

These can include fatigue, oedema, ascites and hepatic pain as the liver capsule is stretched. On examination there may be giant 'v' waves in the JVP. There may be a right ventricular heave. A pansystolic murmur will be audible at the lower sternal edge, best heard on inspiration. The clinical findings of tricuspid regurgitation are summarized in Fig. 30.27.

Management

Treat any underlying cause, then treat the consequences of right heart failure with diuretics, digoxin and ACE inhibitors. Valve replacement is an option but is often high risk (20% mortality) if pulmonary hypertension is present.

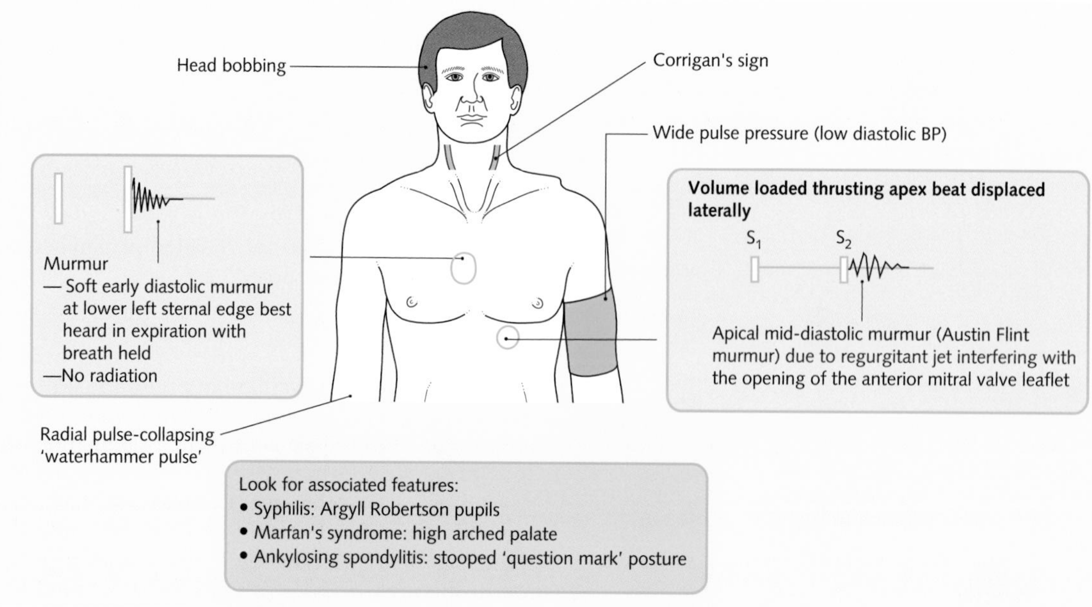

Fig. 30.26 Aortic regurgitation.

Fig. 30.27 Tricuspid regurgitation.

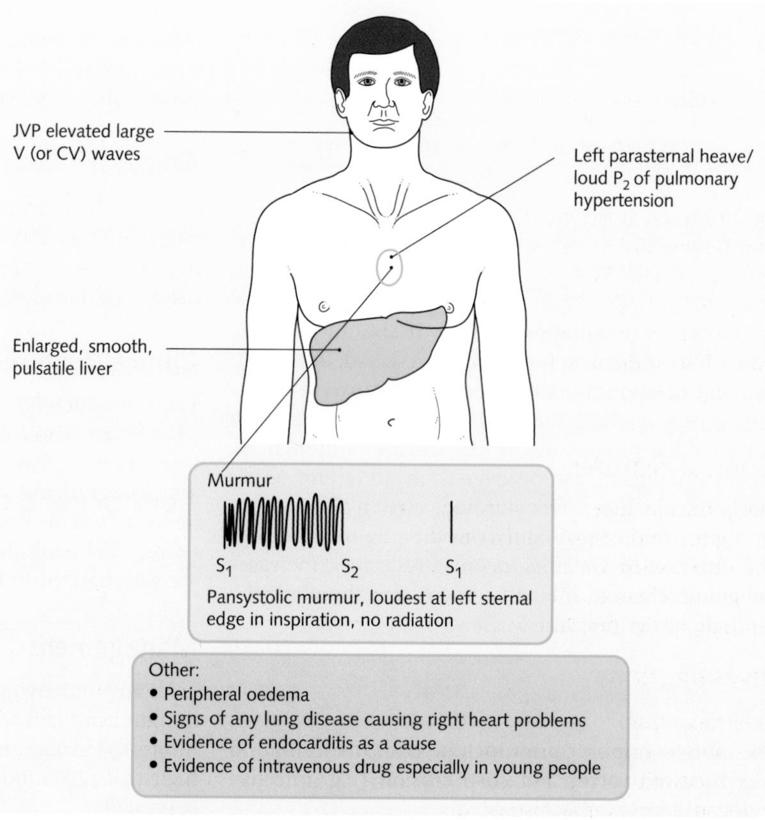

Pulmonary valve lesions

Pulmonary valve lesions are least common. Pulmonary stenosis is often congenital and associated with, for example, Noonan's syndrome. It is also one of the features of Fallot's tetralogy. Pulmonary regurgitation is caused by any cause of pulmonary hypertension and causes a Graham Steell murmur.

HINTS AND TIPS

Left-sided heart murmurs are loudest in expiration and right-sided murmurs loudest in inspiration due to increased blood flow across the valves.

HINTS AND TIPS

There are four things to remember when describing a murmur:
(i) Where is it loudest on the praecordium?
(ii) Where is it in the cardiac cycle?
(iii) What happens on inspiration and expiration?
(iv) Where does it radiate to?

MISCELLANEOUS CARDIOVASCULAR CONDITIONS

Pericarditis and pericardial effusion

Pericarditis is inflammation of the pericardium which may be primary or secondary to systemic disease. Common causes include viruses (e.g. EBV, Coxsackie or HIV), bacteria (e.g. TB), myocardial infarction (Dressler's syndrome), autoimmune disorders such as rheumatoid arthritis or SLE and drugs such as hydralazine or radiotherapy (Fig. 30.28).

Fig. 30.28 Causes of pericarditis.

Idiopathic
Infections – viral (e.g. Coxsackie virus B), bacterial (e.g. *Mycobacterium*), parasitic
Neoplastic (e.g. breast, lung, lymphoma)
Connective tissue disease (e.g. SLE, RA)
Uraemia
Myocardial infarction
Dressler's syndrome following myocardial infarction or cardiac surgery
Radiotherapy
Trauma
Hypothyroidism

RA, rheumatoid arthritis; SLE, systemic lupus erythematosus.

Clinical features

Symptoms include a sharp retrosternal pain relieved by sitting forward. It may radiate to the left arm, or inferiorly. It is worse on lying down, with inspiration and coughing. There may be a 'scratchy' friction rub on examination. Pericardial effusion may be present.

Investigations

Electrocardiography

This shows concave (saddle-shaped) upwards ST-segment elevation, often with PR-segment depression. Inverted T waves may also occur.

Chest X-ray

This is usually normal. If there is an associated pericardial effusion, the heart appears large and globular.

In addition to ECG and CXR, the following investigations should be considered:

- Blood and sputum culture for bacteria.
- Viral titres and viral culture from throat swabs and stools.
- Autoantibodies if there is evidence of connective tissue disease.
- TFTs.

Management

The underlying cause is treated. NSAIDs relieve pain.

Clinical features of an associated pericardial effusion include signs of left and right heart failure. Pericardial tamponade means that the intrapericardial pressure increases, with reduced right heart filling and hypotension from reduced cardiac output. Clinically, there is hypotension, Kussmaul's sign (the JVP increases on inspiration) and muffled heart sounds (Beck's triad), plus pulsus paradoxus and tachycardia. The ECG may show low-amplitude QRS complexes with electrical alternans. Echocardiography is diagnostic. Management is by pericardiocentesis.

Constrictive pericarditis

This is usually idiopathic or secondary to tuberculosis, although it may follow any cause of pericarditis. The heart is encased within a non-expansile pericardium. Clinically the signs are of right heart failure with ascites, hepatomegaly and a raised JVP. There may be pulsus paradoxus and hypotension, and auscultation reveals a pericardial 'knock' due to an abrupt end to ventricular filling. The CXR may show pericardial calcification. Management is by pericardiectomy if constriction is severe.

HINTS AND TIPS

Remember the causes of pericarditis by the mnemonic CARDIAC RIND: Collagen vascular disease, Aortic aneurysm, Radiation, Drugs, Infections, Acute renal failure, Cardiac infarction, Rheumatic fever, Injury, Neoplasms and Dressler's syndrome.

Cardiomyopathy

Cardiomyopathy is a disorder of heart muscle. It is classified into three types as hypertrophic, dilated and restrictive. Fig. 30.29 gives examples of aetiology.

Hypertrophic/obstructive cardiomyopathy

Hypertrophic cardiomyopathy (HOCM) follows an autosomal dominant inheritance, although half of all cases occur sporadically. There is asymmetrical left ventricular hypertrophy, usually of the intraventricular septum.

Clinical features

Symptoms of HOCM are dyspnoea, angina, palpitations, syncope. On examination, there is a jerky pulse, the apex beat has a double impulse, there may be third and fourth heart sounds, and there is a harsh ejection systolic murmur best heard at the left sternal edge when upright or performing a Valsalva manoeuvre. There may also be associated mitral regurgitation.

HOCM may be complicated by atrial fibrillation, systemic emboli, heart failure and sudden death, the risk of which is probably increased by strenuous exercise.

Investigation

Electrocardiography shows left ventricular hypertrophy and sometimes atrial fibrillation, LBBB or ventricular ectopics. The classic echocardiography finding is asymmetrical septal hypertrophy and systolic anterior movement of the mitral valve. 24-h ECG monitoring may identify silent arrhythmias, which are often transient, e.g. PAF or VT. Cardiac catheterization shows a small left ventricular cavity with obliteration in systole. There is a systolic outflow tract gradient within the ventricle.

Management

Beta-blockers or verapamil help with symptoms and are useful for angina or dysrhythmias. Some treat dysrhythmias prophylactically with amiodarone; implantable defibrillators may be indicated. The patient should be anticoagulated if there is atrial fibrillation. If medical treatment is ineffective, the patient should be considered for dual-chamber pacemaker, septal myomectomy, myotomy or cardiac transplantation. Screening of first-degree relatives may be indicated as HOCM is a risk for sudden death in young people.

Fig. 30.29 Causes of cardiomyopathy.

Cause	Examples
Toxic	Alcohol, cyclophosphamide, corticosteroids, lithium, phenothiazines
Metabolic	Thiamine deficiency, pellagra, obesity, porphyria, uraemia
Endocrine	Thyrotoxicosis, acromegaly, myxoedema, Cushing's disease, diabetes mellitus
Collagen diseases	Systemic lupus erythematosus, polyarteritis nodosum
Infiltrative	Amyloidosis, haemochromatosis, neoplasia, sarcoidosis, mucopolysaccharidosis, Whipple's disease
Infective	Viral, rickettsial, mycobacterial
Genetic	Hypertrophic cardiomyopathy, muscular dystrophies
Fibroplastic	Endomyocardial fibrosis, Lôffler's endomyocardial disease, carcinoid
Miscellaneous	Ischaemic heart disease, postpartum

Dilated cardiomyopathy

The ventricles are dilated and contract poorly. There are a number of possible heterogeneous causes, which include alcohol, infiltrative disorders, collagen diseases, infective, toxic, metabolic, postpartum and genetic conditions. However, IHD remains the leading UK cause.

Clinical features

There are usually signs and symptoms of right and left heart failure, cardiomegaly and atrial fibrillation with emboli. Patients may have a permanent tachycardia with a low blood pressure. The apex beat may be diffuse, with an S3 gallop rhythm and potential mitral and/or tricuspid valve regurgitation. More dangerous arrhythmias and conduction defects occur.

Echocardiography shows a globally hypokinetic and dilated heart. Coronary arteriography is usually normal.

Management

Underlying conditions are treated as appropriate. Heart failure should be treated as for ischaemic cardiomyopathy with diuretics, ACE inhibitors, etc. Anticoagulants and maintenance of sinus rhythm to reduce the risk of emboli are standard. The prognosis is variable. Patients should be considered for cardiac transplantation. The mortality of this condition is 40% at 2 years.

Restrictive/infiltrative cardiomyopathy

This is due to endomyocardial stiffening and includes fibroplastic and infiltrative conditions as shown in Fig. 30.29. The commonest cause in the UK is amyloidosis. It results in impaired diastolic function. Clinically restrictive cardiomyopathy presents with features of right ventricular failure. The ECG may show small voltage complexes. The differential diagnosis includes constrictive pericarditis. Myocardial biopsy may be indicated. Treatment is that of the cause.

Infective endocarditis

Infective endocarditis is an illness caused by microbial infection of the cardiac valves or endocardium. The annual incidence in the UK is approximately 7 in 10 000. It follows invasion of the bloodstream by microorganisms from the mouth, gastrointestinal and genitourinary tracts, respiratory tract or skin. Platelets adhere to endothelial breaks and form 'vegetations', which are then colonized by circulating bacteria. Common sites of infection are bicuspid aortic valves and mitral valves, with prolapse and regurgitation.

Risk factors for infective endocarditis are abnormal or prosthetic heart valves (although 50% of cases occur on normal valves), intravenous drug use and immuncompromise.

Streptococcus viridans is the commonest pathogen; others include *Streptococcus faecalis*, *Staphylococcus aureus* and *Staphylococcus epidermidis*, especially in intravenous drug users.

Clinical features and complications

The diagnosis should be suspected in a patient with fever and a new or changing heart murmur. The clinical features are:

- Infection: malaise and lassitude, sweats, myalgia, arthralgia, weight loss, finger clubbing, anaemia and splenomegaly. Fever is often low grade.
- Heart disease: listen for murmurs. In tricuspid endocarditis the patient may be murmur-free. The patient may present with embolic pneumonia, pleurisy or haemoptysis, or later with a raised venous pressure, jaundice and a pulsatile liver.
- Embolism: this is the most common cause of death in endocarditis. Most emboli are sterile but large fungal mycelia may embolize.
- Immunological phenomena: examples include vasculitic skin lesions, splinter haemorrhages, Roth spots in the retina and Osler's nodes. They are classic signs of infective endocarditis but are often absent in cases detected relatively early.
- Urine: this is normal in uncomplicated endocarditis. There may be mild proteinuria resulting from fever, or haematuria as a result of embolism with infarction.

Fig. 30.30 Duke criteria for the diagnosis of infective endocarditis.

Major criteria	Positive blood culture Typical organism in 2 separate blood cultures Persistently positive blood culture Endocardium involvement Positive echocardiogram (vegetation, dehiscence of prosthetic valve, abscess) New valvular regurgitation
Minor criteria	Predisposition (e.g. mechanical valve) Fever >38°C Vascular/immunological signs (e.g. splinter haemorrhage) Positive blood culture that does not meet major criteria Positive echocardiogram that does not meet major criteria

For a diagnosis of infective endocarditis the patient must meet either 2 major criteria or 1 major with 3 minor criteria or all 5 minor criteria

Investigations

Blood cultures

Numerous sets of blood cultures from different sites at different times are the essential investigation. Positive blood cultures are part of the diagnostic criteria (Fig. 30.30).

Inflammatory markers

The erythrocyte sedimentation rate, CRP and white cell count are usually raised. There is a normochromic normocytic anaemia.

Chest X-ray

A CXR with right-sided endocarditis may show multiple shadows due to an embolic pneumonia with infarction.

Electrocardiography

The ECG may show changes of MI due to coronary embolism, or conduction defect due to the development of an aortic root abscess.

Echocardiography

Echocardiography may show vegetations or paravalvular abscess formation. A negative transthoracic echo does not exclude the diagnosis of endocarditis; transoesophageal echocardiography is preferred.

Management

Antibiotics

When there is a high degree of suspicion treatment should be started after blood has been taken for culture but before obtaining confirmation of a positive culture, because valve destruction can occur rapidly and vegetations may grow and embolize.

Patients with endocarditis require a prolonged course of intravenous antibiotics. The exact regime depends on the positive cultures plus local resistance patterns. Benzylpenicillin and gentamicin plus flucloxacillin, if *Staphylococcus aureus* is suspected, is good empirical therapy. If the likelihood of penicillin resistance is high, vancomycin should be given.

Surgery

This is needed for haemodynamic complications with acute severe valvular regurgitation, for valve obstruction by vegetations, for intractable heart failure, for cardiac abscess formation and for resistant infections.

The role of antibiotic prophylaxis

Recent NICE guidelines (March 2008) have suggested a change in practice. At-risk patients (i.e. mechanical valve, known valvular heart disease, previous IE) no longer receive prophylactic antibiotics for dental procedures, GI or genitourinary surgery, bronchoscopy or ENT procedures.

Culture-negative endocarditis

Possible causes of culture-negative endocarditis are given in Fig. 30.31. The addition of broad-spectrum antifungal therapy is indicated if continuing sepsis is likely.

HINTS AND TIPS

Symptoms in infective endocarditis may be very non-specific in older patients. They may complain just of tiredness or weight loss. Maintain a high degree of suspicion in patients found to have cardiac murmurs.

Rheumatic fever

Acute rheumatic fever is a multisystem immune disease following infection with a group A beta-haemolytic streptococcus. Antibodies generated against the bacteria also bind to and damage valvular tissue. The multisystem involvement reflects the vasculitic nature of the underlying disease. It is rare in the developed world because of use of antibiotics for pharyngeal infection. It usually affects children aged 5–15 years but no age or race is immune. Risk factors include crowding and low socioeconomic status.

Fig. 30.31 Possible causes of endocarditis in the event of negative culture.

Coxiella burnetii (Q fever)
Fungi, e.g. *Aspergillus*, *Histoplasma*
Partially treated bacterial endocarditis
Systemic lupus erythematosus
Atrial myxoma
Non-bacterial endocarditis associated with carcinoma

The diagnosis of acute rheumatic fever is based on clinical findings organized by the Jones criteria. The presence of two major or one major and two minor criteria indicates a high probability of rheumatic fever (Fig. 30.32). Evidence of a preceding streptococcal infection greatly strengthens the diagnosis of rheumatic fever.

Major Jones criteria for rheumatic fever

Carditis (40–50%)

There may be myocarditis (tachypnoea, dyspnoea, pulmonary oedema), endocarditis (listen regularly for transient murmurs – the mitral valve is most commonly affected), or pericarditis (friction rub, effusion). It is more evident in children and may be asymptomatic or result in death in the acute stage, and it can lead to heart failure and chronic valvular heart disease (the classic exam cause of mitral stenosis).

Arthritis (80%)

This is the most common major criterion and usually presents as migratory joint pain affecting larger joints. The onset is sudden with signs of inflammation and limitation of movement. It responds well to anti-inflammatory drugs and rarely leaves any residual deformity. Symptoms last for 3–6 weeks.

Fig. 30.32 Revised Jones criteria for guidance in the diagnosis of rheumatic fever.

Major criteria	Polyarthritis Carditis Chorea Erythema marginatum Subcutaneous nodules
Minor criteria	Fever Arthralgia Previous rheumatic fever or rheumatic heart disease Raised acute phase reactants (ESR, CRP, WCC) Prolonged PR interval in ECG

For a diagnosis of rheumatic fever, there must also be supporting evidence of preceding streptococcal infection (i.e. increased antistreptolysin O or other streptococcal antibodies, positive throat culture for group A streptococcus, or recent scarlet fever). CRP, C-reactive protein; ECG, electrocardiogram; ESR, erythrocyte sedimentation rate; WCC, white cell count.

Sydenham's chorea (10%)

Movements are choreoathetoid and involuntary, involving mainly the face and limbs, and may be unilateral. It is associated with emotional lability. There can be a latent period of 2–6 months. Symptoms last for approximately 6 months. It is commoner in girls. There may be no other signs of rheumatic fever.

Erythema marginatum (5%)

This is a painless rash appearing as large, pink macules that spread quickly to give a serpiginous edge with a fading centre.

Subcutaneous nodules (rare)

These are round, firm and painless, ranging from 0.5 to 2 cm. They are mobile and occur mainly over bony prominences.

Diagnosis of streptococcal infection

Evidence of recent streptococcal infection should be sought and is indicated by a positive throat swab, increased antistreptolysin O or anti-DNAse B titres or recent scarlet fever.

Management

Anti-inflammatory drugs relieve the pain and swelling of joints and possibly the later development of valvular heart disease. Treatment is usually for a prolonged period of time (months).

Aspirin or a short course of corticosteroids in severe carditis are the drugs of choice. They reduce the arthritis, although evidence of their effectiveness in changing overall disease progression is lacking. Diazepam is given to control choreiform movements. Intramuscular penicillin G is given in the acute stages and is followed by continued penicillin.

Prognosis

The initial mortality rate is low at 1%. The long-term risk is of structural valve disease, both stenosis and regurgitation. The mitral and pulmonary valves are the most and least affected valves, respectively. Standard management of valve disease applies.

Atrial myxoma

These are rare, benign, primary tumours, usually in the left atrium, which are twice as common in women as men. They present with vague symptoms (e.g. fever, weight loss, general malaise, atrial fibrillation, left atrial obstruction or systemic emboli). Auscultation may reveal a diastolic 'tumour plop'. The erythrocyte sedimentation rate is characteristically raised. They are diagnosed by echocardiography and treatment is by surgical excision.

Congenital heart disease in adults

Introduction

Congenital heart disease is any defect of the heart present at the time of birth. The disease may cause impairment of flow, contraction or electrical conduction. Broadly speaking, congenital heart disease affecting blood flow can be divided into acyanotic (left-to-right shunt) or cyanotic (right-to-left shunt).

Acyanotic conditions

Atrial septal defect

Atrial septal defect (ASD) accounts for 10% of congenital heart defects and is more common in women than in men. There are two types: ostium secundum (the more common type) and ostium primum. The communication between the atria allows for left-to-right atrial shunting. Atrial arrhythmias are common. In ostium primum defects, there may be involvement of the mitral and tricuspid valves producing regurgitation.

Most patients are asymptomatic; a few have dyspnoea and weakness. The patient may have palpitations secondary to atrial arrhythmias, and right heart failure may develop later in life. Auscultation reveals wide, fixed splitting of the second heart sound. The increased right heart output gives rise to a pulmonary systolic flow murmur. There may be a tricuspid diastolic flow murmur with large defects. There may be a left parasternal heave of right ventricular hypertrophy.

On ECG, there may be evidence of atrial arrhythmias (e.g. atrial fibrillation). In ostium secundum defects, there may be right axis deviation and right ventricular hypertrophy. In ostium primum defects, there is RBBB, left axis deviation and right ventricular hypertrophy. Chest radiography shows prominent pulmonary arteries and the lung fields are plethoric. The right atrium and ventricles are enlarged. Echocardiography reveals dilatation of the right-sided cardiac chambers. Doppler studies allow visualization of the left-to-right shunt across the atrial septum. Cardiac catheterization demonstrates a step-up in oxygen saturation at the right atrial level due to shunting of oxygenated blood from the left atrium to the right atrium. The catheter can be directed across the defect into the left atrium.

Ventricular septal defect

Ventricular septal defect (VSD) is the most common congenital heart lesion, accounting for approximately one-third of all malformations. Blood moves from the high-pressure left ventricle to the right ventricle. If the defect is large, pulmonary flow increases, leading to obliterative pulmonary vascular changes and an increase in pulmonary vascular resistance. The pulmonary arterial pressure may then equal the systemic pressure, reducing or reversing the shunt, and central cyanosis may develop (Eisenmenger's syndrome).

A small defect (maladie de Roger) may cause no symptoms but there is a loud pansystolic murmur at the left sternal edge; it may close spontaneously. Larger VSDs produce dyspnoea and fatigue, and the pulse volume may be decreased. The apex beat is prominent as a result of left ventricular hypertrophy, and there may be a left parasternal heave if there is right ventricular hypertrophy with pulmonary hypertension. There is a thrill at the left sternal edge, as well as a pansystolic murmur in the same place. A mitral diastolic flow murmur implies a large shunt.

ECG can show no changes in small VSDs and features of right and left ventricular hypertrophy. Chest X-ray may be normal if the defect is small. Prominent pulmonary arteries are present in pulmonary hypertension. There may be left atrial and ventricular enlargement. Echocardiography is diagnostic if the defect can be imaged. Doppler studies identify abnormal flow across the septum. Cardiac catheterization will show a step-up in oxygen saturation at the right ventricular level due to shunting of oxygenated blood from the left ventricle to the right ventricle. Left ventricular angiography produces opacification of the right ventricle through the defect.

Moderate and large defects should be closed surgically to prevent pulmonary hypertension and Eisenmenger's syndrome.

Patent ductus arteriosus

Patent ductus arteriosus (PDA) accounts for approximately 10% of congenital heart defects and is more common in women. The ductus arteriosus connects the pulmonary artery to the descending aorta but should close off at birth. Because the aortic pressure is higher than the pulmonary artery pressure throughout the cardiac cycle, the PDA produces continuous shunting from the aorta to the pulmonary artery, leading to increased pulmonary venous return to the left heart and an increased left ventricular volume load.

There are usually no symptoms. Large defects lead to left ventricular failure with dyspnoea. The pulse is collapsing. There may be left ventricular hypertrophy. There is a continuous 'machinery' murmur with systolic accentuation loudest in the first or second left intercostal space.

Electrocardiography shows features of left atrial and left ventricular hypertrophy and on chest X-ray the aorta and pulmonary arteries are prominent. The lung fields are plethoric. At echocardiography, there is dilatation of the left-sided cardiac chambers and Doppler studies identify the abnormal flow across the ductus. Cardiac catheterization demonstrates a step-up in oxygen saturation at pulmonary artery level. The catheter can sometimes be passed across the ductus into the descending aorta.

Indometacin given within the first few days of birth may stimulate duct closure by inhibiting prostaglandin synthesis. If this fails, the duct can be ligated surgically or with an umbrella occlusion device.

Aortic coarctation

This accounts for 5–7% of congenital heart defects. It is twice as common in men and is associated with Turner's syndrome, Marfan's syndrome and berry aneurysms. There is a narrowing of the aorta at or just distal to the ductus arteriosus; the vast majority are distal to the origin of the left subclavian artery. The condition is a cause of secondary hypertension. It encourages the formation of a collateral arterial circulation involving the intercostal arteries. In 30% of patients, there is an associated bicuspid aortic valve.

In adults, the condition is often asymptomatic until long-standing hypertension becomes apparent. When present, symptoms include headache, left ventricular failure, stroke and endocarditis. On examination, the femoral pulses are weak or absent and there is radiofemoral delay. The upper limbs may be hypertensive or have unequal blood pressure, and the lower limbs have a low pressure. There may be features of left ventricular hypertrophy. There is a mid- or late systolic murmur over the upper praecordium or back due to turbulent flow through the coarctation. Collateral murmurs may be heard over the scapulae and there may be an aortic systolic murmur of an associated bicuspid valve.

There may be left ventricular hypertrophy on ECG, and chest radiography shows tortuous and dilated collaterals that may erode the undersurface of the ribs to produce 'rib notching'. There may be a double aortic knuckle due to stenosis and poststenotic dilatation. Cardiomegaly may indicate left ventricular enlargement. MRI and aortography confirm the diagnosis.

Treatment is by surgical resection. Angioplasty is an alternative.

Aortic and pulmonary stenosis

Aortic stenosis and its clinical features and management has been covered previously in this chapter. The commonest congenital abnormality is a bicuspid valve (1–2%) which results in chronic turbulent flow resulting in calcification of the leaflets. Supravalvular aortic stenosis is also associated with Williams syndrome.

Pulmonary stenosis is rare and often asymptomatic until severe when symptoms include exertional dyspnoea, light-headednessand and eventually symptoms of right heart failure. It is associated with Noonan's syndrome and Alagille syndrome. In general, invasive intervention is recommended, and often valvotomy is very effective.

Cyanotic conditions

Tetralogy of Fallot

This represents 6–10% of cases of congenital heart disease. The four features comprising the tetrad are as follows:

- VSD.
- Right ventricular outflow obstruction (pulmonary stenosis – infundibular or valvar).
- The aorta is positioned over the ventricular septum ('overriding aorta').
- Right ventricular hypertrophy.

Because there is right ventricular outflow obstruction, the shunt through the VSD is from right to left. This results in central cyanosis.

Children may present with deep cyanosis and syncope. Squatting helps to decrease the right-to-left shunt by increasing systemic resistance. Signs include cyanosis and finger clubbing. There is a parasternal heave and systolic murmur in the pulmonary area (second left intercostal space), P_2 is soft or absent, and there may be growth retardation.

ECG features include right atrial and ventricular hypertrophy. The heart is boot-shaped ('coeur en sabot') and the pulmonary artery is small with oligaemic lung fields. Echocardiography can be diagnostic but it may be necessary to proceed to cardiac catheterization studies to confirm the diagnosis. Look for the horizontal thoracotomy scar towards either axilla.

Management is by total surgical correction. There are palliative procedures for the very young as holding measures (e.g. the Blalock shunt, which produces an anastomosis between a subclavian artery and a pulmonary artery to increase pulmonary blood flow).

Further reading

The American College of Cardiology publishes guidelines and reviews on all aspects of cardiology. They are available on its website: www.acc.org.

Evans, J., 2012. Crash Course: Cardiovascular system 4th edition. Mosby, London.

National Institute for Health and Clinical Excellence (NICE), 2006. The management of atrial fibrillation. Clinical guideline CG36. Available online at: http://www.nice.org.uk/CG36.

National Institute for Health and Clinical Excellence (NICE), 2010. Chronic heart failure – Management of chronic heart failure in adults in primary and secondary care. Clinical guideline CG108. Available online at: http://www.nice.org.uk/CG108.

National Institute for Health and Clinical Excellence (NICE), 2010. The early management of unstable angina and non-ST-segment-elevation myocardial infarction. Clinical guideline CG94. Available online at: http://www.nice.org.uk/CG94.

National Institute for Health and Clinical Excellence (NICE), 2011. Hypertension: Clinical management of primary hypertension in adults. Clinical guideline CG127. Available online at: http://www.nice.org.uk/CG127.

National Institute for Health and Clinical Excellence (NICE), 2011. Management of stable angina. Clinical guideline CG126. Available online at: http://www.nice.org.uk/CG126.

Scandinavian Simvastatin Survival Study Group. Randomized trial of cholesterol lowering in 4444 patients with coronary heart disease: the Scandinavian Simvastatin Survival Study (4S). 1994. Lancet 344, 1383–1389.

ISIS-2 Collaborative group. Randomized trial of intravenous streptokinase, oral aspirin, both or neither among 17,187 cases of suspected acute myocardial infarction: ISIS-2. 1988. Lancet 2, 349–360.

Ross, R., 1999. Atherosclerosis – an inflammatory disease. N. Engl. J. Med. 340, 115–123.

Respiratory disease

Objectives

The key learning points for this chapter:

- Define type I and type II respiratory failure and understand the causes.
- Understand the underlying pathology in asthma and its 'stepwise' management.
- Describe how bronchitis differs from emphysema.
- Assess who would benefit from long-term oxygen therapy.
- Know how community- and hospital-acquired pneumonia differ and how to assess severity.
- Understand who is at risk of pulmonary emboli.
- Know the main types of primary lung cancer and why this knowledge is important for treatment.
- Investigate a patient with suspected tuberculosis.
- Understand when a pneumothorax should be aspirated and when a chest drain is indicated.

RESPIRATORY FAILURE

Definition

Respiratory failure is defined as a dysfunction of gas exchange resulting in abnormalities of oxygenation or ventilation (carbon dioxide (CO_2) elimination) severe enough to impair or threaten the function of vital organs such as the brain and heart.

Respiratory failure is said to be present in a patient breathing air at sea level when the P_{O_2} is less than 8.0 kPa. If hypoxia is combined with a normal or low P_{CO_2} (<6.0 kPa), this is type I respiratory failure. The primary cause for type I respiratory failure is ventilation/perfusion ($\dot{V}/\dot{Q}$) mismatch. When hypoxia is combined with a raised P_{CO_2}, type II respiratory failure is present. The underlying cause for type II respiratory failure is alveolar hypoventilation, with or without ($\dot{V}/\dot{Q}$) mismatch. Measurement of the arterial blood gases (ABGs) is thus essential to the diagnosis of respiratory failure.

In a healthy subject a rise in arterial P_{CO_2} causes an increase in ventilation by central stimulation of the respiratory centres in the medulla, resulting in an increase in minute ventilation to lower P_{CO_2}. In type II respiratory failure, this mechanism fails and there is effective alveolar hypoventilation from one of several causes.

Clinical features of respiratory failure can be thought of as those due to hypoxaemia (present in both type I and II) and those due to hypercapnia (type II). Hypoxia causes dyspnoea, restlessness, central cyanosis and eventually impaired consciousness. Hypercapnia causes headache, tachycardia with bounding pulse, tremor, clouding of consciousness and, rarely, papilloedema.

Type I respiratory failure

Causes

This is hypoxaemia without CO_2 retention. Physiological causes include:

- A low inspired oxygen concentration (F_{iO_2}), e.g. at high altitude.
- $\dot{V}/\dot{Q}$ mismatch through, for example, a right-to-left shunt

In medical practice, the common causes of type I respiratory failure include:

- Pneumonia.
- Asthma.
- COPD (predominantly emphysema – 'pink puffers').
- Pulmonary thromboembolism.
- Acute respiratory distress syndrome (ARDS).
- Pulmonary oedema.
- Pulmonary fibrosis.

Investigations

Blood tests

- Full blood count; look for anaemia, polycythaemia, neutrophilia.
- Arterial blood gases.
- U&Es.
- CRP.
- Blood cultures if pyrexic.

Imaging

- CXR.
- CT pulmonary angiogram if pulmonary embolism suspected.

Other tests

- Sputum microbiology.
- Spirometry.

Management

The main therapeutic objective in acute hypoxaemic respiratory failure is to ensure oxygen delivery to vital organs. Severe hypoxia is life-threatening and oxygen therapy is indicated to maintain saturations of >92% (>8 kPa). The patient may be cyanosed, confused and delirious.

While high concentrations of inspired oxygen (F_iO_2 >50%) are safe in patients with type I respiratory failure, pulmonary oxygen toxicity is a risk if the F_iO_2 concentration remains over 60% for more than 48 h continuously.

Continuous positive airway pressure (CPAP) via a face mask can improve oxygenation and allow intubation to be avoided.

Therapeutic objectives include:

- Specific therapy of the underlying cause (e.g. antimicrobial therapy for pneumonia, bronchodilators and steroids for asthma, or chest drain insertion for pneumothorax).
- General supportive care: adequate hydration, nutrition and electrolyte balance, endotracheal intubation if needed.

Type II respiratory failure

Causes

Type II respiratory failure can be broken down anatomically as dysfunction somewhere between the brainstem and the chest wall:

- Reduced central drive (e.g. sedation and brainstem disorders).
- Neuromuscular disease (e.g. spinal cord lesions, poliomyelitis, myasthenia gravis and diaphragmatic palsy).
- Thoracic wall abnormalities (e.g. kyphoscoliosis and obesity).
- Intrinsic lung disease (e.g. asthma, COPD, pneumonia and lung fibrosis).

Management

As in type I failure, the main therapeutic objective is to ensure adequate oxygen delivery to vital organs by administering oxygen therapy. However, in the most common clinical setting (an acute exacerbation of COPD), some patients may have chronic CO_2 retention. In the past, the teaching was that because this patient group was reliant on their 'hypoxic drive' for ventilation, oxygen therapy could be harmful. As a result oxygen was (and is) often withheld. The reason why high-flow oxygen could potentially be dangerous and should indeed be administered with care is not 'hypoxic respiratory drive' but due to oxygen-driven pulmonary vasoconstriction causing $\dot{V}/\dot{Q}$ mismatch. Oxygen therapy must be carefully controlled to ensure that sufficient oxygen is supplied, usually 24% via a Venturi mask, to prevent death from hypoxaemia (remember that saturations of 88–92% are adequate) but without worsening the respiratory acidosis. This needs repeated monitoring of ABGs. (See *British Thoracic Society Guidelines on emergency oxygen use in adult patients*, Oct 2008.)

Other therapeutic objectives include:

- Specific therapy of the underlying cause (e.g. antimicrobial and bronchodilator therapy for an infective exacerbation of COPD).
- General supportive care as for type I failure.

In certain circumstances, non-invasive ventilation (NIV) via a face or nasal mask can augment minute ventilation enabling control of CO_2, allowing the underlying disease to be treated and endotracheal intubation and its negative consequences to be avoided. However, NIV is not a substitute for formal mechanical ventilation if it is needed but cannot be provided. Chemical stimulants to breathing such as doxapram are rarely used now.

HINTS AND TIPS

Beware! Some patients with type II respiratory failure may deteriorate if given uncontrolled high-flow oxygen. The underlying physiology causing this is oxygen-sensitive pulmonary vasoconstriction rather than 'dependence on hypoxic drive'

HINTS AND TIPS

Remember to always note the inspired oxygen concentration when taking an arterial blood gas sample.

Prognosis in acute respiratory failure

The course of the disease and its prognosis depend to a great extent on the underlying pathology and the premorbid condition of the patient. In patients with COPD who do not require mechanical ventilation, the immediate prognosis is good. Patients developing acute respiratory distress syndrome associated with septicaemia have a very poor prognosis, with mortality rates of approximately 90%. In general, patients requiring ventilation for respiratory failure have survival rates of approximately 60% to weaning off the ventilator, 40% to discharge from hospital and approximately 30% 1-year survival.

ASTHMA

Introduction

Asthma is a disease of the airways characterized by an increased responsiveness of the tracheobronchial tree to many different stimuli, resulting in episodes of reversible airway obstruction. It manifests as episodes of shortness of breath, cough, chest tightness and wheeze. These symptoms may resolve spontaneously or be relieved by treatment.

Asthma is episodic, with acute, exacerbations interspersed by symptom-free periods. Typically, most attacks are short (minutes to hours) and, clinically, the patient appears to recover completely after an attack.

In more severe asthma, patients can experience some degree of airway obstruction daily, with accompanying symptoms.

Asthma is common, with a prevalence of approximately 10% of the population in the UK. It appears to be increasing worldwide for reasons that remain uncertain. Bronchial asthma occurs at all ages but peaks in childhood and is more common in boys. However, in adult asthma, the sex ratio is approximately equal by the age of 30 years. In the UK, 1000–2000 people die from acute asthma attacks every year.

Aetiology

Asthma is likely to be a combination of multiple environmental and genetic factors.

Many asthmatics are atopic, with the production of IgE in response to an antigenic challenge. Atopic asthma can be associated with a personal or family history of allergy such as hay fever, urticaria and eczema. There may also be increased levels of IgE in the serum and a positive response to provocation tests (e.g. methacholine challenge).

The 'hygiene hypothesis' is supported by epidemiological evidence and much debated. It suggests that early exposure to allergens reduces the allergic response and hence blunts allergen sensitivity in later life, reducing the likelihood of asthma. Our more hygienic lifestyles reduce childhood allergen exposure and may have contributed to the increase in asthma.

Intrinsic asthma is a term used to describe patients with no personal or family history of allergy, negative skin tests and normal serum levels of IgE. Many develop typical symptoms following an upper respiratory infection, which leads to paroxysms of wheezing and shortness of breath that can last for months.

In general, asthma that occurs in childhood or early adult life tends to have a strong allergic component, whereas asthma that develops late tends to be non-allergic.

However, many patients do not fit into either category but fall into a group with a mixture of allergic and non-allergic features.

Pathophysiology

Many theories have been proposed to explain the increased airway reactivity of asthma. The relationship between atopy and environment in the airway inflammation of asthma is uncertain. Many theories and mediators are proposed as the mechanisms for asthma. The role of IgE, various cytokines and chemokines, mast cells, histamine, eosinophils, leukotrienes, cell adhesion molecules and activated T lymphocytes – in particular the balance between Th1 and Th2 cells – provides much academic debate and has provided new therapeutic targets such as monoclonal antibodies against IgE.

The clinical features of asthma probably derive from chronic airway inflammation causing denuded airway epithelium, inflammatory cell infiltrate, mast cell activation plus smooth muscle and mucous gland hypertrophy. Acute events produce an intense immediate inflammatory reaction involving bronchoconstriction, vascular congestion and oedema formation – the pathological hallmarks of asthma.

A number of factors interact with normal airway responsiveness and provoke acute episodes, including:

- Allergens (e.g. house dust mites and animal dander).
- Drugs (e.g. beta-blockers and non-steroidal anti-inflammatory drugs).
- Environmental (e.g. climatic conditions and air pollution).
- Occupations (e.g. exposure to industrial chemicals, drugs, metals, dusts).
- Infections (e.g. viral and bacterial).
- Exercise.
- Emotion.
- Cigarette smoke.

Clinical features of asthma

The classic symptoms of asthma consist of shortness of breath, wheeze, chest tightness and coughing. In its most typical form, asthma is an episodic disease and the symptoms coexist.

At the onset of an attack, patients experience tightness in the chest, often with a non-productive cough. Breathing becomes audibly harsh, speech is difficult, wheezing becomes prominent, expiration is prolonged as airflow is reduced, and patients frequently have both tachypnoea and tachycardia. If the attack is severe or prolonged, there may be a loss of breath sounds and the wheeze becomes either very high-pitched or inaudible as airflow is severely compromised. Accessory muscles of respiration are used and pulsus paradoxus can develop.

Less typically, a patient with asthma may present with intermittent episodes of non-productive cough or shortness of breath on exertion. These patients often have a normal physical examination but may wheeze after repeated forced exhalations or may show evidence of airways obstruction with spirometry. Occasionally, a provocation test may be required to make the diagnosis of airway hyperresponsiveness.

Confirming the diagnosis of asthma

Diagnosing asthma is usually not difficult, especially if the patient is seen during an acute attack. In addition, a history of episodic symptoms and a history of eczema, hay fever or urticaria is valuable. Nocturnal symptoms (e.g. awakening short of breath, coughing or wheezing) are very common features.

Investigations

The diagnosis of asthma is established by demonstrating reversible expiratory airflow obstruction. Reversibility is traditionally defined as >15% or a 400 mL increase in the forced expiratory volume in 1 s (FEV_1) following administration of a beta-2-agonist or a greater than 20% diurnal variation on more than 3 days in a week for 2 weeks in a peak expiratory flow rate diary. Peak flow diary may be combined with a 2-week trial of oral prednisolone. Once the diagnosis is confirmed, peak expiratory flow rates (PEFR) at home, or the FEV_1 in the clinic, can be used to monitor the course of the illness and the effectiveness of therapy. Blood eosinophilia, high serum IgE levels may be supportive but are not specific for asthma. Very high serum IgE or eosinophilia is not typical for asthma and may indicate asthma plus another diagnosis, e.g. allergic bronchopulmonary aspergillosis (ABPA). Similarly, a chest X-ray (CXR) showing hyperinflation is not diagnostic of asthma.

Differential diagnosis

In a small minority of patients the diagnosis can cause some difficulty and differential diagnoses should be considered:

- Chronic obstructive pulmonary disease (COPD).
- Upper airway obstruction: tumour, vocal cord dysfunction and laryngeal oedema.
- Endobronchial disease: foreign body aspiration, neoplasm, bronchial stenosis.
- Left ventricular failure.
- Carcinoid tumours.
- Recurrent pulmonary emboli.
- Eosinophilic pneumonias.
- Systemic vasculitis with pulmonary involvement.

Management of asthma

Chronic asthma requires long-term management (see *British Thoracic Society guideline on the management of asthma*, January 2012). Ideally, the model of care that characterizes all chronic diseases should be applied (i.e. patient education and empowerment, pharmacological therapy and liaison between different professional groups in hospital and the community).

The therapeutic targets of medications used for asthma include:

- Drugs that inhibit smooth muscle contraction (e.g. beta-2-agonists, anticholinergics and methylxanthines such as theophylline).
- Drugs that prevent or reverse airway inflammation (e.g. corticosteroids and mast cell stabilizing agents).
- Drugs that modify the action of leukotrienes (e.g. leukotriene antagonists or 5-lipoxygenase inhibitors).

In clinical practice, the two most common settings in which patients require treatment are emergency treatment of acute severe asthma and chronic therapy.

Chronic therapy

This is aimed at achieving a stable, asymptomatic state with the best pulmonary function possible, recognizing and treating exacerbations appropriately while limiting quality of life as little as possible. The first step is to educate patients to function as partners in their management. This includes identifying triggers and avoiding precipitants (e.g. smoking). The severity of the illness needs to be assessed and monitored with objective measures of lung function (PEFR diaries). Adjusting therapy guided by non-invasive measures of airway inflammation such as sputum eosinophil counts or exhaled nitric oxide levels may become more common outside of research settings. Regular follow-up care is mandatory. This should involve doctors, both in hospital and GPs, asthma specialist nurses, pharmacists and physiotherapists.

HINTS AND TIPS

If asthma control is poor, do not forget to assess inhaler technique.

Drug therapy should be kept as simple as possible. Many patients find the division of drugs into 'preventers' and 'relievers' useful to understand their disease and its treatment.

There is consensus worldwide that the stepwise management of asthma is effective. In the UK guidelines are produced by the British Thoracic Society – for a summary see Fig. 31.1. Treatment is stepped up when symptoms

Fig. 31.1 Stepped care plan for the management of chronic asthma.

Step	Measures
1. Mild intermittent asthma	Inhaled short-acting beta-2-agonist as required
2. Regular preventer therapy	Start inhaled steroid regularly 200–800 μg/day (e.g. beclometasone, budesonide or fluticasone)
3. Initial add-on therapy	Add long-acting beta-2-agonist (LABA) regularly Increase dose of regular inhaled steroid Add third medication, theophylline or leukotriene receptor antagonist Slow-release beta-2-agonist tablets may also help
4. Persistent poor control	Trial of high dose of regular inhaled steroid Addition of medications not used in step 3
5. Oral steroid	Add lowest dose of oral steroid to achieve control of symptoms Continue maximum dose inhaled steroid Must be under care of a respiratory physician

Treatment is started at the step most appropriate to initial severity, and a 'rescue' course of prednisolone can be given at any time and with any step to cover an exacerbation. Move up the ladder if relief bronchodilators are needed frequently or night-time symptoms occur. Check compliance and inhaler technique, and consider the use of spacer devices. (After British Thoracic Society.)

(e.g. nocturnal wakening, morning dips) are not controlled. Short-acting beta-2-agonists are the first step, then inhaled corticosteroids, which can then be combined with long-acting beta-2-agonists, anticholinergics, oral steroids, leukotriene modifiers and theophyllines added in varying combinations. When control is obtained, the treatment should be reduced to the lowest feasible level.

COMMUNICATION

Asthma control can be greatly improved with a clear self-management plan enabling the patient to lead in their symptom control. Asthma nurse specialists and physiotherapists can be crucial in promoting independence – involve them!

Emergency treatment

Emergency treatment of acute asthma is one of the most common emergencies seen in medical practice and its life-threatening nature can be underestimated by the less experienced. Senior help should be involved earlier rather than later.

Features indicating severe asthma include the inability to speak in sentences, tachypnoea, tachycardia, very poor PEFR, low oxygen saturations, the use of accessory muscles (sternocleidomastoid and scalene muscles) and marked hyperinflation of the thorax with absent breath sounds, cyanosis, absence of wheeze and a tiring patient. Measurements of arterial blood gases (ABGs) and the PEFR or FEV_1 help in assessing severity and will guide management. A checklist for the assessment and treatment of these patients is shown in Fig. 31.2.

Generally, there is a direct correlation between the severity of the obstruction with which the patient presents and the time it takes to resolve it. If the patient is drowsy, not tachypnoeic, making little respiratory effort with a silent chest (no wheeze) and a normal $P\text{CO}_2$ (which is a bad indicator in any patient who presents with an asthma attack), they are NOT improving and, in fact, respiratory arrest may be imminent and intubation and intensive care are required.

CHRONIC OBSTRUCTIVE PULMONARY DISEASE

Introduction

Chronic obstructive pulmonary disease (COPD) is a term used to cover several distinct entities including both chronic bronchitis and emphysema. It is defined by expiratory airflow limitation with an FEV_1 to forced vital capacity (FVC) ratio of less than 70% and limited reversibility to bronchodilators. The percentage of the FEV_1 compared to the predicted normal allows classification of the disease severity.

Chronic bronchitis is defined by excessive mucus production sufficient to cause cough with sputum for at least 3 months of the year for more than two consecutive years in the absence of another condition known to cause sputum production. Emphysema is permanent, abnormal distension of the air spaces distal to the

Fig. 31.2 Checklist for the emergency assessment and treatment of acute severe asthma.

Tasks to consider	Comment
Assessment	Clinical features indicating severe attack: • inability to speak sentences in one breath • respiratory rate >25/min • heart rate >110 bpm • peak flow rate 33–50% best or predicted Features indicating life-threatening attack: • peak flow rate <33% best or predicted • oxygen saturation <92% • Po_2 <8 kPa • Pco_2 normal or high • cyanosis • poor respiratory effort and silent chest • confusion, coma or exhaustion • pulsus paradoxus
Immediate treatment	High concentration oxygen – aim for saturations 94–98% Frequent nebulized salbutamol (5 mg) with ipratropium bromide (0.5 mg q.d.s.) if severe attack. Use oxygen-driven nebulizers if possible Systemic corticosteroids (hydrocortisone 100 mg IV or prednisolone 40–50 mg orally) Magnesium sulphate intravenously as a bronchodilator (1.2–2 g IV over 20 min) Intravenous bronchodilators (aminophylline or salbutamol)
Criteria for hospital admission	Any life-threatening attack All severe attacks that do not respond to initial treatment If peak flow >75% best 1 h after treatment consider discharge from A&E Consider short-stay observation wards for other patients Do not discharge patients in late evening if recent presentation and apparently better as may have early morning dip unless completely better!
Referral to intensive care	Persisting or worsening hypoxia Worsening peak flow despite treatment Exhaustion, poor respiratory effort Hypercapnia or acidosis on ABG Coma or respiratory arrest
Further investigations	CXR (not routine): • if severe or life-threatening attack • if other pathology is considered (pneumothorax, consolidation) Regular ABGs (irrespective of pulse oximetry saturations) FBC, U&Es, ECG (older patients)
Duration of hospital stay	Until symptoms and lung function stable Peak flow >75% best or predicted Peak flow diurnal variation <25% No nocturnal symptoms
Drugs on discharge	Oral steroids for 1–3 weeks Inhaled steroid therapy Inhaled short-acting beta-2-agonist Other medications as per stepwise plan
Treatment changes on discharge	On inhaled medications (no nebulizers) for 24–48 h prior to discharge GP review within 48 h of discharge Inhaler technique reviewed Appropriate lifestyle advice given Clinic follow-up arranged Patient action plan to promote self-management Drug level monitoring if needed

ABGs, arterial blood gases; CXR, chest X-ray; ECG, electrocardiogram; FBC, full blood count; Pco_2, *partial pressure of carbon dioxide;* Po_2, *partial pressure of oxygen; U&Es, urea and electrolytes.*

terminal bronchioles with destruction of alveolar walls. It is ultimately a histological diagnosis.

Aetiology

Cigarette smoking

Cigarette smoking is the most commonly identified factor associated with both chronic bronchitis during life and extent of emphysema at postmortem (remember this is a histological diagnosis). It is the causative agent in 90% of patients with COPD. Prolonged cigarette smoking impairs ciliary movement, inhibits function of alveolar macrophages (dust cells) and leads to hypertrophy and hyperplasia of mucus-secreting glands. It is probable that smoke also inhibits antiproteases and causes polymorphonuclear leucocytes to release elastase. Smoking tobacco and marijuana synergistically increases the risk of COPD. An accurate smoking history should be taken and expressed as a pack year history (20 cigarettes per day for one year equates to one pack year).

Alpha-1-antitrypsin deficiency

Patients homozygous (1/625–2000) for a deficiency of the protease inhibitor alpha-1-antitrypsin have a greatly increased incidence of early-onset emphysema. The protein is a protease inhibitor that protects cells against protease such as neutrophil elastases. The gene is on chromosome 14 and the defect is in release from the liver where it is synthesized. Patients with the ZZ genotype have blood levels of 10% of those with the normal MM genotype. As well as being at increased risk of developing emphysema, patients with the ZZ genotype are also at risk of chronic liver disease.

The importance of heterozygosity for this condition in patients, both smokers and non-smokers, is not fully established. Nevertheless, it is prudent to advise against smoking.

Air pollution

Air pollution with particulate matter is associated with exacerbations of COPD, and the incidence and mortality rates for chronic bronchitis and emphysema are probably higher in heavily industrialized urban areas and in those areas where open fires are used indoors for cooking and heating purposes.

Occupation

Occupational exposure to a variety of dusts and fumes (e.g. gold and coal mining) may contribute to the development of COPD, particularly in non-smokers, and results in a higher prevalence of chronic bronchitis among employees.

Acute respiratory infections

These have been hypothesized as a factor associated with both the aetiology and progression of COPD.

Pathophysiology

The hallmark of chronic bronchitis is hypertrophy of the mucus-producing glands found in the submucosa of large cartilaginous airways. In lungs studied at postmortem, there is goblet cell hyperplasia, mucosal and submucosal inflammatory cells, oedema, peribronchial fibrosis, intraluminal mucous plugs and increased smooth muscle in small airways.

Inflammation in chronic bronchitis occurs at the alveolar epithelium and differs from the predominantly eosinophilic inflammation of asthma by the predominance of T lymphocytes and neutrophils.

Emphysema is classified according to the pattern of involvement of the gas-exchanging units (acini) of the lung distal to the terminal bronchiole. In centriacinar emphysema, the distension and destruction is mainly limited to the respiratory bronchioles, with relatively less change peripherally in the acinus; these are the changes found in smokers. They are more prominent in the upper lobes. Panacinar emphysema involves both the central and peripheral portions of the acinus; these changes are those seen in alpha-1-antitrypsin deficiency and occur more commonly in the lower lobes.

When emphysema is severe, with large emphysematous 'bullous' air spaces, it may be difficult to distinguish between the two types because they can coexist in the same lung.

The chronic airflow limitation that is the hallmark of COPD is a consequence of small airways disease. There is narrowing and blockage of small airways by an inflammatory bronchiolitis and airways collapse in expiration due to the loss of elastic recoil and radial traction to balance the positive transmural pressure. This limits airflow and results in the air trapping and hyperinflation seen on CXR and lung function tests.

Clinical features of COPD

The most common feature of COPD is dyspnoea – initially during activity but progressively at rest. Other symptoms include cough, sputum production (particularly in chronic bronchitis), wheeze, prolonged expiratory phase and tiredness. Patients with severe COPD may develop respiratory failure. Most patients have features of both chronic bronchitis and emphysema. It remains traditional for teaching purposes to categorize patients as having predominant features of one or the other and to use the terms 'pink puffer' and 'blue bloater'. The usefulness of such classifications in clinical practice is limited.

An acute exacerbation of COPD is a common cause for hospital admission and is defined as a sudden worsening of symptoms (increased cough, sputum production and dyspnoea) often, but not always, caused by bacterial or viral infections.

HINTS AND TIPS

Ask about exercise tolerance (e.g. climbing stairs, walking distance to the shop), home nebulizers, long-term home oxygen therapy, and number of previous hospital admissions for acute exacerbations to aid in establishing disease severity.

Investigations

Establishing the diagnosis

History and physical examination should be supplemented by tests of lung function performed during a chronic stable period, pulse oximetry and chest radiography. Post brochodilatory spirometry is essential for diagnosis and severity assessment. The CXR is not diagnostic, although hyperexpansion is certainly in keeping with COPD, but is necessary to rule out alternative diagnoses. A full blood count should routinely be performed to identify anaemia or polycythaemia. The body mass index needs to be calculated for all patients. In severe disease spirometry, lung volumes, transfer factor and ABGs should be measured. Reversibility testing is controversial due to the natural variability of FEV_1, the presence of significant reversibility (>0.4 L) suggesting an asthmatic component to the disease. It may be difficult to differentiate COPD and asthma. The two may also overlap each other. Fig. 31.3 lists the characteristic features of both.

Fig. 31.3 Clinical features to help differentiate COPD and asthma.

Features	COPD	Asthma
Smoker or ex-smoker	Nearly all	Possibly
Chronic productive cough	Common	Uncommon
Symptoms at age <35	Rare	Often
Dyspnoea	Persistent and progressive	Variable
Nocturnal waking with cough or breathlessness	Uncommon	Common
Significant diurnal or day-to-day variability of symptoms	Uncommon	Common

The acute exacerbation

Patients who present with an acute exacerbation of symptoms require a CXR, serial ABGs, a full blood count, U&Es, CRP and an ECG. The patient may be too unwell to perform peak expiratory flow measurements or spirometry. If the patient is pyrexic, and an infective cause for the exacerbation is suspected, blood cultures should be performed in an attempt to isolate the causative organism and thus guide antibiotic therapy. Sputum cultures should be sent.

Management of COPD

Management of patients with COPD is based on an accurate diagnosis, assessment of severity of symptoms and degree of airflow obstruction, smoking status, the extent of disability and ensuring optimal medical therapies are in place (NICE guideline on chronic obstructive pulmonary disease, June 2010). Assessment of severity is based on the FEV_1, as measured by spirometry, which is compared to the predicted value (based on age, sex, height) and expressed as a percentage (FEV_1 % predicted). Stage 1 (mild) disease is defined as >80%, stage 2 (moderate) as 50–79%, stage 3 (severe) as 30–49% and stage 4 (very severe) as <30%.

Treatment strategies for COPD are varied and a multidisciplinary approach to the patient is often required. A treatment plan should consider:

- Smoking cessation.
- Patient education.
- Optimizing pharmacological therapies.
- Pulmonary rehabilitation.
- Nutritional and psychological support.
- Treatment of acute exacerbations.
- Treatment of cor pulmonale, if present.
- Home oxygen therapy and home non-invasive ventilation (NIV) if indicated.

Long-term treatment of COPD

Smoking cessation

This remains the single most important intervention by the healthcare team to modify the natural course of the disease. It should be reinforced repeatedly. Help from

COMMUNICATION

The importance of smoking cessation in COPD cannot be stressed enough. It is the single biggest change a patient can make to prolong life. While it should be reinforced in all consultations, do not antagonize the patient. It can be useful to express understanding as to how hard it is, how addictive smoking is and to not let them become despondent after one attempt fails.

smoking cessation specialists and pharmacological assistance with nicotine replacement, varenicline or bupropion may improve effectiveness.

Bronchodilators

These are important in symptom relief from COPD, and long-acting agents reduce exacerbations. They are commonly given to patients regardless of objective reversible airflow obstruction. They can reduce dynamic hyperinflation not measurable by changes in FEV_1 and exertional dyspnoea. Patients may still find them useful for symptom relief and often become psychologically attached to them. They include:

- Short-acting beta-agonists, e.g. salbutamol and terbutaline.
- Long-acting beta-agonists, e.g. salmeterol and formoterol.
- Anticholinergics, e.g. ipratropium and tiotropium (a long-acting once-daily drug).
- Phosphodiesterase inhibitors, e.g. theophyllines.

Drugs can be delivered through inhalers, spacer devices or home nebulizers.

Corticosteroids

Inhaled corticosteroids in patients whose FEV_1 is <50% predicted reduces exacerbations and improves health status. There may be a small effect on the decline in FEV_1 compared with placebo; as yet, the drugs have not been shown to improve mortality. Fluticasone and budesonide are examples. Combined use with a long-acting beta-agonist is preferred.

Oral steroids are used in exacerbations of COPD and some patients take them long term; this should be discouraged.

Pulmonary rehabilitation

This is an organized programme of graded exercise, nutritional advice and patient education. It improves symptoms and exacerbations and can increase exercise ability.

Domiciliary oxygen therapy

Short bursts of oxygen for symptomatic relief may help some patients. Long-term (>15 h per day) oxygen therapy (LTOT) is to be recommended in certain COPD patients as it has a survival benefit. They include:

- Stable non-smokers with Po_2 <7.3 kPa and FEV_1 <1.5 L.
- Stable non-smokers with Po_2 between 7.3 and 8.0 kPa and pulmonary hypertension.
- Oxygen can be prescribed to terminally ill patients

Assessment should be done when the patient is stable, not during an acute exacerbation. ABGs should be done to achieve the correct Po_2 and ensure the Pco_2 is stable during oxygen supplementation. LTOT is contraindicated if the patient is a smoker due to the potential fire risk.

Surgery

Some patients may be suitable for bullectomy or lung volume reduction surgery (LVRS) to improve symptoms. A variety of bronchoscopic techniques for LVRS are in trials. In end-stage disease, lung transplantation is an option for some, often younger, patients.

Other therapies

There is little evidence to suggest that prophylactic antibiotics, either systemic or nebulized, alter disease progression or prevent exacerbations. Vaccination against influenza and pneumococcal pneumonia should be offered to patients with COPD. Regular assessment of nutritional and psychological status is recommended. Mucolytic agents can help alleviate symptoms if patients have a chronic productive cough. They do not reduce the of exacerbation.

Acute exacerbation of COPD

Treatments include nebulized beta-agonists and anticholinergics, antibiotics if infection is suspected, systemic steroids, controlled oxygen to maintain saturations of 88–92% (if CO_2 retainer) or 94–98% (if non-CO_2 retaining), chest physiotherapy and theophylline if appropriate. Endotracheal intubation may be indicated for severe respiratory failure if a reversible pathology is thought present.

NIV has been shown to be effective in certain patients with COPD and acute type II respiratory failure, with a benefit over intubation. This may be a consequence of avoiding the side effects of mechanical ventilation rather than NIV per se.

Acute exacerbation of COPD often requires admission to hospital. Some less severe cases may be discharged home by an intensive community team. This reduces admission rates and the burden on the secondary care provider while promoting independence and self-reliance for the patient.

Prognosis

In severe disease this is poor, with considerable symptomatic discomfort as the disease process and lung dysfunction become more severe. The involvement of palliative medicine services should be considered. No single therapy changes the natural time course of the disease; in milder disease the importance of smoking cessation cannot be overemphasized. It will not repair damaged lung tissue but the rate of decline in FEV_1 with time will revert to that of a non-smoker.

HINTS AND TIPS

Discussing the patient's wishes with regards to resuscitation status in severe COPD is difficult. It is, however, an important part of the management plan and should be done at an appropriate time using sensitive language.

PNEUMONIA

Introduction

Pneumonia is an infection of the pulmonary parenchyma (i.e. the functional lung tissue) causing fever, chest signs and symptoms and air space consolidation on a CXR. It is a common condition with an incidence of 5–10/1000 population. Many bacterial species, viruses, fungi and parasites can cause pneumonia. As such, it is not a single disease but a group of specific infections, each with a different epidemiology, pathogenesis, clinical presentation and clinical course. Identification of the aetiological microorganism should be of primary importance to enable appropriate antimicrobial therapy. However, empirical antimicrobial therapy is often started without identification of the organisms since pneumonia has a 10% mortality for those admitted to hospital.

Aetiology

Community-acquired pneumonia (CAP)

This occurs out of hospital or within 48 h of admission and may be primary or secondary to existing disease. Causes include *Streptococcus pneumoniae* (most common), *Haemophilus influenzae* and *Staphylococcus aureus*. Viruses are implicated in approximately 10% of cases. In pre-existing lung disease (e.g. COPD/bronchiectasis), organisms such as *Pseudomonas aeruginosa* and *Moraxella catarrhalis* are more common.

Atypical pneumonia

This is caused by organisms such as *Mycoplasma*, *Legionella* and *Chlamydia* species. They can be acquired in the community or in institutions. Detailed travel and occupational and social history are important in identifying risk factors.

Hospital-acquired pneumonia (nosocomial)

This is new-onset pneumonia occurring more than 48 h after admission to hospital. It can be caused by all of the above agents, but Gram-negative organisms such as *Pseudomonas* and *Klebsiella* are much more common.

Aspiration pneumonia

This occurs as a result of the aspiration of gastrointestinal material because of an inability to protect the airway such as after a cerebral vascular event or with a decreased consciousness level. Anaerobic organisms may be implicated. Stroke patients are at particular risk of aspiration pneumonia and involvement of speech and language therapists (SALT) is vital in preventing this potentially fatal complication.

Opportunistic pneumonia

Certain groups of patients are of increased risk of pneumonia. Individuals with cystic fibrosis are at increased risk of *Pseudomonas* pneumonia due to changes in the composition of airway surface mucus. Patients who have an impaired immune system (e.g. HIV positive) may be at increased risk of fungal (e.g. *Aspergillus*), *Pneumocystis jiroveci* (formerly PCP) or viral (e.g. CMV, HSV) pneumonia. Lastly, patients on respiratory support (e.g. ventilated in intensive care) are at increased risk of ventilator-associated pneumonia (VAP) commonly caused by *Pseudomonas or Klebsiella*.

Clinical features of pneumonia

Typical

The 'typical' symptoms of pneumonia are fever, tachypnoea, dyspnoea, cough productive of purulent sputum and, in some cases, pleuritic chest pain. Signs of pulmonary consolidation (dullness, increased vocal resonance, bronchial breath sounds and coarse crepitations) may be found on physical examination and coincide with abnormalities on the CXR.

Atypical

It was traditionally stated that 'atypical' pneumonia has a more gradual onset, a dry cough and extrapulmonary symptoms (headache, muscle aching, fatigue, sore throat, nausea, vomiting and diarrhoea). It is not possible to accurately predict the causative organism from the symptoms. The term 'atypical pneumonia' remains in use but it is the organisms that are 'atypical' and not the symptoms.

Diagnosis of pneumonia

Imaging

- A CXR can confirm the presence of the diffuse or lobar pulmonary infiltrates and assess the extent of infection. Air bronchograms may be seen within the areas of consolidation. Other features that may be present include pleural effusions, pulmonary cavitation or hilar lymphadenopathy. Cavitating lesions may be caused by oral anaerobic bacteria, enteric Gram-negative bacilli, *S. aureus*, *Pseudomonas*, *Legionella*, TB and fungi.
- CT is not commonly used as a first-line imaging modality. However, if the CXR is suggestive of a space-occupying lesion, a CT scan would be indicated.

Blood tests

- Full blood count may show a neutrophilia.
- ABG: assess oxygenation, hypercapnia and pH.
- U&Es: raised urea is indicative of dehydration and is part of the CURB65 score (see later) which assesses severity.
- C-reactive protein: may be raised and can help in assessing response to treatment.
- Blood cultures if pyrexic (and prior to commencing antibiotic therapy, but should not delay antibiotics).
- Serology for atypical organisms should be taken if clinical suspicion is present and then repeated in 10–14 days.

Other tests

- Sputum microscopy and culture is important in severe bacterial pneumonia and those with chronic lung disease. Unfortunately, sputum is frequently contaminated by potentially pathogenic bacteria that colonize the upper respiratory tract without causing disease.
- Pleural tap: pleural effusion, if present and thought to be parapneumonic, should be aspirated to assess for infection or empyema and drained if needed. Microscopy, culture and sensitivity should be performed. If there is any suggestion there may be a more sinister cause for the effusion a sample should be sent for cytology.
- The urine can be tested for streptococcal and *Legionella* urinary antigen. These can remain positive even after antibiotics have been commenced.

Bronchoscopy

- Fibreoptic bronchoscopy is rarely performed for pneumonia but has become the standard invasive procedure used to obtain lower respiratory tract secretions from seriously ill or immunocompromised patients. Samples are collected with a protected double-sheathed brush, by bronchoalveolar lavage or by transbronchial biopsy at the site of the pulmonary consolidation. It may be indicated too if there is evidence of collapse due to airway obstruction/ tumour or mucous plug.

Severity

- The management of community acquired pneumonia is guided by the severity. The CURB65 score is a validated tool to assess severity. Each component (confusion, urea, respiratory rate, systolic blood pressure and age) scores 1 point. A score of 0 or 1 means home treatment is possible, a score of 2 warrants hospital treatment and a score of 3 or above indicates severe pneumonia requiring admission and aggressive management. Increasing score is associated with increasing mortality.
- Confusion: new confusion, abbreviated mental test score <8.
- Urea >7 mmol/L.
- Respiratory rate >30 per min.
- Systolic blood pressure <90 mmHg and/or diastolic blood pressure <60 mmHg.
- Age >65.

Management

The mainstay treatment for pneumonia is antibiotics, oxygen (aiming for saturations of 94–98%), adequate hydration and analgesia for potential pleuritic pain. However, pneumonia is a leading cause of sepsis, particularly in the elderly. Sepsis is a very common cause for hospital admission and has a high mortality. Recent awareness campaigns (e.g. surviving sepsis) have stressed the importance of recognizing sepsis early and treating promptly. All patients who are septic (defined as systemic inflammatory response syndrome, SIRS, in the presence of suspected or proven infection) must receive the 'sepsis six' care bundle. This consists of blood cultures, lactate and Hb measurement, urine output monitoring (potentially through urinary catheterization), fluid resuscitation, oxygen therapy and antibiotic therapy. Antibiotic therapy will often be empirical. It is important antibiotics are given early and as a junior doctor simply prescribing the drug is not sufficient – make sure it is given. The appropriate antimicrobial treatment of pneumonia is shown in Fig. 31.4. However, check with your local microbiology department for their guidelines as local antibiotic sensitivities vary.

HINTS AND TIPS

SIRS – two from: heart rate >90, temperature >38°C or <36°C, respiratory rate >20, WCC >12 or <4.

Sepsis – SIRS in the presence of proven or suspected infection.

Fig. 31.4 Drug choice for pneumonia (this will vary between countries and hospitals and is intended as a guide only).

Community-acquired pneumonia	
Uncomplicated	Broad-spectrum penicillin, e.g. amoxicillin Macrolide, e.g. clarithromycin if penicillin-allergic or if atypical organism suspected Flucloxacillin if *S. aureus* suspected
Severe	Third-generation cephalosporin, e.g. cefuroxime or co-amoxiclav IV and macrolide for atypical organisms Flucloxacillin if *S. aureus* suspected
Atypical	Erythromycin or other macrolide Tetracycline for *Chlamydia* or *Mycoplasma* Give for 10–14 days
Hospital-acquired pneumonia	Broad-spectrum cephalosporin or co-amoxiclav plus increased Gram-negative cover, e.g. aminoglycoside, ciprofloxacin Vancomycin or teicoplanin if MRSA pneumonia
Aspiration pneumonia	Cover for anaerobic organisms Cephalosporin plus metronidazole Co-amoxiclav often sufficient

MRSA, methicillin-resistant Staphylococcus aureus.

PULMONARY EMBOLISM

Pulmonary embolism (PE) is a common, potentially fatal and frequently missed diagnosis. It results from thrombus formation in the venous circulation that embolizes to the lungs, obstructing a pulmonary artery, causing hypoxia and circulatory collapse.

Risk factors include immobility, including 'economy class syndrome' with air travel, surgery, malignancy, obesity, pregnancy, the contraceptive pill and one of the increasingly described thrombophilic conditions (e.g. factor V Leiden or the prothrombin 20210A gene mutation).

Clinical features

Dyspnoea is the most frequent symptom and tachypnoea is the most frequent sign in PE. Dyspnoea, syncope, hypotension or cyanosis indicate a massive PE, while pleuritic pain, cough or haemoptysis often suggest a small embolism located near the pleura. On examination, young or previously healthy individuals may simply appear anxious but otherwise seem well, even with a large PE.

Diagnosis

Risk scoring

First perform an assessment of the clinical risk of PE, e.g. the modified Well's criteria (Fig. 31.5).

Blood tests

- ABGs: often normal, hypoxaemia.
- D-dimer: its main value is as a negative result to exclude thromboemboli in low-risk patients.

ECG

- Electrocardiogram: tachycardia is most common, RBBB and right ventricular strain are further indicative. The $S_1Q_3T_3$ pattern is 'textbook' but uncommon.

Imaging

- CXR: usually normal but may show atelectasis or a small wedge shadow.
- CT pulmonary angiogram (CTPA): the recommended initial lung imaging modality and particularly useful for diagnosing PE in more proximal pulmonary arteries and those with pre-existing lung disease. A negative good-quality CTPA is sufficient to rule out PE.
- $\dot{V}/\dot{Q}$ scanning looking for the classical mismatch defect used to be the traditional method of investigating a potential PE. This methodology requires a normal CXR.

Fig. 31.5 Well's score to assess probability of pulmonary embolism.

Clinically suspected DVT	3.0
Alternative diagnosis is less likely than PE	3.0
Tachycardia	1.5
Immobilization/surgery in previous 4 weeks	1.5
History of DVT or PE	1.5
Haemoptysis	1.0
Malignancy (either treated within 6 months or palliative)	1.0

Score >6.0, high (probability 59% based on pooled data); 2.0–6.0, moderate (probability 29% based on pooled data); <2.0, low (probability 15% based on pooled data).

- Pulmonary angiography is now rarely performed other than in certain circumstances (e.g. pregnancy or acutely ill patients who may require embolectomy).

Other tests

- Echocardiography may show evidence of acute right ventricular dysfunction, especially in large haemodynamically significant PEs in which thrombolysis is considered.
- Thromboembolism from deep vein thrombosis is assessed with compression ultrasound or venography.

Management

Current BTS guidelines are based on 2003 recommendations and NICE is in the process of producing their recommendations. The majority of patients are treated with low-molecular-weight heparin or IV heparin followed by oral warfarin for a variable period. Oral anticoagulation should only be commenced once VTE has been reliably confirmed. The target international normalized ratio (INR) should be 2.0–3.0; when this is achieved, heparin can be discontinued. The standard duration of oral anticoagulation is 4–6 weeks for temporary risk factors, 3 months for first idiopathic, and at least 6 months for other. The risk of bleeding should be balanced with that of further VTE. Monitoring of maintenance warfarin treatment is performed regularly in clinical practice, aiming to keep the INR in the range 2.0–3.0.

HINTS AND TIPS

Many drugs interact with warfarin to enhance or diminish its effect. Ask the patient to report any changes in treatment. Certain dietary factors can also lead to INR changes.

Patients who have recurrent or a strong family history of thromboembolic events should be screened for recognized hypercoagulable states. They are may need lifelong anticoagulation and should be considered for a venacaval filter if warfarin fails to prevent further emboli.

Large acute PEs with severe hypoxia and circulatory failure may require inotropic support and thrombolysis. The same contraindications apply as for acute myocardial infarction.

LUNG CANCER

Lung cancer is the second most common malignant disease in Western countries (after breast cancer). In the UK, 40 000 new cases are diagnosed every year. One-quarter of all cancer deaths are attributed to lung cancer; only 5% of patients are cured. The term 'lung cancer' is usually reserved for primary tumours arising from the respiratory epithelium (bronchi, bronchioles and alveoli) rather than metastases from distant malignancies. Four major cell types make up 90% of all primary lung neoplasms:

- Squamous cell carcinoma (35–45%): from the large airways, it grows slowly and spreads late.
- Adenocarcinoma (including bronchioloalveolar cell carcinoma) (20–30%): peripheral and more common in non-smokers.
- Large cell (anaplastic) carcinoma (5–10%): heterogeneous group of undifferentiated tumours.
- Small cell (oat cell) carcinoma (15–20%): from central airways, it grows rapidly and spreads early.

The first three are commonly grouped together as 'non-small-cell lung cancer' as they share common prognoses and treatment strategies.

The remainder includes undifferentiated carcinomas, carcinoids and rarer tumour types (e.g. mesothelioma arising from the pleura following asbestos exposure). All cell types have different natural histories and responses to therapy, and therefore making a correct histological diagnosis is the mandatory first step to correct assessment and treatment.

Aetiology

The vast majority of lung cancers (non-adenocarcinoma) in the UK (approximately 95%) are attributable to cigarette smoking. Cigarette smoke contains numerous well-documented carcinogens. There is a clear link to both the quantity of cigarettes smoked and the duration over which they are smoked. The more somebody smokes and the longer they smoke for, the more likely they are to develop lung cancer (Fig. 31.6). The converse is that if smokers stop smoking the risk of cancer steadily declines over time.

Fig. 31.6 The risk of death from lung cancer related to number of cigarettes smoked.

Pattern of smoking	Deaths per 100 000 people	Relative risk
Never smoked	14	1
Ex-smoker	58	4
Current smoker		
1–14 cigarettes/day	105	7.5
15–24 cigarettes/day	208	15
>25 cigarettes/day	355	25

The role of passive smoking in cancer risk for non-smokers is still debated and will continue to be so. Current wisdom is that there is a small but important increase in the risk of lung cancer if exposed to passive cigarette smoking.

Other risks are much less common and include radon exposure in certain parts of the UK (e.g. Cornwall), asbestos exposure and fibrotic lung disease.

Pathology

Like other carcinomas, it is thought that lung cancer is not caused by a single insult but follows the pattern of cellular dysplasia progressing to carcinoma and spread as the burden of genetic damage accumulates and key oncogenes are mutated. For example, the K-ras proto-oncogene is implicated in 10–30% of all adenocarcinomas.

Clinical features of lung cancer

Although 5–15% of patients are detected while asymptomatic, usually on a routine chest radiograph, the vast majority of patients present with signs or symptoms.

Systemic features

Anorexia, cachexia and weight loss are common. The patient may have digital clubbing and tar staining of the fingers.

Local invasion

- Endobronchial growth: this may result in cough, haemoptysis, wheeze, stridor, dyspnoea and post-obstructive pneumonitis (fever and productive cough).
- Invasion of the chest wall: this could cause pain (pleural or chest wall involvement), cough, dyspnoea and symptoms of lung abscess due to tumour cavitation.
- Transbronchial spread: transbronchial spread (especially bronchioloalveolar carcinoma) produces growth along multiple alveolar surfaces with resultant impairment of oxygen transfer, dyspnoea, hypoxia and the production of copious sputum.
- Invasion of other thoracic structures: this may lead to airway obstruction, oesophageal compression with dysphagia, recurrent laryngeal nerve paralysis with hoarseness, phrenic nerve paralysis with elevation of the hemidiaphragm and dyspnoea, and sympathetic nerve paralysis with Horner's syndrome (ptosis, miosis, enophthalmos and ipsilateral facial loss of sweating). Pancoast's tumour growing in the apex of the lung extends locally with involvement of the eighth cervical and first and second thoracic nerves of the brachial plexus. There is shoulder pain, which characteristically radiates in the ulnar distribution of the arm, often with destruction of the first and second ribs seen on CXR. Other problems of regional spread include superior vena cava syndrome from vascular obstruction, pericardial and cardiac extension with resultant effusion or tamponade, lymphatic obstruction with resultant pleural effusion, and lymphangitic spread through the lungs with hypoxaemia and dyspnoea.

Paraneoplastic syndromes

These syndromes describe symptoms and signs resulting from extrapulmonary organ dysfunction unrelated to space-occupying metastases. They occur in 15–20% of lung cancer patients and are commonly due to tumour secretory products. Important paraneoplastic syndromes associated with lung cancer are listed in Fig. 31.7. Occasionally, resection of the primary tumour may result in resolution of the syndrome.

Diagnosis and further investigation

The diagnosis and treatment of lung cancer is dependent on the appropriate investigations (see NICE guidelines on lung cancer, April 2011). Only 10–15% of patients are picked up as asymptomatic patients (incidental finding on CXR). The majority of patients present with symptoms, most commonly persistent cough, haemoptysis and/or dyspnoea. The following are the appropriate investigations.

Imaging

- CXR: abnormal in most cases. Common findings include hilar masses (squamous and small cell), peripheral masses (adenocarcinoma), atelectasis, infiltrates, cavitation (squamous cell) and pleural effusions. Remember to compare to old films if available.
- CT: contrast-enhanced should include the neck, chest, liver and adrenal glands to enable staging to take place.
- PET-CT, MRI or plain X-ray films can be helpful in assessing metastatic spread.

Blood tests

- Full blood count.
- Liver function test.
- U&Es (including calcium).

Obtaining tissue

- Fibreoptic bronchoscopy: endobronchial disease.
- Percutaneous needle aspiration: peripheral lesions.
- Mediastinoscopy.
- Lymph node biopsy – ultrasound guided if needed.
- Biopsy of other metastatic site (e.g. the skin).
- Open lung biopsy via thoracotomy: when simpler investigations are negative.

Fig. 31.7 Important paraneoplastic syndromes associated with lung cancer.

Organ/system	Syndrome	Lung cancer histology
Endocrine and metabolic	Cushing's	Small cell
	SIADH	Small cell
	Hypercalcaemia	Squamous cell
	Gynaecomastia	Large cell
Connective tissue and bone	Clubbing and HPOA	Squamous cell, adenocarcinoma and large cell
Neuromuscular	Peripheral neuropathy	Small cell
	Subacute cerebellar degeneration	Small cell
	Eaton–Lambert (myasthenia)	Small cell
	Dermatomyositis	All
Haematology	Anaemia	All
	DIC	All
	Eosinophilia	All
	Thrombocytosis	All
Cardiovascular	Thrombophlebitis	Adenocarcinoma
	Non-bacterial thrombotic endocarditis (NBTE)	Adenocarcinoma

DIC, disseminated intravascular coagulation; HPOA, hypertrophic pulmonary osteoarthropathy; SIADH, syndrome of inappropriate antidiuretic hormone secretion.

Extent of disease and tumour–node–metastasis (TNM) staging

Eighty per cent of patients have inoperable disease at the time of presentation. Small-cell cancer is nearly always disseminated at presentation. Diagnosis of this histological type excludes surgical resection, except in very rare circumstances where there is a single, small, peripheral lesion. In all other cell types, surgery is possible and the extent of disease is recorded by the TNM classification as shown in Fig. 31.8. The staging of disease using the TNM classification also helps to estimate the prognosis with treatment.

Fig. 31.8 TNM classification for lung cancer.

TNM	Stage	Characteristics
Primary tumour (T)	T1	<3 cm diameter surrounded by lung or pleura
	T2	>3 cm diameter and/or collapse extending to hilum, invading pleura and more than 2 cm beyond the carina
	T3	Any size extending to chest wall but not involving mediastinal structures (e.g. heart and great vessels); tumour within 2 cm of carina
	T4	Any size invading mediastinum; malignant pleural effusion
Lymph nodes (N)	N0	No involvement
	N1	Ipsilateral hilar and peribronchial nodes
	N2	Ipsilateral mediastinal and subcarinal nodes
	N3	Contralateral mediastinal or hilar nodes; or any scalene or supraclavicular nodes
Metastases (M)	M0	None known
	M1	Distant metastases outside thorax

Preoperative assessment

This is in two stages, firstly by assessing whether the cancer is potentially curable. CT remains the most common method of assessing potential resectability. Positron emission tomography (PET) is now widely available for all surgical candidates.

Secondly, the fitness of the patient to undergo surgery is vital as many have such marked cardiorespiratory disease that surgery is contraindicated. This is done by assessing performance status and thorough physiological measurement such as cardiopulmonary exercise testing. If the patient is a current smoker, smoking cessation advice should not be forgotten as it will help reduce intra- and postoperative complications.

Management

Major treatment decisions are made on the basis of whether a tumour is classified histologically as a small-cell carcinoma or as one of the non-small-cell varieties (Fig. 31.9). In general, small-cell carcinomas have already spread at the time of presentation so that curative surgery cannot be performed, and they are managed primarily by chemotherapy, usually cisplatin, with or without radiotherapy.

In contrast, non-small-cell cancers that are found to be localized at the time of presentation should be considered for curative treatment with either surgery (pneumonectomy or lobectomy) or radiotherapy. Where possible, open or thorascopic lobectomy is the surgical treatment of choice. Hilar and mediastinal lymph node sampling en bloc is always performed where surgery with curative intent is performed. Curative radiotherapy is offered to those patients with poorer respiratory reserve. Chemotherapy, in particular in combination with radiotherapy, is increasingly used to treat both curative and palliative lung cancer.

If the tumour is inoperable, palliative care is essential as unpleasant dyspnoea and respiratory distress may develop as the disease progresses. Palliative care should be provided by general and specialist palliative care providers in line with 'Improving supportive and palliative care for adults with cancer' (NICE cancer service guidance). Radiotherapy may improve endobronchial obstructive symptoms, bone pain secondary to metastases or superior vena cava obstruction. Dexamethasone or whole-brain radiotherapy can be used to treat symptomatic brain metastases. Malignant pleural effusions can be tapped for symptomatic relief.

Prognosis

Fig. 31.10 gives 5-year survival rates in treated lung cancer patients. Perhaps because of the nihilistic view of lung cancer they remain poor in the UK, where overall 5-year survival is approximately 5%, less than half that in the USA.

> **COMMUNICATION**
>
> Patients are rarely surprised when the final diagnosis of lung cancer is explained to them. Ask open questions and seek their opinion as to what might be wrong with them; this can enable cancer to be discussed more easily as they have used the word first.

TUBERCULOSIS

Tuberculosis (TB) is a chronic granulomatous disease caused by a cell-mediated immune response to bacteria belonging to the *Mycobacterium tuberculosis* complex (MTB). The disease usually affects the lungs, although in up to a third of cases other organs are involved. If properly treated, TB caused by drug-susceptible strains is curable in virtually all cases. Transmission usually takes place through the airborne spread of droplets produced by patients with infectious pulmonary TB.

Of the pathogenic species belonging to the MTB, the most frequent and important agent of human disease is

Fig. 31.9 Treatment strategies for lung cancer.

Histology	Extent of disease	Treatment modality
Non-small-cell lung cancer	Stage 0–IIIa	Surgery and/or postoperative radiotherapy (e.g. for node involvement)
	Stage IIIb–IV	Palliative radiotherapy for local complications or pain from bony metastases
Small-cell lung cancer	Proven single peripheral lesion (rare)	Curative surgery attempted
	Limited stage	Combination chemotherapy and radiotherapy
	Disseminated at presentation (usual)	Combination chemotherapy

Fig. 31.10 Estimates of 5-year survival of treated patients with lung cancer.

	Stage	5-year survival
Non-small-cell lung cancer	0 (T1 N0 M0); carcinoma in situ	70–80%
	I (T1–2 N0 M0); no nodes or metastases	50%
	II (T1–2 N1 M0); ipsilateral local nodes only	30%
	IIIa (T1–3 N0–2 M0); more than T2 with ipsilateral mediastinal nodes	10–15%
	IIIb (any T, any N, M0); invading vital mediastinal structure, or non-resectable nodes but no extrathoracic spread	<5%
	IV (any T, any N, M1); extrathoracic distant metastases	<2%
Small-cell lung cancer	Patients rarely live for 5 years after diagnosis – median survival with combined chemotherapy, e.g. with cisplatin-containing regimens, is 40–70 weeks, compared with 6–20 weeks if untreated	

M. tuberculosis itself. Closely related organisms that can also infect humans include *Mycobacterium bovis* (the bovine tubercle bacillus, once an important cause of TB transmitted by unpasteurized milk).

M. tuberculosis is a rod-shaped, non-spore-forming, aerobic bacterium measuring 0.5–3 μm. Although strictly Gram-positive, it may not stain readily and is often neutral on the Gram stain. However, once stained, the bacilli cannot be decolorized by acid alcohol, a characteristic justifying their classification as acid–alcohol-fast bacilli (AAFB).

In most developed countries the incidence of TB fell until the 1980s. It then reached a plateau and is now increasing again in the UK (Fig. 31.11). This is due to an increase in susceptible groups. These include the elderly, immigrants, people from ethnic minorities, alcoholics, the homeless and immunocompromised groups (both iatrogenic and pathological; human immunodeficiency virus (HIV) is the most important group of the latter). Worldwide, 9 million people contract the infection and 2 million people die each year. TB is the cause of death for most people with HIV and recent increases in drug resistance have been alarming. Even in the UK the incidence of multi-drug resistant (MDR) and extremely-drug resistant (XDR) strains of TB are increasing with associated morbidity and mortality.

Fig. 31.11 Notification of TB in the UK, from the HPA.

Year	Number of cases notified
1920	73 332
1930	67 401
1940	46 572
1950	49 358
1960	23 605
1970	11 901
1980	9142
1990	5204
1995	5606
2000	6572
2005	7628
2009	7240

HPA, Health Protection Agency.

Pathogenesis and pattern of disease

TB is usually classified as pulmonary or extrapulmonary. Before HIV infection, 80% of all cases of TB were limited to the lungs; now two-thirds of HIV-infected patients with TB have both pulmonary and extrapulmonary disease, or even extrapulmonary disease on its own.

Pulmonary tuberculosis

Pulmonary TB can be classified as primary or reactivation (postprimary or secondary).

Primary pulmonary tuberculosis

Primary pulmonary TB results from an initial infection with tubercle bacilli. The bacterium is taken up by alveolar macrophages and is either contained or progresses to primary disease, particularly if the host immune system is impaired. The lesion is usually peripheral and associated with hilar or paratracheal lymph node enlargement. In most cases, immunity develops, the lesion heals spontaneously and may later be seen as a small calcified nodule (Ghon focus).

Patients with impaired immunity who develop primary pulmonary TB may progress rapidly to clinical illness. This may result from spread of infection by:

- Pleural effusion: which may lead to tuberculous empyema.
- Necrosis and acute cavitation of the primary lesion: known as progressive primary TB.

- Bloodstream dissemination: resulting in granulomatous lesions in various organs, or even miliary TB with tuberculous meningitis.

Reactivation tuberculosis

Reactivation disease is sometimes termed adult, post-primary or secondary TB. It results from reactivation of latent infection due to any form of debility or immunocompromise and is usually localized to the apical and posterior segments of the upper lobes. Chest radiographic changes can vary from small infiltrates to extensive cavitation. Widespread involvement of the lung with coalescing lesions produces tuberculous pneumonia.

The pathogenicity of TB varies, with a third of untreated patients dying from severe pulmonary TB within weeks or months while the rest undergo spontaneous remission or proceed along a chronic course often involving lung fibrosis.

Extrapulmonary tuberculosis

This most commonly involves lymph nodes, the pleura, genitourinary tract, bones and joints, meninges, liver, gut and peritoneum.

Clinical features

Systemic

- B-symptoms: night sweats, fevers and weight loss.
- Fatigue.
- Anorexia.
- Clubbing.

Pulmonary

- Cough: chronic and productive.
- Chest pain.
- Dyspnoea.
- Haemoptysis.
- Crepitations: involved areas during inspiration.
- Wheeze: partial bronchial obstruction.

Extrapulmonary

This is dependent on the organ system affected. Common sites include

- Meningism, photophobia and reduced conscious level – TB meningitis.
- Lymphadenopathy.
- Abscesses.
- Dysuria, frequency, epididymitis.

Diagnostic tests for tuberculosis

The key to the diagnosis of TB is a high index of suspicion, especially in at-risk groups. It should form part of the differential diagnosis in patients with febrile illnesses, cervical lymphadenopathy, or focal infiltrates on CXR.

The CXR may show the typical picture of upper lobe infiltrates, with or without cavitation. The diagnosis is initially based on the finding of AAFB by microscopy of a diagnostic specimen such as sputum or tissue (e.g. lymph node biopsy) using either auramine staining and fluorescence microscopy or the more traditional light microscopy of specimens using the Ziehl–Neelsen stain.

Patients with suspected pulmonary TB normally require three sputum specimens for AAFB smear and mycobacterial culture and sensitivity. 'Smear-positive' patients have AAFB on sputum smear; they should be considered infectious and isolated. Those without AAFB on sputum smear ('smear-negative') are not infectious and do not need isolation, even if the sputum subsequently grows MTB. Specimens are inoculated on to Löwenstein–Jensen medium. Most species of mycobacterium, including *M. tuberculosis*, are slow-growing so that 4–8 weeks may be required before growth is detected and antibiotic sensitivity can be assessed. Newer molecular biological techniques can confirm *M. tuberculosis* more quickly and give drug sensitivities.

Other diagnostic tests for pulmonary TB include:

- Induced sputum by ultrasonic nebulization of hypertonic saline for patients unable to produce a sputum specimen spontaneously.
- Fibreoptic bronchoscopy with bronchial lavage or transbronchial biopsy (especially with miliary TB).

When extrapulmonary TB is suspected, specimens of involved sites may include:

- Cerebrospinal fluid: tuberculous meningitis.
- Pleural fluid and pleural biopsy samples: pleural disease.
- Bone marrow and liver biopsy culture: good diagnostic yield in disseminated (miliary) TB.
- Early morning urine: renal TB.

In all cases specimens are sent for AAFB microscopy, stain and culture.

Positive tuberculin testing indicates exposure to mycobacteria or vaccination and not active disease per se and is best used in contact tracing and public health screening. The Mantoux and Heaf tests are the two most common methods. They involve intradermal injection of purified protein derivative (PPD) and then observation of the response. Recent developments in interferon-gamma release assays have been approved by NICE (NICE guidelines on clinical diagnosis and management of tuberculosis, and measures for its prevention and control – March 2011), particularly if the Mantoux test is positive.

False negatives are possible in active TB, especially in miliary TB or if the patient is immunosuppressed, e.g. HIV (a defect in cell-mediated immunity).

Management

Uncomplicated TB is treated in the initial phase using at least three drugs (rifampicin, isoniazid and pyrazinamide) for 2 months, then a continuation phase using two drugs (rifampicin and isoniazid) for another 4 months. If drug-resistant TB is suspected, ethambutol should be included until sensitivities are known. Treatment of extrapulmonary and drug-resistant TB requires specialist involvement. Pyridoxine is usually started to minimize the neurological side effects of isoniazid.

Second-line drugs available for infections caused by resistant organisms, or when first-line drugs cause unacceptable side effects, include cycloserine, newer macrolides (e.g. clarithromycin) and quinolones (e.g. ciprofloxacin and ofloxacin).

HINTS AND TIPS

Rifampicin turns urine red. Useful to assess compliance with treatment.

TB is 'notifiable'; you should contact the appropriate public health authorities for contact tracing.

If adherence to treatment is a possible issue, then directly observed therapy, short course (DOTS) should be employed in which medications are taken three times per week under supervision.

Not all patients with TB need to be isolated. All patients with suspected drug-resistant TB should be isolated. Most hospitals would also isolate patients with smear-positive sputum until 2 weeks of effective treatment has been given. Care should be taken to ensure that TB patients do not come into contact with immunocompromised patients.

Monitoring treatment

Isoniazid, rifampicin and pyrazinamide are associated with liver toxicity, and therefore hepatic function should be checked before treatment with these drugs. If this is normal, routine monitoring of hepatic function is not needed. Renal function should also be checked before treatment with antituberculous drugs and appropriate dosage adjustments made. Visual acuity should be tested before ethambutol is used because it can cause loss of visual acuity and visual field defects. Ishihara charts can be used to assess red/ green colour blindness due to optic neuropathy. All TB should be treated by a specialist, usually a respiratory physician.

Control of tuberculosis

By far the best way to prevent TB is the rapid diagnosis of infectious cases with appropriate treatment until cure. Additional strategies include bacille Calmette–Guérin (BCG) vaccination and preventive chemotherapy.

Vaccination

BCG was derived from an attenuated strain of *M. bovis* and was first administered to humans in 1921. Many BCG vaccines are now available worldwide; all are derived from the original strain but the vaccines vary in efficacy. The vaccine is safe and rarely causes serious complications. It should not be given to HIV-positive patients.

BCG vaccination induces PPD reactivity but the magnitude of PPD skin test reactions after vaccination does not predict the degree of protection afforded. In the most recent NICE guidelines (2011), the UK Department of Health recommends 'vaccination of all neonates at higher risk of TB, with opportunistic vaccination of older children as necessary'. Routine BCG is no longer offered to all PPD-negative children at the age of 12 years.

Preventive chemotherapy

A major component of TB control involves contact tracing, skin testing and the administration of isoniazid to contacts at high risk of active disease.

PNEUMOTHORAX

Introduction

A pneumothorax is the presence of air in the pleural space (i.e. between the visceral pleura covering the lung and the parietal pleura covering the inside of the chest wall). It has UK hospital admission rates of 6 in 100 000 and 17 in 100 000 for women and men, respectively. Risk factors for pneumothorax include smoking, increased height, male sex, increasing age and underlying lung disease. The following distinctions are made between the different types of pneumothorax:

- Spontaneous pneumothorax: occurs without trauma to the thorax.
- Primary spontaneous pneumothorax: occurs in the absence of lung disease.
- Secondary spontaneous pneumothorax: occurs in the presence of pre-existing lung disease.
- Traumatic pneumothorax: penetrating or non-penetrating chest injuries.
- Tension pneumothorax: the pressure in the pleural space is positive throughout the respiratory cycle.

Primary spontaneous pneumothorax is usually due to the rupture of an apical pleural bleb that lies within or immediately under the visceral pleura. Approximately 25% of patients with an initial primary spontaneous pneumothorax will have a recurrence.

Clinical features

The patient may be in extremis if a large tension pneumothorax is present or it may be seen on routine chest radiography in a patient with mild chest pain.

Clinical features of pneumothorax include:

- Pleuritic chest pain on the affected side.
- Shortness of breath.
- Tachycardia.
- Decreased expansion, vocal fremitus, hyperresonance and diminished breath sounds which may be detected if the pneumothorax is large.

A CXR will confirm the diagnosis by demonstrating a line of visceral pleura with absent lung markings beyond the line. The diagnosis may prove more difficult in secondary pneumothorax, especially if emphysematous bullae are present. In this case lateral X-rays or CT may be indicated. The most recent UK guidelines classify pneumothoraces as large or small, based on the presence of a visible rim of air <2 cm or >2 cm between the lung and chest wall on plain CXR.

Management

The initial treatment for primary spontaneous pneumothorax is aspiration. If the lung does not expand with aspiration, or if the patient has a recurrent pneumothorax, chest drain insertion with underwater seal drainage is indicated. Small-diameter Seldinger chest drains are preferred for non-traumatic pneumothorax. Pleurodesis or surgery by thoracoscopy or thoracotomy plus pleural abrasion is almost 100% successful in preventing recurrence. Treatment algorithms are shown in Figs 31.12 and 31.13.

HINTS AND TIPS

The top five causes of iatrogenic pneumothoraces are transthoracic needle aspiration, subclavian central line insertion, thoracocentesis, pleural biopsy and mechanical ventilation.

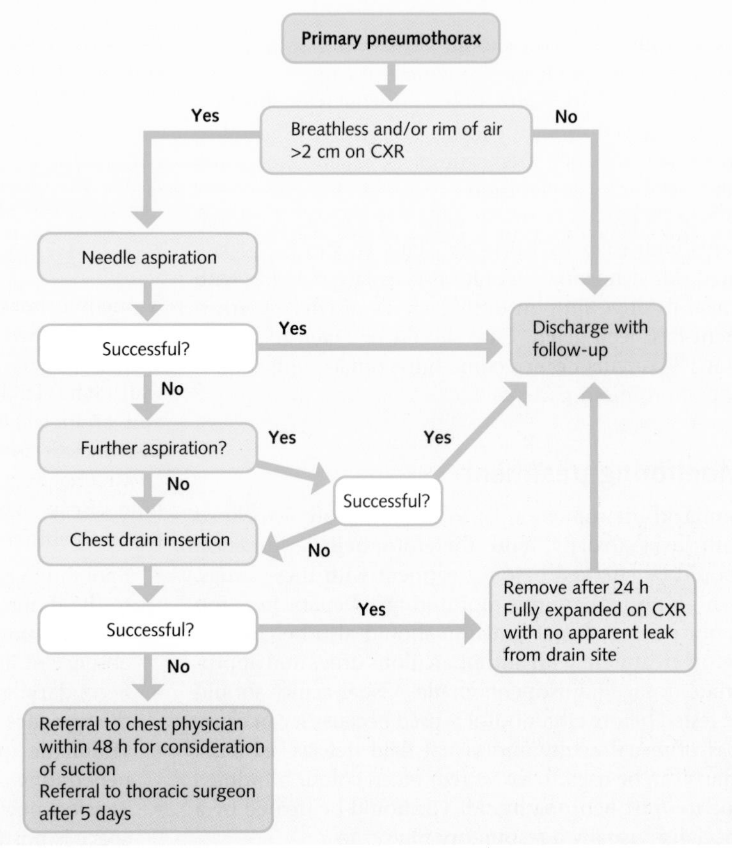

Fig. 31.12 Algorithm for treatment of primary pneumothorax. CXR, chest X-ray. (After British Thoracic Society.)

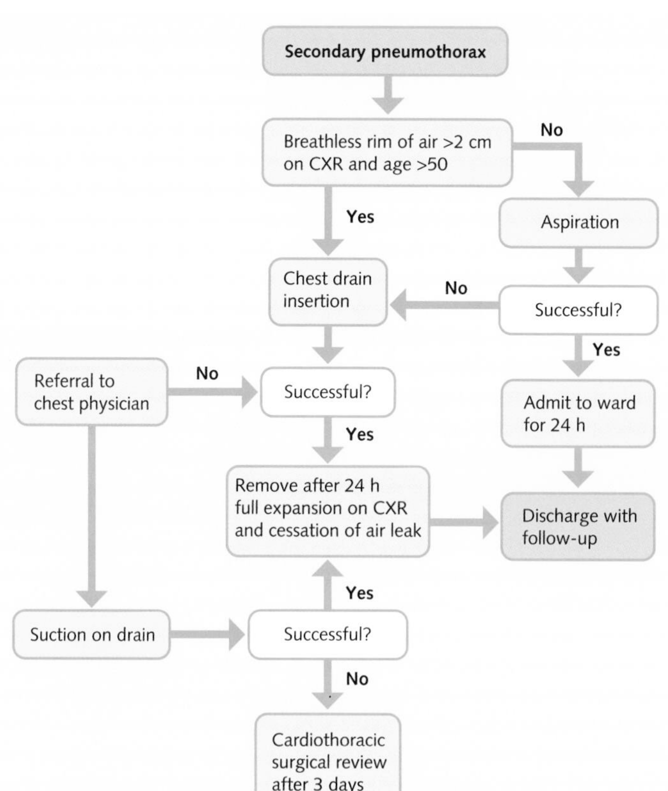

Fig. 31.13 Algorithm for treatment of secondary pneumothorax. CXR, chest X-ray. (After British Thoracic Society.)

PLEURAL EFFUSION

A pleural effusion is an accumulation of fluid in the pleural space. The fluid is often described as being an exudate or transudate, depending on its composition.

Aetiology

Exudative effusions are due to increased capillary leak and diminished fluid resorption:

- Parapneumonic effusion: 'simple' if pH >7.2 and 'complicated' if pH <7.2; empyema if frank pus on aspiration.
- Malignancy.
- Pulmonary emboli.
- Rheumatoid arthritis.
- Mesothelioma.
- Pancreatitis.

Transudative effusions are due to decreased oncotic pressure or elevated hydrostatic pressure:

- Left ventricular dysfunction.
- Cirrhotic liver disease.
- Hypoalbuminaemia.
- Constrictive pericarditis.
- Hypothyroidism.
- Meigs' syndrome – in conjunction with ovarian fibroma.

Clinical features

The accumulation of fluid within the pleural space will be asymptomatic until it is large enough to cause respiratory compromise or unless other symptoms lead to respiratory assessment. Symptoms are breathlessness, particularly on exertion, and sometimes chest pain. The examination findings include decreased breath sounds, stony dull percussion note, and decreased expansion on the affected side. History should cover:

- Evidence of cardiac failure and ischaemic heart disease.
- Evidence of recent pneumonia: empyema and a reactive effusion may develop, especially if symptoms of infection persist.
- Evidence of malignancy: lung primary, metastatic disease and mesothelioma. Always ask directly about asbestos exposure.

Investigations

Imaging

- CXR will confirm the presence of an effusion and whether it is bilateral or unilateral. It may show underlying malignancy, pleural plaques/thickening or heart failure. A repeat CXR should be performed after aspiration or chest drain insertion.
- Ultrasound is a useful tool in visualizing pleural fluid. Further to this, the British Thoracic Society strongly recommends inserting chest drains under direct ultrasound vision. The practice of 'X marks the spot', where tap sites are marked in the Radiology Department, is now discouraged.
- Contrast CT scanning may be required to further determine the underlying cause of the effusion.

Pleural fluid

A sample of the effusion should be obtained by pleural aspiration. Its gross appearance should be noted and then sent for the following tests:

- pH: this can be done on a blood gas machine. A pH of <7.2 in conjunction with pneumonia implies an infected pleural space.
- Protein and lactate dehydrogenase (LDH): this should be done with paired serum samples. Traditionally, effusions are divided into:
  - exudative: protein >30 g/dL
  - transudative: protein <30 g/dL. If the serum protein is low then this is a less useful cut-off and Light's criteria are more sensitive and specific. These state that if one of the following is true then the fluid is exudative:
    - pleural fluid protein:serum protein >0.5
    - pleural fluid LDH:serum LDH >0.6
    - pleural fluid LDH >2/3 the upper serum reference range.
- Gram stain, culture and sensitivities: for bacterial infection. If there is suspicion of TB, then stain and culture for *Mycobacterium* spp. should be requested.
- Cytology: for malignancy and differential cell count.

Further investigations may include pleural biopsy, thoracoscop and bronchoscopy and is likely to need specialist involvement.

Management

The underlying diagnosis should be sought and then treated. Many effusions will resolve with this alone, particularly if due to cardiac failure. If the history and fluid analysis suggest either empyema or complicated parapneumonic effusion then it should be drained in addition to antibiotic therapy. Drainage is usually achieved by inserting a chest drain (Seldinger technique) in the safe triangle (4th to 6th intercostal space anterior to mid axillary line). Fluid should be drained in a controlled fashion at a rate no faster than 2 L/24 h. If malignancy is confirmed and the effusion is causing symptoms then drainage and pleurodesis with talc should obliterate the pleural space, preventing reaccumulation.

CYSTIC FIBROSIS

Cystic fibrosis (CF) is an autosomal recessive disorder that presents as a multisystem disease, and occurs in 1 in 2500 live births in Caucasians; 1 person in 25 is a carrier. Signs and symptoms typically occur in childhood but up to 5% of patients are diagnosed as adults. Improvements in supportive therapy mean that the median survival is now 40 years. The CF transmembrane conductance regulator gene is on chromosome 7; it regulates chloride and water movement across cell membranes. Whilst there are more than 1500 known mutations the Δ508 mutation accounts for over 70% of cases.

CF is characterized by chronic airway infection that ultimately leads to bronchiectasis, exocrine and endocrine pancreatic insufficiency, intestinal and hepatic dysfunction, abnormal sweat gland function and urogenital dysfunction.

Diagnosis

The diagnosis of CF rests on a combination of clinical criteria, analysis of sweat chloride (the 'sweat test') and increasingly by genotyping. Faecal elastase is a useful screening test for exocrine pancreatic function impairment.

Treatment

This is best done by a multidisciplinary team based in a specialist centre. Treatment strategies for CF are to promote clearance of secretions and reverse bronchoconstriction (physiotherapy, mucolytics and bronchodilators), control infection in the lung (prophylactic nebulized and IV antibiotics), vaccinate against influenza and pneumococcus, ensure adequate nutrition (pancreatic enzyme and fat-soluble vitamin supplements), screen for diabetes and prevent intestinal obstruction.

As irreversible complications arise, heart–lung transplantation may be an option for some. Gene therapy remains elusive and far from clinical use.

COMMUNICATION

The transition from paediatric to adult care is difficult for both patients and their parents. Teenage years are a challenge without living with a condition such as cystic fibrosis. Patients need to build relationships with a new medical team at a time when they are becoming independent adults. This may be hard for parents, who have often spent most of their time caring for their child and now feel they have no clear role. They may need support in this transition.

BRONCHIECTASIS

Bronchiectasis is an abnormal and permanent dilatation of the bronchioles secondary to chronic infection associated with the production of copious amounts of purulent sputum. It can be focal, involving airways supplying a limited region of the lung, or diffuse, involving airways in a more widespread distribution.

Aetiology

Bronchiectasis can be congenital. For example it is associated with conditions causing poor mucociliary clearance such as cystic fibrosis, Kartagener's syndrome or primary ciliary dyskinesia. In the past, bronchiectasis was a complication of measles or pertussis infection. Modern vaccination programmes have reduced the incidence of these diseases and the complications dramatically. It is more common in those with impaired immune systems; adenovirus and influenza are the main viral causes and infections with necrotizing organisms (e.g. TB or anaerobes) remain important. Localized bronchial obstruction can also lead on to bronchiectasis.

Clinical features

Patients typically present with persistent or recurrent cough and purulent sputum production. Intermittent haemoptysis occurs in more than half of cases and can cause massive bleeding. Physical examination of the chest overlying an affected area may reveal any combination of coarse crepitations and wheeze, reflecting the damaged airways containing significant secretions. As with other chronic intrathoracic infections, clubbing may be present.

Patients with severe disease and chronic hypoxaemia may develop cor pulmonale and right ventricular failure. Amyloidosis can result from chronic infection and inflammation, but it is now seldom seen.

Diagnosis

Chest radiography may show 'tramline shadows' due to bronchial wall thickening. High-resolution CT (HRCT) has replaced bronchography for definitive diagnosis. Lung function and reversibility should be done by spirometry and sputum culture should guide antibiotic therapy.

Management

Treatment involves regular (preferably twice-daily) postural drainage. Antibiotics should be used according to organism sensitivities. Surgery is occasionally effective for localized bronchiectasis. Appropriate treatment should be started when a treatable cause is found (e.g. antituberculous drugs for TB or steroids for ABPA).

INTERSTITIAL LUNG DISEASE

Interstitial lung disease (ILD), also known as diffuse parenchymal lung disease (DPLD), is a heterogeneous group of disorders that have been variously classified. Some of the terms used are idiopathic pulmonary fibrosis, cryptogenic fibrosing alveolitis, interstitial pneumonitis and diffuse parenchymal lung disease. They share the fact that damage is a result of an inflammatory insult to the lung that then leads to cellular proliferation and scarring with chronic loss of lung function.

Aetiology

One way to begin thinking about this group of disorders is to separate them into those with and those without a known cause.

Known cause

- Environmental agents: asbestosis, silicosis, pneumoconiosis.
- Drugs: sulfasalazine, gold, amiodarone, methotrexate, oxygen, nitrofurantoin.
- Systemic disease: connective tissue disorders (systemic lupus erythematosus, rheumatoid arthritis, systemic sclerosis), neoplasia, vasculitides (Wegener's granulomatosis, Churg–Strauss syndrome, microscopic polyangiitis), sarcoidosis, inflammatory bowel disease.

Unknown cause

- Cryptogenic fibrosing alveolitis (usual interstitial pneumonia (UIP)).
- Cryptogenic organizing pneumonia.

Clinical features

Most present with non-productive cough, slowly progressive dyspnoea, fatigue, weight loss and occasionally haemoptysis. The chest radiograph may show reticular nodular shadowing and loss of lung volume. Careful questioning of occupational and environmental risks, travel, medications, past illness, smoking and family history is important to find a cause. Examination may show cyanosis, finger clubbing and bilateral fine end inspiratory crackles. As the disease progresses cor pulmonale may develop.

Investigations

These should include full blood count, ESR, urea and electrolytes, calcium, liver function tests, serum angiotensin-converting enzyme (ACE) and autoantibodies to look for a cause. If any are abnormal they should be followed up.

CXR is often the first modality of imaging. In sarcoidosis the stages of the disease are classified according to the appearance on the CXR (Fig. 31.14). Beyond this, HRCT provides more detailed diagnostic and prognostic information. Other tests include pulmonary function tests (usually restrictive pattern), bronchoalveolar lavage or lung biopsy. Lung biopsy should be considered to differentiate between the various subtypes of interstitial pneumonia. Only UIP can be accurately diagnosed from HRCT.

Fig. 31.14 CXR stages of sarcoidosis.

Stage 1	Bihilar lymphadenopathy
Stage 2	Bihilar lymphadenopathy and reticunodular shadowing
Stage 3	Bilateral pulmonary infiltrates
Stage 4	Fibrocystic sarcoidosis typically with upward hilar retraction, cystic and bullous change

Management

If a disorder is found then the underlying cause must be addressed. If 'honeycomb' changes are seen on the HRCT then fibrosis is permanent. If 'ground glass' changes are seen then high-dose immunosuppression with steroids and cyclophosphamide may be indicated to attempt to prevent irreversible fibrosis. Treatment of complications is as they develop and when end-stage referral for transplantation may be indicated.

Occupational lung disease

Many acute and chronic lung diseases are directly related to occupational exposure to inorganic and organic dusts. A number of different clinical syndromes may result and these are listed in Fig. 31.15. They are important as they are largely preventable through increased awareness and improved workplace conditions. Patients with asbestosis, silicosis, pneumoconiosis and mesothelioma may be entitled to compensation.

Fig. 31.15 Common occupational lung diseases.

Disease	Aetiology	Lung injury
Chronic fibrotic lung disease	Coal workers' pneumoconiosis Silicosis Asbestosis	Diffuse nodular infiltrates on CXR
Hypersensitivity pneumonitis	Mouldy hay (farmer's lung) Avian proteins (bird fancier's lung)	Restrictive pulmonary dysfunction
Obstructive airways disorders	Grain dust Wood dust Tobacco Pollen Synthetic dyes Formaldehyde	Occupational asthma
Toxic lung injury	Irritant gases	Pulmonary oedema Bronchiolitis obliterans
Lung cancer	Asbestos	Mesothelioma
	Arsenic	All lung cancer types
	Chromium	All lung cancer types
	Hydrocarbons	All lung cancer types
Pleural diseases	Asbestos	May cause benign effusions and plaques
	Talc	May cause benign effusions and plaques

Aspergillus and the lung

Aspergillus is a genus of fungi consisting of more than several hundred of species. The fungi is responsible for causing allergic bronchopulmonary aspergillosis (ABPA), which is a combined type I and III hypersensitivity disorder. It occurs in patients with asthma, cystic fibrosis or sinusitis. It is characterized by bronchospasm, peripheral blood eosinophilia, *Aspergillus* precipitins and raised IgE levels with pulmonary infiltrates. It can lead on to bronchiectasis. Treatment for exacerbations is with corticosteroids. The cause is the fungus *Aspergillus fumigatus*.

ABPA is the most common example of the allergic bronchopulmonary mycoses and is sometimes confused with hypersensitivity pneumonitis because of the presence of precipitating antibodies to *Aspergillus fumigatus*. However, ABPA is an obstructive rather than a restrictive lung disease and is associated with allergic (atopic) asthma. The bronchiectasis associated with ABPA is thought to result from a deposition of immune complexes in proximal airways. Adequate treatment usually requires the long-term use of systemic glucocorticoids.

Aspergillus fumigatus can also cause invasive aspergillosis in immunosuppressed patients, e.g. neutropenia post chemotherapy or HIV. Treatment is with amphotericin, itraconazole or voriconazole.

In the immunocompetent, pre-existing lung cavities, for example secondary to TB or sarcoidosis, can be colonized to form aspergillomas. Surgical resection remains the most effective treatment.

Aspergillus clavatus causes a type of extrinsic allergic alveolitis (EAA) also referred to as malt-worker's lung. Treatment is with oral steroids; if left untreated pulmonary fibrosis may develop.

HYPOVENTILATION SYNDROMES AND SLEEP-RELATED RESPIRATORY DISORDERS

Apnoea is defined as an intermittent cessation of respiratory airflow during sleep, lasting at least 10 s. The most common cause of sleep-disordered breathing is obstructive sleep apnoea (OSA); other hypoventilatory disorders are much less common.

Classification

Sleep apnoea is divided into three types:

- Central sleep apnoea: apnoea with a patent upper airway. The cause can vary, e.g. where the neural drive to all the respiratory muscles is transiently abolished.
- Obstructive sleep apnoea: apnoea despite continuing respiratory effort because of pharyngeal airway occlusion.
- Mixed apnoeas, which consist of a central apnoea followed by an obstructive component.

Obstructive sleep apnoea–hypopnoea syndrome

This is the combination of OSA and excessive daytime sleepiness. The symptoms include snoring, poor concentration, unrefreshing restless sleep, daytime somnolence, morning headaches, poor libido, and reduced cognitive function. Risk factors are increasing age, male gender, obesity, neck circumference, sedative drugs and alcohol.

COMMUNICATION

The history from patients with suspected obstructive sleep apnoea is best obtained with their partner present. The patient may be untroubled by their own snoring. Partners may be affected more than patients; you can gauge the impact of the problem on their combined life. They also often describe apnoeas with great accuracy!

Management

Treatment of mild obstructive sleep apnoea is by weight reduction, avoidance of alcohol, improvement of nasal patency, intraoral mandibular advancement devices and avoidance of sleeping supine. Sleep hygiene advice should be given by the clinician, helping encourage a more restful night's sleep. Moderate-to-severe cases are best treated by nasal CPAP to splint open the upper airway during sleep and rarely with surgical intervention.

Other conditions

Obesity hypoventilation syndrome

This condition is characterized by hypoventilation associated with shallow inspiration (Pickwickian syndrome). The condition is often associated with obstructive sleep apnoea. The resulting episodes of hypoxia and hypercapnia (defined as an increase of 1.3 kPa whilst asleep) cause poor night-time sleep and in the long term may cause cor pulmonale in one-third of patients.

Congenital central hypoventilation syndrome

Congenital central hypoventilation syndrome, or Ondine's curse, is a respiratory condition that, if left untreated, is fatal. It normally presents at birth but may be secondary to significant neurological trauma. The condition is characterized by episodes of central apnoea with cyanois secondary to autonomic failure at the level of the brainstem. It is a rare condition (1/200 000 live births) and may be associated with Hirschsprung's disease, neuroblastoma and dysphagia. Treatment used to involve tracheostomy and mechanical ventilation. More recently biphasic cuirass ventilation and phrenic nerve pacing have been successfully used to manage the condition.

ACUTE RESPIRATORY DISTRESS SYNDROME

Acute respiratory distress syndrome (ARDS) is characterized by severe respiratory failure due to marked lung inflammatory response and capillary leak.

Aetiology

The most common stimulus is sepsis; others include trauma, burns, pancreatitis, disseminated intravascular coagulopathy, blood transfusions, cardiopulmonary bypass, emboli and near drowning. Hypoxaemia results from non-cardiogenic pulmonary oedema.

It is defined by four criteria:

- Acute onset.
- New bilateral infiltrates on chest radiography (see Fig. 31.16).
- No evidence of heart failure or pulmonary artery occlusion pressure <18 mmHg.
- Refractory hypoxaemia: Po_2: F_io_2 <200.

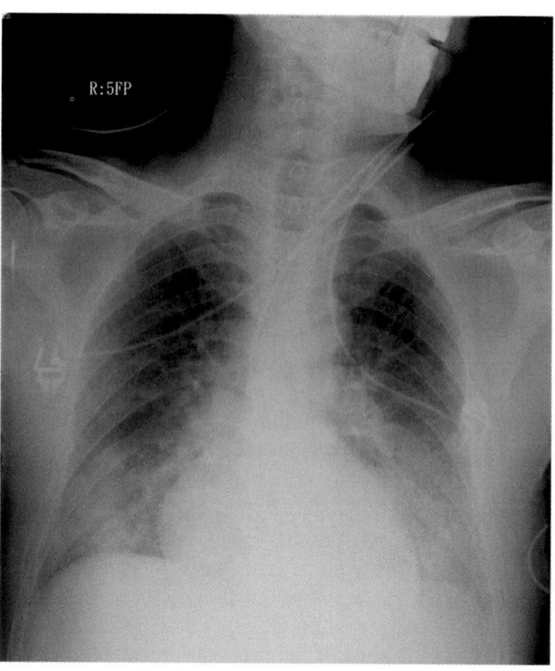

Fig. 31.16 Chest radiograph showing bilateral infiltrates in ARDS. (Reprinted from Yu-Jen Su, Chia-Te Kung, Chih-Hsiung Lee et al. 2010 An Industrial Worker Hospitalized With Paralysis After an Aerosolized Chemical Exposure. *American Journal of Kidney Diseases* 56:A38–A41, with permission from Elsevier.)

Management

ARDS should always be managed on intensive care and should be divided as follows.

- Respiratory support: in early ARDS CPAP may be sufficient although more often than not patients will require intubation and mechanical ventilation. Recent advances include 'lung protective' ventilation by minimizing tidal volumes and airway pressures; this may mean accepting hypercapnia. Positive end-expiratory pressure improves oxygenation and allows the F_io_2 to be lowered. Fluid balance is controlled to try to maintain Po_2 by limiting extravascular lung water without affecting other organ systems. Other strategies, including prone positioning, high-frequency oscillatory ventilation, inhaled nitric oxide and the place of corticosteroids, remain the subject of research and debate.
- Cardiovascular support: ARDS is often associated with multiorgan distress syndrome (MODS or multiorgan failure). Invasive haemodynamic monitoring such as arterial and central venous lines are used to monitor fluid balance, blood pressure and potentially cardiac output (PICCO). If persistent hypovolaemia exists in the presence of adequate fluid resuscitation, ionotropes such as noradrenaline (norepinephrine) or dobutamine may be indicated.
- Sepsis: ARDS is most commonly triggered by sepsis. The 'sepsis six' care bundle should have been started at the time of admission. Antibiotic treatment should be guided by sensitivities. Remember that that the source does not have to be from the lungs to cause ARDS – a patient presenting with sepsis secondary to an *E. coli* urinary tract infection may develop ARDS.

Prognosis

This remains poor: overall mortality is approximately 41–46% (Intensive Care National Audit & Research Centre). It depends on the nature of the precipitating event and the degree to which organ failure develops. Most survivors have residual impairment of lung function, both mechanical and diffusing capacity with diminished exercise capacity.

Further reading

British Thoracic Society: publishes guidelines and reviews on all aspects of respiratory medicine. Available online at: http://www.brit-thoracic.org.uk.

Corne, J., Pointon, K., 2009. The chest X-ray made easy, third ed. Churchill Livingstone Elsevier, Edinburgh.
Decramer, M., Janssens, W., Miravitlles, M., 2012. Chronic obstructive pulmonary disease. Lancet 379, 1341–1351.
Goldstraw, P., Ball, D., Jett, J.R., et al., 2011. Non-small-cell lung cancer. Lancet 378, 1727–1740.
Hunt, J.M., Bull, T.M., 2011. Clinical review of pulmonary embolism: diagnosis, prognosis and treatment. Med. Clin. North Am. 6, 1203–1222.
National Institute for Health and Clinical Excellence (NICE) guidelines. Available online at: http://www.nice.org.uk.
Patel, H., Gwilt, C., 2007. Crash Course: Respiratory System, third ed. Mosby, London.

Gastrointestinal and liver disease

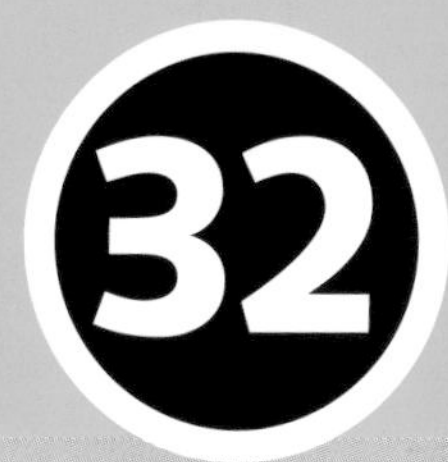

Objectives

The key learning points for this chapter:

- Describe the complications of gastro-oesophageal reflux disease.
- Describe the differences in the management of gastric and duodenal ulcers, and their rationale.
- Describe the emergency management of a patient with a large haematemesis.
- Be familiar with a range of conditions affecting the small bowel including coeliac disease.
- Understand the differences between Crohn's disease and ulcerative colitis.
- Understand the role of genetic factors in the development of colorectal cancer.
- Describe the clinical syndromes that may result from the presence of gallstones.
- List the causes of acute pancreatitis.

OESOPHAGEAL DISORDERS

Hiatus hernia

This is the herniation of part of the stomach, commonly the proximal part, into the chest cavity. Hiatus hernias are generally asymptomatic but may be associated with acid reflux causing dyspeptic symptoms (see below and Ch. 9). Since hiatus hernias are associated with increased body mass index (BMI), weight loss is advised. They rarely require treatment other than symptomatic management for acid reflux (see below). Occasionally surgery is indicated, which involves wrapping the fundus of the stomach around the lower oesophageal sphincter (Nissen's fundoplication procedure). There are two types of hiatus hernia.

Sliding hiatus hernia

Very common (30% of over-50s). Gastro-oesophageal junction 'slides' through oesophageal hiatus into the thorax. Sliding hiatus hernias account for 80% of hiatus hernias.

Rolling (or para-oesophageal) hiatus hernia

The lower oesophageal sphincter (LOS) remains below the diaphragm but part of the stomach rolls up into the chest next to the oesophagus. Occasionally, this results in gastric volvulus, resulting in severe pain and requiring surgery.

Gastro-oesophageal reflux disease

The LOS normally prevents significant acid reflux into the oesophagus. Other anti-reflux mechanisms include the intra-abdominal section of the oesophagus, the diaphragmatic crura and the folds of gastric mucosa. These mechanisms fail in gastro-oesophageal reflux disease (GORD). The factors predisposing to reflux are outlined in Ch. 9.

Clinical features

These are described in Ch. 9. It is important to note particularly how the presentation may be difficult to distinguish from that of angina (including non-specific ECG changes), and how atypical symptoms such as nocturnal asthma or laryngeal discomfort may occur. Severe oesophagitis may be associated with occult and/or overt gastrointestinal (GI) bleeding and iron-deficiency anaemia.

Investigations

These are outlined in Ch. 9. Endoscopy is useful for demonstrating oesophagitis, peptic strictures and Barrett's oesophagus (see below) and allows biopsies to be taken. Endoscopy is indictaed in those >55 years of age, symptoms lasting >4 weeks, dysphagia, persistent symptoms despite treatment, and weight loss. To confirm the diagnosis, 24-h intraluminal pH monitoring is the definitive test, but it is not often required, as explained in Ch. 9. NICE guidance on the management of GORD is in development.

In adhering to the guidelines summarized in Fig. 9.3, a number of patients with GORD (without a firm diagnosis) will undergo *Helicobacter pylori* eradication. However, *H. pylori* infection is just as common in the normal population and probably has no specific role in this condition. As a matter of fact eradicating *H. pylori* in GORD may make symptoms worse; *H. pylori* is not implicated in GORD.

Management

Patients should avoid tight clothes, stop smoking, avoid aggravating foods and drinks, and lose weight if overweight. Patients should be advised to prop themselves up in bed with pillows or put a block under the end of the bed to avoid slipping down. Drugs that affect oesophageal motility (e.g. nitrates or tricyclic antidepressants, calcium channel antagonists) should be avoided if possible.

A number of drugs can be used: antacids (including alginate preparations that form a 'foam raft'), H_2-receptor antagonists (e.g. ranitidine), proton pump inhibitors (PPIs; e.g. omeprazole) and prokinetics such as metoclopramide. Therapy aims to provide symptom relief. Treatment for 4 weeks is a reasonable starting course and then therapy should be titrated to an agent that controls the symptoms at the lowest cost.

Surgery is only indicated if symptoms are severe despite maximum medical management and there is pH monitoring evidence of active acid reflux during symptomatic episodes. Careful candidate selection is absolutely crucial.

Complications

Benign oesophageal stricture

This usually occurs in patients aged over 60 years old and causes intermittent dysphagia. The stricture is usually dilated endoscopically but surgery is rarely required. Acid secretion is controlled pharmacologically.

Barrett's oesophagus

This is intestinal metaplasia from squamous to columnar epithelium following long-standing acid reflux and, although visible macroscopically, is confirmed histologically following endoscopic biopsy. It is particularly significant as it is premalignant for oesophageal adenocarcinoma (see below).

Eosinophilic oesophagitis

This is a hypersensitive inflammatory condition of the oesophagus. The condition more commonly affects children and young adults and presents with symptoms of dyspepsia, dysphagia and food impaction. The diagnosis is based on the histological appearance of endoscopic biopsies. Treatment involves allergy testing and allergen avoidance. Swallowed liquid cortisone may help. Recent evidence suggests a role for proton pump inhibitors in symptom control and potential remission of the underlying pathology. Severe strictures may require endoscopic balloon dilatation. GORD also leads to eosinophil infiltrate, so can be difficult to distinguish.

Oesophageal motility disorders

These can give rise to dyspepsia (see Ch. 9), pain, dysphagia and odynophagia, and regurgitation. Causes include old age, diabetes mellitus, neurological disorders affecting the brainstem, systemic sclerosis, achalasia and diffuse oesophageal spasm. The diagnosis can be suggested by chest X-ray or barium swallow appearances, but oesophageal manometry is the definitive investigation. Treatment options include anti-spasmodic drugs, botulinum toxin injection, balloon dilatation and surgery.

Achalasia

Achalasia is failure of relaxation at the distal end of the oesophagus due to an underlying neuromuscular problem, commonly the ganglionic cells in the myenteric plexus. Because there is a functional obstruction distally, it causes progressive dilatation, tortuosity, incoordination of peristalsis and often hypertrophy of the proximal oesophagus. The condition affects males and females equally and has a peak incidence in the third and fourth decades of life. Diagnosis is on barium swallow (or a water contrast swallow if there is risk of aspiration) and motility studies using monometry probes. The condition is incurable but management with botulinum toxin or endoscopic balloon dilatation can provide symptomatic relieve. Occasionally surgery (Heller's cardiomyotomy) can be performed to permanently dilate the lower 3–4 cm of the oesophagus. This procedure, however, may lead to reflux oesophagitis.

Oesophageal cancer

The incidence in the UK is 5–10 in 100000 and rising (unlike gastric carcinoma) but is higher in China and parts of Africa. It is commoner in men, heavy drinkers and smokers. Predisposing factors include Plummer–Vinson syndrome, achalasia, coeliac disease and tylosis (hyperkeratosis of the palms and soles).

In general, squamous cell carcinomas occur in the upper and mid-oesophagus. Adenocarcinoma typically arises in columnar epithelium of the lower oesophagus. Barrett's oesophagus increases the risk of adenocarcinoma by 40-fold.

Clinical features

The incidence peaks in the seventh decade. General features of malignancy include weight loss, anorexia and lassitude. Local features include dysphagia (initially to solids progressing to liquids), retrosternal pain and odynophagia. Direct invasion of surrounding structures and regional lymph node involvement are common. Metastases to other organs and distant lymph nodes may occur.

Investigations

Endoscopy with biopsy, and barium swallow are the main diagnostic investigations. CT and/or MRI scanning, liver ultrasound and bronchoscopy are commonly performed as part of the staging process. Occasionally a staging laparoscopy is performed if there is a significant infra-diaphragmatic component.

Management

Surgery is considered, depending on the tumour stage/grade and the fitness of the patient, but it carries a high morbidity and mortality. Radiotherapy and chemotherapy may play a role. Often palliation is the only option, and this may include endoscopic dilatation, stent placement, laser photocoagulation and/or radiotherapy with the aim of maintaining patency of the oesophageal lumen. Overall survival is poor, at around 5% at 5 years.

GASTRODUODENAL DISORDERS

Gastroduodenitis and peptic ulcer disease

Acute gastritis and ulceration can result from non-steroidal anti-inflammatory drug (NSAID) use, steroids, alcohol, smoking, or severe stress or burns (Curling's ulcer). Chronic gastritis complicates *H. pylori* infection, autoimmune gastritis (e.g. pernicious anaemia) and chronic NSAID use. Most chronic gastritis is asymptomatic but may be a risk factor for malignant change. Erosive duodenitis is part of the spectrum of duodenal ulcer disease.

Peptic ulcer disease most commonly occurs in the duodenum, followed by the stomach, oesophagus and jejunum in Zollinger–Ellison syndrome or after a gastroenterostomy. It may occur in a Meckel's diverticulum with ectopic gastric mucosa. Its prevalence is 15–20% and it is commoner in men. The incidence increases with age.

Duodenal ulceration is associated with *H. pylori* infection in 95% of cases and NSAIDs are implicated in most others. Eighty per cent of gastric ulcers are *H. pylori*-associated and the remainder are usually due to NSAIDs. It is important to remember that gastric ulceration is a mode of presentation of gastric cancer.

HINTS AND TIPS

Make sure to specifically ask about over-the-counter medicine; aspirin and NSAIDs are an important cause of gastroduodenitis and peptic ulcer disease.

Clinical features

Dyspepsia is the commonest mode of presentation and the symptoms are described in Ch. 9. They are unreliable for separating duodenal ulcer from gastric ulcer. Anorexia, vomiting and weight loss should lead to the suspicion of gastric carcinoma. If there is persistent and severe pain, complications such as perforation or penetration into other organs should be considered.

Examination reveals epigastric tenderness. A mass suggests carcinoma, and a succussion splash may suggest pyloric obstruction.

Investigations

These are described in Ch. 9. Gastroscopy (or rarely a barium meal) is the investigation of choice. All gastric ulcers should be biopsied to exclude malignancy but duodenal ulcers are nearly always benign; biopsies should be taken for *H. pylori* at endoscopy. Acid secretion status may be assessed if Zollinger–Ellison syndrome is suspected, by measuring fasting gastrin level, ideally off PPI.

Management

The patient should be advised to modify exacerbating factors such as smoking, diet and alcohol. NSAIDs should be stopped if not absolutely necessary and the use of cyclooxygenase 2 (COX-2) antagonists may be considered in accordance with national guidelines (see Further reading). Antacids, H_2-antagonists and proton pump inhibitors all help with symptomatic relief. More specific therapies aimed at cure are described below.

Duodenal ulcer

H. pylori eradication should be undertaken using a locally approved regime. If the patient is rendered asymptomatic, no further follow-up is required. If symptoms recur, the breath test should be repeated; if positive, re-eradication is attempted; treatment failure may indicate poor compliance or antibiotic resistance; if negative, clinical re-evaluation and investigation is required. In the minority of patients who are *H. pylori-negative*, culprit drugs such as NSAIDs should be stopped where possible and antisecretory therapy titrated to symptoms. Patients who are persistently *H. pylori*-positive can be cultured and sensitivities determined to successfully eradicate.

Gastric ulcer

If *H. pylori*-positive, eradication should be undertaken followed by antisecretory therapy for 2 months. If *H. pylori*-negative, 2 months of antisecretory therapy should be given. In all cases, NSAID use should be discontinued. If this is not possible, consideration should be given to the use of maintenance therapy with a proton pump inhibitor, and the use of COX-2 inhibitors (see Further reading).

All gastric ulcers should be followed up with endoscopy/biopsy until completely healed due to the risk of an underlying malignancy. If present for longer than 6 months, surgery should be considered.

Surgery

Surgery is usually considered when medical treatment has failed, or for complications that include persistent haemorrhage, perforation or pyloric stenosis. Operations include partial gastrectomy or highly selective vagotomy and pyloroplasty (hardly ever done now). Haemorrhage may be controlled endoscopically by injection with adrenaline (epinephrine) or diathermy, laser photocoagulation or heat probe and application of endoscopically placed clips. Perforations are usually oversewn with an omental plug.

Complications of surgery include:

- Recurrent ulceration.
- Abdominal fullness.
- Bilious vomiting.
- Diarrhoea.
- Dumping syndrome: fainting and sweating after eating, possibly due to food of high osmotic potential being dumped into the jejunum and causing hypovolaemia because of rapid fluid shifts. 'Late dumping' is due to hypoglycaemia and occurs 1–3 h after taking food. This is a result of partial gastrectomy, which is rarely performed now.

Metabolic complications include:

- Weight loss.
- Malabsorption.
- Bacterial overgrowth (blind loop syndrome).
- Anaemia, usually due to iron deficiency following hypochlorhydria and stomach resection.

Complications

The three main complications secondary to peptic ulceration are bleeding, perforation and pyloric stenosis. Perforation is more common in duodenal ulcers than in gastric ulcers. Pyloric stenosis may also be prepyloric or in the duodenum. It occurs because of oedema surrounding the ulcer or from scar formation on healing. The patient often has projectile vomiting with food ingested up to 24 h previously. There may be visible peristalsis and a succussion splash. Vomiting may lead to dehydration and a metabolic alkalosis.

Fluid and electrolyte replacement is needed, as is gastric aspiration with a nasogastric tube. Surgery is indicated if the patient does not settle with conservative management.

Upper gastrointestinal haemorrhage

HINTS AND TIPS

A careful history may help with the diagnosis in haematemesis. In Mallory–Weiss oesophageal tears, violent retching or vomiting occurs and the first contents are usually free of blood.

Upper gastrointestinal (GI) bleeding presents commonly with melaena and/or haematemesis. The pathology can range from insidious loss from gastritis with no apparent blood loss to catastrophic, life-threatening oesophageal variceal bleeding. Emergency resuscitative measures may therefore be needed before a full assessment is made. The approach to taking an appropriate history, examination and developing a complete differential diagnosis is discussed in Ch. 10. This section discusses the emergency management of significant upper GI bleeding. All patients with a significant bleed should be admitted to hospital. The vast majority will stop bleeding spontaneously within 48 h.

Management

General

It is essential to establish early whether or not the patient is haemodynamically compromised. In the shocked patient, fluid resuscitation to correct haemodynamic instability is a priority:

- Ensure the airway is protected and administer high-flow oxygen. Two large-bore cannulae should be inserted into large veins (e.g. antecubital fossa); this enables blood samples to be taken as advised in Ch. 10.
- IV crystalloid or colloid should be given while awaiting cross-matched blood. If bleeding is profuse, O-negative blood may be used.
- Clotting should be corrected with platelets, vitamin K or fresh frozen plasma as required.
- Insert a urinary catheter to monitor urine output. Consider central venous pressure (CVP) monitoring if the patient is unstable – but be aware of the risks of this procedure if clotting is deranged.
- Fluid resuscitation should be titrated to the pulse rate, blood pressure, urine output, CVP and clinical assessment of fluid status.

If there are no signs of shock and the patient is not anaemic, they may be managed 'conservatively' (i.e. bed rest, nil by mouth and close monitoring of the pulse, blood pressure and fluid balance). Blood should be grouped and saved, and normal saline should be given intravenously.

Once the patient is stable, endoscopy should be carried out within 4 h if variceal bleeding is suspected or within 12–24 h if the patient was shocked on admission or has significant comorbidity. Other patients can wait longer; there is no evidence that these individuals will benefit from starting a PPI prior to endoscopy. The cause for the bleed will be apparent in over 80% of cases on endoscopy.

If there is active bleeding, adrenaline (epinephrine) can be injected, or bleeding vessels coagulated with a heat probe or with laser therapy. Proton pump inhibitors are given to patients with bleeding ulcers and then they are managed as described above.

Surgery is indicated if it is not possible to control the bleeding with medical management, especially for persistent or recurrent bleeding, although this is now becoming less common. It is more often carried out in the elderly and for those with gastric ulcers compared to duodenal ulcers.

Bleeds from gastric ulcers carry twice the mortality of bleeds from duodenal ulcers. The Rockall score is used as a prognostic indicator that has a pre- and post-endoscopy component (see Fig. 10.4). Patients must be monitored very closely for re-bleeding as this has a mortality of 40% and is often an indication for surgery.

Management of bleeding oesophageal varices

The cause of oesophageal varices is discussed later in this chapter. Resuscitative procedures, correction of coagulation and endoscopy should be carried out as above:

- Fluid resuscitation should aim to maintain a systolic blood pressure of 80–90 mmHg (and urine output greater than 30 mL/h). Over-aggressive fluid replacement may increase the chance of a re-bleed.
- Prophylactic antibiotics should be commenced and continued for 1 week.
- Vasoconstrictor therapy is used to reduce splanchnic blood flow and therefore portal pressure. Terlipressin (vasopressin analogue) is the agent of choice.
- Urgent endoscopy allows acute variceal banding (or occasionally sclerotherapy). This arrests bleeding in 80% of cases and reduces early re-bleeding.
- Measures to prevent hepatic encephalopathy should be started, which include emptying the bowel with enemas or lactulose.
- If the bleeding continues, a Sengstaken–Blakemore tube can be passed through the oesophagus, with balloons to compress the varices at the oesophagogastric junction. The patient ought to be intubated and sedated for this, to minimize risk, and its use should be restricted to those in whom massive bleeding is not controlled by initial therapy and who are awaiting definitive treatment.
- Options in patients who continue to bleed include transjugular intrahepatic portosystemic shunt, which is performed by interventional radiologists/hepatologists to lower portal pressure by creating a shunt to the systemic circulation, or surgery. Surgical procedures include oesophageal transection with anastomosis, transthoracic transoesophageal ligation of varices, and gastric transection with reanastomosis. These operations are hardly ever done these days.

Approximately 20% of those bleeding from varices for the first time will die. The risk of recurrence is approximately 80% in the next 2 years. Adverse prognostic factors are jaundice, ascites, hypoalbuminaemia and encephalopathy (i.e. other features of decompensated liver failure).

Gastric carcinoma

The incidence of gastric carcinoma is 23 in 100 000 and it is commoner in men and the elderly. There is a link between gastric cancer and *H. pylori*, which may explain the higher prevalence in lower socioeconomic groups. Suggested dietary links include alcohol, spicy foods and nitrates, which are converted to nitrosamines by bacteria. It occurs more often in Japan because of the higher fish intake resulting in a high level of nitrosamines. It is commoner in smokers, in patients with achlorhydria and in patients with blood group A.

Other predisposing conditions include pernicious anaemia, chronic gastritis with atrophy, areas of intestinal metaplasia and partial gastrectomy.

Most cancers are adenocarcinomas and affect mainly the pylorus and antrum. They are polypoid or ulcerating lesions with rolled edges. Less common are leather-bottle-type adenocarcinomas (linitis plastica).

Clinical features

General features of malignancy may be present (weight loss, anorexia, etc.). Local features may include dyspeptic symptoms (see Ch. 9), nausea and vomiting, GI bleeding or iron-deficiency anaemia, and a palpable epigastric mass or tenderness. Metastatic features include Virchow's node in the left supraclavicular fossa and metastases to liver, bones, brain and lung. Transcoelomic spread may occur (e.g. to ovaries, Krukenberg's tumour). Paraneoplastic features include dermatomyositis and acanthosis nigricans.

Investigations

Blood tests include a full blood count (FBC) to look for signs of chronic blood loss, and liver function tests (LFTs) for possible metastases. Diagnosis is made on gastroscopy with multiple biopsies. Endoscopic ultrasound and CT/MRI scanning is used for staging. Occasionally, a diagnostic laparoscopy is indicated to assess spread from locally advanced tumours.

Management

Surgery is the only curative option. Depending on the position and extent of the tumour the patient may have a partial or total gastrectomy. More recent developments have allowed for endoscopic mucosal resection for early-stage cancers. Nonetheless, the overall 5-year survival is poor at approximately 10%. The 5-year survival with gastrectomy is around 20%. Metastases contraindicate curative surgery in up to 60% of cases and palliation may involve the use of drugs, surgery and radiotherapy.

Gastrointestinal stromal tumour

A gastrointestinal stromal tumour (GIST) is a mesenchymal tumour of the GI tract that is commonly benign (70–80%), but may be malignant. The tumours are mostly solitary and can occur anywhere in the GI tract from the oesophagus to the rectum. Malignant spread tends to be intra-abdominal and to the liver; very rarely the tumour metastases to lungs or bone. Clinical features are dependent on tumour size and location, but often include nausea, pain and occult bleeding. GIST is unusual under the age of 50 and is associated with neurofibromatosis type I. Treatment is surgical local excision with or without imatinib (a monoclonal antibody to the tumour-specific antigen c-kit protein). Two-year survival with advanced disease is now 80% due to advances in monoclonal technologies.

SMALL BOWEL DISORDERS

Malabsorption

The clinical features of malabsorption have been outlined in Ch. 11 and include anorexia, weight loss and lethargy, abdominal distension and borborygmi, steatorrhoea, wasting, clubbing, petechiae (vitamin K), anaemia (iron, vitamin B_{12}, folate), paraesthesia, bone pain and tetany (hypocalcaemia), oedema, leuconychia and ascites (hypoproteinaemia) and peripheral neuropathy (vitamin B deficiency). There may also be signs of the underlying disease (e.g. jaundice or lymphadenopathy with lymphomas). Causes of malabsorption are given in Fig. 32.1.

The range of investigations to be considered has been dealt with in Ch. 11.

Chronic pancreatitis

This is a common cause of malabsorption and is discussed later in this chapter.

Coeliac disease

Coeliac disease is a gluten-sensitive enteropathy. Gluten is present in wheat, barley and rye. In this disease, there is an abnormal duodenal and jejunal mucosa leading to malabsorption. The condition improves with a gluten-free diet but relapses when gluten is reintroduced.

Coeliac disease is commoner in Europeans, with an incidence of approximately 1 in 100 in the UK. It is commoner in females and can occur at any age. There is an increased incidence within families, and it is associated with HLA-B8 and DR3. It is also associated with a blistering subepidermal eruption of the skin (dermatitis herpetiformis). The aetiology is thought to be due to alpha-gliadin, a peptide present in gluten, which is injurious to the small bowel mucosa. Immunogenic mechanisms and possibly environmental factors (e.g. viral infections) may also play a role.

Fig. 32.1 Causes of malabsorption.

Cause	Examples
Biliary insufficiency	Primary biliary cirrhosis, biliary obstruction, cholestyramine, ileal resection (impaired enterohepatic circulation)
Pancreatic insufficiency	Chronic pancreatitis, pancreatic carcinoma, cystic fibrosis, Zollinger–Ellison syndrome (pancreatic enzymes inactive at low pH due to gastric acid hypersecretion)
Abnormalities of the small bowel mucosa	Coeliac disease, Whipple's disease, tropical sprue, radiation enteritis, small bowel resection, brush border enzyme deficiency (e.g. lactase deficiency), drugs (e.g. metformin), amyloid, hypogammaglobulinaemia (also predisposes to infection), intestinal lymphangiectasia, lymphoma, abetalipoproteinaemia, ischaemia
Bacterial overgrowth	Especially in diverticula and postoperative blind loops. Also in dilated areas of small bowel in systemic sclerosis
Infection	Giardiasis, diphyllobothriasis, strongyloidiasis, tuberculosis
Intestinal hurry	Postgastrectomy dumping, postvagotomy, gastrojejunostomy, short bowel syndrome (multiple resections, e.g. Crohn's disease)

Clinical features

Symptoms may be non-specific (e.g. lethargy and malaise). There is usually a history of diarrhoea or steatorrhoea, with abdominal discomfort, and there may be weight loss. Other features include mouth ulcers, anaemia and less commonly tetany, osteomalacia, neuropathies, myopathies and hyposplenism. Nonetheless, the disease is mainly picked up by blood testing in patients with anaemia or 'IBS'.

There is an increased incidence of autoimmune disease (e.g. thyroid disease and insulin-dependent diabetes). Coeliac disease may be complicated by GI lymphoma and gastric or oesophageal carcinoma.

Investigations

The following investigations are important in the patient with coeliac disease:

- Anti-tissue transglutaminase (TTG) and anti endomysial antibodies are tests of choice, mainly TTG.
- Duodenal biopsy: villous atrophy with chronic inflammatory cells in the lamina propria.
- FBC: may show anaemia (folate or iron deficiency – vitamin B_{12} deficiency is rare as the stomach and terminal ileum are not involved).
- Blood film may show Howell–Jolly bodies or other signs of hyposplenism.
- Serum albumin: hypoalbuminaemia.
- A DEXA scan is required once diagnosed, as patients are at risk of osteopenia/osteoporosis

Management

NICE have published guidelines on the management of coeliac disease (May 2009). The condition improves on a gluten-free diet. Deficient vitamins are replaced. If symptoms persist, it may be that the patient is not complying with the diet. Occasionally, steroid treatment is added to reduce the inflammatory response. A high index of suspicion for the complications mentioned above should be maintained.

Crohn's disease

Crohn's disease is a common cause for malabsorption and is discussed in detail later in this chapter.

Bacterial overgrowth

Although bacterial overgrowth may occur spontaneously, especially in the elderly, it is normally associated with a structural abnormality of the small intestine (e.g. in diverticula or postoperative blind loops). Aspiration of jejunal contents reveals *Escherichia coli* or *Bacteroides* spp. in concentrations greater than 10^6/mL as part of a mixed flora. The bacteria can deconjugate bile salts, which can be detected in aspirates; this deficiency of conjugated bile salts leads to steatorrhoea. The bacteria also metabolize vitamin B_{12}, leading to its deficiency.

Management

Underlying small bowel lesions should be corrected if possible. The condition may respond to intermittent courses of metronidazole or ciprofloxacin. Vitamin B_{12} should be given (1 mg intramuscularly for 5 days).

Tropical sprue

In this condition, there is severe malabsorption, usually accompanied by diarrhoea and malnutrition. It occurs in most of Asia and the Caribbean. The aetiology is unknown but it is thought to be infective, potentially caused by enterotoxigenic *E. coli*. Jejunal histology shows partial villous atrophy.

Management

Severe cases may need IV fluids and electrolytes, and replacement of nutritional and vitamin deficiencies. Patients often improve when they leave an endemic area. Patients may be helped with tetracycline 250 mg 6-hourly and folic acid.

Whipple's disease

This is a rare cause of malabsorption, usually affecting men over 50 years old. As well as steatorrhoea, there is fever, weight loss, arthralgia, lymphadenopathy and sometimes involvement of the heart, lung and brain. Histologically, cells of the lamina propria are replaced by macrophages that contain periodic acid–Schiff positive glycoprotein granules. The organism responsible is *Tropheryma whippelii*. Treatment is with antibiotics (e.g. tetracycline or co-trimoxazole).

Neuroendocrine tumours of the bowel

Although these are all very rare, they are sometimes discussed in examinations. Carcinoid tumours often occur in the small bowel, and the other tumours discussed below arise in the pancreas. They are discussed in this section for convenience and because they often affect the small bowel.

They arise from APUD (amine precursor uptake and decarboxylation) cells, which secrete a number of hormones, e.g. gastrin, glucagon and vasoactive intestinal peptide (VIP). Pancreatic endocrine tumours may occur with other endocrine tumours as part of MEN syndromes (see Ch. 35).

Carcinoid tumours

These tumours originate from the enterochromaffin cell (neural crest) of the intestine. They may appear in the appendix (45%), terminal ileum (30%), rectum (20%) or other site in the GI tract, ovaries, testis or the lung. They have malignant potential; 80% of large tumours produce metastases. Presentations include appendicitis, GI obstruction and, in 5% of cases, the carcinoid syndrome.

Carcinoid syndrome

This only occurs when liver metastases are present as the level of the metabolites is otherwise controlled by first pass metabolism in the liver. Clinical features include flushing (which may be prolonged and lead to telangiectases), abdominal pain, diarrhoea, bronchospasm, and oedema associated with pulmonary stenosis or tricuspid regurgitation. Symptoms are due to the release of pharmacologically active mediators (e.g. 5-hydroxytryptamine (5-HT), prostaglandins and kinins).

Diagnosis

This is by measurement of 5-hydroxyindoleacetic acid (5-HIAA) in 24-h urine collection. More recent developments include plasma chromogranin A measurements to assess tumour size and ^{111}indium ocreotide scitigraphy or PET scans to aid in tumour localization. Abdominal CT scan or laparoscopy/laparotomy may be needed to localize the tumour.

Treatment

Food and drink that precipitate flushing should be avoided (e.g. alcohol, coffee). Surgery is best for localized tumours and may be curative. Octreotide alleviates flushing and diarrhoea. Other useful drugs include cyproheptadine (an antihistamine with 5-HT and calcium channel blocking properties) and methysergide (which also blocks 5-HT). Other procedures include enucleation of liver metastases, hepatic artery ligation, embolization and 5-fluorouracil injection.

Prognosis

The median survival is 5–8 years after diagnosis; 3 years of metastases are present. However, some patients survive for >15 years, even with metastases.

Gastrinoma

This is usually due to a gastrin-secreting pancreatic adenoma, which stimulates excessive acid production, leading to multiple recurrent ulcers in the stomach and duodenum. Approximately half are malignant and 10% are multiple. It is usually part of Zollinger–Ellison syndrome.

Patients commonly get diarrhoea due to the low pH in the upper intestine and steatorrhoea due to the inactivation of lipase by the low pH. The diagnosis is made from a raised fasting serum gastrin level; the gastric acid output is also raised. Treatment is by removal of the primary tumour (provided there is no evidence of metastases) and omeprazole or octreotide.

Insulinomas

These are tumours of the pancreatic islet beta cells; 5% are malignant and 5% are multiple. The patient presents with recurrent or fasting hypoglycaemia, which may manifest in bizarre behaviour, epilepsy, dementia or confusion. The diagnosis is confirmed by the demonstration of hypoglycaemia in association with inappropriate and excessive insulin secretion. Raised C-peptide levels are found in insulinoma but not in exogenous insulin injection. Treatment is by surgical excision of the tumour. If surgery is not feasible, diazoxide or octreotide are useful. Fasting hypoglycaemia is discussed in Ch. 35.

VIPomas

These tumours release VIP, which produces intestinal secretions leading to watery diarrhoea, hypokalaemia and sometimes achlorhydria. Diagnosis is by high serum levels of VIP. The tumour should be resected if possible. Octreotide is useful for controlling symptoms.

Glucagonomas

These are tumours of the alpha cells of the pancreas, which release glucagon. Symptoms include diabetes, diarrhoea, a necrolytic migratory erythematous rash, weight loss, anaemia and glossitis.

INFLAMMATORY BOWEL DISEASE

HINTS AND TIPS

Extraintestinal manifestations of inflammatory bowel disease are A PIE SAC: Aphthous ulcers, Pyoderma gangrenosum, Iritis, Erythema nodosum, Sclerosing cholangitis, Arthritis and Clubbing.

Ulcerative colitis and Crohn's disease are collectively termed idiopathic inflammatory bowel disease (IBD). It is likely that these conditions represent a spectrum of disease resulting from a combination of genetic and environmental factors, although they typically differ in their natural history and response to treatment (Fig. 32.2).

Fig. 32.2 Features of Crohn's disease and ulcerative colitis.

Feature	Crohn's disease	Ulcerative colitis
Pathology	Transmural inflammation	Only mucosa and submucosa inflamed
	Fissuring ulcers: cobblestone mucosa	Mucosal ulcers: pseudopolyps
	Non-caseating granulomata	Crypt abscesses
	Can involve whole GI tract. Skip lesions	Continuous involvement proximally from rectum to affect variable length of colon
Clinical	Diarrhoea ± rectal bleeding	Diarrhoea: often with blood and mucus
	Abdominal pain and fever prominent	Abdominal pain less prominent. Fever may be present
	Anal/perianal and oral lesions	
	Stricturing causing obstructive symptoms	
Associations	Increased incidence in smokers	Decreased incidence in smokers
	Cholelithiasis	Increased primary biliary cirrhosis, sclerosing cholangitis, chronic active hepatitis
	Extraintestinal manifestations of IBD (see below)	Other extraintestinal manifestations of IBD are less common than in Crohn's
Complications	Fistulae (entero-enteral, -vaginal, -vesical, perianal)	No fistulae
	Strictures causing bowel obstruction	Toxic megacolon (in acute colitis)
	Carcinoma (related to colitis)	Carcinoma
	Iron-deficiency anaemia	
	Abscess formation	
	Vitamin B_{12} deficiency (terminal ileum commonly involved)	Iron-deficiency anaemia

IBD, inflammatory bowel disease.

Aetiology and pathogenesis

The primary cause of ulcerative colitis is unknown, although 10% of patients have a first-degree relative with ulcerative colitis or Crohn's disease. It may result from a genetically determined, inappropriately severe and/or prolonged inflammatory response to a dietary or microbial product. Abnormalities of colonic epithelial cell metabolism have also been reported in ulcerative colitis, and there are associations with certain drugs such as NSAIDs and antibiotics, and with stress, although the significance is uncertain.

There may be a history of atopy, autoimmune disease (e.g. chronic active hepatitis and systemic lupus erythematosus) and the presence of circulating immune complexes and antibodies to colonocytes and neutrophils (pANCA) in ulcerative colitis.

Ulcerative colitis

This is an idiopathic chronic relapsing inflammatory disease that always involves the rectum and extends proximally in continuity to affect a variable length of colon. Although the small bowel is spared there may be some 'backwash ileitis'. It is commoner in the Western world, with a prevalence of approximately 150 in 100 000 and an incidence of about 10 in 100 000 annually, and is maximal at 15–40 years of age. There is no major sex difference.

Clinical features

The disease may present with a single mild episode followed by remission for a prolonged period, or progressive symptoms over months with general ill health and chronic diarrhoea, or as an acute severe episode. In general, the severity of diarrhoea and systemic upset depends on the extent of the disease and depth of mucosal ulceration.

Active subtotal or total ulcerative colitis causes frequent bloody diarrhoea, often with fever, malaise, anorexia, weight loss, abdominal pain, anaemia and tachycardia. With proctitis, characteristic symptoms are rectal bleeding and mucus discharge, but the stool is well formed and general health is maintained. The patient may present with a complication. Between relapses, the patient is usually symptomless.

Complications

Local

Toxic megacolon, perforation or rarely massive haemorrhage can occur. There is an increased risk of colonic carcinoma in patients with subtotal or total ulcerative colitis. The cumulative incidence is 10–15% at 20 years.

Extraintestinal

Extraintestinal complications of inflammatory bowel disease include the following:

- Skin: erythema nodosum, pyoderma gangrenosum, vasculitis.
- Eyes: uveitis, episcleritis, conjunctivitis.
- Joints: large joint arthropathy, sacroiliitis, ankylosing spondylitis.
- Liver: pericholangitis, sclerosing cholangitis, cirrhosis, autoimmune hepatitis, cholangiocarcinoma.
- Vasculature: arterial and venous thrombosis.
- Renal stones and gallbladder stones: in Crohn's disease.

Investigations and diagnosis

Sigmoidoscopy and rectal biopsy show inflamed mucosa. If the disease is active there may be pus and blood, visible ulceration and contact bleeding. Other types of colitis should be excluded, and stool microscopy and culture is needed to exclude infection. Blood tests may show anaemia, raised white cell count and a raised ESR and/or CRP.

Histology shows inflammatory cells infiltrating the lamina propria with crypt abscesses. There is little involvement of the muscularis mucosa and there is a reduction of goblet cells.

Colonoscopy will show the extent of the disease. Ulcers and pseudopolyps may be seen, oedema of the colonic wall produces widening of the presacral space, and there may be narrowed areas secondary to carcinoma. In the patient with acute colitis a plain abdominal X-ray should be performed to look for colonic dilation and evidence of mucosal oedema. An erect chest X-ray is often performed in the acute setting to exclude perforation (60–80% sensitive).

Management

General measures

A multidisciplinary approach is preferred with gastroenterologists, nursing staff, counsellors and stoma therapists in collaboration with primary healthcare teams. Liaison with the colorectal surgical team at an early point is encouraged. Specific nutritional, haematinic and electrolyte deficiencies may require correction. NSAIDs should be avoided.

The acute relapse

The mortality of patients with acute colitis climbs sharply if they perforate. Therefore, management is directed at stratifying patients in terms of severity (and therefore risk of perforation), treating them accordingly to induce remission and carefully selecting those patients requiring emergency colectomy, hopefully before they perforate (Fig. 32.3).

The mainstay of therapy in the acute phase is steroids with bone protection with the addition of a 5-aminosalicylic acid (5-ASA).

In mild ulcerative colitis (less than 4 motions/day, systemically well), oral prednisolone 30–40 mg o.d. with bone protection is the mainstay of treatment. A 5-ASA (e.g. mesalazine) may help further in achieving remission. The steroid dose should be decreased by 5 mg per week. In moderate disease (4–6 motions/day) oral prednisolone (and bone protection) should be started at 40 mg o.d. and reduced by 5 mg weekly. A 5-ASA should be considered in addition. If patients are systemically unwell (tachycardia, hypotension, fever, dehydration, tender colon) and passing more than 8 motions/day, they should be admitted to hospital:

- Nil by mouth, IV fluids, close monitoring of observations, stool chart.
- Daily blood tests and regular plain abdominal X-ray to monitor progress.
- 400 mg IV hydrocortisone/day in divided doses with steroid enemas. Prophylactic subcutaneous heparin is given.
- Antibiotics for any accompanying septicaemia (usually Gram-negative).
- If improved at 5 days, commence oral therapy.
- If failing to respond, some advocate the careful use of ciclosporin or infliximab to induce remission.

Fig. 32.3 Truelove and Witts classification for severity of ulcerative colitis.

Activity	Mild	Moderate	Severe
No. of bloody stools/day	<4	4–6	>6
Temperature (°C)	Normal	37–37.8	>37.8
Heart rate (bpm)	Normal	Intermediate	>90
Hb (g/dL)	>11	10.5–11	<10.5
ESR (mm/h)	<20	20–30	>30

ESR, erythrocyte sedimentation rate; Hb, haemoglobin.

- Indications for emergency colectomy: continuing deterioration despite medical therapy; toxic dilation of the colon; perforation.

Maintaining remission

The 5-aminosalicylates help maintain remission, reducing annual relapse rates from 70% to 30%. They are also available as enemas and suppositories. There are different preparations with different methods of releasing the active component (5-ASA) in the colon. Sulfasalazine is an example. This consists of 5-ASA, linked by an azo bond to sulfapyridine. The 5-ASA is released in the colon by bacterial action. Approximately 20% of patients cannot tolerate sulfasalazine because of adverse effects, mostly related to the sulfapyridine. These include headache and fever, blood dyscrasias, bone marrow suppression, rashes and oligospermia, making newer compounds preferable in young men.

Mesalazine contains 5-ASA alone and may have fewer side effects. It is a delayed-release preparation.

Azathioprine may be used in patients who relapse repeatedly on steroid withdrawal after an acute episode, or in whom aminosalicylates are ineffective for maintaining remission; it may take up to 3–4 months to effect a noticeable clinical benefit. Serious adverse effects include bone marrow suppression and cholestatic jaundice, necessitating blood checks fortnightly for 1 month, then monthly for 2 months, then 2–3 monthly. Long-term risk appears to be low.

Surgery

Surgery is curative for colonic disease, although not for extraintestinal complications. Options include panproctocolectomy with ileoanal pouch, permanent ileostomy or rarely subtotal colectomy with ileorectal anastomosis. It may be considered electively for chronic intractable ulcerative colitis, colonic carcinoma, persistent mucosal dysplasia or growth retardation in children. The emergency indications are summarized above. Advances in laparascopic procedures means many cases can now be done laparascopically. But the majority of patients are managed medically.

Monitoring and prognosis

Approximately 70% of untreated patients relapse annually and up to 30% eventually require surgery, although the overall mortality is close to that of the general population. The main risks to life are severe attacks of ulcerative colitis and colonic cancer. Patients with extensive ulcerative colitis of 10 years' duration or more used to be offered colonoscopy every 1–2 years to prevent colonic cancer by taking multiple biopsies to look for mucosal dysplasia (i.e. detection of cancer at a curable stage), and by offering elective colectomy if appropriate. British Society of Gastroenterologist's guidelines now recommend frequency of colonoscopy should be guided by the extent and degree of disease activity instead.

Crohn's disease

Crohn's disease can affect any part of the GI tract from the mouth to the anus. The involvement is not confluent ('skip lesions') (Fig. 32.2). It most frequently presents with ileocaecal disease followed by colonic, ileal alone, diffuse small intestinal, gastric and oesophageal involvement. The overall prevalence in the Western world is approximately 1 in 1000 and it is more common in Caucasians than in Afro-Caribbeans.

Clinical presentation

The patient has diarrhoea and abdominal pain. There may be a fever, anaemia and weight loss. The patient may be clubbed and there may be associated complications (e.g. joint, skin or eye complications, as with ulcerative colitis).

The presentation depends on the site of disease and on the tendency to perforate or fistulate rather than to fibrose and stricture, which is probably determined by genetic factors. Terminal ileal disease presents with right iliac fossa pain, often with an associated mass. This may present acutely, mimicking appendicitis, or chronically, mimicking irritable bowel syndrome.

Colonic Crohn's disease is distinguishable from ulcerative colitis by the presence of skip lesions (multiple lesions with normal bowel in between), rectal sparing, perianal skin tags or fistulae with or without granulomata on biopsy, although the distinction is unclear in up to 10% of patients.

Complications

Local

Strictures cause partial or complete GI obstruction. Entero-enteric, enterovesical, enterovaginal and perianal fistulae may develop. Prolonged disease increases the risk of small and large bowel cancer. Abscesses may form. Iron, folate and vitamin B_{12} deficiency can all occur.

Extraintestinal

As for ulcerative colitis above. Fig. 32.2 summarizes the few differences between ulcerative colitis and Crohn's in terms of their extraintestinal manifestations.

Investigations and diagnosis

Diagnosis is made by endoscopy and biopsy of lesions. Histology demonstrates transmural inflammation with an inflammatory cell infiltrate and non-caseating granulomata (in 30%). CT (or MRI) of the small and large bowel is performed. This shows skip lesions, a coarse cobblestone appearance of the mucosa and, later, fibrosis producing narrowing of the intestine with proximal dilatation. Capsule endoscopy and MRI are increasingly used to help in diagnosis – MRI is particularly useful for evaluation of fistulae and abscesses and pelvic disease. Blood tests may show anaemia (potentially due to terminal ileum involvement and a resulting inability to absorb vitamin B_{12}). Serum C-reactive protein can be elevated in cases with active disease. ESR is a good measure of response to treatment and a baseline measurement should be available. Stool samples should be sent for microscopy and culture to exclude infection.

Management

In most cases of active Crohn's disease, there are three therapeutic alternatives: drugs, diet and surgery. These options should be discussed with the patient.

Medical management

Some patients manage on symptomatic therapy alone (e.g. loperamide or codeine phosphate) provided there is no evidence of obstruction. Cholestyramine (ion exchange resin) is useful for diarrhoea due to terminal ileal disease or resection as it prevents conjugated bile acids from entering the colon. However, it should not be given at the same time as other medications as it impairs their absorption. Haematinics may require replacement although anaemia often improves as disease activity falls.

Acute attacks are often treated with corticosteroids (e.g. prednisolone 30–40 mg o.d.), but these have no effect on reducing the rate of relapse. Their inappropriate use must be avoided because of their side-effect profile. Budesonide is a corticosteroid analogue with rapid hepatic conversion, and therefore reduced systemic side effects, and is useful in mild attacks. Azathioprine (or its active metabolite 6-mercaptopurine) is often started during the acute attack. It is helpful in maintaining the steroid-induced remission but takes several weeks to be effective.

Patients with colonic involvement may benefit from a 5-ASA compound (see above). Antibiotics also have a role. Metronidazole is effective in colonic and perianal disease and in prevention of recurrence following bowel resection. If used for longer than 3 months, there is a risk of peripheral neuropathy. Other antibiotics are also used.

Elemental diets are useful for inducing remission in small bowel disease but are expensive and unpalatable; therefore compliance is often poor. Except in children where elemental diets are frequently used.

Some patients can be maintained in remission without drug therapy – the importance to Crohn's disease patients of stopping smoking must be emphasized. However, some patients require immunosuppressive therapy – azathioprine and other agents are used. NICE supports the expert use of infliximab and adalimumab (monoclonal antibodies against tumour necrosis factor-alpha) in severe cases resistant to other drugs.

Surgery

A significant proportion of patients will require an operation at some stage but surgery should be avoided if possible. It is indicated for:

- Failure of medical therapy with acute or chronic illness causing ill health.
- Complications: abscess, obstruction, perforation, toxic dilation, fistulae not responding to conservative treatment with antibiotics.
- Failure to grow (children).

Small bowel strictures can be widened (stricturoplasty), whereas those elsewhere need resection. Postoperative fistulae used to be a common complication but are now rare, partly because of the use of perioperative antibiotics, particularly metronidazole. After surgical resection, approximately half the patients remain symptom-free for 5 years and half require further surgery within 10 years.

Prognosis

Around 10–20% of patients remain asymptomatic for 20 years after the first or second episode of symptomatic disease. Around 50% patients need at least one surgical resection within their lifetime, particularly if small and large bowel are involved.

COLORECTAL DISEASE

Colorectal neoplasia

Benign disease

Colonic polyps are common and are often found incidentally during investigation of coincidental GI symptoms such as pain, altered bowel habit or bleeding haemorrhoids. They may be non-neoplastic or neoplastic (commoner) and may be sessile or pedunculated, vary from a few millimetres to up to 10 cm in diameter and be solitary or multiple.

Adenomatous polyps (neoplastic) are usually asymptomatic. They may bleed and lead to iron-deficiency anaemia. Sessile villous adenomas of the rectum may present with profuse diarrhoea and hypokalaemia. Most colonic carcinomas originate from adenomas. Once a polyp is found, it is therefore removed endoscopically and, as further polyps may develop, a programme of continuous colonoscopic surveillance every 3–5 years is recommended by the British Society of Gastroenterology.

Familial adenomatous polyposis is mendelian dominant. Patients have multiple polyps throughout the GI tract. In high-risk patients, colectomy with ileorectal anastomosis may be performed, with continued surveillance of the rectal stump.

Peutz–Jeghers syndrome consists of mucocutaneous pigmentation and hamartomatous polyps (non-neoplastic) anywhere along the GI tract, most commonly in the small bowel. It has a mendelian dominant inheritance.

Colorectal cancer

Colonic adenocarcinoma is the second commonest tumour in the UK, causing approximately 20 000 deaths per year, with a lifetime incidence of approximately 1 in 27. It is commoner in the elderly and less common in Africa and Asia. It may be related to diets low in fibre and high in animal fat. Predisposing conditions include colitis in inflammatory bowel disease and familial adenomatous polyposis. Genetic factors also play a role, with a two- to threefold increased risk of developing colon cancer with one first-degree affected family member. At the upper end of this risk spectrum is hereditary non-polyposis colon cancer. This is a dominantly inherited mutation of a DNA mismatch repair gene. Affected family members develop right-sided cancers at an early age and therefore colonoscopic surveillance is commenced from 25 to 35 years.

Ninety per cent of colon cancer occurs in patients without a strong family history. Over half of these tumours occur in the rectosigmoid area. Two-thirds of tumours occur with ulceration and spread by direct infiltration, invading the lymph nodes and blood vessels, leading to metastases.

Clinical features

General features of malignancy include weight loss, anorexia and lethargy. Local features depend on the location of the tumour. Left-sided tumours present with altered bowel habit and abdominal pain. Rectosigmoid tumours commonly bleed. Right-sided carcinomas can become large and remain asymptomatic (as the stool has a liquid consistency here). They may present with iron-deficiency anaemia alone. The elderly often present with bowel obstruction. Any persistent change in bowel habit or rectal bleeding must be investigated.

Examination should always include a digital rectal examination and sigmoidoscopy. The tumour may be detected as an abdominal mass and hepatomegaly may be felt with liver metastases.

Investigations and staging

Faecal occult blood (FOB) test

FOB testing is now fully established in the UK for people aged 60–69. These home tests potentially detect faecal blood which may be an early sign of colorectal cancer. If the test is positive a colonoscopy is performed to rule out carcinoma. Although it has shown to reduce mortality by up to 20%, the high false-positive rate (10%) has been a problem. One-off flexible sigmoidoscopy screening is soon to be introduced too.

Blood tests

- FBC for microcytic anaemia (blood loss).
- U&Es to detect electrolyte abnormalities with diarrhoea.
- LFTs may indicate liver metastases.
- Tumour markers (CEA) to monitor response to treatment.

Imaging and tissue diagnosis

- Colonoscopy and biopsy is essential for tissue diagnosis and tumour grading (in fit patients).
- Flexible sigmoidoscopy and CT scan (or perhaps CT colonography).
- CT pneumocolon can be used as an alternative to colonoscopy, providing a virtual intraluminal view of the colon.

Staging

- Contrast-enhanced CT of chest, abdomen and pelvis for all colorectal cancers – modified Duke's classification (Fig. 32.4).
- Additional MRI for patients with rectal cancer to assess surgical margins and lymph nodes.
- Endorectal ultrasound for rectal cancers.

Fig. 32.4 Modified Duke's classification of colorectal carcinoma.

Tumour stage	Definition	Percentage of cases	Five-year cancer-related survival (%)
A	Confined to bowel wall	10	90–100
B	Beyond bowel wall/no metastases	35	65–75
C	Involves lymph nodes	30	30–40
D	Distant metastases/ residual disease after surgery	25	<5

Management

NICE recently published guidelines on the management of colorectal cancer (Nov 2011). All new cases are discussed at a multidisciplinary team (MDT) meeting. Over 90% of primary tumours can be resected surgically. Adjuvant radiotherapy and chemotherapy may be used such as adjuvant chemotherapy for Duke's C colonic cancers and preoperative radiotherapy considered for operable rectal cancer. The prognosis is summarized in Fig. 32.4.

HINTS AND TIPS

Adjuvant chemotherapy is given after surgery to reduce the statistical chance of relapse due to occult disease. Neoadjuvant chemotherapy is given prior to surgery, often to shrink or downstage the tumour.

Diverticular disease

A diverticulum is an outpouching of the wall of the gut. Diverticula can occur anywhere in the gut but are most common in the colon, especially the sigmoid colon. Diverticulosis implies the presence of diverticula, and diverticulitis implies that there is inflammation within a diverticulum. They are due to high intracolonic pressure with weakness of the colonic wall. The mucosa therefore herniates through the muscle layers of the gut. The incidence increases with age and affects up to one-third of the population, although most people are asymptomatic. It is more common in women than in men.

Clinical features

There may be colicky left-sided abdominal pain and tenderness, nausea and flatulence. The pain may be relieved with defecation and there may be a change in bowel habit with constipation or diarrhoea. With diverticulitis, pain is more severe and the patient is pyrexial. Diverticula may perforate and lead to localized or generalized peritonitis or fistula formation. Rectal bleeding may occur and is usually sudden and painless. Subacute obstruction may occur due to stricture formation. Fistulae may communicate between the colon and bladder (vesicocolic fistula), leading to pneumaturia and recurrent urinary tract infection. They may also form between the colon and vagina or small bowel.

Investigations

In the acute setting an FBC, U&Es, LFTs, amylase and an arterial blood gas are all indicated as these patients tend to present with an 'acute abdomen'. If the patient is pyrexial blood cultures should be sent. If there is any rectal bleeding proctoscopy may be indicated. Plain abdominal and chest X-rays should be performed (to rule out obstruction and/or perforation), but a CT scan is the imaging modality of choice. Colonoscopy is contraindicated in the acute setting as it may cause colonic perforation; instead this can be performed as an outpatient once the acute episode has resolved.

Management

In acute diverticulitis, treatment is analgesia, adequate hydration and antibiotics. The patient may have to be kept nil by mouth and given IV fluids. Abscesses may need to be drained, and peritonitis following perforation or obstruction may necessitate resection and colostomy. Patients with profuse rectal bleeding may require transfusion and colonic resection. Treatment of fistulae is surgical.

For diverticulosis, a high-fibre diet is recommended, and soluble fibre supplements and bulk-forming agents can be prescribed. Antispasmodics may provide symptomatic relief when colic is a problem. Drugs that slow intestinal motility (e.g. codeine and loperamide) could exacerbate symptoms and are contraindicated.

Clostridium difficile and pseudomembranous colitis

Clostridium difficile is an anaerobic bacterium that can cause anything from mild diarrhoea to severe inflammation and potential perforation of the colon (pseudomembranous colitis). Colonization by *C. difficile* is encouraged by broad-spectrum antibiotic therapy (e.g. broad-spectrum beta-lactams or third-generation cephalosporins), which eliminates other normal gut bacteria. This is a important contributing factor to the incidence of *C. difficile* infection in hospitals. There should be a suspicion of any in-patient who develops diarrhoea after a period of antibiotics. It is usually of acute onset but may run a chronic course. Sixty per cent of those affected are over 75 years of age. Spread is through the faecal–oral route and handwashing with water and soap is of paramount importance to stop the spread of infection

Clinical features include diarrhoea, fever and abdominal cramps. As with all causes of colitis, if severe, toxic dilation of the colon can occur. *C. difficile* infection has become more common and hospitals are taking measures to reduce antibiotic use and stop cross-infection. The most frequently implicated antibiotic is clindamycin but few antibiotics are free of this side effect.

Diagnosis

Diagnosis is by demonstration of *Clostridium difficile* toxin in faeces using either cell culture assay or immunoassay. Sigmoidoscopy reveals an erythematous, ulcerated mucosa, which is covered by a membrane. However, the appearances are not essential for the diagnosis.

Management

Suspected antibiotics should be stopped and patients should be isolated for infection control. Oral vancomycin or metronidazole are used as specific treatments. If the patient is postoperative and has an ileus, IV metronidazole is indicated. Careful attention should be paid to fluid and electrolyte management.

Lower gastrointestinal bleeding

The differential diagnosis of lower GI bleeding is shown in Fig. 32.5.

Resuscitation should be carried out as for upper GI bleeds, and further investigations are carried out when the patient is stable. Examination should include a rectal examination to exclude carcinoma, sigmoidoscopy and colonoscopy. Barium enema may add to information and CT and angiography can be carried out if vascular abnormalities are suspected. Stool samples must also be sent to microbiology to exclude an infectious cause.

Lower GI bleeding may be occult and chronic, presenting with iron-deficiency anaemia and general lethargy and fatigue. If the history does not suggest a particular site in the GI tract responsible for the blood loss, a sensible working plan is upper GI endoscopy followed by colonoscopy. CT and/or MRI ± capsule endoscopy are now the preferred means of investigating small intestinal pathology. Isotope-labelled red blood cell studies may localize the site of bleeding, but this is rarely done. Note that both angiography and isotope-labelled red blood cell studies require active bleeding in order to provide useful information (see Ch. 10).

Fig. 32.5 Differential diagnosis of lower gastrointestinal bleeding.

Anal fissure
Haemorrhoids
Inflammatory bowel disease
Infective colitis
Gastrointestinal carcinoma: sigmoid, caecum, rectum
Ischaemic colitis
Diverticulitis
Intestinal polyps
Vascular abnormalities: angiodysplasia, arteriovenous malformations
Meckel's diverticulum
Peutz–Jeghers syndrome
Osler–Weber–Rendu disease
Endometriosis

Ischaemic colitis

Acute ischaemia of the bowel may occur and is often embolic (e.g. due to atrial fibrillation). This is a surgical emergency. It is suggested by severe abdominal pain, haemodynamic shock and a relative absence of clinical signs with a metabolic acidosis.

Chronic intestinal ischaemia usually relates to low flow in the inferior mesenteric artery and therefore affects the descending colon. Severe postprandial pain occurs ('gut claudication') with rectal bleeding and diarrhoea. There is often a pyrexia, tachycardia and leucocytosis. It usually settles with conservative management. Diagnosis is difficult but revascularization may be attempted following angiography. Occasionally gangrene of the affected gut segment occurs – surgical resection is necessary and mortality is high.

Microscopic colitis

This diagnosis is defined by the triad of chronic watery diarrhoea, normal colonoscopy and histopathological evidence of increased inflammatory cells within colonic biopsies. The condition is associated with other autoimmune conditions such as Sjögren's syndrome and coeliac disease and commonly affects middle-aged females. Treatment is symptomatic is with budesonide.

INFECTIVE ENTERITIS

Infective enteritis is an infectious illness predominantly affecting the small intestine. It can be caused by bacteria, viruses or toxins such as heavy metals or mushrooms.

Aetiology

Bacterial enteritis is frequently a result of infection of water or food sources.

Bacterial gastroenteritis

Bacteria can affect the GI tract by means of direct invasion of the mucosal barrier, releasing toxins or through adherence and disruption of the enterocyte brush border. It is often the case in bacterial infections, fever is a common feature in bacterial gastroenteritis. The time from infection to symptoms is variable depending on the pathological mechanism. For example, *S. aureus* gastroenteritis may be toxin mediated (preformed) and symptoms will occur within 1–6 h of ingestion. In contrast, *Shigella* infection has an incubation time from 1 to 7 days as its pathogenesis is mediated through direct destruction of the intestinal mucosal epithelium causing dysentery. Bacterial causes of bloody diarrhoea include *Campylobacter, Shigella, C. difficile* and *Salmonella* infection.

Viral gastroenteritis

More than half of cases of gastroenteritis are viral, particularly in children. Rotaviruses are the most common. Another, very relevant, cause for healthcare professionals is gastroenteritis due to norovirus. This virus causes profound diarrhoea and vomiting. Usually symptoms last only 24-48 h, but its highly infective nature means it is a frequent cause of ward closure in hospital (the 'winter vomiting bug'). Good hand hygiene is vital in preventing spread. Management is entirely symptomatic.

Clinical features

Symptoms are usually of acute onset. Diarrhoea and/or vomiting are a prominent feature. Diarrhoea is often watery, but may also be bloody. Associated symptoms may include fever and abdominal cramping. Very rarely seizures may be a feature. If symptoms persist and the patient is unable to effectively rehydrate, hypovolaemia and its consequences may ensue.

Investigations

Stool culture and microscopy may reveal the causative organism. If IV fluids are considered U&Es should be measured prior to starting these. Blood cultures are indicated if the patient is pyrexial.

If there is bloody diarrhoea then blood cultures, U&Es and FBC should be performed. If the haemoglobin is low then haemolytic uraemic syndrome (HUS) should be considered and a blood film should be requested to look for fragmented red blood cells

Management

Management is usually symptomatic and the infection self-limiting. Oral fluid intake, with rehydration solution containing salt and sugar, should be encouraged to minimalize losses. Occasionally IV fluids and anti-emetics may be required if symptoms are severe and persistent. Antidiarrhoeals or not normally encouraged as it stops eradication of the causative agent. Antibiotics are only indicated in a few situations (*Salmonella, Cholera, Shigella* and *Campylobacter*). Food poisoning is a notifiable disease in the UK.

IRRITABLE BOWEL SYNDROME AND NON-ULCER DYSPEPSIA

Irritable bowel syndrome

Irritable bowel syndrome (IBS) is the commonest diagnosis made in GI clinics. It is a symptom-based diagnosis and the ROME III criteria are used to classify the disorder in terms of gastrointestinal anatomy and predominant symptoms. Most frequently there is intermittent colicky abdominal pain, which is relieved by bowel action, diarrhoea or frequent passage of small amounts of stool, and bloating. The diarrhoea may alternate with periods of constipation. Some people have a sense of incomplete evacuation or 'rectal dissatisfaction'. Symptoms may be precipitated by certain foods, drugs (e.g. antibiotics) or stress. Other features such as tiredness, nausea, backache and bladder symptoms are common in people with IBS, and may be used to support the diagnosis. Note that rectal bleeding is not a feature and that prominent nocturnal symptoms point away from the diagnosis.

Investigations

The term 'diagnosis of exclusion' is not encouraged now as it belittles symptoms. However, it is important not to miss more serious disease, e.g. inflammatory bowel disease or malignancy. It is prudent to check the FBC and erythrocyte sedimentation rate, CRP, and perform a sigmoidoscopy. Faecal calprotectin, a biochemical test commonly positive in inflammatory bowel disease, has a valuable role in helping exclude this diagnosis. Older patients, or patients in whom colonic carcinoma is suspected, warrant a CT or colonoscopy.

Management

NICE published guidelines on the management of IBS in adults (Feb 2008). Symptoms may improve with a high-fibre diet, or with other agents that increase stool bulk. Specific aggravating foods should be avoided. In some patients there may be important psychological aggravating factors that respond to reassurance. Antimotility drugs such as loperamide may relieve diarrhoea, and antispasmodic drugs (e.g. mebeverine 135 mg t.d.s.) may relieve pain. Opioids with a central action such as codeine are best avoided because of the risk of dependence. Some patients derive benefit from low doses of tricyclic antidepressant drugs or a FODMAP (fermentable oligo-, di-, monosaccharides and polyols) diet in collaboration with a dietician.

Non-ulcer dyspepsia

This term encompasses a heterogeneous group of patients with dyspeptic symptoms (see Ch. 9) and no macroscopic mucosal abnormality. Only a minority of them actually undergo endoscopy (see Fig. 9.3).

The cause of their symptoms is unclear but is likely to be multifactorial and include acid, dysmotility, *H. pylori* infection and depression. Management is often unsatisfactory. Lifestyle advice is given regarding smoking, alcohol, obesity, etc. Culprit drugs, such as NSAIDs, should be withdrawn if possible. Antisecretory therapy is used and is titrated to the lowest-cost preparation that achieves symptom control. Those who are *H. pylori*-positive should receive eradication and patient reassurance is an important part of their management.

HINTS AND TIPS

In irritable bowel syndrome it is important to gain the patient's confidence. Investigations should be sufficient to exclude other important diagnoses. The diagnosis should then be made with appropriate explanation and advice, otherwise patients may move from doctor to doctor seeking further investigation.

DISEASES OF THE GALLBLADDER

Gallstones

The incidence of gallstones rises with age, body mass index and parity, and gallstones are more common in females. Gallstone-related pathology is responsible for a significant proportion of hospital admissions with abdominal pain.

Bile contains cholesterol, bile pigments and phospholipids, and it is the relative concentrations of these that determine the kind of stone that is formed. Pigment stones are small and radiolucent, and they are occasionally associated with haemolytic anaemia due to increased formation of bile pigment from haemoglobin.

Cholesterol stones are large, often solitary, and are radiolucent. Mixed stones contain calcium salts, pigment and cholesterol; 10% are radio-opaque. (Compare with renal stones, of which approximately 90% are radio-opaque.)

Gallstones are often asymptomatic but may cause acute or chronic cholecystitis (see below), biliary colic (stone impacted in neck of gallbladder or cystic duct) or obstructive jaundice. Other presentations include cholangitis (infection of the bile ducts causing right upper quadrant pain, jaundice, and fever with rigors – Charcot's triad), pancreatitis, empyema and gallstone ileus, where the gallstone perforates the gallbladder, ulcerates into the duodenum, and passes on to obstruct the terminal ileum. The long-term presence of gallstones may be associated with gallbladder carcinoma as a consequence of chronic inflammation.

Investigations

- Liver function tests may show a cholestatic picture (see Ch. 13).
- Prothrombin time prolongation may occur over a longer period because of vitamin K (fat-soluble) malabsorption.
- Ultrasound examination may demonstrate stones in the gallbladder or bile ducts.
- In the presence of duct dilation or stones, endoscopic retrograde cholangiopancreatography (ERCP) is usually performed. This is therapeutic, allowing sphincterotomy and the removal of stones.
- Magnetic resonance cholangiopancreatography (MRCP) and endoscopic ultrasound help to image the biliary tree but have no therapeutic use. Hepatic iminodiacetic acid scintigraphy can demonstrate a blocked cystic duct, but is rarely used.
- Haemolysis screen: if pigment stones are suspected or found operatively.

HINTS AND TIPS

Courvoisier's law: 'If the gallbladder is palpable in painless jaundice, the cause unlikely to be gallstones' (because gallstones cause fibrosis and shrinkage of the gallbladder).

Management

Stones in the gallbladder itself can cause various syndromes (see above). If the patient is symptomatic of gallstones (and this is not always easy to ascertain – see 'Chronic cholecystitis' below), treatment is by cholecystectomy, which may be performed acutely or after a delay (see 'Acute cholecystitis' below).

Stones in the biliary tree can cause obstructive jaundice, cholangitis and pancreatitis. These patients require resuscitation and IV antibiotics for infection – notably in cholangitis. Sphincterotomy via ERCP may release stones in the common bile duct preoperatively if these are present. Other options include exploration of the ducts at open operation or laparoscopic exploration in the case of laparoscopic cholecystectomy if there is a reason to suspect stones in the duct.

Acute cholecystitis

This disease is most common in overweight, middle-aged women but may occur at any age. It usually follows the impaction of a stone in the cystic duct or Hartmann's pouch, which causes right upper quadrant or epigastric pain. It is distinguishable from biliary colic by the presence of inflammation leading to fever, rigors, vomiting, local peritonism or a gallbladder mass. If the stone moves to the common bile duct, jaundice may occur. Murphy's sign may be positive; this is pain on inspiration when two fingers are placed over the right upper quadrant, due to an inflamed gallbladder impinging on the examiner's fingers.

Differential diagnosis

The differential diagnosis of acute cholecystitis includes the following:

- Appendicitis in a highly situated appendix.
- Right basal pneumonia.
- Perforated peptic ulcer.
- Pancreatitis.
- Myocardial infarction.
- Biliary colic.
- Cholangitis.

Investigations

The white cell count is elevated and inflammatory markers raised (unlike in biliary colic). A chest X-ray (CXR), ECG, serum amylase and cardiac enzymes should be taken to help exclude differential diagnoses. Ultrasound will commonly show a thickened gallbladder wall and stones with or without common bile duct dilatation.

Management

Management is usually initially conservative, unless complications ensue (e.g. perforation of the gallbladder). The patient should be on bed rest, nil by mouth with IV fluids, and analgesia and antibiotics (e.g. Tazocin and metronidazole) should be given. Either cholecystectomy is performed after 48 h (a 'hot lap chole') or the inflammation is allowed to settle and the gallbladder is removed after 2–3 months.

HINTS AND TIPS

Acute ascending cholangitis is infection of the biliary tree. The causative organisms are commonly Gram-negative and can lead to overwhelming sepsis if not treated promptly.

Chronic cholecystitis

Recurrent episodes of cholecystitis are usually associated with gallstones, leading to intermittent colic and chronic inflammation. There is abdominal discomfort, bloating, nausea, flatulence and intolerance of fats.

The differential diagnosis includes myocardial ischaemia, hiatus hernia and oesophagitis, peptic ulcer disease, irritable bowel syndrome, chronic relapsing pancreatitis and tumours of the GI tract. It can be very difficult to be sure that the symptoms relate to the gallbladder and stones and therefore the decision to perform a cholecystectomy should be made cautiously.

Biliary tract cancer

Cholangiocarcinoma

This is a cancer that arises from the bile duct epithelium, commonly extrahepatic. Patients usually present with obstructive jaundice or cholangitis. The cancer is usually primary, but can be associated with sclerosing cholangitis, chronic inflammation and chronic cholecystolithiasis. Surgery is the only curative option, but prognosis is poor (15% at 5 years). ERCP and stenting is used for palliation.

Gallbladder cancer

Adenocarcinoma of the gallbladder is rare and risk increases with age. The tumour typically arises in the fundus. They are usually associated with gallstones and often discovered incidentally (during cholecystectomy). Curative treatment requires radical cholecystectomy, which includes resecting segment IV of the liver. Prognosis is very poor, unless the cancer is identified incidentally before metastatic spread.

Cancer of the ampulla

This rare condition affects the ampulla of Vater. The tumour arises in the last 1 cm of the common bile duct. Patients present with anorexia, nausea, vomiting, jaundice, pruritus, or weight loss. Because of the location of this cancer, patients present relatively early (compared to pancreatic cancer for example). A Whipple's procedure, with curative intend, is often the preferred option. Prognosis is relatively good for those that undergo surgery; 60–80% at 5 years.

DISEASES OF THE PANCREAS

Carcinoma of the pancreas

The incidence of pancreatic carcinoma is increasing. Risk factors include age, smoking, chronic pancreatitis and familial cancer syndromes (e.g. BRCA2 mutations). Approximately three-quarters of tumours occur in the head, the rest occurring in the body or tail. Secondary diabetes is uncommon. Pancreatitis may occur due to obstruction of the pancreatic duct.

Clinical features

General features of malignancy include anorexia, weight loss and lethargy. Local features are dyspepsia or epigastric pain radiating to the back and obstructive jaundice with an enlarged gallbladder. There may be hepatomegaly from biliary obstruction or metastases.

Thrombophlebitis migrans is a paraneoplastic feature in 10% of patients. Fever may occur. In any patient that presents with painless jaundice the diagnosis of pancreatic cancer must be excluded.

Investigations

Blood tests for anaemia (FBC) and liver metastases or biliary obstruction (LFTs) should be performed and, if a diagnosis of pancreatic cancer is suspected, the tumour marker Ca19-9 should also be measured. Ultrasound may identify a mass and dilated bile ducts. CT scan may define resectability of the tumour and help to stage it. ERCP may confirm the diagnosis, and allow for biopsies to be taken. MRCP and endoscopic ultrasound can provide valuable information, in particular regarding local bile duct involvement. Occasionally, laparoscopy is used to further stage the disease.

Management

A minority of patients may be suitable for operative treatment commonly because pancreatic cancer presents late and the tumour has invaded vital structures (e.g. portal vessels). Patients with ampullary carcinoma often present early with jaundice, and surgical removal may therefore be more successful. If surgery is possible a Whipple's procedure is usually performed. There is no role for (neo)adjuvant chemotherapy. Patients who are deemed suitable for surgery still have a poor prognosis of 10% at 5 years (commonly due to local recurrence).

Without treatment, survival is usually only a few weeks to months after diagnosis. Palliative procedures may include bypass surgery for obstructions (e.g. gastrojejunostomy to bypass duodenal obstruction) or stent insertion to relieve obstructive jaundice (either percutaneously or by ERCP).

Acute pancreatitis

Acute pancreatitis is an acute inflammatory condition of the pancreas causing local and systemic reactions. The incidence is approximately 3 cases per 10 000 population in the UK. Although commonly managed conservatively, general surgeons also manage this condition.

> **HINTS AND TIPS**
>
> The causes of pancreatitis can be recalled from the mnemonic GET SMASHED: Gallstones, Ethanol, Trauma, Steroids, Mumps, Autoimmune diseases, Scorpion stings, Hypertriglyceridaemia, ERCP and Drugs, e.g. azathioprine or diuretics.

Aetiology

Over 80% of cases are secondary to either gallstones or alcohol. Other causes include ERCP, surgery or trauma, toxins and drugs, hyperglyceridaemia, scorpion venom and autoimmune. A careful alcohol history must be taken and evidence of gallstone disease should be sought.

Clinical features

The clinical features of pancreatitis should be thought of in terms of local, pancreatic, effects and systemic effects. Locally, pancreatitis causes pain. The pain is often progressive, severe, epigastric, radiating through to the back. Nausea and vomiting are common. In terms of systemic symptoms the patient may be short of breath due to adult respiratory distress syndrome (ARDS), tachycardic as part of the systemic inflammatory response (SIRS).

On examination, there is abdominal tenderness with guarding and rebound tenderness. There may be a tachycardia, fever, jaundice, hypotension and sweating. There may be bruising around the umbilicus (Cullen's sign) or in the flanks (Grey Turner's sign).

Differential diagnosis

This includes any cause of an acute abdomen (e.g. cholecystitis, mesenteric ischaemia, intestinal perforation, etc.). Myocardial infarction and dissecting aortic aneurysm should also be excluded.

Investigations and prognostic scoring

The following investigations are required in anyone presenting with acute pancreatitis. The reasons are twofold: (1) they make the diagnosis and rule out alternative causes of the acute abdomen, and (2) they help in prognosis as they are required for prognostic scoring systems.

Blood tests

- Serum amylase: often markedly raised (over 1000 IU/mL). Beware though, a negative amylase test does not exclude pancreatitis (this is especially true in acute attacks on a background of previous episodes) Amylase is also raised with cholecystitis, perforated viscus (e.g. a duodenal ulcer) and even in ectopic pregnancy, but usually to a lesser extent. Serum lipase is a more sensitive and specific, but not always available
- Serum calcium: may be low.
- FBC: white cell count usually raised.
- U&Es: raised urea is an indicator of severity.
- LFTs: if aetiology gallstone will show obstructive picture.
- Fasting serum glucose: often raised in pancreatitis.
- Arterial blood gases: metabolic acidosis. It also measures po_2, important in prognosis.

Imaging

- Abdominal X-ray: gallstones, pancreatic calcification indicating previous inflammation, an absent psoas shadow due to retroperitoneal fluid, and a distended loop of jejunum ('sentinel loop').
- Erect CXR: widened mediastinum in aortic dissection; gas under the diaphragm in perforated peptic ulcer.
- Abdominal ultrasound: should be performed in all patients within first 48 h of admission. It allows visualization of gallstones and duct dilatation.
- Contrast-enhanced abdominal CT scan: within 48 h for severe pancreatitis, within 7 days for those failing to improve (suspected pancreatic necrosis), delayed for detection of pseudocyst.

Other tests

- ECG: to exclude myocardial infarction.

Prognosistic scoring systems have been validated to determine severity, guide management and predict mortality. Multiple scoring systems are used, but the modified Glasgow (Imrie) severity score is most commonly used (Fig. 32.6). An alternative prognostic scoring system is APACHE-II, which also considers chronic health problems. Any patient with severe pancreatitis should be discussed with ICU/HDU as multiple organ dysfunction syndrome (MODS) can quickly evolve.

Mortality is 5–10% but recurrence is uncommon in patients who recover. Death may be from shock, renal failure, sepsis or respiratory failure. Other complications include hypocalcaemia due to the formation of calcium soaps, transient hyperglycaemia, pancreatic abscess requiring drainage and pseudocyst (i.e. fluid in the lesser sac presenting as a palpable mass), persistently raised serum amylase or liver function tests, and fever. Patients should be investigated to exclude gallstones, and alcohol should be avoided.

Fig. 32.6 Modified Glasgow severity scoring in acute pancreatitis.

Mnemonic	Crohn's disease	Ulcerative colitis
Po_2	Arterial Po_2	<8 kPa
Age	Age	>55 years old
Neutrophils	WCC	>15 × 10^6/L
Calcium	Corrected calcium concentration	<2.0 mmol/L
Renal	Urea concentration	>16 mmol/L
Enzymes	LDH >600 u/L	AST >125 mmol/L
Albumin	albumin concentration	<32 g/L
Sugar	Fasting glucose concentration	>10 mmo/L

Each element scores 1 point: 0–1, mild pancreatitis; 1–2, moderate pancreatitis; 3 or more, severe pancreatitis.
AST, aspartate transaminase; LDH, lactate dehydrogenase; Po_2, partial pressure of arterial oxygen; WCC, white cell count.

Management

Management is usually conservative. IV fluids should be given to maintain the circulating volume and hourly urine output should be measured (preferably by means of a urinary catheter). In severe pancreatitis a central venous catheter may be helpful for assessing the volume of fluid required. Supplementary oxygen should be given, aiming for saturations between 94 and 98%. Nutritional support is key and early enteral feeding is now recommended

Pain relief is with IV opiates. If the patient has persistent vomiting a nasogastric tube should be inserted. Blood tests, especially U&Es, glucose and calcium, should be monitored daily.

Surgery should be considered for suspected haemorrhagic necrosis of the pancreas. Some give H_2-receptor antagonists, prophylactic antibiotics or peritoneal lavage, although these measures are of unproven value.

Chronic pancreatitis

The main cause of chronic pancreatitis is chronic excessive alcohol intake. Other causes include cystic fibrosis and haemochromatosis. The patient is generally ill with weight loss and has recurrent abdominal pain radiating to the back. Steatorrhoea is secondary to malabsorption from pancreatic insufficiency. Diabetes may occur due to involvement of pancreatic islet beta cells, and there may be intermittent or persistent obstructive jaundice.

Investigations

These are similar to those for acute pancreatitis, although serum amylase is not helpful in the diagnosis as it is usually only slightly raised. In addition the following investigations should be performed:

- Plasma glucose: raised in diabetes.
- CT scan: may show dilated ducts.
- ERCP: outlines the anatomy of the ducts and shows calculi.

Investigations of consequences or complications of pancreatitis should also be carried out (e.g. tests of malabsorption, jaundice and pancreatic exocrine function).

Management

Alcohol should be avoided, and the patient should be advised to follow a low-fat diet because of malabsorption. Fat-soluble vitamins, calcium and pancreatic enzymes are given. Insulin is required if the patient develops diabetes, and gallstones should be removed.

For recurrent attacks causing unremitting pain, pancreatectomy should be considered, although this procedure has a high mortality. Patients often have chronic persistent pain and can become addicted to opiates and there is an increased rate of suicide.

DISEASES OF THE LIVER

Acute hepatitis

Acute hepatitis is inflammation of a previously healthy liver lasting less than 6 months. It has multiple aetiologies (Fig. 32.7). Treatment and prognosis is dependent on the underlying cause (see below). However, certain co-morbidities will affect overall recovery and disease progression. These include chronic infection with, for example, HIV or hepatitis C virus, chronic alcohol abuse, necessary drug therapy (e.g. methyldopa) or genetic disorders (e.g. haemachromatosis). Fulminant hepatic failure is a syndrome that is due to overwhelming hepatocyte necrosis, leading to severe impairment of liver function.

Established chronic liver disease

Chronic liver disease is the result of cycles of destruction and regeneration of liver parenchyma resulting in scarring by means of fibrosis eventually causing cirrhosis. The results of this are portal hypertension, biosynthesis impairment (e.g. clotting factors, albumin), potentially hepatocellular carcinoma and eventually death. Often patients may have no or few symptoms, but the degree of hepatocyte destruction reduces hepatic reserve and minimal events may precipitate hepatic decompensation (Fig. 32.8), the features of which are discussed below.

Fig. 32.7 Causes of acute hepatitis.

Cause	Example
Infection	Hepatitis A, B, C, EBV, CMV
Drugs	Paracetamol, beta-lactams
Toxins	Alcohol, carbon tertrachloride
Autoimmune	Autoimmune hepatitis, SLE
Metabolic disease	Wilson's disease
Ischaemia	Portal vein thrombosis (70% of oxygen is delivered through portal vein)

Fig. 32.8 Factors that can precipitate hepatic decompensation.

Constipation
Vomiting and diarrhoea
Gastrointestinal bleeding
Intercurrent infection
Alcohol
Morphine
Surgery
Electrolyte imbalance

Chronic liver disease

Chronic liver disease can be a result of many underlying pathologies; a number of which are discussed in this chapter. Clinical features include leuconychia, clubbing, Dupuytren's contracture, bruising, gynaecomastia, spider naevae and caput medusa. Liver size is not a reliable sign as end-stage cirrhotic livers are commonly not palpable. Progression is often over years, but patients may present acutely with decompensated liver failure. Symptoms of this are variceal bleeding, ascites, encephalopathy, coagulopathy and hepatorenal syndrome. The principal problems in severe chronic liver disease are the degree of hepatocellular failure and the complications of portal hypertension. Hepatocellular dysfunction causes hypoglycaemia, failure of synthesis of clotting factors and hypoalbuminaemia.

Varices

Oesophageal varices result from portal hypertension – a portal–systemic shunt between the left gastric vein (portal) and lower oesophageal veins (systemic). The increased pressure in these varices makes them prone to rupture and consequently bleeding. The management of variceal bleeding was discussed previously in this chapter.

Ascites

Ascites is the presence of free fluid within the peritoneal cavity. Factors leading to the formation of ascites include salt and water retention as a result of cirrhosis, hypoalbuminaemia resulting in decreased plasma colloid pressure, portal hypertension and increased hepatic lymph production.

Clinically, there may be abdominal distension, shifting dullness and a fluid thrill, if the ascites is tense. Associated features include hernias, divarication of the recti, abdominal wall venous distension, ankle oedema and distension of the neck veins.

Investigations include diagnostic paracentesis. The ascites is clear and yellow unless it is infected, when it appears turbid. If the tap is non-traumatic, blood signifies intra-abdominal malignancy. The protein content is usually less than 15 g/L. Higher values indicate infection, hepatic venous obstruction, or malignancy. Fluid should be sent for cytology to look for malignant cells and for culture.

The patient should be on bed rest with restricted salt and fluids. The first choice of diuretic is spironolactone 100–200 mg/day. This can cause painful gynaecomastia in men, and amiloride can be substituted. If there is a poor response to spironolactone, furosemide is added. Fluid balance, weight and U&Es should be monitored daily. Ascites can also be treated with therapeutic paracentesis and albumin infusion.

Overdiuresis may result in dehydration, uraemia and hyponatraemia, and may precipitate hepatic encephalopathy, oliguria and hepatorenal syndrome.

Encephalopathy

Encephalopathy can either be reversible and episodic or lead to coma and death (Fig. 32.9). Liver failure results in diminished hepatic metabolism of substances derived from the gut, which can cause neurotoxicity. Clinical features include impaired conscious level, personality disturbances, inversion of the normal sleep pattern, slurred speech, constructional apraxia, flapping tremor (asterixis), hepatic fetor, brisk tendon reflexes, increased muscle tone and rigidity, and hyperventilation in deep coma.

Initial treatment aims to correct or remove the precipitating causes. These may include electrolyte abnormalities, sepsis, hypovolaemia, hypoxia, bleeding and constipation. Diuretics, sedatives and opiates should be stopped, and intracranial pathology should be excluded, especially in alcoholic patients. CT scanning of the brain may be appropriate to exclude subdural haematomas.

Measures should then be instituted to remove nitrogenous material and bacteria from the bowel. Oral laxatives and rifaximin, a new antibiotic, are used. The patient is put on a high-calorie diet. In alcoholics, IV thiamine is given to treat possible Wernicke's encephalopathy.

Fig. 32.9 Grading of conscious level in hepatic encephalopathy.

Grade	Features
1	Confusion, altered behaviour, psychometric abnormalities
2	Drowsy, altered behaviour
3	Stupor, obeys single commands, very confused
4	Coma responding to painful stimuli

Once over the acute phase, routine measures include lactulose to ensure two soft bowel motions/day. The patient is educated to avoid precipitating causes, including alcohol. Recurrent acute-on-chronic encephalopathy is an indication for liver transplantation.

Hepatorenal syndrome

Hepatorenal syndrome is discussed in Ch. 33.

Acute viral hepatitis

Hepatitis A

Epidemiology

Hepatitis A virus (HAV) is a member of the picornavirus family. Transmission is by the faecal–oral route. The incubation period varies from 2 to 6 weeks. Fever, fatigue, abnormal liver function and jaundice occur in adults. Clinical disease is uncommon in infants and young children, and the infection may go unnoticed. It may be acquired by eating partially cooked shellfish from estuaries contaminated by sewage.

Serology

At the onset of symptoms, immunoglobulin (Ig)M anti-HAV antibody is present in serum. High titres persist for 3–12 months, so a positive test in a patient with acute hepatitis indicates recent acute infection. Previous infection, and therefore immunity, can be diagnosed by the presence of IgG anti-HAV without IgM anti-HAV. IgG is detectable for life.

Prognosis

The disease is usually self-limiting and treatment is symptomatic. Relapses and cholestatic jaundice may occur but hepatitis A does not progress to chronic hepatitis.

Prevention and control

Prophylaxis can be obtained by immune serum immunoglobulin or active immunization. The latter induces higher levels of anti-HAV.

Hepatitis B

Epidemiology

Hepatitis B (HBV) is a DNA virus. The complete infectious virion (Dane particle) consists of the following:

- Hepatitis B surface antigen (HBsAg): the outer lipoprotein 'surface' envelope.
- Hepatitis B core antigen (HBcAg): the internal core, which surrounds the viral genome of DNA.
- Hepatitis B e antigen (HBeAg): a subunit of HBcAg; it can be detected in serum and is a useful marker of circulating virions and infectivity.

Transmission is parenteral through cutaneous and mucosal routes, across breaks in the skin or mucous membranes, and the mean incubation period is 75 days. In developed countries hepatitis B occurs sporadically.

Those at risk are IV drug users, healthcare workers, haemophiliacs or those on haemodialysis, babies of HBsAg-positive mothers, adopted children from endemic areas, sexual promiscuity, individuals in residence in institutions. Infection is characteristically anicteric, asymptomatic and chronic.

Serology

Following exposure to HBV, HBsAg can be detected throughout the prodromal phase and is not usually cleared from the serum until convalescence. Other early markers include anti-HBc and HBeAg. A positive IgM anti-HBc test typically distinguishes acute from chronic hepatitis B. The presence of HBeAg implies high infectivity but it is often no longer detectable by the time the patient consults the doctor.

The loss of HBeAg is a good prognostic sign, indicating that the patient will clear HBsAg and is unlikely to develop chronic infection. The disappearance of HBeAg is usually followed by the appearance of serum anti-HBe. Anti-HBs is the last marker to appear in serum.

Prognosis

Acute infection rarely leads to fulminant hepatic failure. Treatment is normally supportive and patients are advised to avoid alcohol. The disease may progress to chronic hepatitis, particularly in males and older people, which NICE recommends should be treated with antiviral treatment (e.g. entecavir, adefovir dipivoxil or alpha-interferon). Progression to chronic hepatitis occurs in less than 5–10% of people with clinically apparent hepatitis B. Cirrhosis and hepatocellular carcinoma are complications of chronic hepatitis.

Prevention and control

Infection can be prevented by active immunization.

Hepatitis C

Epidemiology

Hepatitis C (HCV) is an RNA virus, and can be divided into many major types and subtypes. It is a slowly progressive liver disease with a varied clinical picture, ranging from asymptomatic to rapidly progressing cirrhosis with hepatocellular carcinoma. Transmission is through blood, and sexual contact. The mean incubation period is 9 weeks. There is a high prevalence in haemophiliacs, thalassaemics, haemodialysed patients, transplant recipients and IV drug abusers.

Serology

Anti-HCV develops 1–3 months after the onset of clinical illness and, in some patients, will not be detected for up to 1 year afterwards. Identification of the viral RNA in serum is possible using the polymerase chain reaction. HCV antigens cannot be detected in serum.

Prognosis

The acute disease is often asymptomatic and leads to chronic infection in over 50% of patients. In about 20% of patients, cirrhosis may develop insidiously within 10 years, and patients may develop a clinical picture resembling autoimmune hepatitis. Systemic manifestations include cryoglobulinaemia, porphyria cutanea tarda and membranous glomerulonephritis. Hepatocellular carcinoma is recognized with chronic infection. Untreated HIV infection accelerates the progression of HCV-induced cirrhosis. This particular cohort may benefit from treatment using ribavirin with peginterferon-alpha, although NICE also recommends it for moderate and severe chronic HCV if PCR positive.

Prevention and control

Unlike HAV and HBV there is no effective vaccination. Prevention of transmission is therefore the mainstay of infection control. Blood bank screening for anti-HCV and genetically engineered factor VIII preparations for haemophiliacs limit the occurrence of hepatitis C.

Hepatitis D

Hepatitis D (delta) virus (HDV) is an RNA virus. The virion particle is encapsulated by the coat protein of HBV (i.e. HBsAg). Thus infection by HDV only occurs in patients affected by hepatitis B. Transmission is similar to HBV and the incubation period is 35 days. In developed countries, infection occurs mainly in drug addicts, haemophiliacs and institutionalized persons. Diagnosis is through IgM anti-HD, IgG anti-HD, and HDAg detection. The disease is not usually progressive but outbreaks of fulminant hepatitis caused by HBV plus HDV are described. Chronic infection can occur. The prevention of HBV infection will also prevent HDV infection as HDV cannot replicate in the absence of HBsAg.

Hepatitis E

This RNA virus is transmitted via the faecal–oral route with a peak of epidemic infection 6–7 weeks after primary exposure and low secondary attack rate. Serum IgG and IgM to anti-HEV can be detected by ELISA. The condition is usually self-limiting and progression to chronic hepatitis does not occur. There is a high mortality (20%) particularly in pregnancy. Prevention and disease control is dependent on high standards of public sanitation and sewage elimination.

Other viruses

Viral hepatitis can be caused by non-hepatic, systemic viruses. Examples include EBV, CMV, herpes simplex, Q fever and arbovirus (yellow fever). Clinical features vary enormously from asymptomatic mild hepatitis to rapidly progressive fulminant fatal hepatitis. Diagnosis is through specific viral assays using techniques such as PCR or ELISA. If virology is negative, alternative causes such as autoimmune hepatitis or Budd–Chiari syndrome must be considered.

Clinical features of hepatitis

The clinical features of the various forms of acute viral hepatitis are similar. In the pre-icteric phase, the main symptoms include malaise, fatigue, listlessness and lack of energy. Anorexia, nausea and vomiting occur, which may be induced by fatty food. There is often a distaste for cigarettes. There may be right upper quadrant pain, change in bowel habit, myalgia, fever and headaches.

In 10% of patients, acute hepatitis B may be accompanied by a serum-sickness-like syndrome, which is characterized by low-grade fever, urticarial rash and arthralgia.

The prodromal symptoms become less severe as jaundice appears. The urine darkens and the stools are pale. During the first week, the jaundice may deepen, and anorexia and fatigue may worsen in this period. There may be accompanying weight loss.

During recovery, symptoms gradually resolve although malaise and fatigue may persist and mild relapses can occur in 1–5% of patients. Exercise tolerance is generally depressed for some weeks; depression may be a prominent symptom.

Physical signs are usually minimal. Common findings are jaundice, hepatic tenderness, hepatomegaly, splenomegaly and occasionally lymphadenopathy. Skin rashes may be noted.

Fulminant hepatitis leads to hepatic encephalopathy with severe jaundice, ascites and oedema and is usually accompanied by haemorrhage caused by coagulopathies. The disturbance of consciousness reflects a combination of hepatic coma, hypoglycaemia and cerebral oedema.

Investigations

The following investigations are important in the patient with acute viral hepatitis:

- Liver enzymes, alanine aminotransferase (ALT) and aspartate aminotransferase: these are markedly elevated. Bilirubin concentration is also increased. During recovery, liver enzymes return to normal. A persistently raised ALT 6 months after the acute onset of hepatitis usually indicates progression of the disease.
- Prothrombin time: may be prolonged if fulminant hepatic failure occurs.
- Serum albumin concentrations: may fall slightly during the course of hepatitis, and serum globulin may rise.
- Hypoglycaemia: may occur with fulminant hepatic failure.
- Serum alpha-fetoprotein values: increased transiently in patients with acute viral hepatitis.

Management

The aetiology of hepatitis ranges from infective (e.g. viral or bacterial), to drug-induced, to autoimmune, to alcohol. Management of the cause may therefore be different. In terms of the management of hepatitis per se this depends on the severity. Mild disease can be managed at home with simple analgesia, alcohol avoidance and good nutrition. Cholestyramine may alleviate itching. Conversely, severe disease may progress to liver (and further organ) failure requiring intensive care unit admission and potentially organ support. Patients should be barrier nursed until the cause of the hepatitis is identified. All unnecessary drugs should be stopped.

Alcoholic liver disease

Men who drink over 500 g of alcohol per week (50 units) and women who drink over 350 g per week (35 units) have a significant risk of developing cirrhosis. However, cirrhosis is not inevitable. Only 10–20% of chronic alcoholics develop cirrhosis even though they drink the same amount of alcohol over the same period as other alcoholics. Risk factors for developing cirrhosis include genetics, gender (women develop alcoholic hepatitis and cirrhosis younger, and after less intake, than men), nutrition (alcohol is better tolerated under optimal dietary conditions), and a synergistic effect with hepatotropic viruses.

Pathology

Initially there are fatty changes within the liver. With alcoholic hepatitis, there is liver cell necrosis and an inflammatory reaction. Cells contain alcoholic hyaline or Mallory's bodies. Later there is deposition of collagen around the central veins, which may spread to the portal tracts.

Cirrhosis may result, which is initially micronodular. Extensive fibrosis contributes to the development of portal hypertension. With continued cell necrosis and regeneration, the cirrhosis may progress to a macronodular pattern.

Clinical features

The patient may initially be asymptomatic. With alcoholic hepatitis, there may be fatigue, anorexia, nausea and weight loss. There may be signs of chronic liver disease (see Ch. 13). Ascites may develop and complicating hypoglycaemia can precipitate coma.

Hepatic decompensation leads to encephalopathy and liver failure and can be precipitated by the factors listed in Fig. 32.8.

With advanced cirrhosis, there may be signs of malnutrition, ascites, encephalopathy and a tendency to bleed. Signs include bilateral parotid enlargement, palmar erythema, Dupuytren's contractures and multiple spider naevi. Men develop gynaecomastia and testicular atrophy. Portal hypertension develops, leading to splenomegaly and distended abdominal wall veins. There may be signs of alcohol damage in other organs (e.g. peripheral neuropathy, cardiomyopathy, proximal myopathy or pancreatitis).

Investigations

The mean corpuscular volume (MCV) and gamma-glutamyl transpeptidase are sensitive indices of alcohol ingestion. Important variables for predicting outcome include the prothrombin time, serum albumin, serum bilirubin and haemoglobin.

Ultrasound will demonstrate fatty liver, and histology of liver biopsy will show the pathological changes discussed above.

Management

Patients should abstain from alcohol. General measures for the management of chronic liver disease should be instigated. Patients may need nutritional support including vitamins B and C.

Prognosis

Fatty liver alone carries a good prognosis if the patient abstains from alcohol. If the patient is encephalopathic and malnourished, the mortality is up to 50%. Ascites, peripheral oedema, persistent jaundice, uraemia and the presence of collateral circulation are unfavourable prognostic signs.

Non-alcoholic steatohepatitis

Non-alcoholic steatohepatitis (NASH) is an increasingly common condition as a consequence of the obesity epidemic. The condition is characterized by fatty deposit in the liver in association with inflammation. The condition is typically asymptomatic, although occasionally a smooth enlarged liver may be felt in clinical examination. The diagnosis may be suspected because of chronically elevated aminotransferase levels, typically with an aspartate transaminase:alanine transaminase ratio <1. Liver ultrasound scan will show diffusely increased echogenecity. Alkaline phosphatase and gamma-glutamyl transferase are usually raised. Treatment is predominantly lifestyle-based – increased exercise and weight loss have shown to reverse early disease. Tight glycaemic control, particularly relevant as diabetic patients are at increased risk of NASH, has been shown to be important. Glitazones were shown to be particularly effective. Prognosis is good if lifestyle changes are made, but NASH can progress to liver cirrhosis.

Haemochromatosis

Haemochromatosis is due to excess iron in the tissues. The presence of skin discoloration and diabetes mellitus have led to it being called 'bronze diabetes' in the past.

Haemochromatosis may be classified as hereditary ('primary') or secondary. Hereditary haemochromatosis is autosomal recessive. Secondary haemochromatosis may result from excessive iron administration (e.g. blood transfusion or iron tablets).

Affected organs are the liver, endocrine system, heart and joints. Most patients are asymptomatic or have non-specific symptoms such as arthralgia and lethargy, until the effect of iron overload becomes apparent in the fifth or sixth decade. Joints are involved by chondrocalcinosis.

In the early stages, pain and swelling of the second and third metacarpophalangeal joints is characteristic. There is slate-grey skin, due to melanin, and iron deposition. Symptoms include asthenia, abdominal pain, impotence, arthralgia and amenorrhoea. Signs include hepatomegaly, splenomegaly, jaundice and gynaecomastia. The disease may lead on to cirrhosis.

The prevalence varies from 1 in 200 to 1 in 2000, and men are five to 10 times more likely to be affected than women, indicating that environmental and genetic factors modify disease expression. Women are usually affected at a later age, partly because of loss of iron during pregnancy or menstruation. Alcohol may exacerbate the problem by influencing iron metabolism and absorption.

Total body iron is increased in haemochromatosis from 4 g up to as much as 60 g. There is cellular damage and fibrosis, leading to a rusty colour of the liver, pancreas, spleen and abdominal lymph nodes. The liver is usually enlarged and may be cirrhotic. Iron is found in all liver cell types and in cardiac myocytes, the adrenals, pituitary, pancreas and testes. Chondrocalcinosis in the joints is associated with synovial haemosiderin and loss of intra-articular space.

Complications include diabetes mellitus, cirrhosis, heart disease with arrhythmias, and liver cancer.

Investigations

- Serum iron is elevated and saturation of plasma transferrin is high. Serum iron is reduced in inflammatory conditions and is subject to diurnal variation.
- Serum ferritin is usually high.
- Definitive diagnosis of haemochromatosis depends on histology of liver biopsies.
- CT scanning and MRI can be used to detect increased tissue iron but are not routine.
- Genetic testing can be performed to look for the most common mutations (C282Y and H63D).

Treatment

Patients should be venesected regularly (e.g. 500 mL weekly), until they develop a mild microcytic anaemia. Care is needed in patients with severe hepatic disease because vigorous bleeding may be complicated by hypoproteinaemia. Folate supplementation may be needed to optimize erythropoiesis. Seriously ill patients with overt cardiac haemochromatosis may require high-dose parenteral chelation therapy with desferrioxamine to reverse life-threatening disease.

Patients with established haemochromatosis should be investigated for cardiac involvement and pituitary as well as target organ endocrine failure, and replacement therapy should be instituted when necessary. Patients should be reviewed to monitor diabetic control, to care for joint disease and to search for the development of complications (e.g. hepatocellular carcinoma).

Physical examination and screening tests to search for disordered iron metabolism should be carried out in family members to identify presymptomatic individuals so that iron can be removed before cirrhosis and other complications occur. Genetic studies may be of help.

Life expectancy and hepatic and cardiac function in primary haemochromatosis are improved by iron depletion. The 5-year survival rate increases from 30% to 90% by treatment. Removal of iron does not prevent the development of cancer in patients with established cirrhosis.

Venesection does not improve endocrine failure or joint disease.

Primary biliary cirrhosis

Primary biliary cirrhosis is a disease of unknown aetiology primarily affecting the middle-sized intrahepatic bile ducts as a non-suppurative, destructive cholangitis leading to bile duct damage, cholestasis, fibrosis, cirrhosis and death from liver failure. It is more common in Europe than in Africa and Asia, with a prevalence of 3–35 per 100 000 and an incidence of 6–15 per million per year.

Clinical features

The disease is nine times more common in women. It usually presents in middle age with lethargy and pruritus. Pigmentation and xanthomata may be present, jaundice may develop and portal hypertension may lead to ascites or oesophageal varices. There may be stigmata of chronic liver disease. Approximately 80% have hepatomegaly at presentation, and 50% have splenomegaly. The patient may be asymptomatic at presentation, or present with liver failure.

The average life expectancy is 10 years from diagnosis but varies considerably. If the serum bilirubin is greater than 180 μmol/L, the life expectancy is 18 months without transplantation.

Primary biliary cirrhosis is associated with autoimmune conditions (e.g. Sjögren's syndrome, thyroid disease, Addison's disease, Raynaud's syndrome, systemic sclerosis and coeliac disease). It is also associated with malabsorption, extrahepatic malignancies, particularly of the breast, and hepatocellular carcinoma.

Investigations

LFTs show an obstructive pattern with elevated serum alkaline phosphatase and gamma-glutamyl transpeptidase. As the disease progresses, serum bilirubin rises.

With regard to immunology, HLA-B8 and HLA-DR3 are associated with a threefold increase in the risk of primary biliary cirrhosis. Serum immunoglobulins are raised, especially immunoglobulin M. Antimitochondrial antibody is positive in approximately 90%.

Ultrasound of the liver is important to exclude obstruction. It can also show evidence of portal hypertension and splenomegaly.

Histology of the liver will confirm the diagnosis. Initially, there is asymmetrical destruction of middle-sized bile ducts and surrounding lymphocytic infiltrate. Granulomas may be present. Increasing fibrosis, and eventually cirrhosis, develops.

Treatment

There is no evidence for immunosuppressive agents. Bile salts (e.g. ursodeoxycholic acid) may help with cholestasis, and improve biochemical blood results, but have no proven effect on slowing disease progression. Liver transplantation is indicated for intractable symptoms or end-stage disease.

Patients with jaundice should receive supplementation with fat-soluble vitamins A, D and K. Diarrhoea is treated with a low-fat diet and pancreatic supplements.

Primary sclerosing cholangitis

Primary sclerosing cholangitis (PSC) is characterized by inflammation, scarring and stricturing of the bile ducts, both intra- and extrahepatic. The cause is unknown, but the condition is associated with ulcerative colitis, rarely Crohn's disease, and HIV infection. Immunologically, there is an association with HLA-A1, HLA-B8 and HLA-DR3. Clinical features are due to chronic biliary obstruction and include jaundice, hepatomegaly, pruritus, fatigue and abdominal pain. Patients are at increased risk of ascending cholangitis, cholangiocarcinoma and autoimmune hepatitis.

Investigations

Alkaline phosphatase and bilirubin will be elevated. Test for ANA, SMA and ANCA may be positive. ERCP shows multiple bile duct strictures with a characteristic beaded appearance. MRCP is an alternative, non-invasive, modality to show strictures in the biliary tree. Liver biopsy shows fibrous, obliterative cholangitis.

Management

Ursodeoxycholic acid is used to improve cholestasis. Endoscopic stent insertion can be used for decompression of prominent strictures in larger ducts. Liver transplantation is indicated for end-stage disease

Autoimmune hepatitis

Autoimmune hepatitis (AIH) is caused by autoantibodies against hepatocytes, causing an inflammatory condition of the liver. It predominantly affects young and middle-age women and is associated with thyroiditis, diabetes mellitus, ulcerative colitis and fibrosing alveolitis amongst others. Clinical features may be insidious and include fever, right upper quadrant pain, jaundice, epistaxis and gum bleeding, polyarthritis, urticaria and glomerulonephritis.

Investigations

Liver function tests will usually be abnormal (raised AST/ALT) and IgG levels will be raised. Autoantibodies (anti-LKM, ANA and anti-smooth muscle) may be present. Liver biopsy will show mononuclear cell infiltration of portal and periportal regions with piecemeal necrosis, fibrosis or cirrhosis.

Management

A reducing dose course of oral prednisolone, starting at 30 mg/day, should be commenced and maintained for 2 years. If stopped, relapse is likely. Azathioprine can be used as an alternative immunosuppressant. If decompensated liver cirrhosis is present then liver transplantation is indicated.

Hepatolenticular degeneration (Wilson's disease)

This is an autosomal recessive disorder of copper metabolism leading to deposition of copper in the following:

- Liver: cirrhosis with its ensuing complications.
- Basal ganglia: tremor and choreoathetosis.
- Cerebrum: dementia and fits.
- Eyes: Kayser–Fleischer rings (a brown pigmentation of the periphery of the iris best seen with a slit lamp).
- Renal tubules: renal tubular acidosis.
- Bones: osteoporosis and osteoarthritis.
- Red blood cells: haemolytic anaemia.

Clinical features are usually due to hepatic or central nervous system involvement.

Investigations

There is a high concentration of copper in the blood, and low caeruloplasmin, the copper-binding protein.

Management

The dietary intake of copper should be reduced, and penicillamine is given to aid the elimination of copper ions. Regular blood counts are mandatory because of potential agranulocytosis and thrombocytopenia with treatment. Other side effects include oedema, proteinuria, haematuria, rashes, loss of taste and muscle weakness. Relatives should be screened. The prognosis is generally good.

Hepatic tumours

Benign tumours

Benign tumours of the liver are often an incidental finding on CT or ultrasound scan. Haemangiomas are the most common. Cysts, adenomas, fibromas, focal nodular hyperplasia and leiomyomas are further types of benign liver tumours. Haemangiomas should not be biopsied because of bleeding risk. Tumours are managed conservatively unless they become symptomatic.

Malignant tumours

The most common malignant liver tumours are metastases. Primary tumours that tend to metastasize to the liver are colon, stomach, lung, uterus, breast, pancreas and carcinoid tumours. Lyphoma and leukaemias may also spread to the liver. Primary carcinomas of the liver are less common, although increasing in incidence, and include hepatocellular carcinoma (HCC), angiosarcoma, cholangiocarcinoma and fibrosarcoma. HCC is by far the most common primary liver tumour and is associated with viral hepatitis, cirrhosis, parasite infection and anabolic steroid use. Clinical features of malignant liver cancer, primary or secondary, are weight loss, anorexia, malaise and right upper quadrant pain. The pain is capsular in nature and is clinically difficult to treat. Jaundice is a late feature, if at all, with the exception of cholangiosarcoma. Investigations include FBC and blood film, LFTs, hepatitis serology, alpha-fetoprotein (elevated in 75% of HCC) and CT or MRI scanning. A liver biopsy is taken to get a tissue diagnosis. Treatment and prognosis in metastatic liver cancer depends on the cause and the extend of the disease. For example, in colorectal cancer with liver metastases specialist centres now perform metastectamies with curative intend. Treatment for HCC is surgical resection if the tumour is solitary and <3 cm or liver transplantation. Percutaneous ablation, chemotherapy and tumour immobilization increasingly have a role in the management of HCC.

Miscellaneous conditions

Alpha-1-antitrypsin deficiency

Alpha-1-antitrypsin is a serine protease inhibitor, synthesized in the liver, important in the correct functioning of the inflammatory cascade. The deficiency of this protein is a autosomal recessive disorder (chromosome 14) and causes emphysema, cirrhosis and potentially hepatocellular carcinoma. The diagnosis is made by measuring protease inhibitor concentrations and can be screened for prenatally with oligonucleotides. There is no cure and management is essentially symptomatic. Liver transplantation is performed for end-stage liver failure and has the further effect of halting further emphysema formation.

Liver abscess

Liver abscesses are relatively rare in the UK, but common in the developing world. The infectious organism can be bacterial, parasitic, protozoal or helminthic. Entry to the liver can be direct (penetrating injury), through the portal circulation, the systemic circulation or ascending the biliary tree. The clinical feature is predominantly swinging pyrexia with right upper quadrant pain. There is commonly tender hepatomegaly and if subacute associated with cachexia. Liver function tests will often show a raised alakaline phosphatase and gamma-glutamyl transferase. Blood cultures may yield the causative organism. Ultrasound scan of the liver will show defined areas of hypoechogenicity. CT is an alternative/additional imaging modality in liver abscess. Treatment can be conservative with antibiotics or specific agents against the suspected or proven micro-organism. Surgical drainage, under CT or ultrasound scan guidance, is an alternative option.

Budd–Chiari syndrome

This condition is characterized by hepatic vein obstruction, either through thrombosis or compression, causing hepatomegaly, ascites and abdominal pain. It has multiple aetiologies, including hypercoagulability states, myeloproliferative disorders, hepatocellular tumours and radiotherapy, although 30% are deemed to be idiopathic. The investigations of choice are ultrasound with Doppler or CT scans to show hepatic vein thrombosis and ascites. Management involves treating the underlying cause and draining the ascites. Angioplasty or a surgical shunt may be required to bypass the obstruction. Lifelong anticoagulation is indicated in the absence of varices. In fulminant liver failure transplantation should be considered.

Further reading

British Society of Gastroenterology: Clinical guidelines. Available online at: http://www.bsg.org.uk/clinical/general/guidelines.html.

Griffiths, M., 2012. Crash Course: Gastrointestinal System, fourth ed. Mosby Elsevier, Ediburgh.

National Institute for Health and Clinical Excellence (NICE), 2008. Irritable bowel syndrome. Clinical guideline CG61. Available online at: http://www.nice.org.uk/CG61.

National Institute for Health and Clinical Excellence (NICE), 2009. Coeliac disease. Clinical guideline CG86. Available online at: http://www.nice.org.uk/CG86.

National Institute for Health and Clinical Excellence (NICE), 2010. Crohn's disease – infliximab and adalimumab. Technology appraisal TA187. Available online at: http://www.nice.org.uk/ta187.

National Institute for Health and Clinical Excellence (NICE), 2011. Colorectal cancer. Clinical guideline CG131. Available online at: http://www.nice.org.uk/CG131.

Genitourinary disease

Objectives

The key learning points for this chapter:

- Understand how to investigate and manage acute kidney injury.
- Assess and manage patients with acute and chronic kidney disease.
- Understand the relationship between the various clinical presentations of intrinsic renal disease and their underlying causes.
- Assess and manage patients with urinary tract infections and malignancies.
- Understand the pathophysiology, causes and management of common disorders of fluid and electrolyte balance.

ACUTE KIDNEY INJURY

Acute kidney injury (AKI) has relatively recently replaced the term 'acute renal failure'. AKI is a decline in glomerular filtration rate (GFR) over a period of hours–days. It is defined if one of the following criteria is met:

- Serum creatinine rises by ≥26.4 μmol/L within 48 h.
- Serum creatinine rises ≥1.5-fold from the reference value known to have occurred within one week.
- Urine output is <0.5–mL/kg/h for >6 consecutive hours.

NICE guidelines on the management of AKI are expected in August 2013.

Aetiology

The conventional classification of AKI is into prerenal, renal and postrenal causes (Fig. 33.1). Prerenal causes predominate in hospital and are commonly due to relative hypotension. If poor renal perfusion is allowed to persist, acute tubular necrosis results. This is the most common cause of intrinsic renal failure. In 'real life', however, the aetiology of AKI is often multifactorial. For example, in postsurgical AKI, fluid depletion, systemic inflammatory response syndrome (SIRS) and nephrotoxic drugs may all play a role.

HINTS AND TIPS

Always remember to establish whether the patient is taking drugs that interfere with renal perfusion, e.g. NSAIDs, ACE inhibitors and angiotensin II receptor blockers.

Clinical features

The symptoms of AKI are often non-specific and are commonly detected with routine urea and electrolyte blood tests. A full history should be taken focusing on previous renal disease, a background of diabetes, hypertension, analgesic and ACE inhibitor use, urinary symptoms, recent diarrhoea, vomiting or blood loss and recent operations.

The examination should focus on the cause and consequences of the renal impairment. The most important initial assessment is to gauge the patient's volume status. Skin turgor, jugular venous pressure, postural blood pressure, heart rate, urine output and the presence of peripheral or pulmonary oedema should be noted. If in hospital, the patient's fluid balance chart may be available. There may be palpable kidneys with polycystic kidney disease or hydronephrosis. Renal angle tenderness may be present in renal colic or pyelonephritis (or any other pathology that stretches the renal capsule). The bladder may be palpable with associated suprapubic discomfort with outflow obstruction. If present, a rectal examination for prostatic disease and vaginal examination for masses is indicated. Vasculitic changes can be seen in the skin.

Complications of AKI should be elicited as they may indicate the need for dialysis or haemofiltration. Uraemia manifests as pericarditis, twitching, hiccups and uraemic frost. Kussmaul's deep sighing respiration may indicate acidosis. Respiratory examination may show pulmonary oedema.

Investigations

Urine

- Urine should be dipped for blood, protein, nitrites, leucocytes, glucose and specific gravity.

Fig. 33.1 Causes of acute kidney injury.

Prerenal injury (ischaemic)	Extracellular volume loss: gastrointestinal loss (e.g. severe diarrhoea or vomiting), urinary loss (polyuria with salt-losing kidneys), burns Intravascular volume loss or redistribution: sepsis, haemorrhage (e.g. postpartum or at operation), hypoalbuminaemia Decreased cardiac output: heart failure (e.g. post myocardial infarction), cardiac tamponade, cardiac surgery Miscellaneous: hepatorenal syndrome
Renal injury	Postischaemic acute tubular necrosis: shock, trauma, sepsis, hypoxia Nephrotoxic acute tubular necrosis: antibiotics, analgesics, contrast media, heavy metals, solvents, proteins Glomerulonephritis Acute pyelonephritis Acute interstitial nephritis: antibiotics, analgesics, leptospirosis, *Legionella*, viral infections Vasculitis Intratubular obstruction: myeloma (Bence Jones protein), urate, rhabdomyolysis Coagulopathies: acute cortical necrosis, haemolytic uraemic syndrome, thrombotic thrombocytopenic purpura, postpartum renal failure Miscellaneous: malignant hypertension, hypercalcaemia
Postrenal injury	Renal tract obstruction: stones, tumour (prostatic or pelvic), prostatic hypertrophy, surgical mishap (e.g. accidental ligation of ureters), periureteric fibrosis, bladder dysfunction Major vessel occlusion: renal artery thrombosis, renal vein thrombosis

- A midstream urine (MSU) sample should be sent for microscopy, culture and sensitivity. The presence of red cell casts on microscopy is pathognomonic of glomerulonephritis.
- Assessment of urinary biochemistry may help in distinguishing prerenal failure from established acute tubular necrosis. In prerenal failure the kidney avidly retains salt and water, and hence urinary sodium is below 20 mmol/L; the urine is concentrated (osmolality over 500 mmol/L) with a urine/plasma osmolality ratio over 1.5:1. Patients with established acute tubular necrosis cannot concentrate the urine or conserve sodium. Consequently, urinary sodium is over 40 mmol/L; the urine is dilute (osmolality below 350 mmol/L) with a urine/plasma osmolality ratio below 1.1:1. These parameters are much less reliable in patients on diuretic therapy.
- Test urine for Bence Jones protein or myoglobin levels if indicated.

Blood tests

- Urea, creatinine and electrolytes should be assessed (and monitored daily). This will confirm renal impairment and serve as a useful baseline for monitoring the patient's progress. If the patient is acidotic, serum bicarbonate will be low. It is crucial to check the potassium, as hyperkalaemia can be life-threatening and immediate measures to lower the potassium need to be taken. The anion gap should be calculated. The following equation is used: $([Na^+] + [K^+]) - ([Cl^-] + [HCO_3^-])$.
- Arterial blood gases.
- Full blood count, liver and bone profiles, creatine kinase, ESR and CRP.
- Blood cultures if infection is suspected.
- Serum autoantibodies (e.g. ANCA), complement, antistreptolysin O titres, immunoglobulin levels, serum electropheresis can all be tested to aid in identifying the cause.

Other tests

- Electrocardiogram (ECG) can show the precipitating cause (e.g. myocardial infarction) or complications such as pericarditis or hyperkalaemia.
- CXR if fluid overload suspected.
- If the patient is truly anuric, especially if signs of sepsis are present or if volume depletion is not likely, then an urgent ultrasound scan of the renal tract is indicated. It will show urinary tract obstruction and kidney size and structure.

Management

AKI is associated with significant mortality – 10% if isolated and 50% if associated with multi-organ distress syndrome (MODS) (previously multi-organ failure). As such, diagnosis needs to be prompt, with early senior or specialist input and instigation of a careful management plan. The management of AKI can grossly be divided into (1) addressing serious or life-threatening complications and (2) treating the underlying cause. Commonly, AKI responds well to careful fluid management and blood pressure control, withholding nephrotoxic drugs, adequate nutrition and treating the underlying cause (such as relieving obstruction, treating infection, etc.). If, however, renal function does not improve, renal replacement therapy may be indicated. In the acute setting this is commonly achieved by either haemofiltration or haemodialysis. The details of these techniques are not covered in this book, but the basic differences are as follows: In haemodialysis blood flows on one side of a semi-permeable membrane, allowing for diffusion to create an ultrafiltrate which can be removed. In haemofiltration the blood is filtered by the process of continuous convection through a highly permeable synthetic membrane. Haemofiltration is a more time-consuming process and is more expensive than haemodialyis; it does, however, not require complex vascular access, and is less likely to cause haemodynamic compromise.

HINTS AND TIPS

When assessing a patient with AKI ask yourself the following questions:

- Are there any life-threatening complications?
- Is this renal impairment acute or chronic?
- If acute, is this prerenal, renal or postrenal?
- If intrinsic renal failure, what is the cause?

Life-threatening complications and emergency dialysis

It is important to look for and treat hyperkalaemia, pulmonary oedema, acidosis and symptomatic uraemia (pericarditis, encephalopathy). If these complications do not respond to conservative therapy (see below) emergency haemodialysis or haemofiltration should be considered.

Hyperkalaemia

This may be life-threatening and so the reduction of potassium should be the first priority if it is over 6.5 mmol/L, particularly if ECG changes are present. The management of hyperkalaemia is discussed in detail later in this chapter.

Pulmonary oedema

This may be life-threatening, particularly in patients with a reduced urine output. Conventional therapies may be used – high-flow oxygen, diuretics (high doses may be necessary), nitrates and opiates (low dose as renally excreted). Non-invasive positive pressure ventilation may be helpful. In the absence of a reasonable urine output, renal replacement therapy will be required.

Treat the underlying cause

The precipitating cause(s) of the renal failure should be corrected, e.g. relief of obstruction, treatment of infection. Stop all nephrotoxic drugs and toxins. If the patient is dehydrated stop all diuretics. Treat any intercurrent infection. It is important to correct and maintain the intravascular filling of the patient. In some cases this can be assessed clinically and non-invasively. However, when uncertain, invasive haemodynamic monitoring may be helpful. High-dose diuretics may be used to achieve a urine output if the patient is fluid-overloaded. This can make it easier to give IV drugs and blood products without causing pulmonary oedema but there is no evidence that renal recovery is hastened by diuretics. In patients with severe sepsis or cardiogenic shock, inotropic support may be required.

Supportive management

Patients with AKI require intensive monitoring, particularly of their fluid balance and electrolytes. Particular attention should be paid to oxygenation, nutrition and glycaemic control.

Prognosis

The prognosis of patients with AKI depends on the cause, other organ impairment and premorbid state. Prerenal and postrenal aetiologies usually respond well to prompt treatment and appropriate support and regain independent renal function. Intrinsic renal disease is less predictable. Patients with non-oliguric AKI have a better outcome.

HINTS AND TIPS

Do not give diuretics to patients who are dehydrated – this will worsen their renal impairment!

CHRONIC KIDNEY DISEASE

Chronic kidney disease (CKD) describes an irreversible reduction in renal function. As serum creatinine has its limitations in the estimation of GFR (see section on Glomerular disease), UK laboratories now report estimated GFR (eGFR) values. This procedure has resulted in the identification of many more patients with chronic kidney disease in primary care. The majority of these patients can be managed in primary care as very few will progress to needing renal replacement therapy. Their management is focused on prevention of cardiovascular disease and delaying the worsening of renal failure. The following groups of patients are referred to secondary care:

Fig. 33.2 Classification of chronic kidney disease.

Stage	Description	eGFR (mL/min)
1	Kidney damage with preserved GFR, e.g. proteinuria	>90
2	Kidney damage with mild renal impairment	60–90
3	Moderate renal impairment	30–59
4	Severe renal impairment	15–29
5	End-stage renal failure	<15

eGFR, estimated glomerular filtration rate.

- Severe renal failure (eGFR <30 mL/min).
- Progressive loss of renal function.
- Likely to have intrinsic treatable kidney disease, e.g. blood and protein in the urine.
- Complications of renal failure, e.g. renal anaemia.

eGFR is used to classify patients with chronic kidney disease (Fig. 33.2). It is estimated that about 5% of the population have chronic kidney disease stage 3 or worse; this figure exceeds 20% in the population aged over 70 years.

Aetiology

Identifying the cause of chronic kidney disease is important since early treatment can delay or prevent progression to end-stage renal failure (ESRF). In addition, prognosis will be more accurate, risks of recurrence with renal transplantation can be assessed, and diagnosis of familial disease may benefit other family members. Common causes include the following:

- Diabetes mellitus: both insulin-dependent and non-insulin-dependent diabetes can lead to ESRF.
- Hypertension: the incidence of ESRF seems to be decreasing due to better identification and treatment of hypertension. It is more common in the Afro-Caribbean population.

Diabetes and hypertension are responsible for approximately 80% of all patients entering dialysis programmes. Other causes include:

- Glomerular disease: both primary and secondary (see below).
- Chronic or recurrent infection: mainly due to obstruction or vesicoureteric reflux.
- Obstruction: most cases are due to prostatic hypertrophy and stones.
- Renovascular causes: renovascular atheroma and consequent ischaemia is becoming increasingly recognized, reflecting the ageing population. Risk factors are the same as for all vascular disease.
- Drugs: analgesic nephropathy; HIV-associated nephropathy is increasingly common.
- Interstitial nephritis: this may be idiopathic but may also be secondary to non-steroidal anti-inflammatory drugs (NSAIDs) and chronic furosemide use.
- Inherited disease: the two most common conditions are autosomal dominant polycystic kidney disease (ADPKD) and Alport's disease (type IV collagen defect associated with sensorineural deafness).
- Less common causes are amyloidosis, myeloma, SLE, gout, hypercalcaemia and retroperitoneal fibrosis.

Clinical features

Progressive loss of renal function per se does not cause symptoms until the eGFR falls to very low levels (<30 mL/min; i.e. CKD 4 or 5). Under these circumstances patients may develop fatigue, malaise, thirst, anorexia, nausea and itching. Unfortunately, by this stage the patient is close to needing dialysis.

When evaluating a patient with chronic kidney disease for the first time the history taken should be similar to that taken for patients with AKI or haematuria/proteinuria (see Ch. 16). This will cover symptoms that may reveal an underlying cause. Always remember to evaluate the patient's drug history thoroughly.

Uraemic skin is classically 'lemon yellow' and there may be bruising due to platelet dysfunction. Hypertension is common as both a cause and consequence of chronic kidney disease. Examine for signs of obstruction (e.g. a palpable bladder) and perform a rectal examination for prostatic hypertrophy or pelvic masses. The kidneys are large in polycystic disease. Rarer clinical symptoms or signs include a pericardial rub, pleural effusion, pulmonary oedema and proximal myopathy.

Investigations

The following are important in the patient with chronic renal failure:

- Urine: dipstick and microscopy for casts and culture to exclude infection. If there is proteinuria, send an ACR (albumin:creatinine ratio) or PCR (protein:creatinine ratio) to quantify this (see below).
- GFR may be estimated using a 24-h urine collection; this also enables quantification of 24-h urinary protein excretion.
- A cause should be sought and the tests are common to AKI – autoantibody testing and a myeloma screen help to rule out treatable pathology.
- Once chronic renal failure is established the following are needed to check for complications and progress: regular blood pressure checks, urinary protein

estimation and control of diabetes plus haemoglobin (normochromic normocytic anaemia), calcium, phosphate, parathyroid hormone (PTH) levels, haematinics and lipid profile. Estimation of cardiovascular risk may help to guide intervention (see below).
- Renal ultrasound should be done to exclude obstruction and assess kidney size.
- Renal biopsy should be considered once prerenal and postrenal disease have been excluded, especially if renal size and structure is normal on ultrasound scan, suggesting more acute disease.

Management

The aims of treatment are to minimize further deterioration in renal function and to prevent or treat the complications of renal failure. The most significant complication of chronic kidney disease is premature cardiovascular disease. This accounts for the high mortality in this group and explains why a large proportion of these patients do not survive long enough to develop chronic kidney disease stage 5.

Nephrotoxic drugs should be discontinued and drugs that are renally excreted may need to be stopped or reduced in dose.

Prevention of decline in renal function

Hypertension should be tightly controlled (130/80 mmHg). This usually requires several antihypertensives. Patients with proteinuria derive particular benefit from the use of drugs that inhibit the renin–angiotensin system.

In diabetic nephropathy tight control of glycaemia plus ACE inhibitors or angiotensin receptor blockers slows the decline in renal function.

Prevention of complications

Cardiovascular

Control of hypertension can slow the deterioration of renal function and prevent cardiovascular complications. Patients who have suffered a cardiovascular event should be treated aggressively with antiplatelet and statin therapy as well as aggressive blood pressure lowering for secondary prevention. There is less evidence in terms of primary prevention in this group of patients with chronic kidney disease. Guidelines suggest antiplatelet therapy and a statin in those with an estimated risk of cardiovascular disease of more than 20% over 10 years.

All patients should also receive lifestyle advice, including smoking cessation if appropriate.

Renal osteodystrophy

Renal bone disease is due to a combination of disturbed vitamin D metabolism and secondary hyperparathyroidism. Serum alkaline phosphatase and phosphate levels are raised; serum calcium falls. Dietary phosphate restriction is combined with oral phosphate binders. Serum calcium should be maintained in the normal range and PTH levels controlled with synthetic vitamin D analogues. Parathyroidectomy may be required if tertiary hyperparathyroidism supervenes.

Acidosis

Systemic acidosis accompanies declining renal function. It increases myocardial excitability, accelerates renal bone disease and may contribute to increased potassium levels. Sodium bicarbonate supplements will help to maintain serum bicarbonate levels within the normal range. Preliminary evidence suggests that correction of acidosis may help prevent loss of renal function.

Anaemia

In renal failure there is a normochromic normocytic anaemia. Evidence of blood loss should be sought if there is an inappropriately low haemoglobin. Ferritin, vitamin B_{12} and folate deficiency should be corrected with diet and supplements if needed. Recombinant human erythropoietin has improved the management of anaemia and will increase the haemoglobin and improve symptoms attributable to anaemia but it can cause hypertension.

Hyperkalaemia

Correction of acidosis and dietary restriction help to control potassium levels. This can be particularly important in patients on ACE inhibitors and/or angiotensin receptor blockers. As mentioned above, these agents may reduce the rate of decline of renal function but their use is associated with hyperkalaemia.

End-stage renal failure

End-stage renal failure is identified on biochemical and clinical grounds as that point when, despite conservative measures, the patient will die without the institution of renal replacement therapy. Specific indications for dialysis in ESRF include symptomatic uraemia, hyperkalaemia, metabolic acidosis, peripheral neuropathy, pericarditis, central nervous system disorders and poor control of ESRF by conservative treatment. The need for dialysis should be predictable, allowing for the creation of vascular access and education of the patient well before it is required. Renal replacement can be done through continuous ambulatory peritoneal dialysis (CAPD) using a catheter placed into the abdomen to allow fluid in and out, and the dialysis membrane is the peritoneum. The most common method is thrice-weekly haemodialysis via an arteriovenous fistula or indwelling dual-lumen central venous catheter. Problems with dialysis include loss of vascular access, infection, hypotension and the maintenance of fluid and electrolyte balance.

Renal transplantation is increasingly common and successful (This is largely due to advances in using non-heart-beating donors). Patients are on immunosuppressive drugs (e.g. tacrolimus, prednisolone and mycophenolate mofetil), which have their own problems such as susceptibility to opportunistic infections, and skin malignancies. Other complications of transplantation include acute rejection, obstruction of the ureteric anastomosis and gradual loss of function with time (chronic allograft nephropathy).

Fig. 33.3 Systemic disorders that can involve the glomerulus.

Diabetes
Amyloidosis
Systemic lupus erythematosus
Rheumatoid arthritis
Ankylosing spondylitis
Neoplasia
Myeloma
Vasculitic syndromes
Liver disease
Sarcoidosis
Partial lipodystrophy

GLOMERULAR DISEASE

Glomerular disease may be primary or secondary, i.e. a manifestation of systemic disease (Fig. 33.3). There are many types of glomerular disease, but all affect the glomerular filtration apparatus, commonly leading to a unified set of symptoms.

Clinical features

The clinical features of glomerular disease often relate to the associated reduction in glomerular filtration rate. This results in acute or chronic renal impairment. Glomerular disease may also result in defective filtration and therefore the appearance of blood and/or protein in the urine (see Ch. 16). Like almost all renal pathologies, hypertension can also be a feature (Fig. 33.4). Two distinct syndromes, nephrotic and nephritic, are commonly associated with glomerular disease and are favourites in exams.

Nephritic syndrome

Nephritic syndrome refers to the combination of proteinuria, haematuria and renal failure.

Oliguria and hypertension are often features and this syndrome is classically associated with post-streptococcal glomerulonephritis.

Nephrotic syndrome

Nephrotic syndrome is the triad of significant proteinuria (>3 g/day), hypoalbuminaemia (albumin <20 g/L) and peripheral oedema. The oedema is thought to be due to sodium retention rather than changes in plasma oncotic pressure. The majority of cases are due to primary glomerulonephritis; a minority of patients have a causative systemic disease

Fig. 33.4 Relationship between glomerular pathologies and clinical presentations.

	Proteinuria/nephrotic syndrome	Haematuria/nephritic syndrome	Renal pain	AKI	CKD	↑BP
Minimal change	+	–	–	±	–	–
FSGS	+	–	–	±	+	+
Membranous	+	–	±	–	+	+
IgA nephropathy	±	+	±	±	+	+
MCGN	+	+	–	+	+	+
Diffuse/proliferative	–	+	–	+	–	+
RPGN	–	+	–	+	–	+

Note that any given pathology may present in a number of ways and, conversely, a particular clinical presentation may have a number of possible causes.
AKI, acute kidney injury; ↑BP, hypertension; CKD, chronic kidney disease; FSGS, focal segmental glomerulosclerosis; MCGN, mesangiocapillary glomerulonephritis; RPGN, rapidly progressive glomerulonephritis.

(e.g. diabetes, amyloid, HIV and SLE). Other clinical features include hyperlipidaemia due to increased hepatic synthesis, a prothrombotic tendency due to urinary loss of antithrombin III, protein C and protein S, and increased risk of infection due to urinary loss of immunoglobulins. Renal biopsy is indicated in most adults.

HINTS AND TIPS

The causes of secondary nephrotic syndrome (i.e. not of direct renal origin) are DAVID: Diabetes mellitus, Amyloidosis, Vasculitis, Infections and Drugs.

History

It is important to ask about any urinary symptoms, especially proteinuria and haematuria (e.g. Is there frothy urine? – see Ch. 16). There may also be a history of previous nephritis, urinary tract infections or stone disease. Ask about associated systemic diseases (e.g. arthritis, diabetes, hypertension or evidence of malignancy). A full drug history should be taken including exposure to toxins.

Hearing impairment is present in Alport's syndrome, and there may be a family history of renal disease. Ask about recent upper respiratory tract infections (post-streptococcal glomerulonephritis) and valvular heart disease.

In younger patients ask about enuresis (suggests defective urinary concentrating ability, e.g. in reflux nephropathy) and problems in pregnancy.

HINTS AND TIPS

When taking a drug history be sure to ask directly about illicit drugs, over-the-counter medication and herbal remedies.

Investigations

The following investigations are important in the patient with glomerular disease.

Urine

- Urine dipstick: to detect proteinuria and haematuria. In the presence of proteinuria a urine sample may be sent for ACR or PCR to quantify severity.
- Urine microscopy for red blood cell casts and dysmorphic red cells indicating glomerular disease.
- Urine for Bence Jones protein.
- 24-h urine collection.

Blood tests

- Full blood count, urea and electrolytes, liver function tests and bone profile. Laboratories in the UK now routinely report estimated GFR – this is calculated from serum creatinine levels using an equation. Its use is not validated in AKI when the GFR may be changing rapidly.
- Fasting blood glucose: to exclude diabetes mellitus.
- ESR and CRP.
- Antineutrophil cytoplasmic antibodies (ANCA) are present in microscopic polyangiitis and Wegener's granulomatosis.
- Anti-dsDNA and antinuclear antibodies in SLE.
- Antiglomerular basement membrane (anti-GBM) antibodies for the diagnosis of Goodpasture's disease.
- Hepatitis B and C serology.
- Antistreptolysin O titre and anti-DNase: recent streptococcal infection.
- Serum immunoelectrophoresis: to exclude myeloma.
- Rheumatoid factor.
- Cryoglobulins.
- Blood cultures.
- Serum complement levels: C3 and C4 are classically reduced in active SLE, as well as cryoglobulinaemia and some forms of glomerulonephritis.

Imaging

- Chest X-ray (CXR): this may show pulmonary oedema, malignancy, pulmonary haemorrhage or cavitation in Wegener's granulomatosis or anti-GBM disease.
- Renal ultrasound scan: exclude obstruction and assess renal size/symmetry.

Renal biopsy

- Renal biopsy: to make a histological diagnosis if suspect intrinsic renal disease.

HINTS AND TIPS

Never forget to dipstick the urine in patients with renal disease. The presence of blood and protein in the urine should raise the suspicion of intrinsic renal pathology.

General principles of management

All patients with suspected glomerulonephritis should be seen by a nephrologist. Although the causes of glomerulonephritis are multiple, tight blood pressure control is advocated if proteinuria is >1 g/dL – this is best achieved using an ACE inhibitor and/or an angiotensin receptor blocker. Thereafter, specific management is guided by a firm histological diagnosis, which is also helpful in prognosis.

Nephrotic syndrome is managed by restricting salt intake, aggressive blood pressure control (again with an ACE inhibitor and/or an angiotensin receptor blocker) and prompt treatment of infections. Often diuretics are used, particularly furosemide, metolazone or spironalactone, to reduce fluid overload at a rate of ~1 kg/day. Regular U&Es, weight charting and blood pressure monitoring is an absolute requirement. Hyperlipidaemia and thromboembolism, associated complications of nephrotic syndrome, should be addressed.

Important primary and secondary glomerular diseases

Rapidly progressive glomerulonephritis

Rapidly progressing glomerulonephritis or crescentic glomerulonephritis is usually an aggressive process and presents with renal failure, haematuria, oliguria and hypertension. The biopsy shows severe acute inflammation in the glomerulus with necrotizing 'crescent' formation. It may occur in SLE, anti-GBM disease and vasculitides but can occur in the absence of underlying disease. It is a medical emergency. Treatment is with immunosuppression, commonly high-dose hydrocortisone. The prognosis is usually poor unless treatment is instituted sufficiently early.

ANCA-positive vasculitis

This is typically either Wegener's granulomatosis (cANCA against proteinase-3) or microscopic polyangiitis (pANCA against myeloperoxidase). They are both small-vessel vasculitides causing pulmonary and renal disease, although other sites can be affected. Wegener's causes granulomatous lesions and commonly has upper airway involvement. Both can cause a rapidly progressing glomerulonephritis and AKI.

Symptoms include malaise, fever, haemoptysis, sinusitis and epistaxis. CXR may show transient shadowing due to pulmonary haemorrhage and resolution. They are considered together as treatment is the same: namely, aggressive immunosuppression and possibly plasma exchange. Most enter complete remission with treatment; if the response is incomplete, long-term renal support may be needed.

Antiglomerular basement membrane disease

This condition is associated with the presence of circulating antibodies against collagen resulting in damage to the alveolar and glomerular basement membranes. Goodpasture's syndrome is anti-GBM disease associated with pulmonary haemorrhage. Other 'pulmonary–renal syndromes' include SLE, Wegener's granulomatosis and microscopic polyangiitis.

Treatments with plasma exchange and immunosuppressive drugs remove and suppress the antibody, together with the reversal of its renal and pulmonary effects.

HINTS AND TIPS

Always think of urgent referral to a nephrologist when you see a patient with haemoptysis and renal failure, i.e. pulmonary–renal syndrome. If caught in time, therapy is more likely to be successful.

IgA nephropathy

IgA nephropathy (Berger's disease) is the most common acute glomerulonephritis worldwide. This condition is classically associated with 'synpharyngitic' haematuria, i.e. macroscopic haematuria 1–2 days after an upper respiratory tract infection. In contrast, post-streptococcal glomerulonephritis usually follows a delay of 1–2 weeks. Other presentations include microscopic haematuria, proteinuria and renal impairment.

Steroids and immunosuppression are not very effective. Angiotensin-converting enzyme inhibitors are the mainstay of treatment. Approximately 25% of patients will go on to require dialysis. Henoch–Schönlein purpura has much in common with IgA nephropathy and can be thought of as its systemic cousin.

Lupus nephritis

SLE is a multisystem disease and the kidneys are commonly affected. The changes are classified by the World Health Organization from I–V based on histology. The different types lead to presentations varying from nephritis to nephritic syndrome. Typically, the anti-double-stranded DNA titres and ESR are raised with a normal CRP and C3 and C4 levels are low in active lupus. If treatment is indicated, steroids and cyclophosphamide are the mainstay.

Minimal change nephropathy

This accounts for 80% of children and 20% of adults in the UK who present with nephrotic syndrome. Renal biopsy is therefore not always indicated in children. Light microscopy is normal (hence the name) but electron microscopy shows podocyte foot process fusion. There is usually significant proteinuria, which responds to corticosteroid therapy in the majority of children (90%) and adults (75%). Relapsing episodes are treated with cyclophosphomide or ciclosporin. The development of renal failure is rare (<1%).

Focal segmental glomerulosclerosis

Nephrotic syndrome is the most frequent presentation. It can be idiopathic but is associated with a wide range of systemic diseases. Human immunodeficiency virus (HIV)-associated nephropathy is increasingly common and causes a characteristic 'collapsing' FSGS.

Treatment with high-dose steroids can induce remission but progression to end-stage renal failure is common.

Membranous glomerulonephritis

This condition accounts for about a quarter of all cases of nephrotic syndrome. The cause is often unknown, but diagnosis is made by biopsy which shows characteristic diffuse thickening of the glomerular basement membrane. The condition is associated with malignancy, drugs (e.g. gold), autoimmune conditions such as SLE or rheumatoid arthritis, and infections. If left untreated 40% resolve spontaneously; mainstay medical management is with corticosteroids with cyclophosphamide.

Membranoproliferative glomerulonephritis

This condition, also known as mesangicapillary glomerulonephritis, is characterized be immunocomplex deposits in the glomerular mesangium and basement membrane thickening. It is associated with chronic infections, autoimmune disorders such as SLE and chronic thrombotic microangiopathies It may cause nephritic syndrome. There are three types of membranoproliferative glomerulonephritis (MPGN). Type I is caused by immunocomplex deposition, often in association with hepatitis C infection, and causes activation of the classical complement pathway and immune deposits in mesangium and subendothelial space. Type II (dense deposit disease) is similar to type I but is associated with activation of the alternative complement pathway. Furthermore, type II is associated with drusen, a condition that causes blindness through similar deposition in the Bruch's membrane in the retina. Type III is very rare and is characterized by subendothelial and subepithelial deposits. Treatment of MPGN focuses on symptom control and aggressive immunosuppression and plasmapheresis in severe cases. Prognosis is poor – 50% of patients develop ESRF at 10 years.

Post-streptococcal glomerulonephritis

This condition, also known as acute proliferative glomerulonephritis, is a complication of streptococcal pharyngitis (strep throat) or impetigo. Clinically, it is characterized by sudden-onset haematuria, proteinuria, oedema, hypertension. There commonly is a latent period after the infection; 1–2 weeks for strep throat and typically 6–8 weeks for impetigo. Treatment is symptomatic (i.e. treat hypertension, oedema and hyperkalaemia). Immunosuppression is not indicated. Prognosis is good in children; recovery in adults may be complicated by congestive cardiac failure.

URINARY TRACT INFECTIONS

Urinary tract infections (UTIs) are one of the most common infections encountered in medical practice, and in the elderly population can rapidly cause sepsis. Women are more prone to UTIs than men, except during the first few months of life and in old age. Approximately 25–35% of all women describe symptoms of a UTI at some stage in their lives.

UTI is a general term referring to the presence of microorganisms in the urine. Significant bacteriuria is defined as urine that yields a pure growth of more than 100 000 organisms per millilitre on culture. Predisposing factors for UTI are given in Fig. 33.5. Broadly speaking UTIs are divided into those affecting the lower urinary tract (urethra, prostate, bladder) or upper urinary tract (kidneys). A further distinction is made between uncomplicated (normal renal tract and function) and complicated (abnormal renal or genitourinary tract, impaired host defences or virulent organism) UTIs.

Lower urinary tract infections

Lower UTIs may take the following forms:

- Cystitis: a symptomatic infection of the bladder with significant bacteriuria.
- Asymptomatic bacteriuria: the patient has no symptoms, but urine culture yields a growth of over 100 000/mL.
- Acute urethral syndromes: symptomatically similar to cystitis but the urine culture may be sterile.

Upper urinary tract infections

Upper UTIs may take the following forms:

- Acute pyelonephritis: an inflammatory process within the renal parenchyma, most commonly caused by bacterial infection.

Fig. 33.5 Precipitating causes of urinary tract infection.

Stones
Obstruction
Polycystic kidneys
Papillary necrosis
Diabetes mellitus
Analgesic nephropathy
Sickle cell disease
Sexual intercourse
Pregnancy
Bladder catheterization

- Chronic pyelonephritis: this is usually the result of long-standing or recurrent bacterial infection with eventual parenchymal scarring characteristic of chronic pyelonephritic kidneys. Vesicoureteric reflux and obstruction also contribute. Hypertension and chronic renal failure may ensue. It is more common in children.

Infection usually occurs by ascent of the invading organism from the urethra into the bladder. Colonization of the ureters may occur, and from there to the kidneys. The haematogenous route of infection is less common but may occur secondarily to bacteraemia, septicaemia or endocarditis.

Clinical features

Symptoms of lower UTI are suprapubic pain, frequency, nocturia, dysuria (classically 'burning') and strangury. Upper UTIs such as acute pyelonephritis or renal abscesses present with fever, rigors, loin pain, vomiting and weight loss. Macroscopic haematuria can occur in one-third of severe cases. In the elderly, the presentation may be very non-specific with mild cognitive, behavioural and mobility changes.

Investigations

A clean, midstream urine sample should be obtained and a dipstick test done for blood, protein, leucocytes and nitrites; subsequently it should be sent for microscopy and culture. White cell count and CRP will be raised in infection. Urea and electrolytes may demonstrate poor renal function. Obvious predisposing factors such as pregnancy, diabetes or indwelling catheter should be considered. Indications for further investigations include recurrent infections, childhood onset, male sex, urological symptoms, persistent haematuria, especially if aged over 40 years, unusual organisms (such as *Pseudomonas*) and recurrence of infections.

Renal tract ultrasound should be performed for UTI in children, men, if >2 episodes/year, failure to respond to treatment, pyelonephritis, unusual organism or persistent haematuria. A DMSA scan can be performed to assess renal function and is a reliable test for diagnosing pyelonephritis.

HINTS AND TIPS

The causes of sterile pyuria (a common exam question) include:

- Tuberculosis of the urinary tract.
- Analgesic nephropathy.
- Partially treated UTI.
- Neoplasia.
- Intra-abdominal inflammation.

Management

Treatment should be started *after* urine has been sent for culture and antibiotic sensitivities but, commonly, before results are available. Broad-spectrum antibiotics may then be changed if necessary according to the results. High fluid intake should be encouraged. More than 80% of lower UTIs respond to a short course of an antibiotic such as trimethoprim, nitrofurantoin or amoxicillin. For complicated UTIs a 5–10-day course of therapy is indicated. Follow-up microscopy and culture should be carried out to ensure eradication of organisms and pyuria. Patients with acute pyelonephritis usually require admission to hospital for IV fluids and antibiotics.

Patients with recurrent infections require a high fluid intake; frequent and complete voiding should be encouraged. Long-term, low-dose prophylaxis using rotating antibiotics may be of benefit but the need for continued treatment should be reassessed after 6 months.

If infection is related to sexual intercourse, the patient should void after intercourse and may benefit from a single dose of an antibiotic.

RENAL CALCULI

Renal calculi (kidney stones) are common cause for attendance in the Emergency Department. Men are more likely to be affected than women, with the initial presentation usually in the third and fourth decades of life. Most are calcium containing and most are radio-opaque (80%). They include calcium oxalate, calcium oxalate/phosphate, calcium phosphate and triple phosphate staghorn stones. Urate and xanthine stones are radiolucent.

Aetiology

Predisposing factors are dehydration, infection, hypercalcaemia and hypercalciuria, gout and high oxalate intake (chocolate, instant coffee and spinach).

Clinical features

The classic presenting complaint of renal calculi is colicky pain – severe loin pain radiating to the groin associated with nausea and vomiting. Frank haematuria may occur, but more commonly haematuria is microscopic.

Investigations and management

Renal colic is a typical 'end of the bed' diagnosis – the patient is restless, clutching their loin and often appears pale. Diagnosis is based on a suggestive history, examination and haematuria on urine dipstick. If these are present, a CT KUB (kidney/ureter/bladder) scan should be performed (the gold standard for diagnosis of renal calculi). The scan will also help in determining whether there is any associated hydronephrosis, which may require urgent referral to the urologists. Acute treatment is analgesia with NSAIDs (typically diclofenac), fluids and antibiotics if indicated. Often tamsulosin is advised to relax the ureteric smooth muscle. Urinary tract obstruction needs urological intervention, especially if infection is a possibility. Ureteric decompression is achieved through a double J stent. Most stones, however, pass spontaneously (typically those <4 mm); if they do not then they can be crushed endoscopically or fragmented with lithotripsy. To avoid future stones, the patient should avoid dehydration and excess dietary calcium oxalate or phosphate.

HINTS AND TIPS

Patients with renal colic typically complain of 'loin to groin' pain. They will be unable to lie still and often feel nauseated with the pain. Typically NSAIDs are a better analgesic than morphine.

URINARY TRACT MALIGNANCIES

Renal cell carcinoma

Renal cell carcinoma (hypernephroma) is the commonest renal tumour in adults and is twice as common in men. The peak age of onset is between 50 and 60 years of age. It may be solitary, multiple or occasionally bilateral. The classic triad of haematuria, loin pain and a palpable mass is found in only 10% of patients. Other features may include cough, pyrexia, polycythaemia, anaemia, bone pain with hypercalcaemia, and left-sided varicocele associated with left renal vein obstruction. A tendency to grow into the inferior vena cava (IVC) is a typical characteristic. About a quarter of patients present with metastases. Fifty per cent of renal cell carcinomas are incidental findings on CT.

Investigations include urinalysis for red cells, ultrasound, then CT scan of the kidneys, CXR (cannon ball metastases), bone scan for metastases and magnetic resonance imaging of the abdomen to assess IVC spread.

Treatment is by radical nephrectomy if possible, although nephron sparing surgery and laparoscopic procedures are becoming more common. Metastases may regress after the primary tumour is removed. This can be enhanced with interferon-alpha and interleukin-2 administration. Chemotherapy or radiotherapy has not proven to be very effective, but recent developments in monoclonal antibodies to for example tyrosine kinase and VEGF are looking promising. The overall 5-year survival is approximately 40% but is better if the tumour is confined to the renal parenchyma and worse if there are metastases or lymph node involvement.

HINTS AND TIPS

Tumours presenting with polycythaemia include renal cell carcinoma, hepatoma and cerebellar haemangioblastoma.

Transitional cell carcinoma

This occurs mainly in those aged over 40 years and most commonly affects the bladder, although the ureter and renal pelvis are other sites. It is three times more common in men than women. Predisposing factors include cigarette smoking, exposure to industrial carcinogens, exposure to drugs (e.g. cyclophosphamide) and chronic inflammation (e.g. schistosomiasis).

Patients usually present with painless haematuria, although pain may occur. There may be symptoms similar to UTI. Investigations include urine cytology, IVU, cystourethroscopy and abdominal CT scanning.

Treatment options include local resection with regular follow-up cystoscopy, cystectomy, radiotherapy and local or systemic chemotherapy.

Prostatic carcinoma

Prostatic carcinoma is the second most common malignancy in men. The incidence increases with age and may be very indolent. Patients are often asymptomatic but may present with symptoms of 'prostatism' (e.g. hesitancy, frequency, nocturia and postmicturition dribbling), or with symptoms arising from metastatic spread, especially to bone. There is a hard irregular prostate on rectal examination.

Investigation includes prostate-specific antigen (PSA), transrectal ultrasound and prostatic biopsy (Gleeson score to assess tumour grade), which shows an adenocarcinoma. Evidence of local invasion, nodal spread and metastases should also be sought (staging).

Treatment for local disease may be observation alone, transurethral resection of the prostate, radical prostatectomy or radiotherapy. Testosterone is a growth factor for prostate cancer and therefore it responds well to antagonizing its effect. This can be achieved with orchidectomy, luteinizing hormone-releasing hormone analogues (e.g. goserelin) and antiandrogens (e.g. cyproterone acetate).

Prognosis even with metastases may be excellent if the tumour responds to hormonal treatment.

The PSA is very useful as a tumour marker to allow the response to therapy to be assessed when prostate disease is present. However, how to screen for prostate cancer and how to follow up abnormal PSA tests is a cause of much debate for urologists and public health authorities. Currently it does not meet criteria for a national screening programme.

Testicular cancer

Testicular cancer is the most common malignancy to affect males in their second to fourth decade. Typical presentation is a painless testicular mass. Risk factors include maldescended testicle, infant hernia and infertility. The most common varieties are derived from germ cells and include seminomas and teratomas. Much rarer are tumours derived from cord or gonadal stroma cells which include Sertoli and Leydig cell tumours.

Excision and biopsy allows for histological assessment and guides further investigation and treatment. All patients have a CT scan to rule out metastases. Alpha-fetoprotein and beta-HcG are tumour markers which are particularly helpful in monitoring response to treatment.

Treatment is orchidectomy. Seminomas are extremely sensitive to radiotherapy. Teratomas respond well to combination chemotherapy with bleomycin, cisplatin and etoposide. Five-year survival is >90% for all groups.

MISCELLANEOUS CONDITIONS

Adult polycystic kidney disease

This is an autosomal dominantly inherited disease, the genes (*PKD2* and *PKD1*) lying on chromosomes 4 and 16 respectively. Patients are usually between the ages of 30 and 50 years. Cysts develop in the kidney and lead to progressive renal failure. Approximately 40% of patients also have cysts in the liver. Haematuria, infection, stones or abdominal pain are common presenting features. If due to a new mutation, established renal impairment may be the first sign. There is an association with subarachnoid haemorrhage due to intracranial 'berry' aneurysms (typically at the anterior communicating artery of the circle of Willis).

Examination reveals large irregular palpable kidneys, and the patient is often hypertensive. Mitral valve prolapse, diverticular disease and hernias are also increased in frequency. Ultrasound shows multiple cysts. CT provides greater detail. Blood pressure should be controlled and infections treated. Decline in renal function is progressive and may necessitate dialysis or renal transplantation. Screening of first-degree relatives and genetic counselling is recommended.

Hepatorenal syndrome

Hepatorenal syndrome (HRS) is defined as renal failure in patients with severe liver disease for which no other cause can be found. Hence the exclusion of sepsis, hypovolaemia, nephrotoxic drugs and nephritis is paramount, not least because they may be easily remediable. It is divided into:

- HRS 1: rapidly progressive renal failure often in acute liver failure, alcoholic hepatitis or decompensation of chronic disease.
- HRS 2: more slowly progressive renal failure, often over months.

The aetiology is unknown. It is characterized by renal vasoconstriction and decreased perfusion pressures and peripheral and splanchnic vasodilatation. Resulting activation of the renin–angiotensin axis and release of neuropeptide compounds the problem by causing further renal vasoconstriction. It occurs in ~20% of patients with liver cirrhosis in the presence of ascites. Kidney biopsy is always normal in HRS. This is emphasized in treatment as it is mainly supportive and renal function recovers if the liver recovers, including after liver transplantation. Combinations of octreotide, vasopressin analogues, midodrine and dopamine have all been tried to improve renal haemodynamics but no treatment is especially advantageous. Prognosis is usually poor.

Thrombotic microangiopathies

This term encompasses haemolytic uraemic syndrome (HUS) and thrombotic thrombocytopenic purpura (TTP). HUS is a disorder characterized by microangiopathic haemolytic anaemia, renal failure, thrombocytopenia, normal coagulation and no neurological changes. These separate it from disseminated intravascular coagulopathy and TTP (with which it shares many features; see Ch. 37). It may follow diarrhoea in children (especially from *Escherichia coli* O157:H7), although this is less common in adults. In adults the prognosis is worse. Treatment includes plasma exchange, steroids and renal support. A large proportion of patients will need long-term dialysis even with treatment.

FLUID AND ELECTROLYTE BALANCE

As a house officer you will frequently prescribe IV fluids and be responsible for checking your patients' electrolytes. As such, understanding basic fluid balance and electrolyte homeostasis is important.

In a 70-kg man, the total fluid volume is 42 L (i.e. 60% of the body weight). The intracellular fluid volume is 28 L or two-thirds of the total body fluid, and the extracellular fluid volume is 14 L or a third of the total body fluid. The intravascular component is 3 L (plasma contributing to 5 L of blood).

The average total fluid intake in 24 h is 2500 mL (1500 mL drunk, 800 mL in food and 200 mL via the metabolism of food). The output matches this via urine, insensible loss and stool.

Sodium ingestion is approximately 2 mmol/kg in 24 h and potassium is approximately 1 mmol/kg in 24 h.

Understanding the above requirements will help you in prescribing fluids in a sensible and appropriate manner. Generally speaking, fluids can be divided into crystalloids (e.g. 'normal' saline or Hartmann's solution) or colloids (e.g. Gelofusine or Volulyte).

Sodium and water balance

Disorders of sodium homeostasis are common. Total body sodium is reflected in the extracellular volume and is regulated by baroreceptors and the renin–angiotensin system. Serum sodium concentration is determined by water balance and is regulated by osmoreceptors and antidiuretic hormone (ADH)/thirst.

Hyponatraemia

New-onset hyponatraemia is frequent in hospital practice. It is rarely due to the legion of potential causes, especially the syndrome of inappropriate antidiuretic hormone production (SIADH). It is usually the result of neurohumoral changes in acute illness and the type, volume and route of fluid administered. To evaluate chronic hyponatraemia three questions should be answered:

- What is the patient's volume status?
- What is the urine osmolality?
- What is the urinary sodium value?

For example, in hypovolaemia secondary to dehydration or diarrhoea, the kidneys retain salt and water resulting in low (<20 mmol/L) urinary sodium. Diuretics or mineralocorticoid deficiency will cause hypovolaemia with a high urinary sodium (>20 mmol/L). With this information the diagnostic algorithm shown in Fig. 33.6 can be followed.

Treatment depends on the cause. If the patient is dehydrated then volume replacement with normal saline is required. Fluid restriction for SIADH is correct. Beware of diagnosing it in hospital patients admitted for other reasons, because fluid-restricting a dehydrated patient is a well-recognized cause of AKI. The sodium level should not rise at more than 1 mmol/L/h as central pontine myelinolysis can ensue. This is osmotically induced demyelination. Severe hyponatraemia (<115 mmol/L) can cause confusion and seizures. It is an emergency and treatment with 0.9% or 1.8% saline to raise the levels to >120 mmol/L is sometimes indicated. In reality this is a contentious issue and twice normal saline is infrequently used.

SIADH is characterized by hyponatraemia, low plasma osmolality, inappropriately increased urine osmolality (>500 mOsmol/kg, urinary sodium >20 mmol/L without hypovolaemia, cardiac, renal, adrenal and hepatic disease. Causes are shown in Fig. 33.7.

Hypernatraemia

Hypernatraemia usually results from reduced intake or increased loss of water. Causes include dehydration and diabetes insipidus (Fig. 33.8). Excess saline replacement can be the cause in hospital.

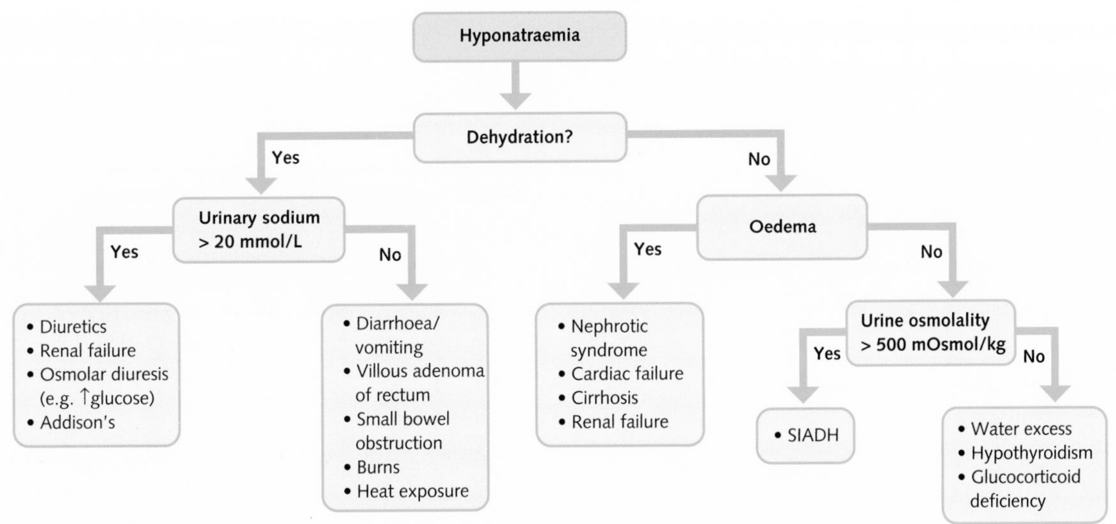

Fig. 33.6 Algorithm for investigation of hyponatraemia. SIADH, syndrome of inappropriate antidiuretic hormone secretion.

Fig. 33.7 Causes of syndrome of inappropriate antidiuretic hormone secretion.

Groups	Examples
Central nervous system	Stroke Subarachnoid haemorrhage Head trauma Brain tumour
Pulmonary	Neoplasms Tuberculosis Pneumonia
Malignancies	Small-cell lung cancer Pancreas Lymphoma
Drugs	Antidepressants Neuroleptics Chlorpropamide Carbamazepine

Fig. 33.8 Causes of hypernatraemia.

Low total body sodium	Extrarenal: e.g. sweating, diarrhoea Renal: osmotic diuresis
Normal total body sodium	Diabetes insipidus
High total body sodium	Steroid excess: e.g. Cushing's, Conn's iatrogenic, e.g. hypertonic sodium infusions Self-induced: e.g. ingestion of sodium chloride tablets

Treatment is again that of the cause and appropriate fluid replacement. The sodium level should be reduced no faster than 1 mmol/L/h to avoid rapid fluid shifts and cerebral oedema. Normal saline can be used as it may have a lower osmolality than the blood and will not abruptly lower the sodium level.

Potassium balance

Hypokalaemia

The causes of hypokalaemia are given in Fig. 33.9. It may be useful to assess the urinary potassium to help distinguish urinary from other losses. The clinical features of hypokalaemia are muscle weakness, confusion, ileus, increased cardiac excitability, augmented digoxin toxicity, thirst, polyuria, renal lesions (e.g. Fanconi's syndrome), interstitial inflammation, and fibrosis in severe prolonged depletion.

Management

The underlying cause should be identified and treated. If hypokalaemia is mild, oral potassium supplements are given. These are rarely required for patients on thiazide diuretics. If the patient is severely hypokalaemic, the infusion of IV potassium should be considered (but not more than 20 mmol/h).

Fig. 33.9 Causes of hypokalaemia.

Cause	Examples
Losses	Gastrointestinal: chronic laxative abuse, diarrhoea and vomiting, villous papilloma of the colon Renal: diuretics (e.g. thiazides and furosemide), hyperaldosteronism, glucocorticoid excess (including treatment with steroids, and ACTH-secreting tumours), renal tubular acidosis, Bartter's syndrome Inadequate replacement: postoperative, diuretic phase of acute kidney injury
Redistribution of potassium	Alkalosis Insulin overdose Familial periodic paralysis
ACTH-secreting tumour	
Secretion of atrial natriuretic peptide	Paroxysmal SVT

ACTH, adrenocorticotrophic hormone; SVT, supraventricular tachycardia.

Hyperkalaemia

The causes of hyperkalaemia are given in Fig. 33.10.

Management

Hyperkalaemia can cause arrhythmias and ventricular fibrillation and must therefore be treated promptly. Rapidly reducing extracellular potassium levels is best

Fig. 33.10 Causes of hyperkalaemia.

Cause	Examples
Excess oral intake	Potassium supplements
Diminished renal excretion	Renal impairment Drugs, e.g. potassium-sparing diuretics, ACE inhibitors, ARBs, NSAIDs
Redistribution of potassium from intracellular compartment	Haemolysis Tissue necrosis, e.g. burns
Artefact	Delay in separation of plasma or serum

ACE, angiotensin-converting enzyme; ARBs, angiotensin receptor blockers; NSAIDs, non-steroidal anti-inflammatory drugs.

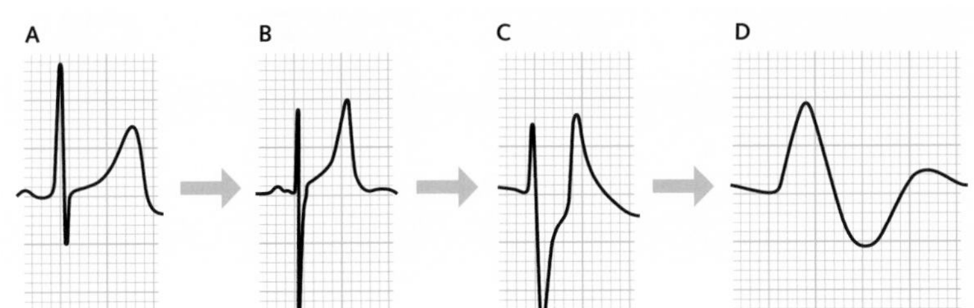

Fig. 33.11 ECG changes in hyperkalaemia.

achieved by utilizing physiological mechanisms: potassium can be temporarily redistributed into cells using an infusion of 50% dextrose and insulin and nebulized salbutamol. This can be repeated if needed. If the patient is acidotic, the use of bicarbonate can help this. Remember that these interventions only redistribute potassium between compartments and provide a window of opportunity for definitive therapy to excrete potassium from the body. The only way of achieving potassium excretion acutely is in the urine. Therefore, oligoanuric patients with severe hyperkalaemia require urgent dialysis to achieve potassium removal.

Significant hyperkalaemia is commonly associated with typical ECG changes (Fig. 33.11). These ECG changes can be reversed temporarily by boluses of 10% calcium gluconate, which acts to stabilize the myocardial membrane.

Calcium resonium resin orally or rectally will help excrete potassium over a period of days. This slow response means that it has no role in the acute management of hyperkalaemia complicating AKI.

Further reading

Chadban, S.J., Atkins, R.C., 2005. Glomerulonephritis. Lancet 365, 1797–1806.

Gines, P., Guevara, M., Arroyo, V., Rodes, J., 2003. Hepatorenal syndrome. Lancet 362, 1819–1827.

Jones, T., 2012. Crash Course: Renal and Urinary Systems, fourth ed. Mosby, Edinburgh.

Lameire, N., van Biesen, W., Vanholder, R., 2008. Acute kidney injury. Lancet 372, 1863–1865.

Renal Association: Clinical practice guidelines. Available online at: http://www.renal.org/Clinical/GuidelinesSection/Guidelines.aspx.

Central nervous system

Objectives

The key learning points for this chapter:

- The characteristic features, differential diagnosis and management of cerebrovascular disease.
- How to assess a patient with headache,
- Common causes of headache and their management.
- The features and management of disabling neurological conditions such as parkinsonism, multiple sclerosis and motor neurone disease.
- How to recognize, investigate and treat meningitis and encephalitis.
- The classification, differential diagnosis and management of epilepsy.
- How to consider neurological problems by logically following the neuromuscular pathway.
- To develop a working knowledge of the common conditions affecting the different parts of this pathway.

CEREBROVASCULAR DISEASE

Stroke and TIA

Introduction and definition

A stroke is a focal neurological deficit, caused by a vascular lesion, that lasts for more than 24 h. Approximately 80% are due to infarction secondary to thrombosis or embolism, and 20% are due to intracerebral haemorrhage. If the symptoms last less than 24 h (though usually much less) they are termed 'transient ischaemic attacks' (TIA). These are usually due to emboli. The annual incidence of stroke is about 150 in 100 000 but rises with age so that the incidence at 75 years is 1000 in 100 000; the incidence of TIA is approximately 50 in 100 000. Around 11% of patients with a TIA have a stroke in the next 90 days, many in the days shortly following the TIA. TIA therefore needs to be investigated carefully.

Aetiology and pathophysiology

Risk factors for stroke are summarized in Fig. 24.3. The main causes of ischaemic stroke are thromboembolism from arteries and emboli from the heart. Uncommon causes of cerebral infarction are vasculitis, arterial dissection, venous sinus thrombosis (which may also cause haemorrhage), polycythaemia and meningovascular syphilis. Thrombus in situ may also occur in perforating arteries, often due to lipohyalinosis as a complication of hypertension. The risk factors for TIA are identical, and the underlying disease process very similar, the main cause being embolism from a distant source. Other possible causes include thrombotic occlusion of small perforating vessels, low flow through stenosed vessels, vasculitis and haematological conditions such as sickle cell disease. Although the symptoms of TIA resolve within 24 h, infarction may have occurred.

Cerebral haemorrhage is usually due to rupture of perforating arteries or intracerebral vessels (primary intracerebral haemorrhage); the main underlying causes are hypertension (causing vessel fragility and microaneurysms) and cerebral amyloid angiopathy. Rarely, cerebral haemorrhage is secondary to other pathologies (e.g. arteriovenous malformations, tumour, abscess or blood dyscrasias).

> **HINTS AND TIPS**
>
> The sudden onset of any symptom usually suggests a vascular aetiology.

Clinical features

Signs and symptoms usually appear rapidly, often over seconds, whereas a gradual progression suggests another pathology (e.g. tumour). The most common presentation of stroke is with hemiplegia due to occlusion of the middle cerebral or internal carotid artery causing infarction of the internal capsule.

The Bamford classification is now widely used in clinical practice and is also a useful guide to prognosis (see Ch. 24, Fig. 24.5). The diagnosis of stroke is made clinically and the physical findings are interpreted to predict which part of the cerebral circulation has been affected. Motor signs are upper motor neurone. Lacunar strokes result from small areas of infarction affecting the internal capsule, basal ganglia, thalamus and pons.

In TIA, as for stroke, the symptoms depend on the size of the emboli and the distribution of the artery affected. The symptoms resolve gradually over minutes to hours, with complete recovery within 24 h. Recurrent TIAs in the same carotid artery territory occurring closely together in time may be due to an unstable plaque, and are often termed 'crescendo TIA'.

HINTS AND TIPS

'Amaurosis fugax' (transient monocular visual loss) is most frequently due to ischaemia – a 'retinal TIA'.

Fig. 34.1 ABCD2 score for TIA.

Feature	Severity	Score
Age ≥60		1
Blood pressure ≥140/90 mmHg		1
Clinical features	Unilateral weakness	1
	Speech disturbance only	2
	Other	0
Duration of symptoms	≤10 min	0
	10–59 min	1
	≥1 h	2
Diabetes		1

Score 0–3, low risk; ≥4, high risk.

Differential diagnosis

Establishing the diagnosis may be difficult, especially in the case of TIA, and the differential includes anything that may cause transient neurological symptoms. Epilepsy is usually distinguished by features such as jerking, and migraine is usually associated with headache, which is rare in TIAs. Hypoglycaemia must be excluded, and in the history any features of multiple sclerosis or intracranial lesions should be sought. Occasionally, phaeochromocytoma or malignant hypertension can mimic TIA. Attacks with loss of consciousness should not be regarded as TIAs.

Investigations

The investigations that should be performed following stroke are detailed below; patients with established stroke should always be admitted. Following TIA, the investigations are very similar due to the risk of further stroke; to help decide whether the patient should be admitted for investigation, or seen with an urgent outpatient appointment, risk stratification is performed using a scoring system such as the ABCD2 score (see Fig. 34.1).

- Full blood count (FBC): polycythaemia or thrombocytopenia. Sickling tests in Afro-Caribbean patients.
- Electrolytes: dehydration.
- Clotting screen: bleeding disorders.
- Erythrocyte sedimentation rate (ESR): vasculitis including giant cell arteritis.
- Blood glucose: hyper- or hypoglycaemia.
- Chest X-ray (CXR): primary tumour, aspiration pneumonia.
- Imaging: CT or MRI should be performed promptly in stroke to distinguish haemorrhage from infarction; MRI is preferred for posterior circulation strokes as it provides better images of the posterior fossa. It is also helpful in cases of diagnostic uncertainty (especially to exclude tumour and subdural haemorrhage). In some cases imaging MUST be performed urgently (see Ch. 24), as urgent intervention may be required. Brain imaging in TIA is helpful to exclude other causes of transient symptoms and to look for areas of previous silent infarction; this may be done at an urgent follow-up appointment.
- Echocardiogram: especially if you suspect a cardiac embolic source (e.g. bilateral infarcts) and the patient is suitable for anticoagulation.
- Carotid Doppler ultrasound scan: performed for anterior circulation events where the patient makes a good recovery and would be suitable for carotid surgery if a significant stenosis (>70%) is found.
- Thrombophilia screen: for patients <55 years, in the absence of other risk factors, following multiple episodes (see Ch. 37).
- Autoimmune screen: if vasculitis is suspected.
- Magnetic resonance (MR) angiography: if arterial dissection or venous sinus thrombosis is suspected.

Management

Treatment

- Thrombolysis in selected patients with ischaemic stroke is beneficial when given up to 4.5 h after symptom onset. Patients need to be quickly and carefully assessed, including an NIHSS score calculation (which is a measure of the severity of the stroke and helps judge whether thrombolysis will be beneficial) and an urgent brain scan is required. There are many contraindications which must be excluded.
- Antiplatelets: evidence of small but significant prognostic benefit if given in first 48 h after stroke. Aspirin (300 mg) should be started immediately and continued for 2 weeks, after which long-term secondary

prevention is implemented (see below). Clopidogrel can be given if aspirin is contraindicated. Studies suggest that if CT is likely to be delayed, the first dose can be given empirically without increased risk if the stroke is found to be haemorrhagic. All patients with TIA should be started on antiplatelet therapy.

- Swallow assessment: required to assess risk of aspiration. Give IV fluids if swallowing is compromised to maintain hydration.
- Stroke unit: management in a specialized unit has been shown to reduce mortality and morbidity.
- Supportive therapy: monitoring of pressure areas, for infection and complications like hydrocephalus; nutrition; physiotherapy; occupational therapy; speech and language therapy.
- Neurosurgical review is required for brain haemorrhage, especially posterior fossa as surgical drainage may be life saving, and for life-threatening cerebral oedema following ischaemic stroke (malignant MCA syndrome) when decompression may be possible.
- Blood pressure should be monitored carefully; hypertension should not be treated unless extreme (systolic ≥220 mmHg) or there are other indications (e.g. encephalopathy, heart failure, significant coronary artery disease) as reduction may worsen infarction due to impaired cerebral autoregulation of blood flow.
- Blood glucose: this should be monitored and controlled if necessary with IV insulin (sliding scale). Hyperglycaemia is associated with a worse outcome.

COMMUNICATION

If the patient is unconscious or severely impaired, a decision on the most appropriate degree of intervention needs to be taken in liaison with relatives, and the patient if possible. Factors to consider include prognosis, quality of life and the patient's wishes.

Prevention

Preventing further strokes (secondary prevention) is critical. These patients are also at elevated risk of cardiovascular events at other sites – it is also important to target this risk.

- Current NICE guidelines advocate the use of clopidogrel as first-line agent for secondary prevention following stroke, and combined aspirin/dipyridamole following TIA. If any single agent is not tolerated, other agents can be tried.
- Anticoagulant therapy should be started for cardioembolic strokes associated with atrial fibrillation, and possibly for those occurring less than 3 months after myocardial infarction (presumed cardioembolic).

Fig. 34.2 CHADS2 score for stroke risk with atrial fibrillation.

Feature	Score
Congestive heart failure	1
Hypertension consistently >140/90 mmHg	1
Age >75	1
Diabetes	1
Previous **s**troke	2

Score ≥2 is generally taken as an indication for anticoagulation.

It should also be considered for primary stroke prevention in patients with atrial fibrillation. The risks and benefits of anticoagulation need to be considered and discussed with the patient; scoring systems such as CHADS2 (Fig. 34.2) or CHADS2-VASc may help. Anticoagulation is avoided in the 10–14 days following infarction due to the risk of bleeding into friable, infarcted brain. For a long time warfarin was the only available agent, but newer direct thrombin/factor Xa inhibitors have been developed. Dabigatran is recommended by NICE as an alternative to warfarin and has better efficacy and side-effect profile.

- Blood pressure and cholesterol (aim for total cholesterol <4 mmol/L, low-density cholesterol <2 mmol/L, or 25% reduction) should be lowered. This applies even if they are not particularly raised as these patients have a high absolute cardiovascular risk (see Chs 30 and 35).
- Carotid endarterectomy: for patients with anterior circulation ischaemic strokes (or transient ischaemic attacks (TIAs) – see below) who make a good recovery and have a stenosis >70% in the culprit artery without near occlusion.
- Advice and help with smoking cessation and other lifestyle measures should be given.

HINTS AND TIPS

Global rather than focal problems (such as dizziness and syncope) are rarely explained by TIAs.

Extra-axial haemorrhage

Subarachnoid haemorrhage

Subarachnoid haemorrhage (SAH) is due to bleeding into the subarachnoid space. The annual incidence is 15 in 100 000. Most cases (about 80%) are due to rupture of a saccular aneurysm in the circle of Willis and its adjacent branches (see Fig. 24.2); 15% are multiple. Estimated population prevalence of aneurysms is around 5%; hence most aneurysms do not rupture. The remaining 20% of SAH are mostly due to perimesencephalic haemorrhage (a relatively benign subtype) or vascular malformations.

Risk factors for aneurysm formation and rupture overlap, and include genetic factors (including the well-defined conditions autosomal dominant polycystic kidney disease and Ehlers–Danlos syndrome), coarctation of the aorta, smoking and hypertension.

Haemorrhage may occasionally be due to ruptured mycotic aneurysm from endocarditis and bleeding diatheses.

Clinical features

The classic history is of a sudden-onset severe headache that feels like a blow to the head or back of the neck. Around 30% are preceded by a less severe headache due to a small 'sentinel' haemorrhage. Severity is maximal at onset or in the following seconds. This is usually followed by faintness, nausea, vomiting and sometimes loss of consciousness or seizures.

On examination, there may be photophobia and features of meningism (see Ch. 18) although this may take some hours to develop. If bleeding continues, the level of consciousness deteriorates. There may be signs of raised intracranial pressure or pressure effects on surrounding structures causing focal neurological deficits. Large arteriovenous malformations occasionally cause an audible bruit over the skull. Deficits appearing later may relate to vasospasm, re-bleeding or hydrocephalus, and seizures may occur. Non-neurological complications include neurogenic pulmonary oedema, cardiac arrhythmia and SIADH.

Investigations

A CT scan shows blood in the subarachnoid space in 90–95% of cases if performed within 24 h, and it can also identify arteriovenous malformations. A lumbar puncture shows xanthochromia (yellow colour due to haemoglobin degradation products), which develops after approximately 12 h and persists for several days. It is present in all cases. Consecutive samples should be equally bloodstained (though this is not a reliable sign), and the CSF pressure is often raised. To identify a causative aneurysm, the gold standard is digital subtraction angiography. However, CT/MR angiography is usually quicker to organize and has fewer complications. Either technique allows planning of the optimal treatment method.

HINTS AND TIPS

Approximately 5% of SAH are missed by CT scan on day 1 and sensitivity decreases over time; therefore an appropriately timed lumbar puncture for xanthochromia is necessary to exclude the diagnosis.

Management

Immediate treatment is bed rest, analgesia and supportive measures. The neurosurgeons should be consulted early. Up to one-sixth of patients re-bleed, most within the first 8 h. If untreated, the risk of re-bleeding may be as high as 50% at 6 months. Angiography should therefore be performed as quickly as possible to identify the culprit aneurysm and plan surgical clipping or endovascular coiling. Blood pressure should be monitored and lowered if severely raised.

Nimodipine, a calcium channel blocker that acts preferentially on cerebral arteries, should be given at 60 mg 4-hourly to prevent vascular spasm following SAH. It should be started within 4 days and continued for 21 days, and is proven to reduce mortality. Fluid intake should be at least 3 L/day to avoid hypovolaemia and hypotension.

Prognosis

The mortality rate of SAH is 50%; 10–15% will die before they reach hospital. Patients who have severe neurological deficits have a poor prognosis. Late re-bleeding and epilepsy are complications that may develop after discharge from hospital and long-term psychosocial dysfunction is common.

Subdural haematoma (SDH)

This is due to bleeding from bridging veins between the cortex and venous sinuses. Acute SDH due to severe trauma is life threatening with a high mortality, and presents shortly following the event. In chronic SDH, an initial small haemorrhage gradually enlarges by absorbing fluid osmotically from the cerebrospinal fluid (CSF). It is more common in those with brain atrophy such as the elderly and alcoholics. Although it is often secondary to trauma, the initial event may not be recalled.

Symptoms of SDH are often global and may develop insidiously. They include headache, confusion, a fluctuating level of consciousness and sometimes a personality change. There may be focal neurological signs (which can develop many days after the initial insult), signs of raised intracranial pressure or secondary epilepsy.

A CT scan should show the haematoma, which may be bilateral (Fig. 34.3). As the clot breaks down at around 7 days post-event it becomes transiently isodense to the brain, making it harder to identify on the scan. Treatment is by removal of the haematoma, which often leads to a full recovery if performed early.

Haematomas may resolve spontaneously, and in those patients carrying a high risk of surgery can be monitored with serial CT scans.

Extradural haematoma

This results from tearing of the middle meningeal artery or its branches following head injury, causing bleeding into the space between the dura and the skull.

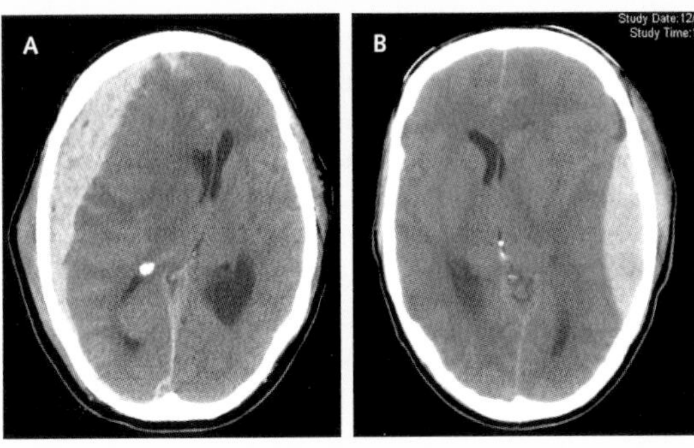

Fig. 34.3 (A) A subdural haematoma, which is concave in appearance. (B) An acute extradural haematoma. Note the characteristic biconvex collection. (Courtesy of Dr Steven Powell and Dr Alex Roberts, Royal Liverpool University Hospital.)

The classic picture is of a sudden brief loss of consciousness followed by a lucid interval. With severe EDH and a rapidly expanding haematoma the patient then develops headache, reduced conscious level and signs of raised ICP. There may be seizures and ipsilateral pupil dilation (a 'false localizing sign'), followed by death due to brain herniation. The location of the bleeding causes a characteristically biconvex haematoma (Fig. 34.3). Treatment is by evacuation of the clot through burr hole or open craniotomy.

HEADACHE SYNDROMES

The approach to the patient with headache is described in Ch. 18. Specific types of headache are considered here. The clinical approach to headache depends on a detailed analysis of symptoms and a thorough general and neurological examination.

> **COMMUNICATION**
>
> History taking is of paramount importance in patients complaining of headache. Listen and allow the story to unfold. There may be hidden fears of an underlying tumour.

Migraine

Migraine affects approximately 10% of the population and is more common in women than in men (ratio of 1.5:1). Approximately 75% of sufferers have their first attack before the age of 20 years.

Clinical features

The frequency of headaches varies from one to two each week to a few attacks scattered over a lifetime. Premonitory symptoms in the 24 h prior to headache occur in around 60% of sufferers and may consist of yawning, euphoria, depression, irritability and sometimes a craving for or a distaste of food.

In 25% of cases an aura is experienced 30–60 min before the headache. It is usually visual, consisting of teichopsias (flashes of light), scotomata and fortification spectra (zigzag lines). Objects may appear small (micropsia) or distorted (metamorphopsia). Paraesthesiae of the hands or face may occur and are often followed by numbness. In hemiplegic migraine, a hemiparesis, sometimes with dysphasia, occurs. Other focal neurological phenomena have been described. The symptoms develop gradually and are fully reversible.

The headache is commonly unilateral. It usually starts during the day and is classically throbbing or pulsating. Commonly associated features include nausea and vomiting, photophobia and phonophobia. The headache is usually worse with movement, and lasts for 4–72 h.

Occasionally, especially in older people, the aura may occur without the headache –'migraine sine cephalgia'. Migraine with aura is a risk factor for stroke.

Pathology

The mechanisms of migraine are not well understood. Human studies provide evidence that migraine aura is associated with a brief period of cortical hyperaemia followed by a longer period of reduced blood flow. It is thought that this is linked to 'cortical spreading depression', a slowly expanding wave of depolarization followed by hyperpolarization. However, it is much debated as to whether this is the cause of the headache itself, which is thought to involve activation of trigeminal nerve afferents from the dura and vascular structures, and release of vasoactive neuropeptides.

The cerebral mechanism is responsive to mood, emotions, tiredness, relaxation, hormonal changes and peripheral stimuli (e.g. bright lights and noise). There is often a seasonal and/or diurnal pattern.

Management

Precipitating factors should be identified and avoided, such as certain foods including cocoa, cheese, citrus fruits and alcohol. Acute attacks should be treated as early as possible with simple analgesia (e.g. aspirin, ibuprofen or paracetamol), combined with an antiemetic (e.g. domperidone or metoclopramide). Sometimes a stronger analgesic such as codeine or morphine is required.

Sumatriptan and other 5HT 1b/1d agonists, which inhibit the release of vasoactive neuropeptides, are of value in the treatment of acute attacks as proven in trials. They can be given orally, intranasally or subcutaneously. They should not be given to patients with ischaemic heart disease, coronary vasospasm or uncontrolled hypertension.

Ergotamine is used occasionally in patients who do not respond to other treatments, but it may worsen nausea and vomiting. It also binds to 5-HT receptors. Common side effects include nausea, vomiting, abdominal pain and muscular cramps, and it should not be used for hemiplegic migraine or in patients with vascular, hepatic or renal disease. The frequency of administration should be limited to no more than twice a month to avoid habituation.

Prophylaxis

Prophylactic drugs are indicated in patients who have two or more attacks each month, and include antihypertensives (especially beta-blockers), amitriptyline and topiramate, as well as several other agents. The need for continuing therapy should be reviewed every 6 months.

Cluster headache

Cluster headache is the most common of the trigeminal autonomic cephalalgias, and is 10 times more common in men than in women. Attacks usually start in adulthood. Headaches are unilateral and of agonizing severity around the eye or temple, and often occur at night. Attacks last from 15 to 120 min, occur up to 8 times per day, and continue for around 4 weeks to 3 months. Total remission usually follows and lasts until the next cluster a year or two later.

The pain may radiate to the face, jaw, neck and shoulder. Autonomic symptoms are prominent: the eye may water and become red, the nostrils may run or feel blocked, and there may be sweating. Miosis and ptosis are common, and in some patients may persist permanently. Attacks can be precipitated by vasodilators, e.g. alcohol, nitrites and calcium channel blockers.

Acute attacks can be aborted by high-flow oxygen. Subcutaneous sumatriptan is also effective, and in some patients intranasal lidocaine many resolve symptoms. Verapamil, lithium, steroids or methysergide may be used to prevent attacks.

Other trigeminal autonomic cephalalgias include paroxysmal hemicrania and the SUNCT syndrome, which also have prominent autonomic features.

Tension-type headache

Tension-type headache is the most common type of primary headache, and may be episodic or chronic. It is slightly more common in women. The classical presentation is of intermittent attacks of diffuse tightness, pressure or heaviness over the vertex, or in the neck or occiput, lasting from 30 min to 7 days. It may occasionally be unilateral. The headache may be relieved by simple analgesia but is not accompanied by vomiting or visual disturbance. Chronic tension-type headache may evolve from the episodic form, and simple analgesia is often of limited use when this occurs. The condition must be distinguished from medication-overuse headache.

Enquiries should be made for the common and often concealed fear of a brain tumour or stroke.

Idiopathic intracranial hypertension

Also known as pseudotumour cerebri, this is not strictly a headache syndrome but is an important cause of headache. The aetiology and pathogenesis is unknown but many medications have been associated with the condition, notably tetracyclines and vitamin A. It occurs mainly in overweight young women. Obesity is the only established association; others, such as irregular menstruation and pregnancy, have not been reliably proven. Common symptoms include headache, visual disturbance and pulsatile tinnitus. There is often marked papilloedema, which, if long-standing, can lead to optic atrophy and infarction of the optic nerve causing blindness.

MRI is preferred to CT and may show flattened sclera and an empty sella turcica. For the diagnosis to be made, other causes of raised ICP must be absent. Lumbar puncture shows raised CSF pressure but normal composition. Mainstays of treatment are weight loss, acetazolamide and diuretics; therapeutic lumbar punctures may be needed in certain cases. In resistant cases, or if visual acuity deteriorates, a ventriculoperitoneal CSF shunt may be necessary.

Trigeminal neuralgia

There are many causes of facial pain, of which trigeminal neuralgia is one of the most common. This condition of unknown cause is seen most frequently in the elderly and is more common in women. Although in many patients the precise cause is never found, compression due to an aberrant blood vessel is thought to account for the vast majority of cases. In young patients, MS should be considered. It is unilateral in 96% of patients and consists of paroxysms of stabbing pain in the distribution of one or more branches of the trigeminal nerve. The face may screw up with pain, hence the alternative name 'tic douloureux'. If motor or sensory deficits are present consider underlying structural disease (e.g. atrioventricular malformation, cerebellopontine angle tumour or MS).

The pain may be brought on by touching a specific trigger zone and is thus provoked by factors such as eating, shaving or talking. If left untreated, the condition usually progresses, with shorter periods of remission.

Treatment is with carbamazepine, phenytoin, lamotrigine or gabapentin. Surgical procedures such as microvascular decompression or thermocoagulation of the ganglion are reserved for when medical therapy fails.

Other neuralgias include glossopharyngeal neuralgia, precipitated by swallowing, and auriculotemporal neuralgia. Postherpetic neuralgia occurs in patients with previous herpes zoster.

Persistent idiopathic facial pain (atypical facial pain)

This refers to episodes of prolonged facial pain for which no cause can be found, and is therefore a diagnosis of exclusion. It is more common in women and may be preceded by facial surgery or injury. It is associated with depression and may respond to tricyclic antidepressants.

MOVEMENT DISORDERS

Parkinsonism

Parkinsonism is a syndrome of tremor, rigidity, bradykinesia and later, postural instability; it has several causes, of which Parkinson's disease is just one. The differential diagnosis is detailed in Fig. 34.4. This section will focus on idiopathic Parkinson's disease.

First described by James Parkinson in 1817, Parkinson's disease (PD) is now known to be due to degeneration primarily affecting dopaminergic neurones in the substantia nigra. Eosinophilic inclusion bodies (Lewy bodies) are characteristic pathological features.

People with PD are less likely to be smokers. The incidence increases with age, with 1 in 100 people aged over 60 years old affected. Most studies suggest a higher incidence in men. PD is generally felt to be sporadic, although there is increasing evidence of genetic factors playing a role, especially in early-onset disease.

COMMUNICATION

It is essential to have an holistic approach to the care of patients and their carers in chronic conditions such as Parkinson's disease. This hopefully culminates in the formation of a supportive therapeutic alliance.

Clinical features

Early on the patient may complain of fatigue, muscular discomfort or restlessness. Fine movements may be difficult. Onset is unilateral, becoming bilateral after months or years, although severity may remain asymmetric for the duration of the disease.

Tremor

Initially, this is intermittent and may only appear when the patient is tired. The frequency of the tremor is 3–6 beats per second and is most marked at rest (whereas

Fig. 34.4 Differential diagnosis of parkinsonism.

Differential diagnosis		Suggestive features
Idiopathic Parkinson's disease		Asymmetry of onset, not ascribable to other cause
Parkinson's plus syndromes	Progressive supranuclear palsy	Vertical gaze palsy, postural instability. Rigidity and bradykinesia are symmetrical in onset
	Multi-systems atrophy	Autonomic, cerebellar or pyramidal involvement. Symmetrical in onset
	Dementia with Lewy bodies	Dementia preceding or simultaneous to movement disorder
Drug-induced parkinsonism	Neuroleptics, antiemetics	Improves on removal of causative agent
Vascular parkinsonism		History of vascular disease, evidence on CT scan
Metabolic disorders	Wilson's disease, neuroacanthocytosis	Young age at onset, features on laboratory investigation
Post-infectious	Encephalitis lethargica	Preceding episode of illness
Toxic	Heavy metals, carbon monoxide	Known history of exposure, often occupational

a cerebellar tremor is more marked on intention). There is a 'pill rolling' movement of the thumb over the fingers.

Rigidity

There is resistance to passive movement, which may be smooth throughout its range ('lead pipe' rigidity). When combined with tremor, resistance to passive movement is jerky and is termed 'cogwheel' rigidity. It is likely that rigidity contributes to the features of stooped posture and reduced arm swing that are commonly seen (Fig. 34.5).

Bradykinesia

Bradykinesia means difficulty in initiating movements. Dexterity is often affected first, and it may be difficult for the patient to rise from a chair. Writing becomes small (micrographia), spidery and cramped. Repeated movements show slowing and reduced amplitude. The face is expressionless and mask-like, the frequency of spontaneous blinking reduces, and the voice is monotonous and unmodulated. There is a shuffling, 'festinant' gait, and gait freezing may occur.

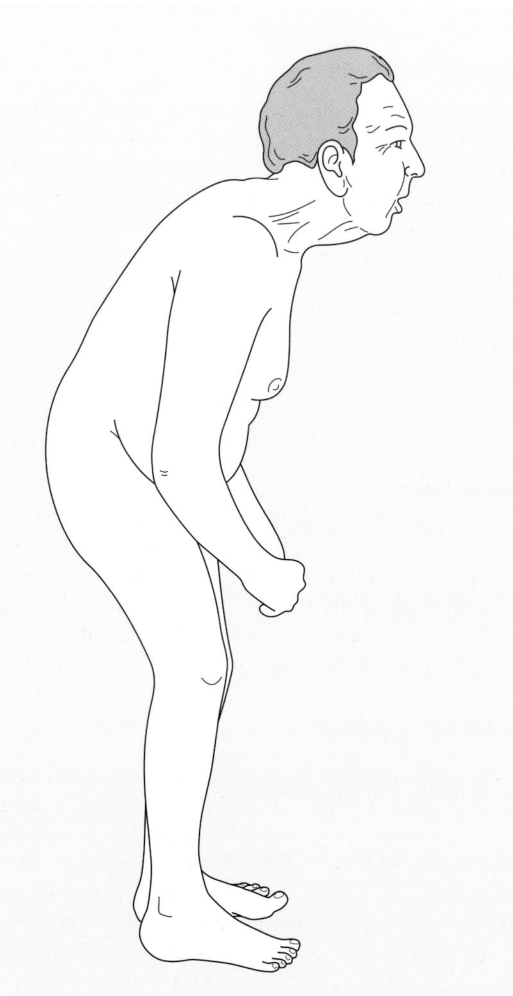

Fig. 34.5 Typical posture in Parkinson's disease. (Courtesy of Dr Kamal, St George's Hospital, Lincoln.)

HINTS AND TIPS

To examine for bradykinesia, ask the patient to unbutton and button their shirt.

Other features

Postural instability occurs late in the disease and results in a significant risk of falls and serious injury. Disordered swallowing causes saliva to gather and drip from the half-open mouth. Autonomic dysfunction is common and may cause constipation and urinary difficulties. Rigidity may be accompanied by pain and sensory disturbance. Late in the disease, dementia may occur. Sleep disorders and mood disorders such as depression are frequently seen.

Differential diagnosis of parkinsonism

Fig. 34.4 describes different causes of parkinsonism. Other conditions that may need to be considered are:

- Essential tremor: this is often straightforward to distinguish but, in some cases, essential tremor can continue at rest, and the tremor of PD may continue on action.
- Other neurodegenerative disorders, such as Huntington's disease and frontotemporal dementia that may have Parkinson-like features.

Diagnosis

The diagnosis of PD is a clinical one. Laboratory investigations may help exclude metabolic causes if there is a degree of suspicion. In difficult cases, SPECT scanning with radioactive iodine (also called DaTSCAN) may help.

Management

The disease is treated symptomatically. Physiotherapy can improve the gait and help build confidence. Physical aids such as high chairs and rails may help with daily activities. Patient and carer information, education and support are very important.

Drugs

The aim of drug therapy is to correct the neurochemical imbalance. This may greatly improve the quality of life but does not prevent progression of the disease, and 10–20% of patients are unresponsive to treatment. Much research is now aimed at developing neuroprotective agents, but none is yet used routinely.

Drugs may cause confusion in the elderly, and it is important to start treatment with low doses and use small increments. There are now a large number of potential pharmacological agents, and the choice of agent has to be made carefully, taking into account individual patient factors.

Levodopa (L-dopa)

L-dopa acts mainly by replenishing depleted striatal dopamine. It helps bradykinesia and rigidity more than tremor. It is generally administered with an extracerebral dopa decarboxylase inhibitor (e.g. benserazide or carbidopa). These prevent the peripheral breakdown of L-dopa to dopamine but, unlike L-dopa, do not cross the blood–brain barrier. Effective brain concentrations of dopamine can thus be achieved with lower doses of L-dopa.

The reduced peripheral formation of dopamine decreases peripheral side effects (e.g. nausea, vomiting and cardiovascular effects). There is less delay in the onset of therapeutic effect and a smoother clinical response. However, there is an increased incidence of abnormal involuntary movements.

L-dopa is the treatment of choice for idiopathic Parkinson's disease. It is less helpful for older patients or those with long-standing disease who may not tolerate the high doses required to overcome their deficit. Side effects of L-dopa include nausea and vomiting, which may be limited by domperidone. Late side effects include the sudden unpredictable swings of the 'on–off' syndrome, dyskinesia and 'end-of-dose' deterioration. In the latter example, the duration of benefit after each dose becomes progressively shorter. This may be improved with modified-release preparations.

In view of the diminishing efficacy of L-dopa with time it is worth delaying the start of drug therapy until the disease is interfering with life, or starting another agent first, thereby saving L-dopa for when symptoms are more disabling. Clearly these decisions should be made in conjunction with patients and carers.

Dopamine agonists

These act at the endogenous neuroreceptor. They may be used as an adjunctive therapy after motor complications have arisen from the long-term use of L-dopa, but may also be used as monotherapy before starting L-dopa, especially in young patients.

The most common side effect of these agents is nausea due to stimulation of the area postrema in the medulla. This can be alleviated with domperidone. Drugs in this group include bromocriptine, pergolide, ropinirole, rotigotine and apomorphine (which may be given by continuous subcutaneous infusion).

Monoamine oxidase B (MAO-B) inhibitors

Selegiline and rasagiline are the MAO-B inhibitors in use. They inhibit the breakdown of dopamine and offer modest symptoms control. They are licensed as a first-line therapy but are more often used as an adjunct.

Catechol-O-methyltransferase (COMT) inhibitors

These reduce the peripheral breakdown of L-dopa and thus reduce the fluctuation in plasma levels and prolong the benefit from each dose. Entacapone is an example.

Anticholinergics

Examples include benzhexol and procyclidine. Tremor and rigidity are improved more than akinesia. They are best avoided in the elderly because of their side effects.

Amantadine

The mechanism of action of this drug is unclear. It improves bradykinesia and rigidity more than tremor. It may be helpful in the late stages of disease as an adjunct.

Other therapy

Surgery (deep brain stimulation of the globus pallidus or subthalamic nucleus) may help in cases with refractory motor complications, but only certain patients are suitable. There is as yet no good evidence for the transplantation of dopaminergic neurones, nor for gene therapy or nerve factor infusion.

Tremor

Tremor is defined as a rhythmic oscillatory movement of a body part, most commonly the hands, although other body parts may be affected. It is a common complaint. The main causes are outlined below. In evaluating a tremor important points to consider are the frequency and amplitude of the tremor, when it is present or most pronounced (at rest, on action or in fixed posture), how disabling it is, and whether the patient has symptoms or signs suggestive of a clear underlying disorder. Differential diagnosis is summarized in Fig. 34.6.

Essential tremor

This is probably the most common movement disorder. Between cases the tremor is variable in frequency and amplitude, but is usually high frequency, most commonly affecting the hands, although the head, trunk or legs can also be affected. It is a postural tremor that is maintained on movement and can be severely disabling. Classically it is alleviated by alcohol, but this is an inadvisable treatment. A proportion of patients will respond to beta-blockers. In severe intractable cases, thalamotomy or deep brain stimulation is sometimes used.

Fig. 34.6 Causes of tremor.

Type	Features	Causes
Resting	Seen when patient relaxed with hands at rest	Parkinsonism
Postural	Seen when hands held outstretched	Benign essential tremor Anxiety Thyrotoxicosis Physiological tremor – often enhanced by adrenergic agonists
Intention	Seen when patients try to touch examiner's finger with their own finger	Cerebellar disease Midbrain lesions

Parkinsonian tremor

This is described above.

Cerebellar tremor

This is classically a low-frequency intention tremor (severity increasing as the movement approaches its end point) although it may be postural or movement related. It is caused by lesions to the cerebellum or its outflow. Other features of cerebellar disease may be present (see Ch. 26).

Huntington's disease

This is an autosomal-dominant inherited disorder caused by a trinucleotide repeat expansion in the gene encoding huntingtin on chromosome 4. The mutation causes a progressive neurodegenerative disease characterized by chorea (irregular, involuntary, 'dance-like' movement) and dementia. It usually starts in middle age, although earlier onset and more severe disease may be seen with successive generations: this is termed 'anticipation'. Neuroleptics or tetrabenazine may help with chorea, but there is no disease-modifying treatment.

Sydenham's chorea

This occurs weeks to months after group A streptococcal infection and is one of the features of acute rheumatic fever. It is occasionally seen in children.

Other movement disorders

For a description of dystonias, tics, myoclonus and akathisisa see *Crash Course: Neurology*.

MULTIPLE SCLEROSIS

Multiple sclerosis (MS) is an autoimmune inflammatory, demyelinating disorder. It is the most common cause of neurological disability in young adults in the UK. The prevalence of MS varies worldwide and is higher in white populations in temperate zones. The overall prevalence in the UK is 1 in 1000, rising to as high as 3 in 1000 in the Shetland and Orkney islands.

There is a female preponderance, with a female-to male ratio of around 2:1. Genetic factors are thought to account for 20–30% of the disease risk, and there may be an association with a previous viral infection such as with Epstein–Barr virus and reduced vitamin D levels. Relapsing/remitting MS has an average onset of 25–29 years, whereas the onset of primary progressive MS is around a decade later.

Pathogenesis

The hallmark of MS is the presence of multiple lesions in the central nervous system (not peripheral nerves) disseminated in location and time. Inflammation, demyelination and axonal loss all play a part in the pathogenesis of MS, but the precise cause remains unknown and is the focus of much ongoing research. It is thought that the disease is started by self-reactive lymphocytes which invade the CNS, causing blood–brain barrier disruption and areas of inflammation and demyelination. Over time and repeated insults, the microglia (resident macrophages of the CNS) become permanently activated and axonal loss occurs. However, the chronicity and contribution of inflammatory and neurodegenerative components is much debated. Sites of predilection include the optic nerve, spinal cord, periventricular areas and brainstem.

Clinical features

The diagnosis depends on obtaining evidence of neurological lesions that have occurred at different sites at different times; this may be clinical or radiological. There is a wide spectrum of disease activity and the course of the disease is extremely variable. It is divided into the following subtypes:

- Relapsing remitting MS is present in 85% of patients. A small number of patients experience progression between relapses ('relapsing progressive' MS)
- Secondary progressive MS: 50% of all relapsing/remitting patients will enter a 'secondary progressive' phase within 10 years of diagnosis.
- In 15% the disease is progressive from the outset and is termed primary progressive MS.

  The onset is monosymptomatic in 85% of patients. Common presentations include optic neuritis, symptoms referable to the brainstem and cerebellum (including diplopia and ataxia), or sensory disturbance of the limbs and leg weakness.

Optic neuritis

This presents as unilateral eye pain (often exacerbated by eye movement) and/or blurred vision, which may progress over a few hours to days to variable visual loss. Central vision is usually more severely affected, with scotomata developing, but complete uniocular blindness may occur. The optic nerve head appears normal unless the lesion is very anterior, when the disc may be swollen. In 90% of patients vision improves over a few months, but colour vision may be permanently affected. Transient blurring of vision lasting minutes, associated with exercise or raised body temperature may occur (an example of Uhthoff's phenomenon – worsening of symptoms with increased temperature). Following an episode of optic neuritis, optic atrophy may ensue with pallor of the disc on fundoscopic examination. Risk of MS following optic neuritis depends on whether lesions are present on MRI.

Diplopia

This is a common symptom caused by a brainstem lesion involving fibres of the 3rd, 4th or 6th cranial nerves, or by a lesion in the medial longitudinal bundle causing an internuclear ophthalmoplegia (see Ch. 2).

Sensory symptoms

These are a common presentation symptom and are very variable depending on the tracts affected. They include paraesthesia and dysaesthesia (altered sensation), diminished proprioception and vibration sense, and reduced pain and light touch sensation. The distribution is also variable and may be limited to the extremities, patchy over the limbs and trunk, or in an 'evolving sensory level' pattern. Flexion of the neck may lead to an electric shock sensation in the back and limbs (Lhermitte's sign), which is associated with a lesion in the cervical cord.

Motor weakness

Lesions of the descending spinal tracts may cause weakness and spasticity in the limbs. The lower limbs are often more affected than the upper limbs. Upper motor neurone signs are present. With an extensive transverse myelitis, sensory and autonomic features may also be present.

Cerebellar signs

Cerebellar signs include nystagmus, incoordination, tremor, dysdiadochokinesia, titubation (continuous rhythmical tremor of the head and trunk) and dysarthria.

HINTS AND TIPS

Cerebellar lesions lead to DASHING: Dysdiadochokinesia, Ataxia, Speech abnormalities (fluctuating, slurring), Hypotonic reflexes, Intention tremor, Nystagmus, and Gait abnormalities.

Other manifestations

Other manifestations include the following:

- Cognitive impairment: especially of memory, sustained concentration and abstract conceptual reasoning.
- Psychiatric abnormalities: most commonly depression; about 10% of patients suffer psychotic symptoms; euphoria may be present in severely disabled patients.
- Pain: this occurs in up to 50% of patients; trigeminal neuralgia is 300 times more common in patients with MS than in the general population.
- Paroxysmal symptoms: these include tonic seizures and rapid flickering contraction in the facial muscles (myokymia). Myokymia may frequently occur in healthy people and is not necessarily pathological.
- Bladder and bowel disturbance: this occurs in 50–75% of patients and is the presenting symptom in 10%; frequency, urgency, incontinence and constipation are the most frequent symptoms; sexual dysfunction is common.
- Uncommon manifestations: 'useless hand' syndrome (an upper limb ataxia), lower motor neurone signs, swallowing and respiratory problems, and extrapyramidal movement disorders.

Diagnosis and differential diagnosis

The diagnosis of MS is based on clinical findings and the exclusion of conditions producing a similar clinical picture. Fulfilment of the revised McDonald criteria (see Further reading) is required after thorough assessment of the patient. There must be evidence of lesions disseminated in space and time. MRI is used to support the diagnosis (see below).

A single episode of disease consistent with MS is termed 'clinically isolated syndrome'. It may present a diagnostic conundrum and compressive, inflammatory and mass or vascular lesions must be excluded. Inflammatory conditions include primary angiitis of the CNS, SLE, primary Sjögren's syndrome, Behçet's disease and PAN, and in children acute disseminated encephalomyelitis.

The differential diagnosis also includes infectious diseases (e.g. Lyme disease, brucellosis, TB, HTLV-1-associated myelopathy), multiple emboli and granulomatous disorders (e.g. sarcoidosis and Wegener's granulomatosis).

Neuromyelitis optica (previously Devic's disease) involves extensive demyelination of the spinal cord and optic nerve and is more common in African and Asian populations.

Familial conditions that may present like MS include adrenoleucodystrophy and CADASIL (cerebral autosomal dominant arteriopathy with subcortical infarcts and leukoencephalopathy).

Investigations

The following investigations are important in the patient with MS:

- MRI is invaluable and shows lesions in the vast majority of patients with clinically definite disease. Gadolinium contrast shows areas of blood–brain barrier disruption, and allows some discrimination between old and new lesions.
- The CSF shows a lymphocytosis and moderately raised protein. Oligoclonal bands of IgG isolated to the CSF are seen in 90% of patients with clinically definite MS but are not specific for MS.
- Delay in the visually evoked response follows optic neuropathy, which may be subclinical. It is useful in providing evidence of a second lesion in patients whose neurological deficits are only attributable to a single lesion. Delays may also occur in auditory or somatosensory evoked potentials depending on the site of the lesions.
- Antibodies to myelin proteins may be present but are of no diagnostic use. Antibodies to aquaporin-4 are 98% specific for neuromyelitis optica.

Prognosis

The progression of MS is very variable and depends on the pattern of disease. Relapsing/remitting disease has a better prognosis. After 5 years, 70% of patients are still employed. After 20 years, only 35% are employed, and 20% are dead from complications. A few patients have 'benign MS' characterized by long periods of remission, infrequent relapses and no functional disability at 15 years' post-diagnosis.

Management

Treatment of MS has two aims: symptom management and disease modification. Pulses of IV methylprednisolone effectively shorten acute relapses but do not alter the course of the disease and should be used sparingly to limit side effects.

Symptomatic treatment is of great importance. Physiotherapy and occupational therapy maintain maximum function. Spasticity may respond to baclofen, dantrolene or vigabatrin. The intention tremor resulting from the involvement of the cerebellum may respond to isoniazid and pyridoxine, or to beta-blockers. Trigeminal neuralgia and paroxysmal symptoms may respond to carbamazepine, and chronic dysaesthetic pain may respond to tricyclic antidepressants.

The management of patients with bladder disturbance has been revolutionized by the introduction of clean intermittent self-catheterization. Anticholinergic agents, particularly oxybutynin, may alleviate urinary frequency. In men with erectile dysfunction, sildenafil or intracorporeal papaverine may be helpful.

Several disease-modifying agents have shown promise in reducing the frequency of relapses and lesions on MRI. However, whether this translates into a reduction in the accumulation of disability and a delay in disease progression is unclear. Beta-interferon and glatiramer acetate remain first-line therapy for relapsing/remitting disease. Natalizumab, a monoclonal antibody directed against alpha-4 integrin, is reserved for patients with highly active disease due to the risk of progressive multifocal leukoencephalopathy. Mitoxantrone is occasionally used for patients who have failed other therapies. Fingolimod has been approved for use in the USA but remains under review in the UK. Several other agents are being assessed in clinical trials.

CENTRAL NERVOUS SYSTEM INFECTION

Meningitis

Meningitis is inflammation of the membranous coverings of the brain and spinal cord. It may be caused by the following:

- Infection: bacteria, viruses and fungi.
- Malignant cells.
- Blood following SAH.
- Inflammatory conditions: sarcoid, lupus, vasculitis.
- Air, drugs or contrast media during encephalography.

The term 'meningitis' is usually reserved for infection of the meninges by organisms. This section will focus on bacterial meningitis.

Causative organisms

This is likely to vary with the patient's age:

- In neonates: *Escherichia coli* and group B streptococci are common.
- In children: meningococcus *(Neisseria meningitidis)* predominate and *Streptococcus pneumoniae* are common. *Haemophilus influenzae* is a less common cause since vaccination was introduced.

- Young adults: prone to meningococcus.
- Older adults: prone to pneumococcus (*S. pneumoniae*).
- Immunocompromised patients and the elderly: prone to pneumococcus, *Listeria*, Gram-negative organisms and *Cryptococcus*.

Predisposing factors

Outbreaks of meningitis tend to occur with overcrowding, poverty and malnutrition. Infection may spread in institutions such as prisons or universities. Secondary meningitis can occur after head injury, sinusitis, mastoiditis or extension of infection from the ears and nasopharynx. Immunocompromised patients such as those with acquired immunodeficiency syndrome (AIDS), with carcinoma, on cytotoxic drugs and following splenectomy are at increased risk. People with congenital meningeal defects or CSF shunts are also prone to infection.

Clinical features

Meningism

The features of meningism are headache and neck stiffness. Kernig's sign (Fig. 34.7) (i.e. pain on passively extending the knee with the hips fully flexed) or Brudzinski's signs may be positive.

Sepsis

High fever is typical. The patient may describe malaise and arthralgia. Any rash may occur, although a petechial/purpuric rash is strongly suggestive of meningococcal disease. Rigors, tachycardia and hypotension may occur.

Raised intracranial pressure

Headache, vomiting, reduced consciousness and seizures may all occur. Later, bradycardia and hypertension can occur (Cushing's reflex).

In tuberculous meningitis, symptoms may initially be non-specific with malaise, anorexia, headache and a variable mild pyrexia. These symptoms may persist for days but gradually an unremitting deterioration occurs. There may be personality changes and intermittent dulling of consciousness before signs of meningism are obvious. The appearance of focal neurological signs suggests a complication (e.g. venous sinus thrombosis, cerebral oedema or hydrocephalus).

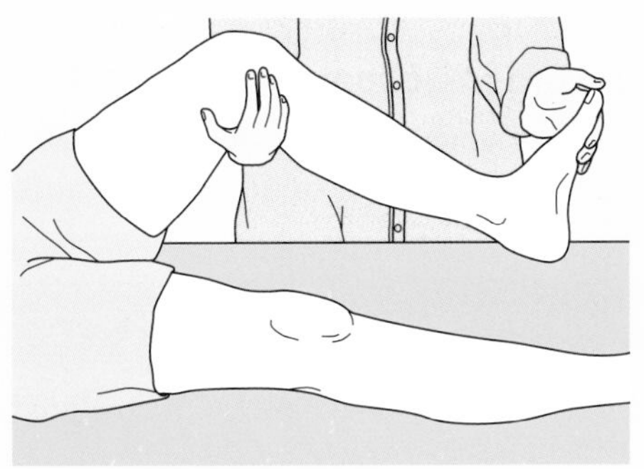

Fig. 34.7 Eliciting Kernig's sign.

Differential diagnosis

Any cause of headache (Ch. 18) or infection should be considered. Of particular note are severe migraine, acute encephalitis and SAH. Unusual organisms should be considered in the setting of immune compromise.

Investigations

HINTS AND TIPS

DO NOT delay therapy in favour of completing investigations in suspected meningitis.

Blood should be taken for FBC, urea and electrolytes (U&Es), CRP, glucose and culture. Blood cultures, throat swabs and a stool sample for viruses should be taken.

Lumbar puncture is the key investigation and should be performed as soon as possible. If the patient is profoundly ill, IV antibiotics should be given first. A CT scan should be performed first if there is any evidence of raised intracranial pressure: reduced consciousness, seizures, focal neurology, papilloedema. Samples should be sent for microscopy and culture, Gram stain, protein estimation, glucose (with simultaneous plasma glucose) and virology. Polymerase chain reaction (PCR) for diagnosis of meningococcus infection should be performed on peripheral blood. PCR for individual organisms can also be performed on CSF. CSF changes in meningitis are summarized in Fig. 34.8 (see also Ch. 26).

Treatment

High doses of appropriate antibiotics should be given as soon as possible. If a lumbar puncture can be performed quickly it may be possible to obtain a sample of CSF first, but this should not delay the administration of antibiotics.

If outside a hospital, give 1.2 g IM of benzylpenicillin. Therapy in hospital is usually empirical initially (consult local policy) (e.g. IV ceftriaxone for patients <50 years and IV ceftriaxone and amoxicillin (to cover *Listeria*) in patients >50 years). Aciclovir IV should also be given if encephalitis is suspected (see below). These treatments may subsequently be modified depending on the results of microbiological analysis.

Fig. 34.8 Changes in the cerebrospinal fluid in meningitis.

	Normal	**Viral**	**Bacterial**	**Tuberculous**
Appearance	Clear	Clear/turbid	Turbid	Turbid/fibrinous
Predominant cell	<5 mononuclear cells/mL	10–100 mononuclear cells/mL	200–3000 polymorphs/mL	10–300 mononuclear cells/mL 0–300 polymorphs/mL
Protein	0.2–0.4 g/L	0.4–0.8 g/L	0.5–5 g/L	0.5–5 g/L
Glucose	>⅔ plasma level	>⅔ plasma level	<⅔ plasma level	<⅔ plasma level

Analgesia and careful monitoring of the patient's haemodynamic status and urine output are important. If the patient is septicaemic involve the Intensive Care Unit early. If meningitic signs predominate the clinical picture give IV dexamethasone before, or at the same time as, antibiotics. This can reduce the risk of long-term neurological sequelae and mortality in pneumococcal meningitis. It is also indicated in tuberculous meningitis. It should be avoided in septic shock, known meningococcal disease and immunocompromised states.

Always remember that meningitis is a notifiable disease and cases must be reported to the Department of Health. Prophylactic antibiotics are recommended for close contacts of the index case.

Encephalitis

This is inflammation of the brain parenchyma. There is usually some inflammation of the meninges in encephalitis and conversely some inflammation of the parenchyma in meningitis.

Encephalitis can be caused by viruses (most commonly herpes simplex – HSV), *Listeria* and *Toxoplasma* if immunocompromised, tuberculosis, and by bacteria where there may be associated abscess formation.

The patient may present with altered mental state, reduced consciousness, seizures, headache or focal neurology. Features of meningism will be present in combined meningoencephalitis. A high index of suspicion is required.

The diagnosis depends on knowledge of local epidemics, unreliable radiological features (such as temporal lobe swelling in HSV encephalitis) and electroencephalogram (EEG) findings (periodic complexes in HSV encephalitis), CSF findings (see Ch. 26), and demonstration of viruses in the CSF by serology or PCR. Often, the diagnosis is not confirmed. The differential diagnosis is wide and includes paraneoplastic and autoimmune encephalitis as well as any cause of encephalopathy.

HSV encephalitis is potentially treatable and therefore if there is any suspicion of encephalitis IV aciclovir should be given (in addition to other empirical treatments for meningoencephalitis) and the CSF should be sent for HSV PCR.

Fig. 34.9 The differential diagnosis of a ring-enhancing lesion on brain CT/MRI.
Primary or secondary tumour
Brain abscess
Toxoplasmosis
Tuberculoma
Aspergilloma
Neurocysticercosis

CNS abscess

This can occur via direct spread, for instance from mastoiditis or sinusitis, or from a distant region, most commonly a site of chronic infection such as subacute bacterial endocarditis or chronic suppurative lung disease. Haematogenous spread often leads to multiple abscesses. There is a wide range of possible causative organisms, particularly in the patient with immune compromise, including aerobic and anaerobic bacteria as well as fungi.

Presentation with headache is most common, although features of meningitis or encephalitis may be present depending on the extent of the inflammation. In large, rapidly expanding abscesses, signs of raised ICP may be present. MRI or CT scan with contrast will show a ring-enhancing lesion (for differential diagnosis see Fig. 34.9). Treatment will require an extended course of IV antibiotics, the choice of which depends on the suspected source and therefore identity of the organism. Surgical aspiration may be required.

Spinal cord infection

This includes epidural abscesses, viral myelitis and tuberculous myelopathy.

EPILEPSY

Epilepsy refers to a group of conditions in which paroxysms of abnormal electrical activity of cerebral neurons result in seizures. A single acute seizure has many possible provoking factors (see Aetiology); a person is considered to have epilepsy if the seizures recur over time. As many as 1 in 20 of the general population have a seizure at some time in their lives and around 200 000 people in the UK are taking antiepileptic drugs (AEDs). In understanding the classification of epileptic disorders, the distinction between seizures and syndromes must be understood; a patient with a epilepsy syndrome may experience several different types of seizure.

Classification

The International League against Epilepsy reviewed the classification in 2010, reclassifying the aetiology (previously idiopathic, symptomatic or cryptogenic) as 'genetic, structural/metabolic, or unknown'. Seizures were previously classified as generalized, simple partial (not affecting consciousness) or complex partial (affecting consciousness), with or without secondary generalization. The new classification advised that with regard to focal seizures, the distinction between 'complex' and 'simple' should be dropped. However, these terms, and the term 'idiopathic generalized epilepsy' remain widely used. There may be a prodrome lasting hours to days before a seizure, where there is a change in mood or behaviour. This is not part of the seizure, unlike an aura (see below). Some common syndromes are outlined in Fig. 34.10.

Generalized seizures

These are not referable to a single hemisphere.

Tonic–clonic (grand mal) seizures

Prior to the seizure, the patient may experience a prodrome with symptoms such as mood change, irritability and anxiety. There is no aura, which would represent an initial partial seizure. The seizure has a sudden onset with sudden loss of consciousness, followed by a tonic phase involving powerful muscular contractions. Teeth are clenched; cyanosis may occur. After about a minute, the clonic phase starts, consisting of convulsive movements – jerking/twitching – as the muscles intermittently relax before clenching again. The patient is often drowsy and confused following the event (postictal confusion).

HINTS AND TIPS

Faecal (as opposed to urinary) incontinence and biting at the side of the tongue (as opposed to the tip) are helpful pointers towards the diagnosis of a seizure.

Absence attacks (petit mal)

These often start in childhood. There are brief interruptions of consciousness, sometimes accompanied by rhythmical blinking of the eyelids. To an observer, the child may appear to be dazed or daydreaming. Recovery is immediate and there are no sequelae.

Myoclonic epilepsy

This is a form of idiopathic epilepsy developing in early childhood. Various types of generalized fit occur, including sudden jerking movements of the limbs (myoclonus). The patient often remains conscious and alert throughout.

Atonic or akinetic epilepsy

During the attack the patient becomes flaccid and falls to the ground.

Fig. 34.10 Some of the common epilepsy syndromes.

Epilepsy syndrome	Age of onset	Features	First-line AEDs
Lennox–Gastaut syndrome	1–7 years	Generalized, multiple seizure types 2–2.5 Hz slow spike-wave pattern on EEG Cognitive impairment	Sodium valproate, lamotrigine
Childhood absence epilepsy	2–14 years; peak age 8	Absences predominate, may be many times/day 3 Hz spike and slow wave on EEG	Ethosuximide, sodium valproate
Juvenile myoclonic epilepsy	10–20 years	Myoclonus (especially in the morning), GTCS and absences 4–6 Hz polyspike and wave discharge on EEG	Sodium valproate, levetiracetam
Mesial temporal lobe epilepsy with hippocampal sclerosis (MTLE with HS)	Peak 4–16 years	Focal Aura, impairment of consciousness, automatisms EEG: build up and rhythmic discharge	Carbamazepine, lamotrigine

Note that MTLE with HS is not yet clearly defined as a syndrome. GTCS, generalized tonic–clonic seizures.

Focal (partial) seizures

The features of partial seizures can be referred to a single hemisphere and are therefore suggestive of underlying structural problems. The nature of the attack varies according to the primary site of the lesion.

Without impairment of consciousness (simple partial seizures)

Consciousness is unimpaired and these attacks are characterized by focal activity related to the site of abnormal electrical activity. This may be motor, sensory (including special senses), autonomic (e.g. sweating) or affecting higher consciousness. In motor seizures, the affected limb may suffer a short-lived weakness after the attack (Todd's paresis).

With impairment of consciousness (complex partial seizures)

These seizures are often derived from the temporal lobes. Hippocampal sclerosis may be present. An aura precedes the loss of consciousness in the majority of cases, and may consist of hallucinations of any of the five senses or of higher function (e.g. memory). Abdominal aura, a 'rising' feeling in the upper abdomen, is common. Gustatory and olfactory hallucinations are usually unpleasant. 'Jamais vu' is a sudden feeling of unfamiliarity while the patient is in their own environment and 'déjà vu' is a vivid sense of familiarity with the current situation.

When consciousness is lost, the patient may still appear awake, and automatisms may occur: semi-purposeful, stereotyped, repetitive movements such as lip smacking or picking at clothing. An abnormal posture may be adopted due to dystonia. The patient cannot remember these events after the attack.

Focal seizure evolving to generalized seizure

The seizure starts off with focal involvement but then spreads widely, causing a generalized seizure.

COMMUNICATION

Take time to discuss and explain this condition to patients. They will often feel stigmatized by the diagnosis and their concerns and worries need to be addressed.

Aetiology

The majority of seizures are 'idiopathic' although it is increasingly understood that genetic disorders underlie a significant number of these syndromes. Structural causes, such as congenital malformations or acquired lesions, are also common causes. When a patient presents with a first seizure, provoking factors must be sought. These include the following:

- Metabolic causes: hypoxia, hyper- or hypoglycaemia, hypocalcaemia, uraemia, alcoholism, hypo- and hypernatraemia, liver failure, pyridoxine deficiency.
- Drugs and toxins: alcohol, lead, both prescription and recreational drugs (e.g. phenothiazines, monoamine oxidase inhibitors, tricyclic antidepressants, amphetamines, lidocaine, nalidixic acid). Acute withdrawal from alcohol or benzodiazepines is associated with seizures.
- Trauma and surgery (e.g. perinatal trauma or head injury).
- Space-occupying lesions: e.g. tumour, abscess, extra-axial haemorrhage.
- Cerebral infarction.
- Other organic brain diseases: SLE, PAN, sarcoidosis, vascular malformations.
- Infections: encephalitis, syphilis, and human immunodeficiency virus.
- Degenerative brain disorders: Alzheimer's disease, Creutzfeldt–Jakob disease.

HINTS AND TIPS

Reflex anoxic seizures following a faint are common, especially if the patient remains in an upright posture.

Precipitants of seizures

In a patient with epilepsy, seizures may be triggered by flashing lights, exercise, strong emotions and hyperventilation (leading to alkalosis). Other conditions that may precipitate seizures by lowering the seizure threshold include fever, irregular meals, menstruation, lack of sleep and pregnancy. Certain medications also lower the seizure threshold.

Differential diagnosis

Seizures can be difficult to distinguish from other causes of collapse. This is discussed in Ch. 22. Non-epileptic attack disorder (psychogenic seizures or pseudoseizures) can be very difficult to distinguish from true epilepsy.

Investigations

NICE guidelines propose that all patients with a recent-onset suspected seizure are seen urgently by a specialist to ensure accurate diagnosis and appropriate therapy.

General tests

The diagnosis is a clinical one and a good witness account of the 'seizures' is vital. After a thorough history and examination to consider differential diagnoses, blood tests should be performed including FBC, U&Es, serum calcium and magnesium, liver function tests and glucose. An ABG taken during or just after the seizure will often show a metabolic acidosis, which will normalize rapidly after cessation of the seizure. It may be necessary to screen blood and urine for drugs/toxins. A CXR and ECG should be performed.

Imaging

A CT scan may be useful in the acute setting to look for large lesions. However, MRI is the modality of choice and may uncover subtle structural abnormalities. It is especially important when epilepsy develops in adulthood or in the very young (under 2 years old), and for focal seizures. It is not always necessary when there is a clear diagnosis of an idiopathic generalized epilepsy syndrome.

Electroencephalogram (EEG)

The diagnosis should not be based solely on the EEG, as 10–15% of the general population may have an 'abnormal' EEG and approximately 15% of people with epilepsy never have specific epileptiform discharges. However, it may help further identify the type of epilepsy.

Treatment

Treatment is recommended after two seizures, but may be started after a single unprovoked seizure in certain circumstances – if EEG or imaging is conclusive, or if the risk of a further seizure is considered too great. The aims of drug treatment are to prevent seizures while keeping the patient free of side effects. Antiepileptic drugs should be prescribed individually, using the lowest dose to obtain complete seizure control with minimum side effects. A single drug will suffice in approximately 80% of patients, the remainder needing a second drug to achieve acceptable control. Partial epilepsy is more likely to be refractory.

Having chosen a drug, the dose is gradually increased until control is achieved, the maximum dose is reached or toxic effects supervene. In the latter two cases, alternatives need to be considered (see below).

Carbamazepine, phenytoin and barbiturates all induce hepatic enzymes and therefore speed up the metabolism of oestrogens and progestogens, making the oral contraceptive pill unreliable. Sodium valproate does not affect oral contraceptive efficacy, but carries a significant risk of teratogenicity.

Treatment is first instituted according to the specific epilepsy syndrome; if this is not clear, it is started according to the seizure type.

First-line drugs

Generalized seizures

The type of seizure must be carefully assessed. Sodium valproate is recommended as the first-line treatment of choice for tonic–clonic seizures or for myoclonic seizures. Lamotrigine may also be used for tonic–clonic seizures, but can worsen myoclonic seizures. Carbamazepine is ineffective for the treatment of absence or myoclonic seizures, but is effective for tonic–clonic seizures. Common unwanted effects of sodium valproate include weight gain, hair thinning and tremor.

Focal seizures

Carbamazepine and lamotrigine are the first-line therapies. Levetiracetam, oxcarbazepine or sodium valproate may also be used. Carbamazepine may cause CNS side effects (e.g. dizziness, nausea, headaches and drowsiness), which may be avoided by slowly increasing the dose. It induces hepatic enzymes and so increases the metabolism of hepatically metabolized drugs.It may increase or decrease serum phenytoin levels depending on the individual

Second-line drugs

Phenytoin is useful but less commonly used because of its unpredictable pharmacokinetics. NICE suggests that the newer AEDs (e.g. lamotrigine, levetiracetam, topiramate, zonisamide, vigabatrin) be used as second-line agents if valproate and carbamazepine are contraindicated or ineffective.

Changing drugs

This may be performed in cases of treatment failure or because of side effects. The new drug is commenced at its starting dose and gradually increased. The old drug is withdrawn slowly.

Withdrawing drugs

Most patients are seizure-free within a few years of starting therapy and 60% remain so after drug withdrawal. Therefore drug withdrawal is considered in some patients after a period of therapy if they have been seizure-free for two years or more. Certain factors increase the risk of seizure recurrence, such as abnormal EEG, abnormalities on neurological exam, or some types of epilepsy (e.g. juvenile myoclonic epilepsy). Therefore the risks need to be assessed on an individual basis and carefully explained.

The role of surgery

Surgery is sometimes needed for refractory, drug resistant epilepsy. It is most effective for focal seizures when the focus of the abnormal electrical activity can be accurately localized and resected.

Ketogenic diet

The use of this high fat, moderate protein, low carbohydrate diet should be considered in children and young adults when seizure control is difficult.

Epilepsy and other issues

Pregnancy

There are several important issues to be considered when an epileptic patient wants to become, or becomes, pregnant. It is important to enlist specialist help in this situation.

- The effect of AEDs on the fetus: several AEDs, including carbamazepine and valproate, are teratogenic. Are the drugs necessary?
- The effect of pregnancy on the mother's seizures and the risk to the fetus from maternal seizures.

It is imperative to counsel the patient regarding these issues so that informed choices can be made. If it is felt that antiepileptic therapy must continue during pregnancy it is important to try to use a single agent at the lowest possible dose.

Driving and work

Current regulations stipulate that after a single unprovoked seizure, the patient must not drive for 6 months. If a diagnosis of epilepsy is made, the patient must be seizure-free for at least one year before driving can be recommenced. Longer periods are necessary for drivers of large commercial vehicles. When a seizure at work would pose a significant risk to the patient or his colleagues, this needs to be carefully discussed.

Convulsive status epilepticus

This is a medical emergency and is defined as prolonged generalized tonic–clonic seizures lasting more than 5 min, or repeated seizures without intervening recovery of consciousness. Both the risk of permanent brain damage and mortality are related to the length of the attack and therefore seizures must be stopped as soon as possible.

Check bedside glucose levels. Once therapy has been instigated, the following tests should be performed: arterial blood gas, electrolytes, serum calcium, ECG, FBC. Consider checking anticonvulsant levels if appropriate, toxicology screen, lumbar puncture and blood/urine cultures, CT scan.

- Priority is basic life support and ABC (Airway, Breathing, Circulation).
- Lay the patient in the recovery position, remove false teeth and insert an oral airway. The patient may require intubation.
- Administer high-flow oxygen and suction.
- Check capillary glucose.
- Gain IV access and take blood for FBC, lab glucose, U&Es, liver function tests, calcium, toxicology screen and drug levels if on anticonvulsant. A blood gas is useful.
- Give a bolus of 20% or 50% dextrose if any suggestion of hypoglycaemia.
- Give slow IV bolus of lorazepam 4 mg (IV diazepam or buccal midazolam are alternatives).
- If seizures persist, commence a phenytoin infusion (with cardiac monitor) or a diazepam infusion.
- If seizures still persist, consider paralysis, ventilation and an urgent EEG.

Post-seizure, consider further investigations: brain scan, ECG, lumbar puncture.

Sudden unexpected death in epilepsy (SUDEP)

Patients with epilepsy are at higher risk of sudden death, termed SUDEP. Certain features, which are mainly relate to the severity of the epilepsy, place patients at higher risk, such as seizure frequency and duration of disease. Patients should be informed and counselled regarding this issue.

INTRACRANIAL TUMOURS

Primary intracerebral tumours account for around 2% of all cancers. Due to their location and threat to health, even if 'benign', they are often classified as high-grade or low-grade tumours rather than benign or malignant. Certain familial conditions, such as neurofibromatosis, predispose to development of brain tumours. Secondary intracerebral tumours (metastases) are more common and occur in up to 30% of cancers, mainly from the bronchus, breasts, kidneys, colon, ovary, prostate or thyroid. The main sites of origin of brain tumours are shown in Fig. 34.11.

Clinical features

Symptoms arise from the direct effects of the mass on surrounding structures, from the effects of raised intracranial pressure or by provoking seizures. Similar symptoms may be produced by any mass lesion (e.g. haematomas, aneurysms, abscesses, tuberculomas, granulomas and cysts).

Fig. 34.11 The origins of brain tumours.

Site	Example of tumour derived
Glia	Astrocytomas (including glioblastomas), oligodendrogliomas, ependymomas
Meninges	Meningiomas (25%)
Blood vessels	Angiomas, angioblastomas
Schwann cells of the cranial nerves	Acoustic neuromas
Pituitary gland	Craniopharyngioma
Lymphocytes	Primary CNS lymphoma

Direct effects depend on the site of the tumour:

- Frontal lobe: personality changes, apathy and impairment of intellectual function. There may be anosmia, contralateral hemiparesis or dysphasia (Broca's area).
- Parietal lobe: contralateral homonymous field defects and hemisensory loss. There may be apraxia, spatial disorientation and dysphasia if the temporoparietal region is affected. Signs include 'parietal drift' or falling of the outstretched contralateral arm, astereognosis (inability to recognize an object placed in the hand) and sensory inattention.
- Temporal lobe: problems with memory, comprehension, emotion. Contralateral superior visual field defects.
- Occipital lobe: contralateral hemianopia.
- Cerebellopontine angle: vertigo and progressive ipsilateral perceptive deafness (8th nerve), numbness of the ipsilateral side of the face (5th nerve), facial weakness (7th nerve) and ipsilateral cerebellar signs.

Raised intracranial pressure

Symptoms include headache (worse in the morning and with stooping, coughing and sneezing), vomiting (possibly without nausea) and papilloedema. Displacement of intracranial contents may cause focal signs similar to direct mass effects or general effects due to herniation; as this occurs there will be impairment of consciousness progressing to coma and respiratory depression. 'False localizing signs' may be present (e.g. a 6th nerve lesion, as it is compressed against the petrous temporal bone).

Investigations

Cross-sectional imaging is the first investigation; plain X-rays are of limited use. MRI provides more detailed images than CT. More advanced techniques such as PET, SPECT or MR spectroscopy may provide additional information about the extent and grade of tumour; this is particularly useful in planning surgery. If metastases are suspected, investigations for the primary neoplasm should be carried out. If a primary intracranial tumour is suspected, stereotactic biopsy is required for definitive diagnosis of type and grade of tumour. It will also rule out other causes, such as abscess or inflammatory lesions, which may be difficult to differentiate on imaging.

Management

Initial management is of the complications: dexamethasone for cerebral oedema and anticonvulsants for seizures. Emergency surgery such as shunt insertion may be required to adequately decompress the brain.

Further treatment depends on type and grade of tumour, and estimates of risk and benefit are often difficult. Surgical resection is preferred if possible. Radiotherapy is usually recommended for gliomas and for radiosensitive metastases. Adjuvant chemotherapy may provide a small but significant survival benefit.

A watch-and-wait policy is sometimes adopted for small, indolent tumours such as low-grade meningiomas.

COMMUNICATION

The multidisciplinary team meeting is extremely important in the management of brain tumours and provides a forum where investigations can be reviewed, and all aspects of care can be discussed.

Prognosis

The overall 1-year survival for patients with primary intracerebral tumours is less than 50%.

There may be complete recovery from meningiomas if they are removed completely.

DISORDERS AFFECTING MUSCLE AND THE NEUROMUSCULAR JUNCTION

Muscle disorders

For more on muscle disorders, see polymyositis and dermatomyositis in Ch. 36.

Myotonic dystrophy (myotonia dystrophica)

This is an autosomal dominant condition characterized by myotonia: the inability of the muscles to relax normally after contraction. The peak onset is between the ages of 20 and 30 years, and the incidence in the UK is approximately 5 in 100 000. There is muscle wasting and weakness of the facial muscles with ptosis, a wry smile or 'sneer' and a 'hang-dog' expression due to the thin face and lax jaw muscles. The neck and distal limb muscles are also affected.

Other associated features include frontal baldness, cataracts, testicular or ovarian atrophy, cardiomyopathy with conduction disturbances, mental impairment and endocrine dysfunction including diabetes. Reflexes are lost. The myotonia is often revealed by shaking the patient's hand (slow to release grip) or by asking patients to repetitively open and close their eyes or fists. It may be elicited by percussing the thenar eminence – the induced depression is slow to fill ('percussion myotonia'). It increases with fatigue, cold and stress. Diagnosis is by genetic testing. The myotonia may improve with procainamide or phenytoin.

Muscular dystrophies (MD)

These are a group of genetically determined diseases characterized by progressive degeneration and weakness of certain muscle groups.

Duchenne and Becker muscular dystrophies (pseudohypertrophic)

These are the commonest types and are X-linked recessive. Both involve mutations of the dystrophin gene. The incidence is around 2 in 10 000 male births. Duchenne MD presents at around 5 years of age with clumsiness in walking and difficulty climbing stairs. Examination reveals a lordotic posture and 'waddling' gait due to proximal muscle weakness. The calves are hypertrophied. When rising from the floor, patients may need to use their hands to bring themselves into an upright position (Gower's sign). Investigations show a markedly raised creatine kinase concentration. Electromyography and muscle biopsy show characteristic changes. Cardiomyopathy is common. Death usually occurs before the age of 20 years from intercurrent illnesses (e.g. chest infection). There is no specific treatment. Becker MD is less severe, with onset usually in the teenage years and survival usually beyond the third decade.

Fascioscapulohumeral dystrophy (Landouzy–Dejerine syndrome)

This is autosomal dominant. The onset is around puberty with wasting and weakness of the upper limb girdle and face. Life expectancy is usually normal.

Limb girdle dystrophy

This describes a group of disorders affecting predominantly proximal muscles. Most are autosomal recessive, and onset is frequently in childhood in the most common types. The condition is progressive, with death in middle age. There may be cardiac involvement.

Neuromuscular junction disorders

Myasthenia gravis

This is an autoimmune disease where muscle weakness is caused by a reduction in the number of functional postsynaptic acetylcholine receptors, and their eventual destruction. Approximately 90% of patients have detectable levels of antibody to the postsynaptic acetylcholine receptor. Most of the remainder have antibodies to muscle-specific kinase (MuSK). It is associated with thymoma and thymus hyperplasia, hyperthyroidism, rheumatoid arthritis and SLE.

Clinical features

In younger patients (<50 years) it is more common in females and associated with other autoimmune conditions. In older patients there is a male preponderance and an association with thymic atrophy/tumour. There is painless muscle weakness, which worsens on repetitive contraction and fluctuates over the day. Over half of patients present with extraocular muscle weakness causing ptosis and diplopia. The facial and bulbar muscles are commonly affected, causing the 'myasthenic snarl' on smiling, dysarthria and dysphagia. Proximal muscles and upper limbs are more often affected than distal muscles and lower limbs. Reflexes are usually normal. In 15%, the disease remains limited to the eyes. Myasthenic crisis is a rare complication with rapidly worsening weakness often precipitated by infection or medication. Respiratory weakness is the concern, and the patient may require intubation and ventilation.

Investigations

Edrophonium 10 mg can be given intravenously (with cardiac monitoring and resuscitation facilities), and in a positive test improves muscle power for 3–4 min. It enhances neuromuscular transmission in myasthenia gravis by inhibiting acetylcholinesterase and thereby prolonging the action of acetylcholine. It is a sensitive test but has a high false-positive rate.

The mainstays of laboratory diagnosis are serological testing for anti-acetylcholine receptor and anti-MuSK antibodies, as well as electromyography which reveals a decremental muscle response to repetitive nerve stimulation. A CT scan of the thymus is performed.

Management

Symptomatic control is with a longer-acting anticholinesterase (e.g. pyridostigmine or neostigmine). The dose is slowly titrated against muscle power. Side effects include nausea, vomiting, increased salivation, diarrhoea and abdominal cramps. Cholinergic crisis can occur and is similar in presentation to myasthenic crisis.

Immunosuppression with prednisolone on alternate days may achieve remission. If there is no remission and weakness is severe, azathioprine may be helpful. In intractable cases, plasmapheresis gives approximately 4 weeks of benefit. The condition is usually relapsing or slowly progressive, and respiratory muscle involvement can lead to death. The 5-year survival with a thymoma is approximately 70%. Resection of the thymus may increase the likelihood of achieving remission.

Lambert–Eaton myasthenic syndrome

This is an autoimmune condition but may be paraneoplastic; around 50% of cases are associated with small-cell lung cancer. Antibodies to the presynaptic voltage-gated calcium channels are present. The resulting weakness diminishes with exertion (opposite of myasthenia). Slowly progressive weakness is typical, particularly affecting the lower limbs. Autonomic involvement and hyporeflexia are characteristic. Therapy with IV immunoglobulin, plasmapharesis or 3,4-diaminopyridine is supervised by experts. Regular chest X-rays are important; the neurological symptoms may predate cancer detection by months or even years

DISORDERS OF THE PERIPHERAL NERVES

Peripheral neuropathy

Peripheral neuropathy is a general term referring to disorders of peripheral nerves; the presentation can be divided into mononeuropathy, mononeuritis multiplex and polyneuropathy. The causes of these are summarized in Ch. 26. The four most common causes are diabetes mellitus, malignancy, vitamin B_{12} deficiency, and drugs (notably alcohol). Treatment is aimed at the underlying cause. Some specific peripheral nerve syndromes are considered here.

Guillain–Barré syndrome (GBS)

This is an acute immune-mediated condition with several subtypes, the most common of which in Caucasians is acute inflammatory demyelinating polyneuropathy (AIDP). It affects motor nerves more than sensory nerves and occurs days or weeks after an infectious illness such as *Campylobacter* sp., cytomegalovirus or Epstein–Barr virus. Clinically there is progressive, relatively symmetrical weakness starting in the legs in 90% of patients and often accompanied by paraesthesia and numbness. The upper limbs, trunk, respiratory and cranial nerves may then become affected. In 10% the weakness starts in the arms or facial muscles, and in the Miller Fisher subtype there is ophthalmoplegia and ataxia. Complications of GBS include respiratory failure, cardiac arrhythmias due to autonomic dysfunction and aspiration due to bulbar palsy. Due to immobility the patients are at high risk of deep vein thrombosis (DVT) and pulmonary embolism.

Most patients with GBS start to improve within a month. A small proportion of patients will continue to progress or suffer relapses; if this continues for more than 8 weeks the illness is termed chronic inflammatory demyelinating polyneuropathy (CIDP).

Investigations

The CSF shows a high protein concentration (up to 10 g/L) with a normal cell count. Nerve conduction studies confirm slowing of conduction. The vital capacity should be measured 4–6-hourly to anticipate respiratory depression. In addition, the patient's swallowing should be monitored closely as should the postural drop in blood pressure (as an indicator of autonomic function).

Management

Supportive

Attention should be paid to fluid balance and nutrition, and prevention of pressure sores, DVT and pneumonia (with physiotherapy). Mechanical ventilation may be necessary if respiratory failure occurs.

Specific

Steroids are not of benefit. However, IV immunoglobulin and plasma exchange have been shown to improve outcome, and are recommended for patients presenting up to 4 weeks after the onset of symptoms.

Around 5% of severely affected patients will die in intensive care. Around 90% of all patients with GBS make a good recovery.

Entrapment/compression neuropathies

These are extremely common syndromes causing mononeuropathy with neurological symptoms and signs in the distribution of a single peripheral nerve. The injury to the nerve may be transient, changing with position, but with chronicity demyelination and axonal degeneration may occur. Some of the most frequently encountered conditions are described here:

- Carpal tunnel syndrome: compression of the median nerve as it passes through the carpal tunnel at the wrist, causing numbness, paraesthesiae and weakness of the hand.
- Radial nerve palsy: compression of the radial nerve, frequently at the spiral groove in the upper arm, causing weakness of wrist and finger extensors, with numbness of the dorsum of the hand and forearm ('Saturday night palsy').

- Meralgia paraesthetica: entrapment of the lateral cutaneous nerve of the thigh as it passes under the inguinal ligament, causing numbness over the lateral aspect of the thigh.

DISORDERS OF THE SPINAL CORD

Spinal cord compression

Spinal cord compression is a medical emergency. Causes are summarized in Fig. 34.12. Symptoms include local or radicular pain, often precipitated by movement or straining, spastic paraparesis with upper motor neurone signs below the level of the lesion and lower motor neurone signs at the level of the lesion, sensory loss with a characteristic 'sensory level', and sphincter disturbances at a later stage. It is important to note that there is a discrepancy between the level of the root lesion and that of the sensory level and spastic paraparesis. This arises because the spinal cord is shorter than the spinal column (it ends at the second lumbar vertebra in the adult) and below the cervical spine the nerve roots travel inferiorly before exiting through the vertebral foramina. For instance, a lesion at the level of the T10 cord segment may be at the T9 vertebra level and hence cause T9 root symptoms but a T10 sensory level. Compression of the cauda equina (the descending lumbar and sacral nerve roots below the level of the L2 vertebra) causes root pain and lower motor neurone pattern weakness in the legs, with saddle anaesthesia (numbness of buttocks and perineum) and sphincter disturbances. If suspected, MRI or CT is required to show the spinal cord. These must be done urgently as early intervention may prevent irreversible paraplegia. Therefore the neurosurgeons must also be informed promptly. Investigations should also include those of the underlying cause.

Treatment is by decompression, which should be performed as soon as possible to prevent irreversible damage. Radiotherapy may be useful in malignant disease. If the patient has a known or suspected malignancy, dexamethasone should be given.

Fig. 34.12 Causes of spinal cord compression.

Cause	Example
Vertebral (extradural)	Collapsed vertebrae, e.g. metastatic cancer (bronchus, breast, thyroid, kidney, prostate), osteoporosis, myeloma Spondylosis with disc prolapse Pott's disease (tuberculosis) Paget's disease Abscess Reticuloses
Intradural, extramedullary	Meningioma Neurofibroma
Intramedullary	Glioma

Subacute combined degeneration of the cord

This is due to vitamin B_{12} deficiency and refers to demyelination of the posterior and lateral columns. The onset is usually insidious and associated with a sensory peripheral neuropathy. Clinical features include the following:

- Loss of vibration and joint position sense, and positive Romberg sign: posterior columns.
- Weakness, hypertonia and extensor plantars: lateral corticospinal tract.
- Absent knee jerks and reduced touch sensation: peripheral neuropathy.

Treatment is with vitamin B_{12} injections intramuscularly.

Syringomyelia and syringobulbia

Syringomyelia is due to a longitudinal cyst in the cervical cord. As it enlarges it may extend into the dorsal horns and white matter. Clinical features are insidious and include the following:

- Dissociated sensory loss in the hand: loss of pain and temperature sensation only. This may involve the trunk and arm ('cape-like distribution').
- Weakness and wasting of the small muscles of the hand.
- Loss of tendon reflexes and arm pain.

As the syrinx expands, it may lead to spastic paraplegia with upper motor neurone signs. Insidious loss of normal sensation may lead to joint destruction (Charcot's joints) or injury.

Treatment is by surgical decompression or aspiration.

If the syrinx extends into the brainstem it is called syringobulbia, and may affect cranial nerves, causing the following symptoms:

- Facial pain or sensory loss: 5th cranial nerve.
- Vertigo and nystagmus: 8th cranial nerve.
- Facial, palatal or laryngeal palsy: 7th, 9th, 10th and 11th cranial nerves.
- Wasting of the tongue: 12th cranial nerve.
- Horner's syndrome: sympathetic tract.

MISCELLANEOUS NEUROLOGICAL DISORDERS

Motor neurone disease

This is a disease involving progressive degeneration of the motor cortex, pyramidal and corticospinal tracts, lower cranial nerve nuclei (hence the external ocular movements are normal) and anterior horn cells of the spinal cord. Both upper and lower motor neurones can be affected but there are no sensory abnormalities.

It is slightly more common in men, with a peak incidence between the ages of 50 and 70 years. The prevalence in the UK is about 6 in 100 000. Familial forms account for 10% and are usually due to mutations in superoxide dismutase-1 (SOD1), although mutations of many other genes have recently been implicated in the pathogenesis of both the familial and sporadic forms. An association with frontotemporal dementia is increasingly recognized.

Clinically there are four main patterns of disease:

- Amyotrophic lateral sclerosis (ALS): combined lower motor neurone wasting and upper motor neurone spasticity and hyperreflexia. Weakness starts in the legs and spreads to the arms.
- Progressive muscular atrophy: anterior horn cell involvement, leading to lower motor neurone weakness, wasting and fasciculation of distal muscles, which spreads proximally.
- Progressive bulbar palsy: LMN weakness and wasting of the tongue and pharynx, leading to dysarthria and dysphagia. UMN features are usually also present, such as stiff tongue, spastic speech and brisk jaw jerk. Long tracts usually become affected.
- Primary lateral sclerosis: disease isolated to upper motor neurones; LMN signs may develop much later. It is usually slower to progress than ALS.

Combinations of the above may occur.

Management

Management is symptomatic. The aim is to help the patient with activities of daily living and to reduce symptoms. Opiates should be considered for joint pains and distress. Difficult decisions regarding nasogastric or percutaneous endoscopic gastrostomy feeding and tracheostomy insertion and artificial ventilation may arise. These interventions may prolong life but also the process of dying. Riluzole, an antiglutamate drug, is licensed in motor neurone disease and offers a small increase in length of life. Other agents are used in trials. Death usually occurs 2–5 years after diagnosis.

Horner's syndrome

This describes the combination of miosis, partial ptosis and ipsilateral loss of sweating (anhydrosis) caused by interruption of the sympathetic nerve supply to the face. The sympathetic nerves may be disrupted anywhere along their course:

- Brainstem: demyelination, vascular disease.
- Cervical cord: syringomyelia.
- Thoracic outlet: Pancoast's tumour.
- Neck (postganglionic): carotid artery aneurysm or dissection, tumours.

Bulbar and pseudobulbar palsy

These two conditions result from disruption of lower cranial nerve motor function, affecting the tongue, muscles of chewing/swallowing (therefore causing an increased risk of aspiration) and facial muscles.

Bulbar palsy is a lower motor neurone syndrome with a flaccid, fasciculating tongue, normal or absent jaw jerk and quiet nasal speech. It is caused by motor neurone disease, Guillain–Barré syndrome, polio, syringobulbia and brainstem tumours.

Pseudobulbar palsy refers to bilateral upper motor neurone lesions affecting the brainstem motor nuclei. The tongue is spastic, jaw jerk is increased, speech is like 'Donald Duck' and there is emotional lability. Pseudobulbar palsy is more common and is usually due to bilateral strokes. Other causes are multiple sclerosis and motor neurone disease.

Bell's palsy

This is an idiopathic unilateral lower motor neurone palsy of the 7th nerve. Other causes must be excluded (see Ch. 2). It is thought that viruses account for most cases.

Rapid onset of facial weakness occurs and may be accompanied by pain below the ear. The characteristic physical signs are described in Ch. 2 and shown in Fig. 34.13.

Most patients recover fully in a few weeks. Approximately 15% have axonal degeneration and recovery may only begin after about 3 months and may be incomplete. Occasionally, aberrant reconnections are formed (e.g. eating may stimulate unilateral lacrimation –'crocodile tears').

High-dose prednisolone may reduce damage and quicken recovery if given within a few days (ideally <24 h) of onset. The role of antiviral drugs remains controversial. The eye must be protected when closure is incomplete: patches and artificial tears are useful.

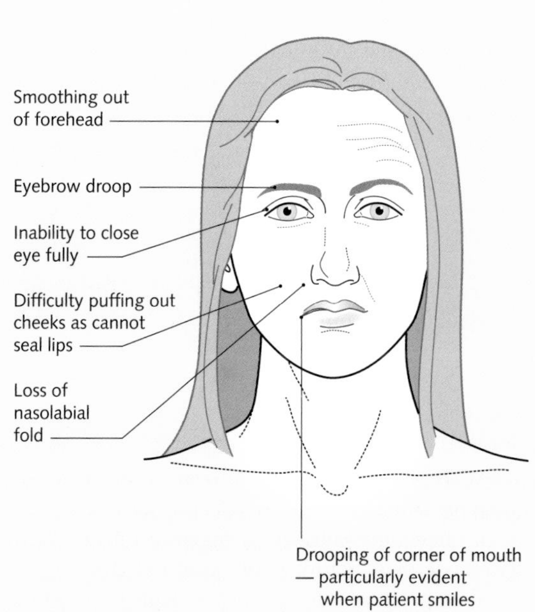

Fig. 34.13 Bell's palsy.

DEMENTIA

The approach to the confused patient and the differential diagnosis of dementia is covered in Ch. 20. For a more in-depth discussion of the topic please see *Crash course: Neurology*.

Further reading

Berg, A., Berkovic, S.F., Brodie, M.J., et al., 2010. Revised terminology and concepts for organization of seizures and epilepsies: report of the ILAE Commission on Classification and Terminology, 2005–2009. Epilepsia 51, 676–685.

Driver and Vehicle Licensing Agency, 2007. About medical standards for drivers. Available on line at: http://www.dvla.gov.uk/medical/about_dri_med.

Jacob, S., Viegas, S., Lashley, D., Hilton-Jones, D., 2009. Myasthenia gravis and other neuromuscular junction disorders. Pract. Neurol. 9, 364–371.

National Institute for Health and Clinical Excellence (NICE), 2003. Multiple sclerosis. Clinical guideline CG8. Available online at: http://www.nice.org.uk/CG8.

National Institute for Health and Clinical Excellence (NICE), 2008. Stroke. Clinical guideline CG68. Available online at: http://www.nice.org.uk/CG68.

National Institute for Health and Clinical Excellence (NICE), 2008. Parkinson's disease. Clinical guideline CG35. Available online at: http://www.nice.org.uk/CG35.

National Institute for Health and Clinical Excellence (NICE), 2010. Bacterial meningitis and meningococcal septicaemia. Clinical guideline CG102. Available online at: http://www.nice.org.uk/CG102.

National Institute for Health and Clinical Excellence (NICE), 2010. Transient loss of consciousness in adults and young people. Clinical guideline CG109. Available online at: http://www.nice.org.uk/CG109.

National Institute for Health Clinical Excellence (NICE), 2012. Epilepsy. Clinical guideline CG137. Available online at: http://www.nice.org.uk/CG137.

Polman, C., Reingold, S., Banwell, B., et al., 2011. Diagnostic criteria for multiple sclerosis: 2010 revisions to the McDonald criteria. Ann. Neurol. 69, 292–302.

Metabolic and endocrine disorders

Objectives

The key learning points for this chapter:

- The assessment and management of patients with type 1 and type 2 diabetes mellitus.
- The management of common diabetic emergencies.
- The growing public health problem of obesity and approaches to tackle this.
- How to approach the management of dyslipidaemia by considering the overall cardiovascular risk of a patient.
- The common causes of metabolic bone disease and their management.
- The common disorders of the parathyroid gland and the management of acute hypercalcaemia.
- The management of patients with crystal arthropathy.
- The endocrine pathways and common disorders of the pituitary, thyroid and adrenal glands.

DIABETES MELLITUS

Diabetes mellitus is a persisting state of hyperglycaemia due to diminished availability or effectiveness of insulin. There were 171 million people in the world with diabetes in 2000 and this is projected to increase to 366 million by 2030. In the UK it is estimated that around 4.5% of the population have diabetes. The rising tide of obesity is responsible for much of this increase (see below) and type 2 diabetes accounts for around 90% of cases.

The World Health Organization (WHO) criteria are used for the diagnosis of diabetes mellitus (Fig. 35.1). In addition to these tests, diabetes can be diagnosed on a random sample if above 11.1 and symptoms are present. Impaired fasting glycaemia and impaired glucose tolerance refer to fasting (no intake of calories for 8 h) and postprandial abnormalities of glucose metabolism, respectively; the terms are not interchangeable. In both cases, patients have an elevated risk of progression to frank diabetes and increased risk of macrovascular disease (see below).

Classification and aetiology

Type 1 diabetes mellitus usually presents in childhood, with a peak age of incidence of 10–15 years, although it can occur at any age. Signs and symptoms develop fairly quickly over days to weeks. Type 1 diabetes is due to autoantibodies directed against the insulin-producing beta cells of the pancreatic islets of Langerhans, causing a low concentration of circulating insulin. These patients always require insulin replacement therapy and there is an association with other autoimmune diseases.

Patients with type 2 diabetes mellitus are usually older and overweight, and the onset is more insidious. Type 2 diabetes is due to a combination of reduced sensitivity of peripheral tissues to circulating insulin (insulin resistance) and failure of the beta cells to produce enough insulin to overcome this resistance. Patients may require insulin if hyperglycaemia persists despite maximal doses of oral hypoglycaemic agents, or in times of physiological stress such as severe infections or after myocardial infarction. There is approximately 80% concordance between identical twins for type 2 diabetes mellitus, suggesting that inherited factors have a significant role. Type 2 diabetes is increasingly seen in children and may be linked with rising levels of childhood obesity. A very small proportion of patients with type 2 diabetes have a familial autosomal dominant form and also present at a young age. This was previously called maturity onset diabetes of the young (MODY) but is now classified according to the genetic defect. Fig. 35.2 demonstrates some of the differences in presentation between type 1 and type 2 diabetes.

Secondary diabetes mellitus may be caused by:

- Drugs (e.g. steroids).
- Gestational diabetes: patients develop impaired glucose tolerance or frank diabetes during pregnancy.
- Pancreatic disease (e.g. pancreatectomy, carcinoma of the pancreas, pancreatitis, cystic fibrosis, haemochromatosis).
- Endocrine causes: Cushing's syndrome, acromegaly, phaeochromocytoma.

Diagnosis of diabetes

In addition to serum glucose testing (Fig. 35.1), the presence of antibodies to pancreatic islet cells, glutamic

Fig. 35.1 World Health Organization (2006) criteria for the diagnosis of diabetes and intermediate hyperglycaemia.

	Fasting plasma glucose (mmol/L)		2-h plasma glucose* (mmol/L)
Diabetes	≥7.0	*or*	≥11.1
Impaired glucose tolerance (IGT)	<7.0	*and*	≥7.8 and <11.1
Impaired fasting glucose (IFG)	6.1–6.9	*and* (if measured)	<7.8

**Venous plasma glucose 2 h after ingestion of oral 75 g glucose load.*

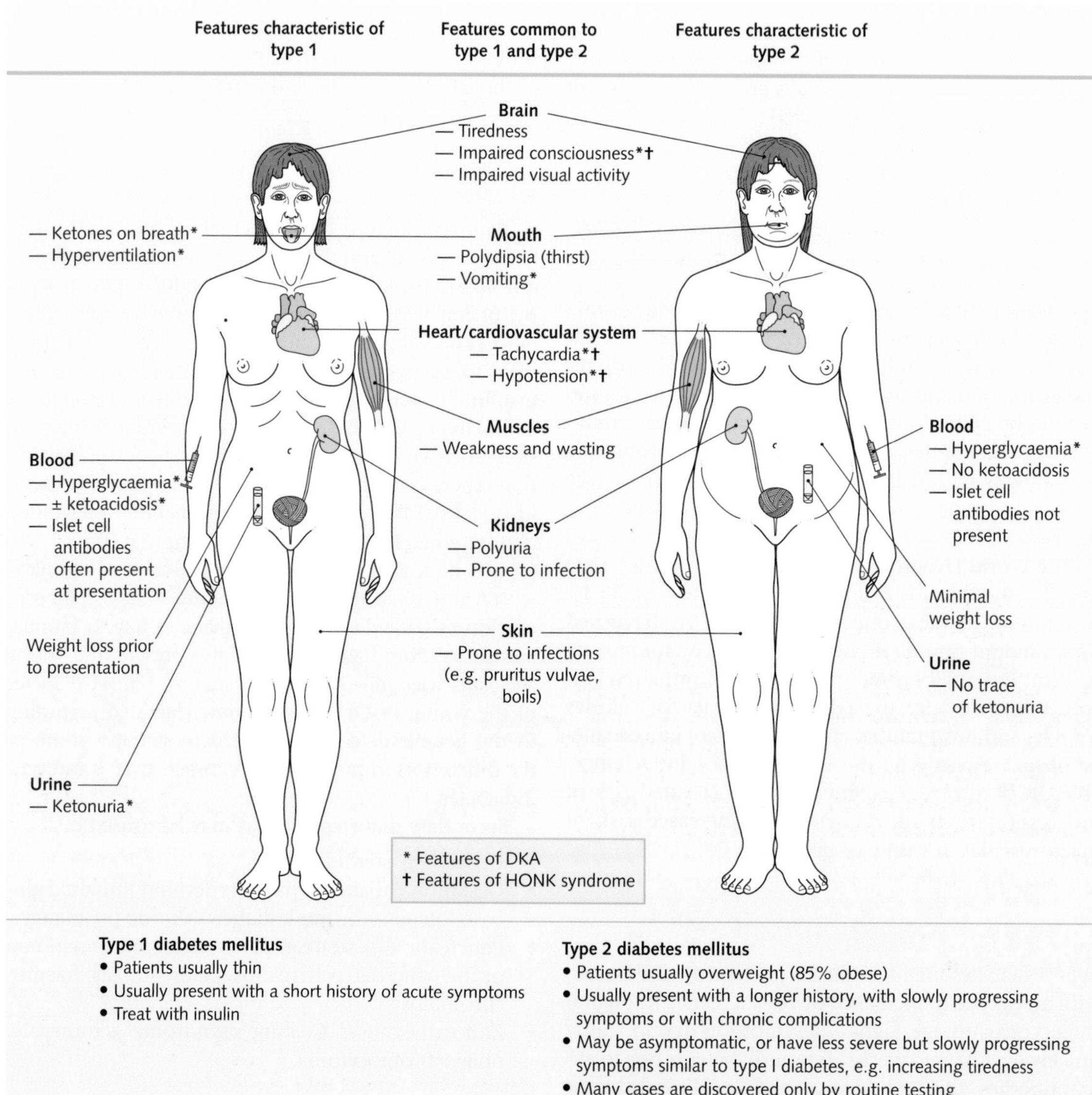

Fig. 35.2 Acute symptoms and signs of diabetes mellitus (types I and II).

acid decarboxylase or insulin can be assessed and may help discriminate between type 1 and type 2 diabetes in challenging cases. Glycated haemoglobin (HbA1c) is often measured at presentation and may be useful in distinguishing patients with diabetes from those with transient hyperglycaemia. It is used more frequently for diagnosis in the USA than the UK, where it is used for monitoring.

Clinical presentation

Diabetes may be asymptomatic and discovered on routine screening where elevated levels of glucose are found in the blood or urine, but approximately half of all type 2 diabetics are undiagnosed.

Patients may present with non-specific symptoms such as weight loss and lethargy, and they are more prone to infection (e.g. carbuncles, thrush, cellulitis). Polyuria and polydipsia are characteristic and relate to the osmotic diuresis caused by the filtered glucose load in the nephrons overcoming their ability to reabsorb it.

A significant proportion of patients presents for the first time with a diabetic emergency: diabetic ketoacidosis (DKA) in the case of type 1 diabetes or, more rarely, hyperosmolar non-ketotic (HONK) syndrome in the case of type 2 diabetes.

Some patients, particularly type 2 diabetics with an insidious onset of disease, may present with chronic complications of their diabetes (see below). Fig. 35.2 summarizes the characteristic presenting features in diabetes mellitus.

Chronic complications

The chronic complications of diabetes are summarized in Fig. 35.3. They can be considered in two broad groups: macrovascular and microvascular. 'Macrovascular' refers to complications related to larger blood vessels (e.g. coronary artery, cerebrovascular and peripheral vascular disease). 'Microvascular' refers to complications related to smaller blood vessels (e.g. diabetic retinopathy, nephropathy and neuropathy). Some complications will arise as a result of both macrovascular and microvascular disease.

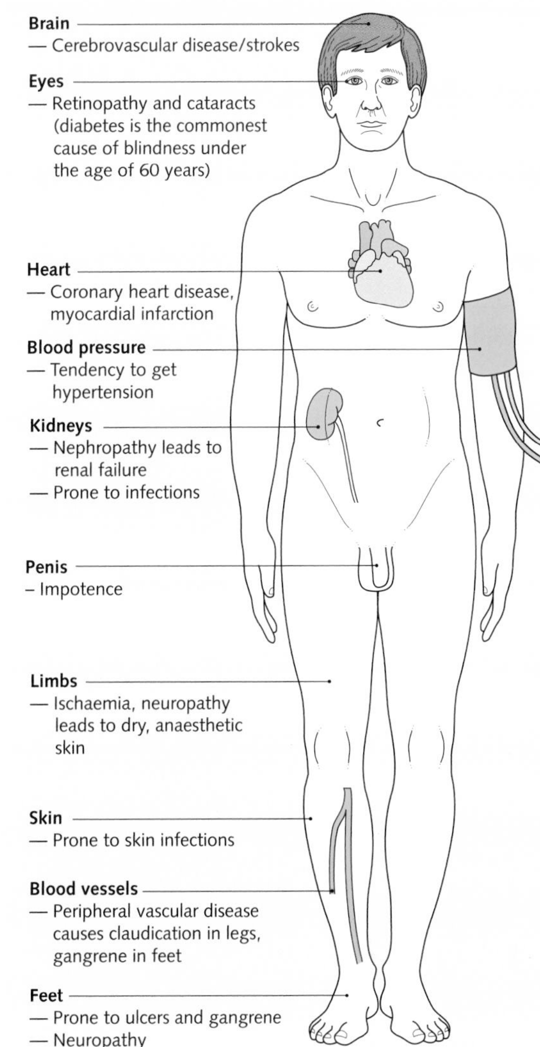

Fig. 35.3 Chronic complications of diabetes mellitus.

HINTS AND TIPS

In a patient with gangrene and a palpable dorsalis pedis pulse, think of microvascular disease.

Macrovascular disease

This is a cause of significant morbidity and mortality among diabetics. A diabetic's risk of myocardial infarction is equivalent to that of a non-diabetic patient who has had a previous infarction. Therefore, it is of paramount importance to assess and address all cardiovascular risk factors when managing diabetic patients (see below).

Eyes

Retinopathy occurs in virtually all patients with type 1 diabetes, and maculopathy occurs in up to 20%. Patients with type 2 diabetes often have a degree of retinopathy at presentation. The stages of diabetic retinopathy are shown in Fig. 2.22. Patients with maculopathy and preproliferative changes must be referred to an ophthalmologist; those with proliferative retinopathy require urgent referral for laser therapy.

Diabetics are also at elevated risk of early cataract formation. Rubeosis iridis is a late complication related to new vessel formation on the iris and may result in glaucoma.

Kidneys

The first sign of renal involvement is microalbuminuria (30–300 mg albumin per 24 h). A negative dipstick test does not exclude microalbuminuria and therefore more sensitive tests must be used to screen diabetics for it (estimation of the albumin:creatinine ratio in an early morning specimen). Microalbuminuria affects 20–40% of diabetics 10–15 years after diagnosis. These patients can progress to macroalbuminuria/clinical nephropathy (albumin excretion >300 mg per 24 h) and the renal function then declines at a rate varying from patient to patient. Diabetic nephropathy is almost always associated with the presence of retinopathy and its absence should prompt a search for an alternative renal diagnosis.

The pathological hallmark of diabetic nephropathy is the Kimmelstiel–Wilson lesion (nodular glomerulosclerosis).

Neuropathies

Diabetic neuropathy can take several forms.

Somatic neuropathies

Somatic neuropathies may take the following forms:

- Distal symmetrical polyneuropathy: this commonly affects the lower limbs first, with numbness and paraesthesiae of the feet, spreading up the leg, before then affecting the hands ('glove and stocking' pattern). Symptoms are predominantly sensory with early loss of vibration sense and absent ankle jerks. In advanced cases, the loss of pain sensation may lead to the development of punched-out chronic ulcers at pressure points in areas of thick callus, and may cause arthropathy (see below). Foot pulses may be easily palpable; the foot may then become infected and eventually gangrenous.
- Mononeuritis: may be due to entrapment or ischaemia. Commonly involved nerves include the third cranial nerve, ulnar nerve and lateral popliteal nerve. More than one nerve can be involved, causing 'mononeuritis multiplex'.
- Diabetic amyotrophy: painful asymmetrical weakness and wasting of the quadriceps muscles due to lumbosacral plexopathy and polyradiculopathy. It may recover.

Autonomic neuropathies

This may lead to symptoms of postural hypotension (i.e. dizziness on standing), impotence, nocturnal diarrhoea and urinary retention. Gastroparesis may occur, causing vomiting. There may be lack of awareness of symptoms of hypoglycaemia, which is also more frequent in patients on beta-blockers.

Diabetic feet

Diabetic foot problems are due to a combination of neuropathy and peripheral vascular disease. Diabetics are also predisposed to infection, which may affect the soft tissue and even bone (osteomyelitis) of ulcerated feet. This is a common reason for presentation and admission.

Sensory neuropathy causes ulcers over pressure points (e.g. metatarsal heads) and can cause joint deformity due to the lack of pain and proprioception (e.g. pes cavus, Charcot's joints). Peripheral vascular disease, which may be due to small and/or large vessel occlusion, affects the toes primarily.

Skin

Complications occurring in the skin include the following:

- Lipoatrophy: this is loss of fat at insulin injection sites. It is much rarer now that human insulin has replaced bovine or porcine insulin. The patient should be advised to vary the injection sites because the absorption of insulin at sites of atrophy is unpredictable.
- Necrobiosis lipoidica diabeticorum: these are yellowish areas on the skin with a violet edge and telangiectasia. Biopsy shows atrophy of subcutaneous collagen.
- Infections, such as boils, are more common.
- Granuloma annulare: annular plaques on the extremities.

Infections

Common infections are of the urinary tract and skin, and candidiasis. Tuberculosis is also more common in diabetics. Susceptibility to infection is due to a number of factors, including a reduced immune response due to hyperglycaemia, tissue ischaemia secondary to vascular disease, and increased portals of entry such as ulcers.

Management of diabetes

General principles

COMMUNICATION

The transition of patients with chronic conditions such as diabetes from paediatric to adult services must be managed sensitively with the involvement of patients and parents. This helps avoid them feeling abandoned during this process.

Successful management of diabetic patients requires a high level of patient education and motivation, and this is achieved through regular follow-up with a multi-disciplinary team involving doctors, nurses, ophthalmologists, dieticians and chiropodists/podiatrists. The aims of continued assessment of diabetics are ongoing education, assessment of glycaemic control and assessment of complications.

The Diabetes Control and Complications Trial (DCCT) in type 1 diabetics and the UK Prospective Diabetes Study (UKPDS) in type 2 diabetics demonstrated that tight control of blood glucose (aiming for an HbA1c of 6.5–7.5%) reduces microvascular complications. This needs to be balanced against the increased risk of hypoglycaemic episodes.

The UKPDS also demonstrated that tight control of blood pressure reduces both macro- and microvascular complications. This and other trials have suggested that the aim should be a blood pressure below 130/80 mmHg. This emphasizes the need for a global assessment of a diabetic's cardiovascular risk factors and aggressive management of all of them.

Many patients now monitor their own blood glucose concentrations using blood glucose strips and an electronic meter. These records should be examined, together with any corresponding hypoglycaemic symptoms. The HbA1c should be checked every 3–6 months depending on the level of control.

Microvascular complications must be monitored:

- Visual acuity checks together with examination of the optic fundi for retinopathy.
- The feet should be examined for neuropathy, ischaemic changes and infection.
- Nephropathy should be sought by monitoring the urea and electrolytes, and by testing for albuminuria.

Type 2 diabetes is usually treated initially with oral hypoglycaemic drugs if dietary measures are unsuccessful, although many of these patients will require insulin at some point. Type 1 diabetes is treated with injectable insulin from the outset.

Diet and lifestyle

The diet should be low in fat (to help delay the progression of atherosclerosis) and low in refined sugars, but high in complex carbohydrates (such as starch) and high in fibre, which among other benefits helps to lower the incidence of postprandial hypoglycaemia. Patients should be encouraged to take regular exercise and reduce energy intake in an attempt to maintain ideal body weight. This often proves to be very difficult. Studies suggest that bariatric surgery for weight loss is an effective therapy in type 2 diabetes, and may lead to remission.

Oral hypoglycaemic agents

These are usually started when diet and lifestyle measures fail to offer adequate control, although some organizations now suggest that metformin should be started at diagnosis. Metformin is the first-line drug as it reduces cardiovascular risk in obese patients and does not cause weight gain. The next step is usually the addition of a sulphonylurea, thiazolidinedione, newer agent (see below) or insulin either alone or in combination. Acarbose is used less frequently. The choice of agent must take into account side effects, contraindications and the patient's lifestyle and circumstances.

Biguanides

Metformin is the only available biguanide and is the first-line therapy for patients without contraindications. It exerts its effect mainly by decreasing gluconeogenesis and increasing peripheral utilization of glucose; some residual islet cell function is required. Gastrointestinal side effects are common including nausea and diarrhoea. There is a risk of lactic acidosis and, although it is rare, metformin should be avoided in patients with predisposing conditions including renal failure, heart failure and liver disease.

Sulphonylureas

These act mainly by augmenting insulin secretion and therefore some residual pancreatic beta-cell activity is required. There are several sulphonylureas but all are probably equally effective, and are used as second-line therapy or first-line therapy when metformin is contraindicated. The most frequent and significant side effect is hypoglycaemia, which may persist longer than expected due to the long half-life of some sulphonylureas. Elderly patients are particularly prone to hypoglycaemia and shorter-acting drugs should be used in this population. Other people with increased risk include the undernourished and those with renal or cardiac impairment.

The sulphonylureas tend to encourage weight gain and this can be a problem in obese patients whose insulin resistance is worsened as a consequence.

Thiazolidinediones

Pioglitazone is currently the only licensed thiazoledinedione, and can be added as second- or third-line therapy. It increases insulin sensitivity. The main side effect is fluid retention and it is contraindicated in heart failure. There is also a slightly higher risk of fractures and bladder cancer.

DPP-4 inhibitors

These include sitagliptin and vildagliptin and may work via several mechanisms including increasing the action of glucagon-like peptide 1 (GLP-1). They are generally well tolerated although gastrointestinal side effects can occur and there may be an increased risk of pancreatitis. They are used as second-line therapy.

GLP-1 agonists

This group of injection-only drugs includes exenatide and functions by mimicking the action of GLP-1. They are used as a third-line therapy.

Acarbose

Acarbose, an inhibitor of intestinal alpha-glucosidases, delays the digestion of starch and sucrose and hence the increase in blood glucose levels that follows a carbohydrate-containing meal. It may be used as an adjunctive therapy but often causes intolerable flatulence.

Insulin

All type 1 diabetics are treated with insulin and many type 2 diabetics require insulin to achieve satisfactory glycaemic control. It is inactivated by gastrointestinal enzymes and is administered by subcutaneous injection; pre-clinical trials are underway to assess the efficacy of inhaled insulin. Mixtures of available insulin preparations may be required to maintain good control, and these will vary for individual patients. Requirements may be affected by variations in lifestyle, other medication and concurrent illness such as infection.

Patients should aim for blood glucose concentrations between 4 and 10 mmol/L for most of the time, while accepting that on occasions they will be above or below these values. They should be advised to look for 'peaks' and 'troughs' of blood glucose and to adjust their insulin dosage only once or twice weekly. Animal insulin, human insulin and insulin analogues are available and the preparations may be rapid-, short-, intermediate- or long-acting. If possible, patients are started on a 'basal-bolus' regime: a once-daily injection of a medium- or long-acting insulin, with short- or rapid-acting insulin injection before or with meals. This most closely resembles the physiological changes in insulin levels, but requires education and commitment. Some patients are best started on twice-daily injections of 'biphasic insulin' – mixtures of a short- and intermediate-acting insulin (Fig. 35.4).

Some patients may require continuous insulin infusion via an insulin pump if usual regimens fail. Pancreatic transplant may be performed if the patient meets criteria; these include if the patient is also undergoing renal transplant, or if the metabolic complications are unacceptable in terms of frequency and severity.

Diabetes and surgery

Diabetic patients should be first on the operating list and fasted on the morning of surgery. Diet-controlled diabetics simply require careful monitoring of glucose levels. Oral agents should be avoided on the morning of surgery and can be recommenced with the first meal postoperatively. If glucose levels are poorly controlled, if oral intake will be problematic postoperatively, or if the procedure is long, IV insulin may be required (see below).

For patients already on insulin, long-acting preparations are usually discontinued the night before surgery.

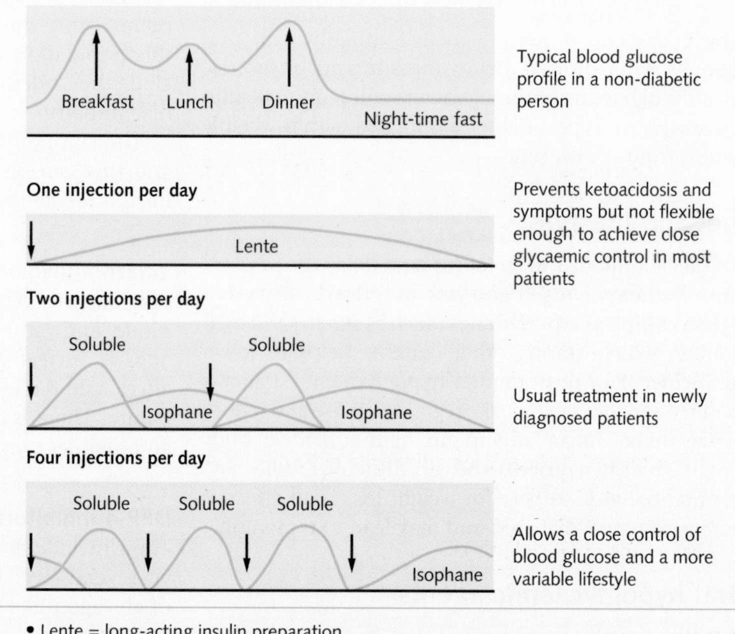

Fig. 35.4 Examples of different insulin regimens.

IV insulin is started early on the day of the operation, and can be given either with potassium and dextrose in the same bag (GKI infusion) or separately ('sliding scale'). The sliding scale regimen usually consists of a 5% dextrose/20 mM KCl infusion given according to the patient's fluid requirements, and runs concurrently with a 1 unit/mL infusion of soluble insulin in 0.9% saline (i.e. 50 U Actrapid in 50 mL 0.9% NaCl). The capillary glucose is checked on an hourly or 2-hourly basis and the rate of insulin infusion changed accordingly. It is important to give both infusions via the same cannula to avoid hyper- or hypoglycaemia if one cannula becomes blocked. When patients start to eat and drink, they may be restarted on the normal insulin regimen.

COMMUNICATION

Patients are often well informed about their diabetes. Ensure that any modifications to their therapy are discussed with and explained to them.

Diabetic emergencies

Hypoglycaemia

Symptoms of hypoglycaemia include sweating, hunger and tremor (autonomic symptoms) and very low glucose concentrations may cause drowsiness, seizures, transient neurological symptoms and loss of consciousness. It is very common in diabetics, but there are many causes as outlined below.

Aetiology

Hypoglycaemia may occur after a meal or after a fast. The aetiology of fasting hypoglycaemia includes the following:

- Drugs: excessive insulin or sulphonylureas. This is usually accidental, but large doses may be taken deliberately, particularly by medical and paramedical staff. Alcohol binges, especially with decreased food intake, may also lead to hypoglycaemia.
- Endocrine causes: pituitary insufficiency, Addison's disease and insulinomas.
- Postgastrectomy and functional hypoglycaemia.
- Liver failure.
- Inherited enzyme defects.
- Non-islet cell tumours: usually large tumours, producing IGF-1 or IGF-2
- Immune hypoglycaemia (e.g. anti-insulin receptor antibodies in Hodgkin's disease).
- Malaria.

Investigations

The cause may be obvious in the case of drug-induced hypoglycaemia in a diabetic patient. In others, simple blood tests may exclude certain causes (e.g. liver function tests, LFTs). Measurement of insulin and C-peptide levels will distinguish between endogenous and exogenous hyperinsulinaemia; C-peptide is produced from the breakdown of pro-insulin and is only raised with endogenous hyperinsulinaemia. Sulphonylurea levels may also be helpful. When the diagnosis is not clear, other investigations may be needed:

- Consider a short synacthen test for Addison's disease.
- Thick and thin blood films for malaria if there is a suggestive history.
- A prolonged inpatient fast with the intention of provoking hypoglycaemia is carried out when a patient reports typical symptoms but the attacks are not witnessed. Frequent measurement of blood glucose, together with insulin and C-peptide levels, is carried out.

Management

If the patient is conscious, dextrose tablets, sugary drinks, or glucose gel should be given, followed by complex carbohydrate. If unconscious, an infusion of 20% or 50% glucose should be given intravenously. Glucagon IM can be given as an alternative – this is a polypeptide hormone produced by the alpha cells of the pancreatic islets of Langerhans. It increases plasma glucose by mobilizing glycogen stored in the liver, and will only be useful in patients with adequate glycogen stores.

For patients who have taken a long-acting preparation, a continuous IV glucose infusion for 24 h may be required. If an underlying cause is found it should be treated on its own merits. In diabetic patients, issues surrounding education and awareness of hypoglycaemia should be addressed.

Diabetic ketoacidosis

Diabetic ketoacidosis occurs in type 1 diabetics. It may be the mode of presentation, or may be precipitated by an inadequate insulin dose or an intercurrent illness (e.g. infection or myocardial infarction). There is usually a gradual deterioration over hours to days.

Symptoms include polyuria, polydipsia, abdominal pain and vomiting. There may be evidence of the underlying cause. Patients often hyperventilate to compensate for the metabolic acidosis (Kussmaul respiration) and their breath smells of ketones (like nail-varnish remover). There are physical signs of dehydration. As the condition worsens, lethargy, confusion, drowsiness and ultimately coma may occur.

Investigations

- Urea and electrolytes, arterial blood gases, full blood count, glucose, blood cultures.

- Urine dipstick and midstream urine. Test urine for ketones. In some centres serum ketone testing is available.
- ECG.

The diagnosis of DKA requires the demonstration of ketosis and acidosis. It is important to look for and treat the underlying cause. After the initial arterial blood gas, venous blood gas or bicarbonate is often sufficient for monitoring.

Management

Correction of dehydration takes precedence. These patients are potassium-depleted overall but the serum concentration may be normal or high as the acidosis causes potassium to move out of the intracellular compartment. Therefore the serum potassium concentration can fall precipitously as acidosis is corrected and it must be monitored closely and replaced.

Some 6–9 L of IV fluid may be required and the first 2 L can be given over the first hour. Initial choice of fluid is usually 0.9% saline unless there is circulatory compromise when colloid may be preferred. Sodium bicarbonate is infrequently used and controversial. An IV infusion of insulin titrated to the blood glucose is commenced. Once the blood glucose drops to around 15 mmol/L, the fluid replacement may be modified to include dextrose until the patient is eating and drinking. In children, fluid requirements need to be calculated more accurately as cerebral oedema may occur with over-aggressive fluid administration.

A nasogastric tube may need to be inserted to reduce the risk of aspiration from the gastric stasis that occurs in this condition. Prophylactic low-molecular-weight heparin is commenced as there is a significant risk of venous thromboembolism.

If there is evidence of infection, broad-spectrum antibiotics are used and attempts should be made to identify the precipitant. The inflammatory markers may rise in the absence of infection. The patient should be observed very closely, with a low threshold for admission to the high-dependency or intensive care unit. IV insulin should be continued until the acidosis is corrected and the patient is eating and drinking.

Hyperglycaemic hyperosmolar non-ketotic coma

Clinical features

This occurs in type 2 diabetes; the patient is often elderly and may not be a known diabetic. Precipitants are as for DKA but onset is gradual, over days. By the time of presentation blood glucose is usually very high (higher than in DKA) and plasma osmolality is increased with significant hypernatraemia. Polyuria leads to severe dehydration. Neurological symptoms such as confusion, seizures and coma may occur. Ketoacidosis almost never occurs as there is enough endogenous insulin remaining to suppress ketone formation. However, an initial check for ketones should be carried out.

Investigations

- Blood tests: full blood count, serum glucose, U&Es, LFTs. Plasma osmolality should be calculated.
- Urine analysis for infection and ketones.
- ECG.
- Further investigations directed to find the underlying cause.

Management

Rehydration is usually with normal saline and patients also require IV insulin, at a lower dose than for DKA. If the sodium concentration is very high it may be tempting to give hypotonic saline. However, this is not used as it can cause cerebral oedema and myelinolysis by lowering the osmolality too quickly, and because these patients are so volume depleted their total body stores of sodium are low and require replacement. Central venous pressure monitoring may be required. Patients are at a very high risk of venous thromboembolism and therapeutic dose anticoagulation with low-molecular-weight heparin is used. The mortality rate is up to 50%.

HINTS AND TIPS

Osmolality can be calculated:
2(Na + K) + glucose + urea.

OBESITY AND METABOLIC SYNDROME

Obesity is defined as a body mass index (BMI) greater than 30. The normal range is 19–25. Central adiposity increased waist circumference:height ratio is associated with greater health risks, including type 2 diabetes mellitus, cardiovascular disease, dyslipidaemia, hypertension, osteoarthritis and cancer. There are several definitions of metabolic syndrome, each comprising a combination of hypertension, low HDL, hypetriglyceridaemia, raised fasting glucose, insulin resistance and obesity.

In 1980, 6% of adult males and 8% of adult females were obese. In 1998, these figures had increased to 17% and 21%, respectively. It is currently estimated that approximately 50% of the adult population is overweight or obese and there is certainly a growing problem among children. This trend constitutes an enormous public health issue with widespread changes in dietary and exercise patterns required.

Management

Patients should be given lifestyle and dietary advice and support. Those patients with a BMI >28 with co-morbid conditions that may benefit from weight reduction, and those with a BMI >30, are considered for drug therapy after exercise, diet and behavioural intervention has been tried. Orlistat inhibits the absorption of fat in the intestine and therefore causes side effects of steatorrhoea, urgency and oily spotting. Sibutramine has been discontinued in the UK due to cardiovascular risk. Orlistat may be continued beyond 3 months if there is evidence of ≥5% weight loss.

Morbidly obese patients with a BMI >40 (or >35 with co-morbidity) in whom there has been a failure to lose weight despite all conservative measures at a specialist clinic may be considered for surgery. This takes two forms: malabsorptive surgery where bypass procedures are performed or restrictive surgery where the size of the stomach is reduced.

THYROID DISORDERS

The control of thyroid hormone production and release is outlined in Fig. 35.5.

Goitre

'Goitre' means an enlarged thyroid gland. It is a clinical sign rather than a diagnosis.

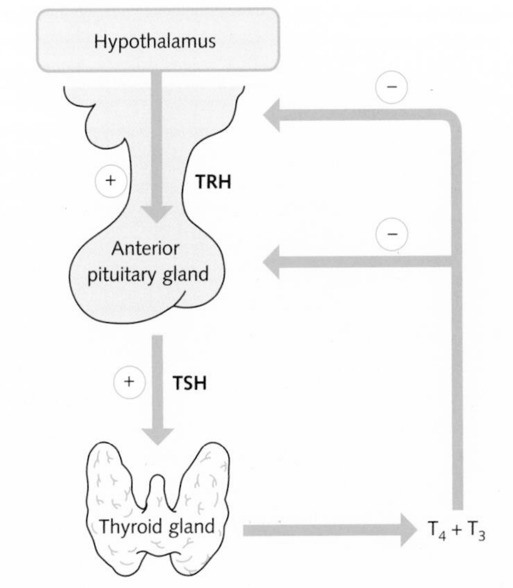

Fig. 35.5 Control of thyroid hormone production via the hypothalamus–pituitary–thyroid axis. TRH, thyrotrophin-releasing hormone; TSH, thyroid-stimulating hormone.

Clinical assessment

Most patients are asymptomatic. The history should cover the following:

- Duration of goitre and rate of change: long-standing goitres suggest benign disease.
- Local symptoms: dysphagia, dyspnoea and hoarseness; all are uncommon.
- Symptoms of hypo- or hyperthyroidism (see below).
- Goitrogenic drugs (e.g. lithium, amiodarone).
- Prior exposure to radiation (medical or environmental) especially in childhood: risk factor for benign and malignant thyroid nodules.
- Age and sex: incidence of thyroid cancer peaks between 30 and 50 and is around 3 times more common in women.
- Family history: ask about a history of goitre (suggesting autoimmune disease) or of thyroid cancer (suggesting familial thyroid cancer or multiple endocrine neoplasia).
- Tenderness: subacute thyroiditis.

Physical examination should look for the following:

- The patient's thyroid status (see below).
- Is the goitre smooth or nodular?
- Are there multiple nodules or a single nodule?
- When assessing a nodule: Is it hard or soft? Regular or irregular? Fixed or mobile? Is there lymphadenopathy?

Differential diagnosis

- Smooth toxic goitre: Graves' disease.
- Smooth non-toxic goitre: congenital, physiological (e.g. in puberty or pregnancy), thyroiditis (e.g. autoimmune, subacute) iodine deficiency.
- Multi-nodular goitre: usually euthyroid, although nodules may become autonomous and cause thyrotoxicosis.
- Single thyroid lump: approximately 10% are malignant. Causes include cyst, adenoma, malignancy, a single palpable nodule within a goitre.

Investigations

The following investigations are important in patients with goitre and thyroid cancer:

- TFTs: hyper- or hypothyroidism. TSH is usually checked first; if abnormal, free tri-iodothyronine (T_3) and thyroxine (T_4) are measured.
- Calcitonin secretion: increased in medullary thyroid cancer and should be measured in patients with a positive family history.
- Thyroid size and nature: assessed using ultrasound, CT or MRI scan. Ultrasound is quick to perform and can differentiate between cystic and solid nodules. It cannot distinguish benign from malignant lesions. CT or MRI are useful in assessing compression or invasion of other structures.

- Respiratory function tests including flow–volume loop: if signs of upper airways obstruction are present.
- Radionuclide imaging (thyroid scintigraphy): can distinguish 'hot nodules' (high uptake of radioisotope) from 'cold nodules' (due to lack of concentration of radioisotope). Unfortunately, there are no specific features that indicate the benign or malignant nature of a thyroid nodule. Malignant nodules are more likely to be cold than hot, although most cold nodules are benign. Even so, the presence of a hot nodule does not exclude malignancy.
- Fine-needle aspiration cytology: performed on nodules where there are suspicious features in the history or examination. It can be performed in outpatients and is well tolerated; cytology is not completely reliable as false-positive and false-negative results occur.

Hypothyroidism

Hypothyroidism results from deficiency of thyroxine (T_4) or tri-iodothyronine (T_3). The prevalence is up to 2% in women; it is around five times less common in men.

Aetiology

Primary thyroid failure may take the forms described below:

- Chronic autoimmune (Hashimoto's) thyroiditis: this is around 5–8 times more common in women than in men and tends to affect the middle aged and elderly. Patients may present with a firm, nontender goitre, hypothyroidism, or both. It is associated with vitiligo, pernicious anaemia, insulin-dependent diabetes mellitus, Addison's disease and premature ovarian failure. Biopsy shows a lymphocytic infiltrate with destruction of follicles and variable fibrosis.
- Idiopathic atrophic thyroiditis: this autoimmune condition may represent progression or a different presentation of chronic autoimmune thyroiditis. The incidence increases with age and it is commoner in women.
- Previous treatment for hyperthyroidism: operative or radioiodine.
- Congenital hypothyroidism: the prevalence in the UK is 1 in 3500–4000 infants and it is diagnosed in the first week of life by routine screening, measuring TSH or T_4. It is usually due to thyroid agenesis, which is mostly sporadic, or dyshormonogenesis, which is due to autosomal recessively inherited enzyme defects. An example is Pendred's syndrome, characterized by congenital hypothyroidism, goitre and nerve deafness in homozygotes.
- Iodine-deficient hypothyroidism: this is a major cause of hypothyroidism and goitre worldwide, although most iodine-deficient people are euthyroid even though they have a goitre.
- Iatrogenic hypothyroidism: long-term iodine therapy, for example in expectorants, may result in hypothyroidism. Other drugs include amiodarone and lithium carbonate.

Secondary thyroid failure is caused by diseases of the hypothalamus or pituitary, resulting in reduced levels of TRH or TSH. These are rare.

Clinical features

The onset is insidious and the symptoms often nonspecific. Common presenting symptoms include tiredness, lethargy, weight gain, cold intolerance, constipation, hoarseness and dryness of the skin. However, virtually any organ system can be affected (Fig. 35.6). Very rarely it presents as myxoedema coma (see below).

Investigations

The following investigations are important in patients with hypothyroidism:

- In primary disease, free and total T_4 are reduced and serum TSH is high.
- In subclinical hypothyroidism, T_4 may be normal, with a high serum TSH.
- In secondary hypothyroidism, the free and total T_4 are reduced and the TSH is usually also low. This picture is also seen in unwell people without thyroid disease ('sick euthyroid') and patients on steroids and anticonvulsants.

Fig. 35.6 Effects of hypothyroidism by body system.

Body system	Effects
Cardiovascular	Bradycardia, hyperlipidaemia, angina, heart failure, pericardial and pleural effusions
Neuromuscular	Aches and pains, carpal tunnel syndrome, deafness, cerebellar ataxia, depression and psychoses, delayed relaxation of reflexes
Haematological	Macrocytic anaemia, iron-deficiency anaemia (due to menorrhagia)
Dermatological	Dry skin, myxoedema (which is local infiltration of the skin with mucopolysaccharides), erythema ab igne, vitiligo, alopecia
Gastrointestinal	Constipation, ileus, ascites
Reproductive	Infertility, menorrhagia, galactorrhoea
Developmental	Growth retardation, mental retardation, delayed puberty

- Antibodies to thyroglobulin or thyroid peroxidase (microsomal antibodies): typically strongly positive in Hashimoto's thyroiditis.
- Cholesterol is often raised.
- FBC: anaemia is often present, possibly with a mild macrocytosis.
- ECG: sinus bradycardia, low-voltage complexes.

Treatment

Thyroxine sodium is the treatment of choice for maintenance therapy. Usual maintenance doses are between 100 μg and 200 μg daily. The initial dose is usually 50 μg, increased as necessary over a few weeks, and even lower doses (25 μg) are started in elderly patients or patients with cardiac disease to avoid worsening angina or precipitating a myocardial infarction. Treatment is monitored by serum TSH and serum T_4 and is nearly always lifelong except in cases of subacute or silent thyroiditis. Current guidelines advise treating subclinical hypothyroidism if the TSH is above 10 mU/L. It is sometimes necessary to rule out adrenal insufficiency (for instance in secondary hypothyroidism) before starting treatment, as giving thyroxine can precipitate an adrenal crisis if there is concomitant glucocorticoid deficiency.

Myxoedema coma

This is uncommon. It is typically seen in the elderly and is precipitated by infection, myocardial infarction, treatment with sedatives, or inadequate heating in cold weather. Most patients have hypothermia and are hypotensive with heart failure, hyponatraemia, hypoxia and hypercapnia.

Treatment is with T_3 intravenously because of its rapid action. IV hydrocortisone is also given, particularly if pituitary hypothyroidism is suspected. Supportive measures are also needed, including IV fluids, antibiotics, ventilation and slow rewarming. T_4 can be substituted after 2–3 days if there is a clinical improvement. Mortality is up to 20%.

Thyrotoxicosis

Thyrotoxicosis is the condition resulting from raised levels of circulating free T_4 and free T_3. It affects approximately 10 in 1000 women and 1 in 1000 men. Hyperthyroidism indicates thyroid gland overactivity, which may cause thyrotoxicosis. However, the two terms are often used interchangeably.

Aetiology

Primary hyperthyroidism

Graves' disease

This accounts for up to 80% of cases of hyperthyroidism. It is caused by the production of autoantibodies that stimulate the TSH receptor. There is a painless diffuse goitre in more than 90% of patients. In addition to the general features of thyrotoxicosis (see below), features specific to Graves' disease may occur, including ophthalmopathy, pretibial myxoedema and thyroid acropachy.

The ophthalmopathy includes grittiness and increased tear production, periorbital oedema, conjunctival oedema (chemosis), proptosis, diplopia, impaired visual acuity and corneal ulceration due to exposure. It is clinically obvious in up to 50% of patients with Graves' disease but subclinical ophthalmopathy can be detected in more than 90% by CT scan or MRI, revealing enlargement of the extraocular muscles caused by lymphocytic infiltration, oedema and later fibrosis.

Pretibial myxoedema occurs in 1–5% of patients with Graves' disease and consists of painless thickening of the skin in nodules or plaques, generally over the shin.

Thyroid acropachy occurs in less than 1% of patients and resembles finger clubbing.

Other causes of primary hyperthyroidism

Toxic multinodular goitre and toxic adenoma account for most of the remaining causes. Less common causes include metastatic thyroid cancer, genetic causes such as the McCune–Albright syndrome and TSH receptor mutations, ectopic thyroid tissue (e.g. struma ovarii) and high iodine load (e.g. in contrast or amiodarone).

Secondary hyperthyroidism

This is very uncommon. Causes include TSH-secreting pituitary adenoma and trophoblast or germ-cell tumours secreting large amounts of human chorionic gonadotrophin, which has mild thyroid stimulating effects.

Thyrotoxicosis without hyperthyroidism

This may occur with destructive thyroiditis such as in postpartum thyroiditis, autoimmune thyroiditis, subacute/de Quervain's thyroiditis (see below) and amiodarone-induced thyroiditis, or with excessive T_4 administration or self-administered T_4.

Clinical presentation

The symptoms and signs of thyrotoxicosis are shown in Fig. 35.7. Occasionally it may present with thyrotoxic crisis (see below). General symptoms include:

- Weight loss.
- Increased appetite.
- Heat intolerance and sweating.
- Fatigue and weakness.
- Hyperactivity, irritability, sleep disruption.
- Tremor.

Less common symptoms include:

- Depression.
- Oligomenorrhoea.

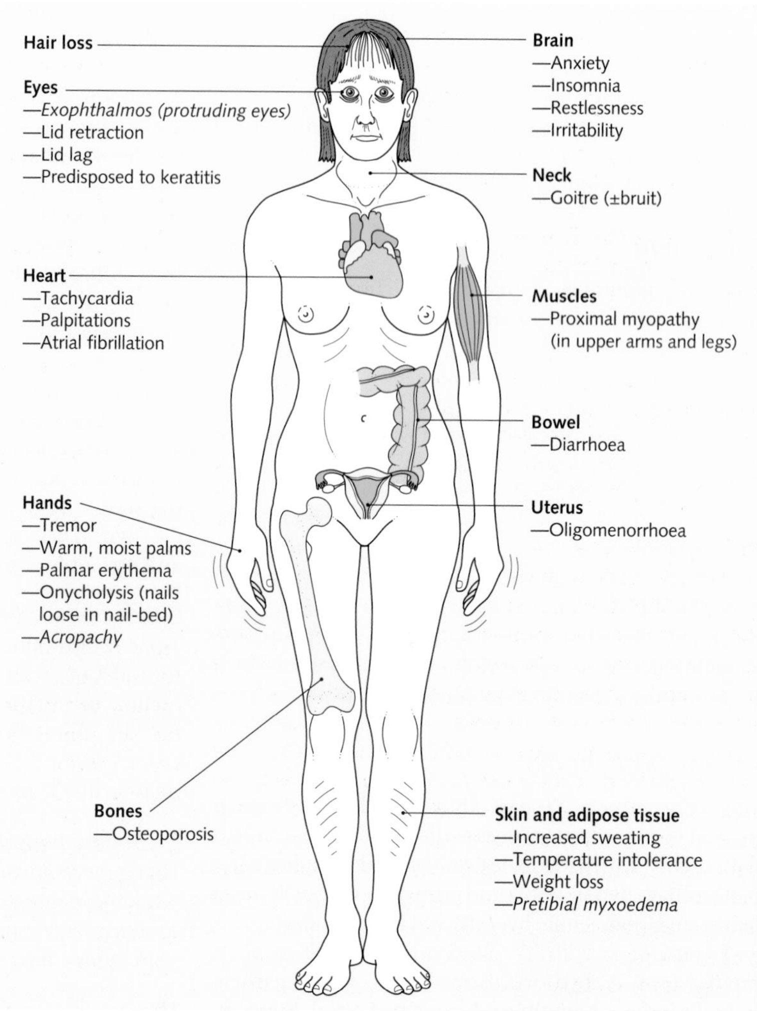

Fig. 35.7 Symptoms and signs of thyrotoxicosis (caused by hyperthyroidism). The features shown in italics are exclusive to thyrotoxicosis caused by Graves' disease.

- Pruritus.
- Diarrhoea and vomiting.
- Polyuria.

Signs include:

- A goitre, possibly with a murmur over it.
- Tremor.
- Tachycardia and atrial fibrillation.
- Warm, moist skin.
- Lid retraction and lid lag.
- Muscle weakness.
- Proximal myopathy.
- Cardiac failure.

Investigations

- Thyroid function tests: secretion of TSH will be suppressed in thyrotoxicosis due to negative feedback (the exception to this being secondary hyperthyroidism). It may also be suppressed in euthyroid patients with Graves' ophthalmopathy, large goitres, recent treatment for thyrotoxicosis or severe non-thyroid illness. T_4 and T_3 are usually both raised, but in some cases only one or the other may be elevated. It is therefore usually prudent to assess levels of both. Excess oestrogens, protein-losing states, drugs and hereditary abnormalities can alter the binding of T_4 to thyroxine-binding globulin, making total T_4 levels inaccurate in these situations. Free T_4 assays are therefore preferable.
- Thyroid autoantibodies: in Graves' disease, TSH-receptor antibodies (TRAb) are elevated, and may be useful where there is confusion about the diagnosis.
- Thyroid imaging: if a toxic nodule or thyroiditis is suspected a radioisotope thyroid scan may be performed. In the case of thyroiditis a low level of uptake is seen; a toxic nodule appears as a 'hot spot'. In Graves' disease there is diffusely increased uptake.

Management

General principles

Treatment options include drugs, radioiodine and surgery. Most patients under 50 years old with Graves' disease receive a course of antithyroid drug as initial treatment. There is a significant risk of relapse after drug treatment, and it is more likely in younger patients and those with a large goitre. Relapse after a period of drug therapy should be treated with iodine-131 (radioiodine) or subtotal thyroidectomy. Subtotal thyroidectomy is often recommended in young patients with large goitres to remove the neck swelling.

Toxic adenoma or toxic multinodular goitre are treated with radioiodine or surgery. All options should be discussed with the patient and a joint decision should be made. Beta-blockers are useful to ameliorate the symptoms of thyrotoxicosis.

Antithyroid drugs

In the UK, carbimazole is the most commonly used drug. It is metabolized to methimazole, the active agent. Propylthiouracil may be used in patients who suffer sensitivity reactions to carbimazole and is preferred in pregnancy. Both drugs act primarily by interfering with the synthesis of thyroid hormones.

Carbimazole is given in a daily dose of 15–60 mg and maintained at this dose until the patient becomes euthyroid, usually after 4–8 weeks. The dose may then be gradually reduced to a maintenance dose of 5–15 mg daily, adjusted according to response. Patients are advised to report any infectious symptoms immediately, as agranulocytosis is a rare complication. Rashes are more common.

If symptoms are profound, a combination of higher-dose carbimazole together with T_4 50–150 μg daily may be used in a 'block and replace' regimen. A euthyroid state may be achieved more quickly with this regimen. Treatment with either regimen is usually for 18 months followed by monitoring.

Iodine may be given 10–14 days before surgery in addition to carbimazole to assist control and to reduce vascularity of the thyroid.

Propranolol is useful for the rapid relief of thyrotoxic symptoms before a euthyroid state is achieved. Beta-blockers are also useful for the control of supraventricular arrhythmias secondary to thyrotoxicosis.

Radioiodine

This is commonly used for adenomas or toxic multinodular goitre. In the USA it is also commonly first-line treatment for Graves' disease. Radioactive sodium iodide ($Na^{131}I$) is concentrated by the thyroid and causes cell damage and cell death. Hypothyroidism may therefore develop at any stage after treatment, and so the patient should be under regular follow-up. Radioiodine is used increasingly for the treatment of thyrotoxicosis at all ages, particularly where medical therapy or compliance is a problem, in patients with cardiac disease and in patients who relapse after thyroidectomy. Contraindications include pregnancy and breastfeeding. Pregnancy is safe 4 months or more after treatment. Radioiodine may worsen the ophthalmopathy of Graves' disease.

Subtotal thyroidectomy

This is more commonly performed for adenoma or multinodular goitre than for Graves' disease, in whom it is reserved for those with a large or obstructive goitre. The aim of surgery is to remove sufficient thyroid tissue to cure hyperthyroidism. One year later, approximately 80% of patients are euthyroid, 15% hypothyroid and 5% have relapsed. Complications include hypoparathyroidism, recurrent laryngeal nerve damage and bleeding into the neck causing laryngeal oedema.

Thyrotoxic crisis ('thyroid storm')

This is an uncommon, life-threatening exacerbation of thyrotoxicosis with a mortality of up to 20% with treatment. Precipitating factors include thyroid surgery, radioiodine, withdrawal of antithyroid drugs, iodinated contrast agents and acute illnesses (e.g. stroke, infection, trauma and diabetic ketoacidosis). In addition to general symptoms, common features are hyperpyrexia, severe tachycardia and psychiatric symptoms including anxiety, delirium or psychosis. It requires emergency treatment with oxygen, IV fluids due to profuse sweating, propranolol (5 mg IV) for control of tachycardia, IV hydrocortisone (which inhibits peripheral T_4 conversion to T_3), oral iodine solution (to block release of thyroid hormone) and propylthiouracil (to prevent new synthesis of thyroid hormones).

Subacute (de Quervain's) thyroiditis

Various viruses (e.g. enterovirus or Coxsackievirus) can cause subacute thyroiditis. Patients present with pain, a small, tender goitre and initially thyrotoxicosis caused by release of stored thyroid hormones. There may be a history of preceding 'influenza-like' illness. Some weeks later, there is a period of hypothyroidism followed by the recovery of normal thyroid function 3–6 months after onset.

The erythrocyte sedimentation rate is raised and there is low radioisotope uptake by the thyroid. LFTs may be abnormal. Treatment is with NSAIDs for mild symptoms and with high-dose prednisolone for moderate or severe thyroiditis. The dose is gradually tailed off in subsequent weeks.

Thyroid malignancy

The incidence of thyroid cancer has risen greatly in the last 50 years. This may be due to improved diagnosis of small tumours. Prognosis is generally good, but worse in older age groups, if metastases are present at presentation, and with anaplastic carcinoma.

Papillary thyroid carcinoma

This accounts for 70–80% of thyroid malignancies and is more common in women; the peak age of onset is 30–50 years. It may be locally invasive or multifocal, treatment is by surgical excision, and the 10-year survival rate is 95%.

> **HINTS AND TIPS**
>
> The most common thyroid carcinoma is Papillary (P-opular). It also has P-sammoma bodies on histology. It causes P-alpable lymph nodes (lymphatic spread).

Follicular thyroid carcinoma

This occurs in older people (peak incidence 40–60 years) and accounts for around 10% of thyroid cancers. Distant metastases develop in around 15% of patients. Treatment is by thyroidectomy and radioiodine ablation of the thyroid remnant. The 10-year survival rate is 80%. Fine needle aspiration biopsy may not be able to distinguish between follicular adenoma and carcinoma, and these patients often undergo surgery with the diagnosis being confirmed on pathology of the excised specimen.

Anaplastic carcinoma

Anaplastic carcinoma is uncommon. The peak incidence is at 60–70 years. The malignant cells are atypical and undifferentiated, and the mean survival is only 6 months from diagnosis.

Medullary thyroid carcinoma

This is rare, accounting for around 4% of thyroid cancer. The cells secrete calcitonin and other hormones. The prognosis is poor. Family members should be screened as it is a feature of multiple endocrine neoplasia (see below).

Primary thyroid lymphoma

Lymphoma arising in the thyroid is almost always non-Hodgkin's lymphoma. There is an increased risk in patients with autoimmune thyroiditis. Most are B-cell tumours, which are treated with chemotherapy, often combined with radiotherapy.

LIPID DISORDERS

Hypercholesterolaemia is widely prevalent in Western societies. In the UK 59% of adults have serum total cholesterol concentrations above 5.0 mmol/L. There is an association between serum cholesterol and cardiovascular (CV) risk. Low-density lipoprotein (LDL) particles are the main carriers of cholesterol to the liver and peripheries; LDL levels are positively associated with CV risk. High-density lipoproteins (HDL) are involved in 'reverse cholesterol transport' from the peripheries to the liver, and levels are inversely related to CV risk.

In assessing patients it is more important to make an assessment of their overall cardiovascular risk to guide your advice and management decisions than to focus on individual risk factors (see below). In this way therapy may be targeted at those with most to gain.

Classification of hyperlipidaemia

The genetics of hyperlipidaemia are complicated; most commonly it is polygenic, with high serum cholesterol concentrations and normal triglyceride concentrations. It is greatly influenced by dietary lipid intake. 'Monogenic' forms are less common; some of these are discussed below.

Primary hyperlipidaemia

Familial combined hyperlipidaemia has a prevalence of 1 in 100 and is associated with high cholesterol and/or high triglyceride concentrations. It is heterogeneous and the causative gene has not been definitely identified.

Familial hypercholesterolaemia is an autosomal dominant condition and is due to LDL receptor deficiency, resulting in an increase in LDL particles in the circulation. The prevalence of heterozygotes is approximately 1 in 500. Homozygotes (prevalence 1 in 250 000) can have serum cholesterol levels of up to 30 mmol/L or more and may develop coronary artery disease in their teenage years.

Familial hypertriglyceridaemia is also an autosomal dominant condition and can cause pancreatitis. Patients may have eruptive xanthomata. Triglycerides may also be raised in diabetes, alcoholism and obesity.

Other types of dyslipidaemia are rare. Cases of primary hyperlipidaemia are generally managed by lipid specialists.

Secondary hyperlipidaemia

Causes include diabetes mellitus, excess alcohol, hypothyroidism, cholestasis (such as in primary biliary cirrhosis), chronic renal impairment, nephrotic syndrome and synthetic oestrogens.

Investigations

A fasting blood sample is required for measurement of total cholesterol, LDL cholesterol, HDL cholesterol and serum triglycerides. The total cholesterol:HDL cholesterol ratio is usually calculated as it is a better indicator of cardiovascular risk than values in isolation.

Management

Causes of secondary hyperlipidaemia should be treated. Where there is no secondary cause, dietary measures should be tried first, including reduction of total energy and saturated fat intake and increasing the consumption of oily fish. However, the average fall in total cholesterol concentration with a general lipid-lowering diet is only 2%. Drug treatment is aimed at high-risk patients, taking into account other cardiovascular risk factors.

Drugs

Statins

The statins competitively inhibit HMG-CoA reductase, an enzyme involved in cholesterol synthesis, especially in the liver. They are usually first-line therapy. There is evidence that statins produce important reductions in CV events in high-risk patients. They should be used with caution in those with a history of liver disease, and LFTs should be checked after starting treatment. Side effects include reversible myositis.

Treatment should be stopped if there are symptoms of myopathy or significantly raised creatinine kinase. Patients should therefore be advised to report unexplained muscle pain, tenderness and weakness. Other side effects include headache, altered LFTs (which occasionally necessitates stopping therapy) and gastrointestinal effects (e.g. abdominal pain, nausea and vomiting).

Fibrates

Their main action is to decrease serum triglyceride but they also tend to reduce LDL cholesterol and raise HDL cholesterol. They can cause a myositis-like syndrome, especially in patients with impaired renal function and those on a statin. They are considered when statins are not tolerated.

Ezetimibe

This drug reduces the intestinal absorption of cholesterol. It may be used when a statin is not tolerated or in addition to a statin to achieve target levels.

Anion-exchange resins (bile-acid sequestrants)

These drugs are rarely used and include cholestyramine and colestipol. They reduce LDL cholesterol but can aggravate hypertriglyceridaemia, and may interfere with the absorption of fat-soluble vitamins. Supplements of vitamins A, D and K and of folic acid may be required when treatment is prolonged.

Side effects are mainly gastrointestinal, including change in bowel habit, nausea, vomiting and abdominal pain. Other drugs should be taken at least 1 h before, or 4–6 h after cholestyramine or colestipol to reduce possible interference with absorption.

Nicotinic acid group

The value of nicotinic acid is limited by its prostaglandin-mediated side effects, including flushing, itch and nausea. In high doses it lowers both cholesterol and triglyceride concentrations by inhibiting synthesis, and increases HDL cholesterol. Troublesome side effects may be improved by the co-prescription of aspirin and gradually increasing the dose.

Dietary supplements

Fish oils lower triglyceride levels but supplementation above dietary intake is not currently recommended. Soluble fibre supplements (such as ispaghula husk) can be used as an adjunct to a lipid-lowering diet in patients with mild hypercholesterolaemia. It probably acts by reducing reabsorption of bile acids. Plasma triglycerides remain unchanged. Plant sterols show promise but further large-scale trials are awaited.

The use of lipid-lowering drugs

The use of lipid-lowering therapy should form part of an integrated approach to the assessment and treatment of CV risk, including interventions directed at smoking, lifestyle, obesity, blood pressure and use of antiplatelet therapy.

Lipid lowering appears to reduce CV risk regardless of baseline serum cholesterol levels. However, the absolute risk reduction is greater if the patient's risk for CV disease is higher. Therefore guidelines aim to target those groups at highest CV risk to maximize gains.

Secondary prevention

This group includes those with known coronary heart disease or 'CHD equivalents' including other atherosclerotic vascular disease, diabetes, renal dysfunction and inherited dyslipidaemias. Therapy aims to achieve a total cholesterol <4 mmol/L and LDL <2 mmol/L.

Primary prevention

Risk is estimated using equations such as the Framingham risk equation. This is incorporated into the Joint British Societies' risk assessment charts which can be found in the *British National Formulary*. These charts may underestimate risk in certain groups such as those with a strong family history, hypertriglyceridaemia, premature menopause, impaired glucose tolerance or fasting glycaemia and in certain ethnic minorities, e.g. those from the Indian subcontinent. Clinical judgement must always be used, but formal assessment and lipid-lowering therapy should be prioritized in those with 10-year risk of greater than 20% to achieve the levels mentioned above.

COMMUNICATION

The communication of levels of risk to patients is difficult. The use of risk prediction charts to illustrate risk may help.

METABOLIC BONE DISEASE

Vitamin D metabolism is shown in Fig. 35.8.

Osteoporosis

Bone normally consists of 60% mineral and 40% matrix or organic matter. In osteoporosis the deposition of calcium salts occurs normally, but there is a loss of bone matrix and a reduction in bone mass per unit volume of anatomical bone. The World Health Organization (WHO) has defined osteoporosis as a bone mineral density (BMD) $\geq$2.5 standard deviations below the mean value for young adults (T-score). Osteopenia is defined as a T score between −1.0 and −2.5.

The prevalence of osteoporosis in white women aged 50–59 years is 4% and the prevalence in those aged 80 years or over is around 25%. Osteoporosis predisposes patients to fractures, commonly of the hip, vertebrae or wrist. It is estimated that almost 200 000 osteoporosis-related fractures occur in the UK each year. These are associated with considerable morbidity and mortality.

Fig. 35.8 Metabolism of vitamin D.

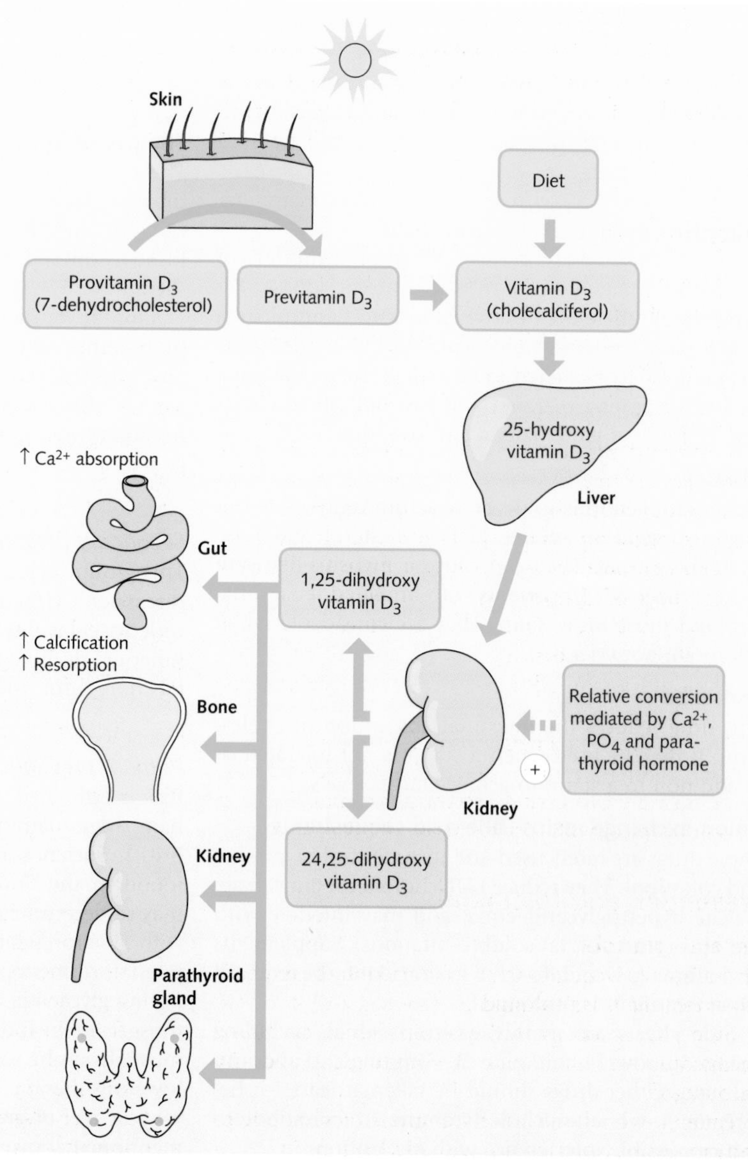

Aetiology and pathogenesis

Involutional or primary osteoporosis

Involutional bone loss commences at age 35–45 years in both sexes but is accelerated in women following the loss of sex steroids at the menopause, explaining the higher incidence in postmenopausal women. Age-related bone loss is increased by smoking, alcohol, inactivity, low BMI and impaired vitamin D production.

Secondary osteoporosis

Causes include steroid therapy, hypogonadism, alcohol abuse, hyperthyroidism, hyperparathyroidism, anticonvulsants and some chronic diseases such as inflammatory bowel disease and cystic fibrosis.

Clinical features

Osteoporosis does not cause pain (or other symptoms) until a fracture occurs. The risk of fracture is related to the BMD but also to conditions predisposing to falls (e.g. stroke, parkinsonism, dementia, visual impairment). These must also be assessed.

Investigations

- Blood tests, including a bone profile (calcium, phosphate, alkaline phosphatase), should be normal. Abnormalities should prompt a search for an underlying cause.
- BMD is estimated by dual-energy X-ray absorptiometry (DXA) scan. There is no evidence for population-based screening. It is performed if there are risk factors and therapy is being considered (e.g. premature menopause, steroid therapy). It may also be done following a fragility (low trauma) fracture, an X-ray demonstrating osteopenia or for monitoring the effect of therapy. As well as the T-score (see above), a Z-score is calculated, which is an age-matched BMD score. It is used in assessment of children and young adults who have not yet reached peak bone density.
- Thyroid function, luteinizing hormone (LH), follicle-stimulating hormone (FSH) and testosterone should be measured to exclude secondary causes. Fifty per cent of males with hip fractures are hypogonadal.

Prevention and treatment

General principles

An holistic approach to the reduction of fracture risk is important. Falls risk should be assessed and interventions implemented, alcohol excess and smoking should be discouraged and a good diet with regular activity encouraged.

Patients with osteopenia are given lifestyle advice and monitored unless they have had a fracture, in which case therapy is instituted. All those with osteoporosis are treated.

Drugs

Treatment options include bisphosphonates, strontium ranelate, denosumab, raloxifene (a selective oestrogen receptor modulator), calcitonin and intermittent parathyroid hormone. Bisphosphonates are first-choice therapy in most cases and are generally well tolerated. In patients who are unable to take them, strontium ranelate or denosumab are considered second line. Raloxifene may be considered for secondary prevention. Other treatments are approved but used less frequently, and hormone replacement therapy (previously used frequently in postmenopausal women) is no longer recommended as first-line therapy. Supplementation of calcium and vitamin D_3 should be considered in all patients.

Patients on long-term steroids are particularly at risk and a low threshold is needed for therapy.

Paget's disease

In Paget's disease, there is uncontrolled bone turnover with areas of increased localized osteoclastic resorption. This is followed by disordered osteoblastic activity, leading to new bone formation that is structurally abnormal and weak (Fig. 35.9). The aetiology is unknown, although viruses have been implicated and genetic factors probably play a role. It is more common in Anglo-Saxons, and the incidence increases with age. Studies in Europe and New Zealand indicate that the overall prevalence has fallen by 50% since the 1970s.

Clinical features

The axial skeleton and femur are most commonly affected. The condition is most commonly asymptomatic but can cause bone pain, tenderness and deformity such as an enlarged skull and bowed (sabre) tibia. Complications include:

- Fractures of long bones.
- Conductive deafness due to involvement of the ossicles.
- Progressive occlusion of the foramina of the skull can cause deafness due to 8th cranial nerve compression, visual impairment due to 2nd nerve compression, or long tract signs due to basilar invagination and cervical cord stenosis.
- High-output cardiac failure (with >20% skeletal involvement).
- Osteogenic sarcoma.
- Osteoarthritis of related joints.

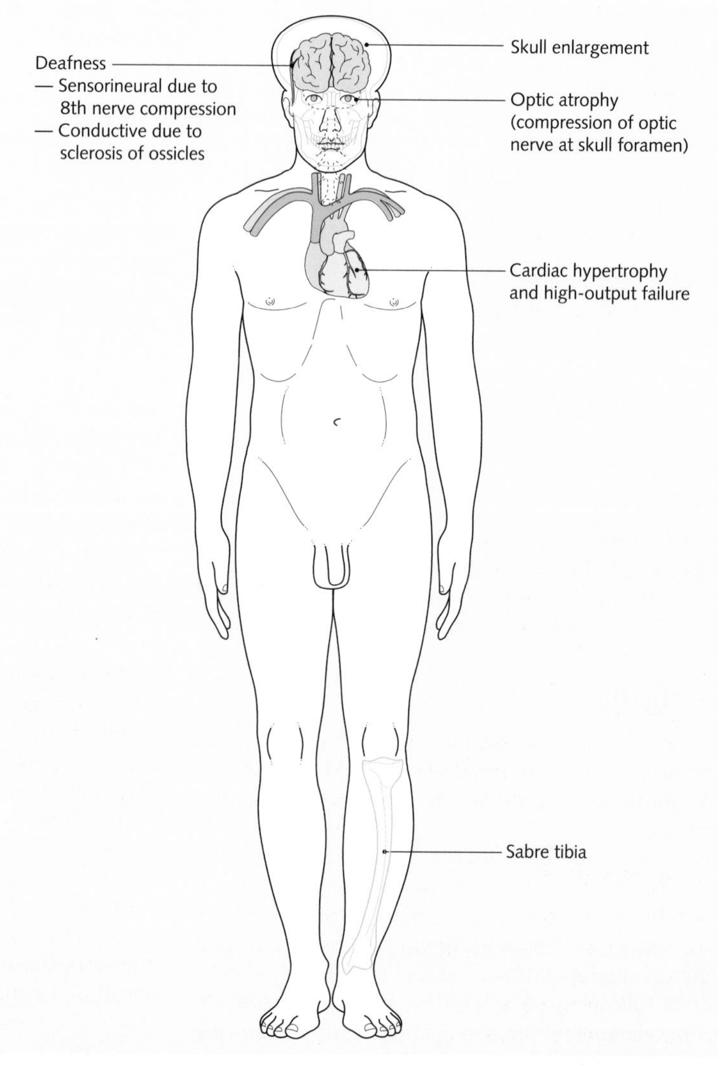

Fig. 35.9 General features of Paget's disease of the bone.

Investigations

Serum alkaline phosphatase is markedly raised but serum calcium and phosphate are usually normal; 24-h urinary hydroxyproline output is raised and reflects the increased bone turnover. There may be mild hypercalcaemia in immobile patients due to unopposed bone resorption.

X-rays of affected bones show a mosaic of osteolytic and sclerotic lesions, thickening of trabeculae and thick cortices with an enlarged irregular outline. Isotope bone scans will demonstrate the extent of skeletal involvement.

Treatment

Asymptomatic patients only require treatment if there is active disease at a site where complications might occur. In addition to standard analgesia, specific treatment is given for bone pain, bone deformities, hypercalcaemia or complications. Drug treatment is with bisphosphonates or calcitonin.

Bisphosphonates

Bisphosphonates are adsorbed on to hydroxyapatite crystals and inhibit osteoclasts, slowing bone resorption and reducing bone turnover. Newer bisphosphonates are preferred, such as oral risedronate (30 mg once daily for 2 months followed by monitoring) or IV zoledronic acid (5 mg as a single dose).

Calcitonin

Calcitonin opposes many of the effects of parathyroid hormone (PTH) and together with PTH regulates bone turnover and calcium balance. It is useful when bisphosphonates are not tolerated but is less effective and has considerable side effects.

Osteomalacia

Osteomalacia results from inadequate mineralization of bone after fusion of the epiphyses has occurred. Rickets is the result if this occurs during the period of bone growth before epiphyseal fusion.

Aetiology

The aetiology of osteomalacia includes:

- Lack of dietary vitamin D.
- Ineffective conversion of 7-dehydrocholesterol (provitamin D_3) to previtamin D_3 by ultraviolet light in the dermis. This is due to lack of sunlight and, in the UK, is most commonly seen in Asians.
- Intestinal malabsorption (e.g. gluten-sensitive enteropathy and postgastrectomy states).
- Vitamin D resistance: commonly this is due to ineffective conversion of 25-hydroxyvitamin D_3 to 1,25-dihydroxyvitamin D_3 in chronic renal disease. Other causes are inherited deficiency of renal 1-alpha-hydroxylase and end-organ receptor abnormality.
- Drug induced: chronic anticonvulsant therapy may induce liver enzymes, leading to the breakdown of 25-hydroxyvitamin D_3.
- Excessive renal phosphate loss due to Fanconi's syndrome or a specific defect in renal phosphate handling.

Clinical features

Bone pain and tenderness are common. Fractures may occur, especially of the femoral neck. There is often a proximal myopathy, which may cause a waddling gait and difficulty in rising from a chair.

In rickets, there are deformities of the legs (bow-legs and knock-knees), the chest (rachitic rosary) and the skull. There may also be features of hypocalcaemia (e.g. tetany).

Investigations

Biochemistry

- Serum calcium and phosphate: tend to be decreased but may be normal.
- Serum alkaline phosphatase activity: increased.
- Urinary calcium excretion: low.
- Plasma 25-hydroxyvitamin D_3: low except in resistant cases.
- 1,25-dihydroxyvitamin D_3: low in renal failure.
- PTH is high because of secondary hyperparathyroidism due to hypocalcaemia.

Imaging

X-rays of bone in rickets show cupped, ragged metaphyseal surfaces. In osteomalacia, there is cortical bone loss and pseudofractures (Looser's zones), which are small translucent bands perpendicular to the bone and extending inwards from the cortex. They are best seen on the lateral border of the scapula, on the femoral neck and in the pubic rami.

Isotope bone scans show a generalized diffuse increase in uptake of isotope.

Treatment

Dietary vitamin D deficiency can be prevented by taking an oral supplement of 10 μg (4000 IU) of ergocalciferol daily. Vitamin D deficiency caused by intestinal malabsorption or chronic liver disease usually requires vitamin D in pharmacological doses, such as calciferol tablets up to 1 mg daily. Calcium supplements may also be required, as may phosphate supplements in hypophosphataemic disease.

The newer hydroxylated vitamin D derivatives (alfacalcidol and calcitriol) have a shorter duration of action and therefore have the advantage that problems associated with hypercalcaemia due to excessive dosage are shorter lived and easier to treat.

In patients with chronic renal impairment, alfacalcidol or calcitriol should be prescribed. All patients receiving pharmacological doses of vitamin D should have their serum levels of calcium checked at intervals and whenever nausea and vomiting are present. Breast milk from women taking pharmacological doses of vitamin D may cause hypercalcaemia if given to an infant.

Renal osteodystrophy

The term 'renal osteodystrophy' is used to cover the various forms of bone disease that develop in chronic renal failure. These include:

- Delayed epiphyseal closure in children and young adults.
- Rickets or osteomalacia.
- Osteitis fibrosa cystica (brown tumours) due to secondary or tertiary hyperparathyroidism.
- Generalized or localized osteosclerosis.

The kidney does not excrete phosphate effectively as its function drops. This hyperphosphataemia stimulates PTH secretion. The impaired hydroxylation of 25-hydroxyvitamin D causes osteomalacia and hypocalcaemia, further stimulating the release of PTH (secondary hyperparathyroidism) and increasing osteoclast activity.

Management

Dietary phosphate intake is reduced and oral phosphate binders are used to help control the hyperphosphataemia. Calcium and hydroxylated vitamin D supplements can be given when the phosphate levels are controlled (reducing the risk of ectopic calcification) to help normalize the calcium and reduce the level of PTH further. Renal replacement therapy in the form of haemodialysis, peritoneal dialysis or transplantation will help restore calcium and phosphate metabolism in end-stage renal failure.

In tertiary hyperparathyroidism (see below), subtotal parathyroidectomy is required.

HYPERCALCAEMIA

The causes of hypercalcaemia are given in Fig. 35.10 and calcium homeostasis is outlined in Fig. 35.11. The two most common causes are primary hyperparathyroidism and malignant disease. Prolonged venous stasis when taking blood can cause spurious hypercalcaemia, and an unexpected result should be verified with repeat measurement.

The physiologically relevant measurement is of ionized (unbound) calcium. This can be determined by correcting serum total calcium levels for serum protein or albumin concentrations. The higher the protein concentration, the more calcium is protein bound, and the lower the proportion of ionized calcium. Add 0.02 mmol/L to calcium concentration for every 1 g/L that albumin is below 40 g/L and perform a similar subtraction for high albumin.

Fig. 35.10 Causes of hypercalcaemia.

Mechanism	Example
Increased calcium intake	Milk-alkali syndrome
Increased vitamin D intake	Self-administered, iatrogenic
Increased activity of vitamin D	Sarcoidosis, lymphoma, Addison's disease
Increased production of PTH	Primary hyperparathyroidism (adenoma, hyperplasia, carcinoma), tertiary hyperparathyroidism (hyperplasia)
Production of PTH-related peptide	Squamous carcinoma, renal cell carcinoma
Increased osteoclastic activity	Osteolytic metastases, multiple myeloma
Increased bone turnover	Hyperthyroidism
Increased renal tubular calcium reabsorption	Familial hypocalciuric hypercalcaemia (autosomal dominant)

PTH, parathyroid hormone.

Clinical features

HINTS AND TIPS

For the clinical features of hypercalcaemia, remember bones (bone pain), stones (renal stones), groans (peptic ulcer) and moans (psychiatric disease).

These include abdominal pain, constipation and vomiting. Polyuria, polydipsia and dehydration are common and may be severe. Depression and confusion may occur. Renal stones may form with chronic hypercalcaemia, and renal impairment may develop due to hypovolaemia or nephrocalcinosis. Arrhythmia has been reported. There may also be features of the underlying cause.

Investigations

- Full blood count, urea and electrolytes, calcium profile and PTH, liver and thyroid function tests. PTH should be suppressed unless hyperparathyroidism is the cause.
- Consider measuring vitamin D levels and PTH-related peptide (PTHrp).
- Chest X-ray – any evidence of malignancy or sarcoidosis?
- Other investigations will be determined by the differential diagnosis (e.g. isotope bone scan, myeloma screen, etc.).

Management

Severe hypercalcaemia is a medical emergency. In the acute phase, it is essential to rehydrate with normal saline as the renal excretion of calcium is dependent on exchange with sodium ions in the nephron. IV bisphosphonate therapy (usually a single dose of pamidronate) is given and can be repeated if necessary. High-dose prednisolone is effective for hypercalcaemia secondary to myeloma, sarcoidosis and excess vitamin D but otherwise is of little value. Calcitonin and loop diuretics are now rarely used.

After the acute phase, it is important to elucidate and treat the underlying cause.

HYPERPARATHYROIDISM

Hyperparathyroidism results from excess circulating PTH, which increases serum calcium by stimulating calcium absorption from the gut, increasing mobilization

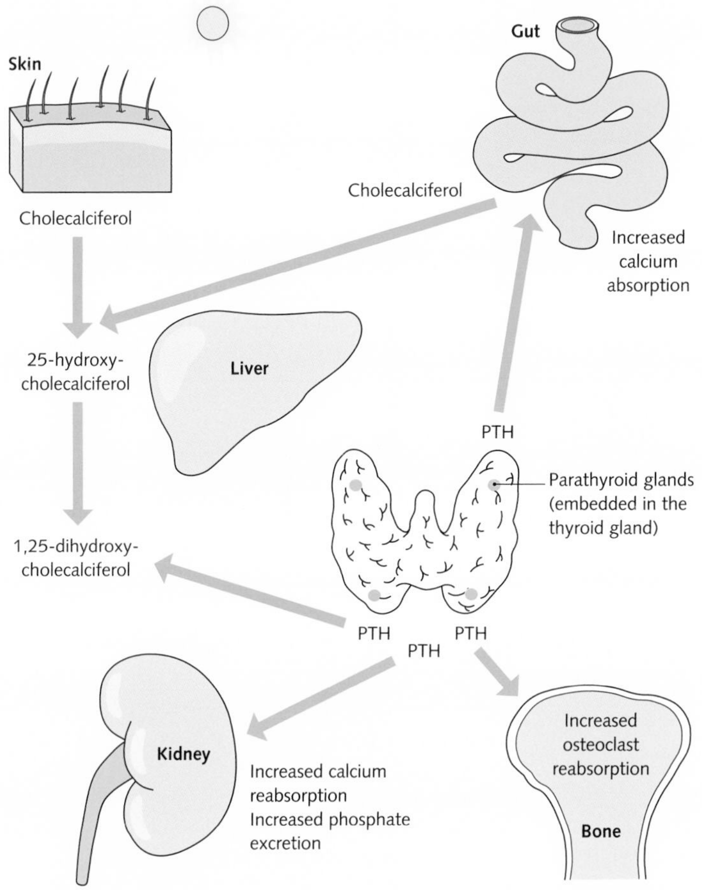

Fig. 35.11 Calcium homeostasis. PTH, parathyroid hormone.

of calcium from bone and reducing renal calcium clearance. Parathyroid hormone (PTH) also increases phosphate release from bone but reduces renal reabsorption, with the overall effect of lowering phosphate concentrations.

Classification and aetiology

- Primary hyperparathyroidism (overproduction of PTH in the absence of other abnormalities) is usually due to a single benign adenoma but less commonly may be due to multiple adenomas, carcinoma or hyperplasia. It may be associated with other endocrine abnormalities as part of the multiple endocrine neoplasia (MEN) syndromes. Ectopic PTH production is very rare; more commonly, cancers of the lung or breast produce PTHrp, which causes a similar picture.
- Secondary hyperparathyroidism occurs when PTH levels are persistently and appropriately raised to maintain calcium concentrations in the face of a disorder that lowers calcium levels. Causes include chronic renal failure and deficiency of vitamin D (e.g. due to inadequate intake or malabsorption).
- Tertiary hyperparathyroidism is the continued secretion of excess PTH after prolonged secondary hyperparathyroidism. The parathyroids act autonomously and cause hypercalcaemia, despite correction of the original cause of the secondary hyperparathyroidism. This occurs in some patients with end-stage renal failure.

Clinical features

Hyperparathryoid bone disease can cause reduced bone density and may result in fractures. In addition, the features of hypercalcaemia discussed above may be present.

Investigations

In primary hyperparathyroidism, serum calcium is raised. Blood samples should be repeated without venous compression to confirm the level. Serum phosphate is low and alkaline phosphatase is high, reflecting increased bone turnover. There may be a mild renal tubular acidosis with a high serum chloride level (i.e. a normal anion gap), and serum PTH is raised.

In secondary hyperparathyroidism of renal failure, serum calcium is low or normal and phosphate is normal or high. Both of these metabolic abnormalities stimulate the secretion of PTH. A 24-h urine collection may be required to rule out familial hypocalciuric hypercalcaemia.

In both, X-rays show subperiosteal resorption, most marked in the hands, and evidence of osteitis fibrosa cystica. A chest X-ray (CXR) should be performed to look for a carcinoma producing PTHrp. A skull X-ray shows a 'pepper pot' appearance.

In tertiary hyperparathyroidism, serum calcium is high and extra-skeletal calcification, including calciphylaxis (calcium deposition in blood vessel walls causing thrombosis and skin necrosis), may occur. Imaging of the neck is only used to plan surgery and not for diagnosis.

Treatment

Parathyroidectomy is indicated for symptomatic disease. The decision is more difficult in asymptomatic patients, many of whom will progress to overt disease. Guidelines suggest surgery when there is persistent hypercalcaemia greater than 0.25 mmol/L above normal, renal impairment, BMD T-score < -2.5 or age below 50. The parathyroid glands may be localized by CT scan, SPECT scan or technetium isotope (sestamibi) scans, which can detect adenomas. The operative procedure may be a full bilateral exploration (if multiple adenomas are present and in certain other situations), or a minimally invasive endoscopic procedure with intraoperative PTH monitoring (when a single adenoma is seen on imaging). All abnormal glands are removed.

If all the glands are hyperplastic, three and a half are usually removed, leaving the last half in situ. Serum calcium and magnesium should be monitored postoperatively, as removal of the glands may lead to rapid and prolonged hypocalcaemia and hypomagnesaemia as the 'hungry bones' recover the minerals lost during the period of hyperparathyroidism.

Asymptomatic patients not meeting the criteria for surgery should be monitored. If surgery is contraindicated, bisphosphonates or calcimimetics, e.g. cinacalcet, may be useful.

HYPOPARATHYROIDISM

Hypoparathyroidism is usually secondary to thyroid surgery. Primary (idiopathic) hypoparathyroidism is an autoimmune disorder associated with vitiligo, Addison's disease, pernicious anaemia and other autoimmune diseases, and it may be part of autoimmune polyendocrine syndrome (see below). Infiltration due to metabolic disease such as Wilson's disease and haemochromatosis can cause destruction of the parathyroid gland, but this is very uncommon. Rare mutations can cause inherited abnormalities of parathyroid development, such as in DiGeorge's syndrome, when it is associated with intellectual impairment, cardiac abnormalities and thymic hypoplasia.

Pseudohypoparathyroidism is a syndrome of variable end-organ (kidney and bone) resistance to PTH. It is associated with intellectual impairment, short stature, a round face and short metacarpals and metatarsals.

Pseudopseudohypoparathyroidism describes the appearance present in pseudohypoparathyroidism but without the calcium abnormalities, and is due to resistance to PTH in bone with normal renal responsiveness.

Other causes of hypocalcaemia include chronic renal failure and osteomalacia. In acutely ill patients, acute pancreatitis and rhabdomyolysis can cause hypocalcaemia. Causes are summarized in Fig. 35.12.

Clinical features

Hypocalcaemia causes circumoral paraesthesiae, cramps, anxiety and tetany, followed by convulsions, laryngeal stridor, dystonia and psychosis. Trousseau's sign (carpopedal spasm when the brachial artery is occluded with a blood pressure cuff) and Chvostek's sign (twitching of the facial muscles when the facial nerve is tapped) may be present.

Fig. 35.12 Causes of hypocalcaemia.

Mechanism	Example
Reduced calcium intake	Dietary deficiency, malabsorption
Reduced vitamin D intake/production	Dietary deficiency, malabsorption, reduced sunlight exposure
Reduced activation of vitamin D	Renal disease, liver disease
Increased inactivation of vitamin D	Enzyme induction by anticonvulsants
Reduced production of PTH	Surgical removal of parathyroid glands, autoimmune, congenital (DiGeorge's syndrome)
Resistance to PTH	Pseudohypoparathyroidism
Hypoalbuminaemia	Shock

PTH, parathyroid hormone.

Investigations

Serum calcium is low, phosphate is high and alkaline phosphatase is normal. Additional tests include serum urea and creatinine, serum PTH level, parathyroid antibodies and vitamin D metabolite levels. Serum PTH will be low in hypoparathyroidism but raised in pseudohypoparathyroidism. Investigations for other endocrinopathies may be required in certain cases.

X-rays of the hands show short fourth metacarpals in pseudohypoparathyroidism.

HINTS AND TIPS

In hypocalcaemia always check magnesium. Hypomagnesaemia often follows hypocalcaemia and magnesium supplementation may be needed for the calcium to respond to treatment.

Treatment

Emergency treatment of hypocalcaemia is with 10 mL 10% IV calcium gluconate, repeated as necessary. IV magnesium chloride may also be required if there is hypomagnesaemia.

Long-term treatment is with alfacalcidol or calcitriol. Serum calcium should be monitored to prevent hypercalcaemia.

PITUITARY DISORDERS

Hypopituitarism

The anterior pituitary produces six hormones – adrenocorticotrophic hormone (ACTH), growth hormone (GH), FSH, LH, thyroid-stimulating hormone (TSH) and prolactin (PRL). Hypopituitarism may be associated with loss of all or some of these hormones. The clinical and biochemical presentation will depend on which hormones are deficient and to what extent. The most common cause is the mass effect of pituitary adenomas (which if functional may cause features of hypersecretion of a particular hormone – see below), with additional loss of pituitary function after surgery and pituitary irradiation. Other causes include hypothalamic tumours and cysts, peripituitary tumours (e.g. gliomas and meningiomas, craniopharyngiomas), infiltrative diseases (e.g. sarcoidosis), pituitary infarction (Sheehan syndrome) or haemorrhage, and metastatic lesions.

HINTS AND TIPS

Sudden haemorrhage or infarction of the pituitary causes headache, diplopia and hypopituarism and is known as 'pituitary apoplexy'.

Clinical features

These can be deduced from knowledge of the effects of the various pituitary hormones. Growth hormone and gonadotrophins are often affected first.

- GH: fatigue, increased abdominal adiposity, and reduced muscle strength and exercise capacity.
- LH and FSH: in women, there is oligomenorrhoea, infertility, dyspareunia, breast atrophy, loss of pubic and axillary hair and hot flushes; in men, there is loss of libido, impotence, infertility, flushes, regression of secondary sexual characteristics, soft testes and fine wrinkles on the face.
- TSH: fatigue, muscle weakness, sensitivity to cold, constipation, apathy, weight gain and dry skin.
- ACTH: fatigue, anorexia, weight loss, postural hypotension, weakness, nausea and vomiting, hypoglycaemia, apathy, reduced libido and loss of pubic and axillary hair.
- Prolactin: inability to lactate.

HINTS AND TIPS

The symptoms of hypopituitarism are non-specific but must not be dismissed. A high index of suspicion may be required to make the diagnosis.

Investigations

Dynamic tests involving stimulation are occasionally needed to assess ACTH or GH; otherwise, basal levels provide all the necessary information. Most pituitary hormones are secreted in a pulsatile fashion and therefore random levels are not very useful.

- Serum thyroxine and TSH: a low thyroxine level together with a low or normal TSH level is suggestive of secondary hypothyroidism.
- To assess ACTH, cortisol should be measured between 8 and 9 a.m. If low or intermediate, serum ACTH should be measured; the sample needs to be taken at 9 a.m. into a cold tube and immediately put on ice. Alternatively, an insulin tolerance test or metyrapone test can be performed but these are rarely done.
- FH/LSH: these should be measured in the morning with a simultaneous serum testosterone level in men and serum oestradiol level in women.
- Growth hormone: as basal levels of GH fluctuate greatly, if deficiency is suspected an insulin tolerance test is required; the normal response is GH release as glucose levels decrease. IGF-1 levels will also be low in GH deficiency.
- Prolactin: this is performed to look for raised levels which would signify a prolactinoma.
- CT/MRI/visual field assessment: see investigations sections below.

Management

Hormone replacement involves the use of multiple hormones. Hydrocortisone is given for adrenal failure, T_4 for hypothyroidism, testosterone for hypogonadal men and oestrogen for hypogonadal premenopausal women. Recombinant human GH is given by injection to patients with significant symptoms. Careful instruction and patient compliance are mandatory for long-term recovery.

Pituitary tumours

Pituitary tumours may be non-functioning or may secrete hormones. Non-functioning and prolactin-secreting are the most common. The incidence of clinically significant pituitary tumours varies from 0.2 to 3 in 100 000 population and the prevalence is about 9 in 100 000. PRL- and ACTH-secreting tumours occur most commonly in 25–35 year olds, GH-secreting tumours in those aged 35–50 years, and non-functioning tumours usually present after the age of 60 years. They can also be classified by their size as microadenoma (<1 cm diameter) or macroadenoma (>1 cm).

Clinical features

The clinical features relate to (i) pressure effects from the tumour mass, (ii) the effects of hypersecretion of any hormone and (iii) the suppression of other pituitary hormones (hypopituitarism).

Pressure effects cause headaches and there may be compression of the optic chiasm causing bitemporal hemianopia. Seizures, other cranial nerve signs and hydrocephalus may occur with large masses. Extension into the hypothalamus affects appetite, sleep and temperature regulation.

The effects of functioning tumours depend on the hormone secreted. They may cause acromegaly via GH, amenorrhoea–galactorrhoea syndrome via PRL, or Cushing's disease via ACTH. Secondary thyrotoxicosis is rare. The features of hypopituitarism have been described above.

Investigations

Endocrinological assessment is performed as described above.

MRI scan is the best modality with which to assess the anatomy of the tumour. Formal visual field assessment is important as many of these tumours have effects on the visual pathways, particularly at the optic chiasm.

Management

Management may be medical, surgical or with radiotherapy. Aside from prolactinomas, surgical resection is the treatment of choice in most cases. The surgical approach is usually trans-sphenoidal, but with larger masses a transfrontal approach may be necessary. Drug therapy includes dopamine receptor agonists (e.g. cabergoline, bromocriptine) for prolactinoma; these inhibit PRL release and induce shrinkage of the tumour in over 90% of cases. Somatostatin analogues inhibit GH release and induce a lesser degree of tumour shrinkage in most GH-secreting adenomas. They are usually used after surgery in acromegaly.

Acromegaly

Acromegaly is an insidious disease resulting from excessive circulating levels of GH in adults. Diagnosis is often made years after symptoms first occur. The incidence is approximately 5 per million per year and the prevalence is 50 per million.

Acromegalic gigantism results from acromegaly in young individuals before epiphyseal fusion, and is very uncommon.

Aetiology

The commonest cause is a benign pituitary tumour secreting GH. Pituitary carcinoma and carcinoid tumours that secrete hypothalamic GH-releasing hormone are uncommon causes.

Clinical features

The clinical features of acromegaly are summarized in Fig. 35.13.

HINTS AND TIPS

The diagnosis of acromegaly may become more obvious by comparing old photographs of the patient with their present appearance.

Cardiovascular problems are often the cause of mortality. Coronary artery disease, hypertension and diabetes are more common than in the normal population. Cardiomyopathy may occur.

Headaches, visual field defects and cranial nerve palsies may occur due to the mass effect of the pituitary tumour. Hyperprolactinaemia (due to compression of the pituitary stalk and therefore loss of tonic inhibitory dopamine from hypothalamus – see below) is common and hypopituitarism can also occur.

Sleep apnoea occurs in up to 50%.

HINTS AND TIPS

Historically, the patient may have noticed a change in their hat size. Now it is more likely they have noticed a change in glove size, or being unable to remove a wedding ring.

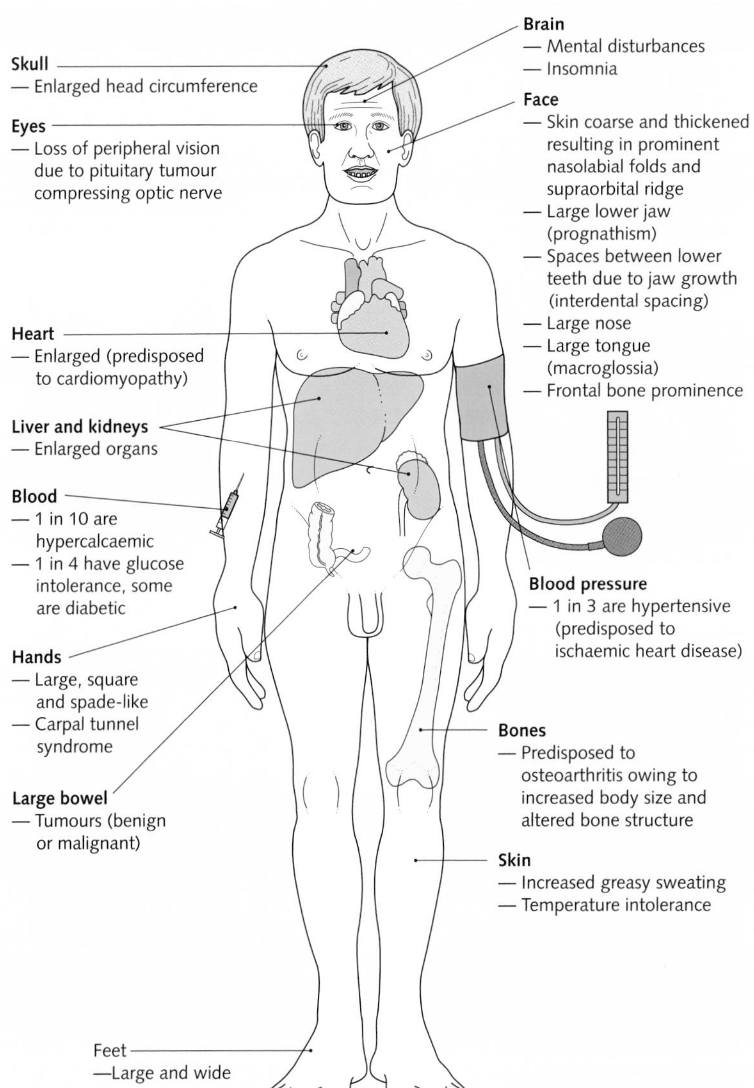

Fig. 35.13 Signs and symptoms of acromegaly (caused by excessive growth hormone secretion in adults).

Diagnosis

GH levels are elevated, although they may rise with stress. Therefore, GH is measured during a glucose tolerance test. In healthy individuals, GH falls to <1 ng/mL in the 2 h following a 75 g glucose load. In some centres, insulin-like growth factor-1 levels are used to provide an estimate of growth hormone levels as this fluctuates less than GH itself.

Other investigations include the following:

- Assessment of visual fields: bitemporal hemianopia.
- Skull X-ray and MRI of the brain.
- Hand X-ray: tufting of the terminal phalanges and increased joint spaces due to hypertrophy of the cartilage. The heel pad is usually thickened.
- CXR, ECG and echocardiogram: left ventricular hypertrophy and cardiomyopathy.

Management

The aim of treatment is to relieve symptoms, reverse somatic changes and reverse metabolic abnormalities. Treatment is by surgery, radiotherapy or drugs.

Surgery

Surgery is the first-choice treatment. The trans-sphenoidal route is usually used. Up to 90% of micro-adenomas are cured, but the success rate is lower for larger tumours. Complications include hypopituitarism, meningitis and intraoperative bleeding.

Radiotherapy

This is often used if attempts at surgery do not reduce GH levels sufficiently. Hypopituitarism may occur, and regular tests of pituitary function should be performed. The effect on GH secretion is slow, but this may be improved with newer techniques such as proton-beam therapy.

Medical therapies

The most effective treatment is with octreotide, a somatostatin analogue. Somatostatin inhibits GH secretion. Side effects include colicky abdominal pain and diarrhoea but this usually settles with continued treatment. Gallstones occur in approximately one-third of patients.

Prognosis

Untreated, the mortality rate is approximately twice that in healthy individuals due to cardiovascular and cerebrovascular disease. There is also an increased risk of colon cancer.

Prolactin disorders

PRL is the hormone most commonly secreted by pituitary tumours. Secretion of PRL is under constant negative control by the action of dopamine produced in the hypothalamus and transported down the pituitary stalk, such that interruption produces hyperprolactinaemia. The causes of hyperprolactinaemia are summarized in Fig. 35.14. It is more common in women.

Fig. 35.14 Causes of hyperprolactinaemia.

Cause	Examples
Physiological	Pregnancy, lactation, stress
Drugs	Antiemetics, e.g. metoclopramide, prochlorperazine Phenothiazines Tricyclic antidepressants
Primary hypothyroidism	
Pituitary tumours	Prolactinoma Growth-hormone-secreting tumours Non-functioning tumours
Polycystic ovary syndrome	
Uncommon	Sarcoidosis
Hypothalamic lesions	Langerhans cell histiocytosis Hypothalamic tumours
Chest wall stimulation	Repeated self-examination of breasts Post herpes zoster
Liver or renal failure	

Clinical features

In premenopausal women, the most common symptoms are oligomenorrhoea, galactorrhoea, infertility and occasionally hirsutism. In men, symptoms include reduced libido, hypogonadism, impotence, infertility and galactorrhoea. Symptoms caused by large tumour size are more common in men and postmenopausal women, and include headache, visual field defects and cranial nerve palsies. Varying degrees of hypopituitarism may be present.

Investigations

Elevated PRL levels should be confirmed on repeat testing. Other blood tests include thyroid function tests (TFTs), renal and liver function, and a pregnancy test in women. A careful drug history should always be taken.

Radiological assessment of the pituitary tumour should be carried out with skull X-rays and MRI scan of the brain. Full assessment of pituitary function should be undertaken if a macroadenoma is suspected, and visual fields should be assessed.

Management

Microprolactinomas are <10 mm on MRI. Dopamine agonist therapy (bromocriptine, cabergoline) should be first line as this is effective in most cases. Transsphenoidal surgery is usually successful for resistant cases, but there is a small recurrence rate. PRL levels are monitored and scans are repeated if there is evidence of tumour growth, e.g. headache, visual field defects.

Macroprolactinomas are >10 mm on MRI. They can be treated with drugs but if there are pressure effects, visual symptoms or pregnancy is considered (25% expand in pregnancy), surgery is usually performed.

Diabetes insipidus

Cranial diabetes insipidus is a rare condition due to deficiency of arginine vasopressin (AVP, also called antidiuretic hormone), one of the hormones released from the posterior pituitary (the other is oxytocin). The differential diagnosis includes nephrogenic diabetes insipidus (i.e. a lack of renal response to adequate circulating vasopressin) and primary polydipsia or excessive drinking. Clinically, the patient presents with polyuria, nocturia and polydipsia. Investigation is outlined in Ch. 15.

Causes of diabetes insipidus

Cranial diabetes insipidus (CDI)

Causes of acquired CDI are given in Fig. 35.15. The most common cause is idiopathic CDI, which may be due to an autoimmune process. Familial CDI is inherited as an

Fig. 35.15 Causes of acquired cranial diabetes insipidus.

Cause	Example
Idiopathic	
Trauma	Head injury and neurosurgery
Tumours	Craniopharyngioma or secondary tumours
Granulomas	Tuberculosis, sarcoid, histiocytosis
Infections	Encephalitis or meningitis

Fig. 35.16 Causes of acquired nephrogenic diabetes insipidus.

Metabolic: hypokalaemia, hypercalcaemia
Chronic renal failure
Lithium toxicity
Post obstructive uropathy
Diabetes mellitus

autosomal dominant trait or as part of the DIDMOAD syndrome (diabetes insipidus, diabetes mellitus, optic atrophy and deafness).

Nephrogenic diabetes insipidus

Familial nephrogenic diabetes insipidus is X-linked recessive or autosomal recessive. It is rare and is due to mutations of the AVP receptor or aquaporin 2 channel protein.

Causes of acquired nephrogenic diabetes insipidus are given in Fig. 35.16.

Treatment

For cranial diabetes insipidus, desmopressin (a vasopressin analogue) is the treatment of choice because it has minimal pressor activity but prolonged antidiuretic potency compared to vasopressin. It may be administered orally, intranasally or parenterally.

For nephrogenic diabetes insipidus, any metabolic and electrolyte disturbances should be corrected and any potential drug causes should be reviewed. In familial forms, thiazide diuretics or indometacin can reduce urine output by up to 50%. NSAIDs may also be useful.

For patients with primary polydipsia, water restriction and treatment of any associated psychiatric disorder is required.

DISORDERS OF THE ADRENAL GLANDS

Histologically, the adrenal glands are divided into the medulla, which secretes adrenaline (epinephrine) and noradrenaline (norepinephrine), and the cortex, which is divided into three zones:

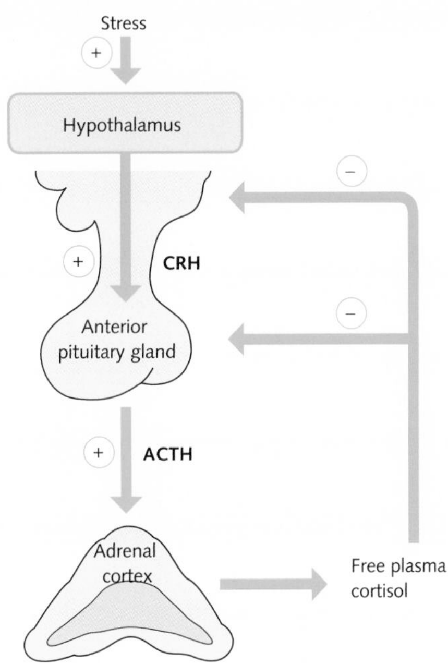

Fig. 35.17 Control of cortisol production via the hypothalamus–pituitary–adrenal axis. ACTH, adrenocorticotrophic hormone; CRH, corticotrophin-releasing hormone.

- The inner zone or zona reticularis produces sex hormones.
- The middle zone or zona fasciculata produces cortisol. Production is stimulated by ACTH released by the pituitary gland. In a negative feedback loop, cortisol reduces both corticotrophin-releasing hormone production in the hypothalamus and pituitary release of ACTH (see Fig. 35.17).
- The outer zona glomerulosa produces aldosterone, which is regulated through the renin–angiotensin system.

Cushing's syndrome

Cushing's syndrome is the result of chronic exposure to excess glucocorticoid. This is most commonly iatrogenic, secondary to glucocorticoid administration given to treat inflammatory diseases. Causes of endogenous Cushing's syndrome include the following:

- Cushing's disease: ACTH hypersecretion by a pituitary adenoma or corticotroph hyperplasia (70%).
- Primary adrenocortical tumours (15–20%).
- Ectopic ACTH syndrome caused by a variety of ACTH-secreting non-pituitary tumours such as small-cell lung carcinoma (10–15%).

The annual incidence of spontaneous Cushing's syndrome is approximately 1 in 100 000 and is three to five times more common in women than men.

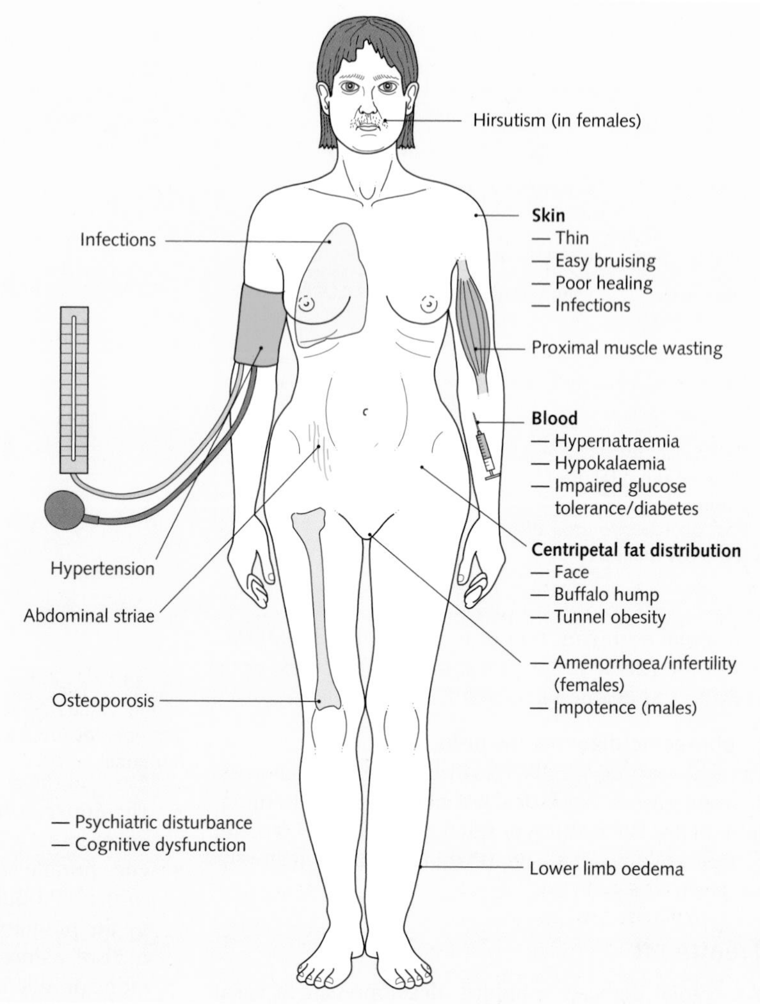

Fig. 35.18 Symptoms and signs of Cushing's syndrome.

Clinical features

The clinical features of Cushing's syndrome are demonstrated in Fig. 35.18. Psychiatric disturbance may range from anxiety to psychosis, and cognitive problems such as short-term memory loss are common.

Investigations

The following investigations are important in Cushing's syndrome.

- Plasma cortisol: this will vary throughout the day in normal individuals and should be measured at 9 a.m. and midnight. Levels will be raised in all causes of Cushing's syndrome.
- 24-h urinary free cortisol: this is a better predictor of Cushing's syndrome than plasma cortisol.
- Plasma ACTH: this will be high in Cushing's disease and ectopic ACTH production, and very low in adrenal cortisol hyperproduction.
- Dexamethasone suppression tests and corticotroph function tests are outlined at the end of the chapter.
- Imaging of the adrenal glands (with CT scan) and the pituitary (with MRI).

A 24-h urinary free cortisol measurement or a low-dose dexamethasone suppression test is the best screening tool but may give false positives in obesity, depression, alcoholism and if the patient is on a hepatic enzyme-inducing drug (as this increases the metabolism of dexamethasone).

Management

Cushing's disease

Trans-sphenoidal surgery is the first line of treatment and is curative in approximately 80% of patients. Pituitary radiotherapy or drugs are used if surgery fails. Metyrapone inhibits steroidogenesis and is the drug of choice. Ketoconazole or mitotane may be used.

Rarely, bilateral adrenalectomy is necessary, although there is a risk of causing Nelson's syndrome, a rapidly enlarging pituitary tumour resulting in hyperpigmentation from excess beta-lipotrophin (see box).

Adrenocortical tumours

Surgical removal of a benign adrenocortical tumour is curative. Bilateral adrenalectomy necessitates replacement therapy with cortisol 20–40 mg daily and fludrocortisone 0.1 mg daily. Carcinomas may recur.

Ectopic ACTH syndrome

Surgical resection of the tumour cures the hypercortisolism, although this is often not possible and medical therapy is used to control cortisol levels.

Addison's disease

Addison's disease is primary adrenocortical failure. The prevalence is approximately 100 per million per year and the incidence is approximately 5 per 1 million per year.

Causes

Causes of Addison's disease include the following:

- Autoimmune adrenal destruction: this accounts for up to 90% of cases in developed countries. Women are affected 2–3 times more often than men. Up to 50% of patients have other autoimmune endocrine deficiencies (see below).
- Infections: worldwide, tuberculosis is a common cause. Cytomegalovirus and fungal infections may cause adrenal failure in the context of HIV/AIDS.
- Adrenal haemorrhage/infarction: this may be associated with sepsis, particularly meningococcal septicaemia – the Waterhouse–Friderichsen syndrome. The presentation is usually acute.
- Metastatic carcinoma: especially from the breast and lung.
- Inherited disorders: there are several familial disorders of adrenal function, which are all rare.

Clinical features

Symptoms and signs of Addison's disease are predominantly caused by cortisol deficiency, although deficiencies of aldosterone and adrenal androgen will also be present to varying extents (Fig. 35.19). The main symptoms are insidious and non-specific: fatigue, weight loss, orthostatic dizziness and anorexia. Patients may present with gastrointestinal symptoms (e.g. abdominal pain, nausea, vomiting and diarrhoea). Hyperpigmentation of the skin and mucous membranes may occur as a result of high beta lipotrophin levels (see box).

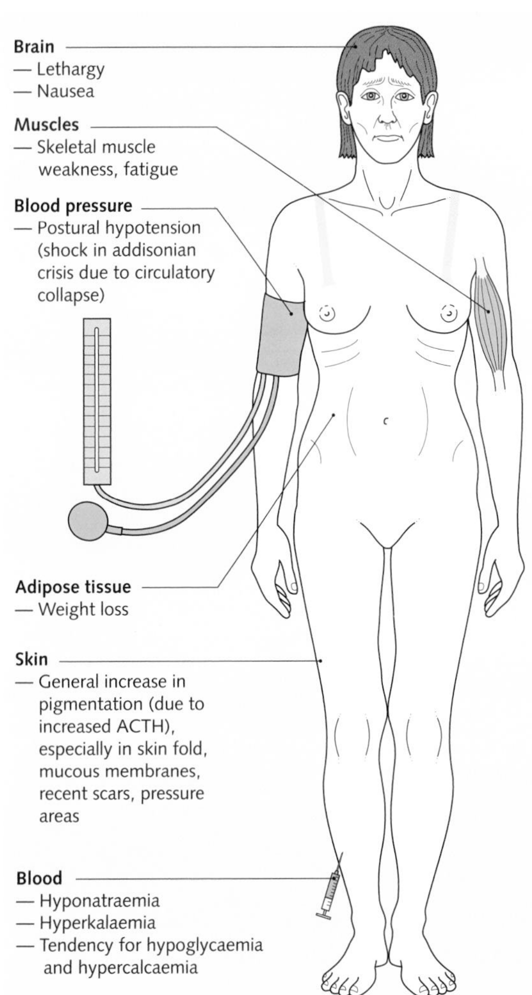

Fig. 35.19 Symptoms and signs of adrenal insufficiency. ACTH, adrenocorticotrophic hormone.

Addisonian crisis may occur with sudden-onset adrenal failure (such as in haemorrhage) or increased cortisol requirements (such as in concurrent infection). There is hypovolaemic shock, often with acidosis and hypoglycaemia as well as the symptoms mentioned above.

HINTS AND TIPS

The ACTH precursor, pro-opio melanocortin, is cleaved to ACTH and beta-lipotrophin, which acts on melanocytes, increasing pigmentation.

Investigations

The following are important investigations in patients with Addison's disease:

- Serum cortisol concentration: low.
- Adrenal autoantibodies are detected in approximately 50% of patients.
- Serum ACTH levels: raised in Addison's disease and low in secondary failure.
- Serum electrolytes: in an impending crisis there may be hyponatraemia, hyperkalaemia and raised blood urea.
- Short and long synacthen tests: described in 'Endocrine investigations' (see below).
- Screening for other autoimmune diseases such as autoimmune thyroid disease.

Management

In emergencies, IV saline and glucose are required. IV hydrocortisone 100 mg 6-hourly is given. Underlying infection must be treated.

Maintenance therapy is with hydrocortisone, usually 20 mg in the mornings and 10 mg in the evenings. The dose of hydrocortisone should be increased during intercurrent illnesses and during surgery. Enzyme-inducing drugs (e.g. phenytoin and rifampicin) may also increase patient requirements for hydrocortisone. Fludrocortisone is used to replace aldosterone because aldosterone taken orally undergoes first-pass metabolism in the liver. The dose is adjusted to maintain blood pressure and potassium levels. The usual dose is about 100 μg daily.

Conn's syndrome (primary hyperaldosteronism)

This is a very rare condition, which is due to a unilateral adrenocortical adenoma in 75% of cases. Other causes include adrenal carcinoma or bilateral hyperplasia of the zona glomerulosa.

Clinical features

The clinical features are due to excess production of aldosterone. Hypertension and hypokalaemia are the principal features. Muscle weakness, polyuria and polydipsia may occur as a result of the hypokalaemia. The diagnosis should be suspected in a patient with hypertension and hypokalaemia when not on a diuretic. Sodium tends to be mildly raised but there is usually no oedema.

Investigations

Serum potassium is low and should be measured while the patient is not on drugs. Urinary potassium is increased for serum blood level. There is usually a metabolic alkalosis. Serum sodium may be mildly raised.

Serum renin is low and serum aldosterone is raised (increased adosterone–renin ratio). Dynamic testing may be required to confirm the diagnosis; a sodium load or fludrocortisone dose is given and the aldosterone levels in serum or urine are measured. Imaging of the adrenals is required following a positive test.

Secondary hyperaldosteronism is a result of high circulating renin. Causes include nephrotic syndrome, heart failure, hepatic failure and bronchial carcinoma.

Management

Tumours should be resected. Spironolactone is an aldosterone antagonist that can be given in primary or secondary aldosteronism.

Phaeochromocytoma

This is a rare tumour arising from the chromaffin tissues of the adrenal medulla, producing catecholamines. Similar tumours may arise from the cells of the sympathetic ganglia. It may be associated with medullary carcinoma of the thyroid, parathyroid adenoma and neurofibromatosis.

HINTS AND TIPS

In phaeochromocytoma 90% are benign and 90% are unilateral.

Clinical features

Symptoms and signs are due to the release of adrenaline (epinephrine) and noradrenaline (norepinephrine). The most common are headache, sweating and hypertension, which may be episodic. Others include pallor, tachycardia and palpitations, nausea, tremor, visual blurring and chest pain. The blood pressure may rise to very high levels and may precipitate a cerebrovascular accident, myocardial infarction or hypertensive encephalopathy. Occasionally, cardiomyopathy occurs with chronic catecholamine exposure.

Investigations

Urine is collected for 24 h for measurement of adrenaline (epinephrine) and noradrenaline (norepinephrine) and metanephrines. An abdominal CT scan may show the tumour. PET-CT or scintigraphy is occasionally used.

Treatment

This is by surgical removal of the tumour. The patient must be fully alpha-blocked with phenoxybenzamine or phentolamine, and beta-blocked with propranolol before surgery to prevent the consequences of release of catecholamines during operation. Changes in pulse and blood pressure should be monitored closely. Alpha-blockade must be achieved before beta-blockade to prevent unopposed alpha-agonism causing severe hypertension.

MISCELLANEOUS ENDOCRINE CONDITIONS

Multiple endocrine neoplasia

There are two main syndromes, both autosomal dominant and both rare. Tumours originate from two or more endocrine glands that produce peptide hormones.

MEN type 1 refers to a predisposition to benign adenomas of parathyroid, pancreatic islet cell/gastrointestinal adenomas and pituitary adenomas. Other tumours are also more common, including thymus, carcinoid and adrenal tumours.

MEN type 2a refers to the association of phaeochromocytoma, medullary carcinoma of the thyroid and parathyroid adenoma or hyperplasia.

In MEN type 2b there is phaeochromocytoma and medullary thyroid cancer, but no parathyroid pathology. There are developmental abnormalities with a marfanoid phenotype and intestinal and visceral ganglioneuromas.

Family members should be screened. In type 1, fasting serum calcium should be measured. In type 2, pentagastrin and calcium infusion tests with measurement of serum calcitonin will detect C-cell hyperplasia. Urinary metanephrines should be measured for phaeochromocytoma.

HINTS AND TIPS

Multiple endocrine neoplasia is a common MCQ question. MEN I is three Ps (Pituitary, Parathyroid and Pancreas), MEN II is two Cs (Catecholamines (i.e. phaeochromocytoma) and medullary Carcinoma of the thyroid) and parathyroid (for MEN IIa) or mucocutaneous neuromas (for MEN IIb).

Autoimmune polyendocrine syndromes

APS type 1 is an autosomal recessively inherited disorder characterized by hypoparathyroidism, adrenal insufficiency and candidiasis. It usually becomes clinically apparent in the second decade. Hypogonadism and gastrointestinal malabsorption also occur frequently.

APS type 2 is more common. Around half of cases are inherited but this may be in a dominant, recessive or polygenic manner. Adrenal insufficiency is the most common feature, often with thyroid disease and diabetes, and there may be a predisposition to non-endocrine autoimmune disease.

Congenital adrenal hyperplasia

These inherited deficiencies of enzymes involved in glucocorticoid synthesis lead to deficiency of cortisol and aldosterone, increased ACTH production and increased synthesis of sex hormones. In children this may present as failure to thrive, ambiguous genitalia in females, and early virilization in males. It may present later with precocious puberty, or in early adulthood with hirsutism and oligomenorrhoea.

Endocrine investigations

Some of the more complex investigations are covered here in more detail.

Diabetes mellitus

Diagnosis

For the interpretation of results of these tests, see Fig. 35.1.

- Random glucose: as the name sounds, a glucose taken at any time. If very high, and symptoms are present, it can diagnose diabetes.
- Fasting glucose: measured in a morning sample following an overnight fast.
- Glucose tolerance test/2-h glucose: a fasting sample is taken first. The patient is then asked to drink a solution with 75 g of glucose, and the blood sample is repeated 2 h later.

Monitoring response to diet or treatment

- Glycated haemoglobin (HbA1c): indicator of glycaemic control over the previous 2–3 months.
- Fructosamine: indicator of overall glycaemic control over the previous 1–3 weeks.

Hypothalamus–pituitary–adrenal axis

Fig. 35.17 summarizes the control of cortisol levels via the hypothalamus–pituitary–adrenal axis. These tests are used to diagnose diseases of glucocorticoid excess (Cushing's disease, ectopic ACTH production, adrenal hyperproduction of cortisol) and glucocorticoid deficiency (pituitary hypoproduction of ACTH and hypoadrenalism).

Dynamic tests for cortisol excess

Overnight dexamethasone suppression test

1 mg oral dexamethasone is taken at midnight; plasma cortisol is measured at 9 a.m. the next morning. In normal patients, ACTH and cortisol production will be suppressed by negative feedback.

In all cases of Cushing's syndrome there is absence of suppression of cortisol. In Cushing's disease the feedback mechanism is less sensitive than normal (see high dose dexamethasone test below). Ectopic ACTH production has no negative feedback mechanism. In adrenocortical tumours, ACTH will already be suppressed and cortisol will remain high.

High-dose dexamethasone suppression test

This is used after other positive tests to differentiate between Cushing's disease and ectopic ACTH production. Plasma cortisol is measured; 2 mg of oral dexamethasone is taken every 6 h for 2 days. After 48 h from the first dose, plasma cortisol is measured again. In normal individuals, the plasma cortisol should be almost undetectable. In Cushing's disease the less sensitive feedback mechanism should be overcome by the high dose, and the cortisol level should fall by at least half. Suppression should not be seen in ectopic ACTH production.

CRH test

Plasma cortisol and ACTH are measured at several intervals shortly following administration of corticotrophin-releasing hormone (CRH). Ectopic ACTH production should not increase, whereas a pituitary adenoma will respond to the CRH, leading to a rise in ACTH and cortisol. This can be used with the high-dose dexamethasone test to improve diagnostic accuracy.

Tests for cortisol deficiency

Short synacthen test

Plasma cortisol is measured and 0.25 mg synacthen (which has the same biological action as ACTH) is given IM or IV. Plasma cortisol is re-measured after 60 min. In normal patients, cortisol will rise by a minimum of 200 nmol/L to at least 500 nmol/L. The response will be poor in any cause of hypoadrenalism.

Long synacthen test

In this test, 1 mg of synacthen is given by IM injection daily for 3 days. Hypoadrenalism due to adrenal gland atrophy as a result of chronic steroid treatment or secondary hypoadrenalism show a response to this level of stimulation. No response will be seen in adrenal hypofunction.

CRH test

This can be used to look for secondary hypopituitarism. There will be a poor response to CRH administration.

Pituitary function tests

If suspected, initial blood tests should include TSH, T_4, T_3, prolactin, growth hormone and insulin-like growth factor-1, luteinizing and follicle-stimulating hormones, testosterone and cortisol. Pituitary fossa imaging is then undertaken (e.g. CT/MRI or lateral skull X-ray). Dynamic tests are sometimes needed:

- Insulin tolerance test: this is used to assess ACTH or GH deficiency. A bolus of insulin is given to cause hypoglycaemia and stimulate ACTH and GH release. A baseline blood sample for GH, cortisol and glucose is taken. A fast-acting insulin is then given and further blood samples taken at intervals. Glucose <2.2 mmol/L must be achieved. Cortisol and GH should rise.

Further reading

Endobible – Advice on endocrine symptoms, diagnosis, treatment: a free online diagnostic and management tool and educational resource authored by a consultant endocrinologist. Available online at: http://www.endobible.com.

Finlayson, A., 2007. Crash Course: Endocrine and Reproductive Systems, third ed. Elsevier Mosby, Edinburgh.

National Institute for Health and Clinical Excellence (NICE), 2004. Type 1 diabetes. Clinical guideline CG15. Available online at: http://www.nice.org.uk/CG15.

National Institute for Health and Clinical Excellence (NICE), 2006. Obesity. Clinical guideline CG43. Available online at: http://www.nice.org.uk/CG43.

National Institute for Health and Clinical Excellence (NICE), 2008. Type 2 diabetes. Clinical guideline CG66. Available online at: http://www.nice.org.uk/CG66.

National Institute for Health and Clinical Excellence (NICE), 2009. Type 2 diabetes – newer agents. Clinical guideline CG87. Available online at: http://www.nice.org.uk/CG87.

World Health Organization, 2006. Definition and diagnosis of diabetes mellitus and intermediate hyperglycaemia. World Health Organization, Geneva.

Musculoskeletal and skin disorders 36

Objectives

The key learning points for this chapter:

- The differentiation of inflammatory arthritis from osteoarthritis.
- The extra-articular problems associated with rheumatoid arthritis.
- The presentation of ankylosing spondylitis and other seronegative arthritides.
- How to differentiate polymyalgia rheumatica from polymyositis.
- The multisystem nature of systemic lupus erythematosus.
- The rationale for and approach to modern therapy in rheumatoid arthritis.
- The diagnosis and management of eczema and psoriasis.
- How to recognize erythema nodosum and the conditions with which it is associated.
- The diagnoses of systemic sclerosis and CREST, their similarities and differences.
- Differentiating the various types of skin malignancy.

RHEUMATOID ARTHRITIS

Rheumatoid arthritis (RA) is a systemic disease producing a symmetrical inflammatory deforming polyarthropathy with extra-articular involvement of many organs. It affects around 1% of Caucasian populations and is three times more common in women than in men. The peak age of onset is between 50 and 70 years, although it can start at almost any age. There is often a family history and there is an association with certain HLA serotypes, particularly HLA-DR4. There is a significant autoimmune component, but the nature of the interaction between genes and environment that triggers the inflammatory process remains unclear.

Pathological features

The classic findings are chronic synovitis, with oedema and inflammatory infiltrate, followed by the formation of pannus, composed of inflammatory T cells, granulocytes, fibroblasts and granulation tissue. Pannus erodes cartilage, bone and tendons. In all phases of RA, soft tissue inflammation surrounds the joint, giving rise to one of its characteristic features. Rheumatoid nodules are granulomata with a central zone of fibrinoid necrosis, surrounded by macrophages, lymphocytes and fibroblasts. These are usually subcutaneous, the most common site being the extensor surfaces, especially the elbows. They can occur in other tissues (e.g. lungs, heart and sclera). They imply that the patient is rheumatoid factor positive. Patients with severe disease are at risk of developing vasculitis, usually of small to medium-sized vessels.

Clinical features

RA usually presents with an insidious onset of pain and stiffness in the small joints of the hands and feet. There is associated joint swelling and there may be progression to involve larger joints. Less common presentations include a relapsing and remitting arthritis of changing joint areas (palindromic rheumatism), a persistent monoarthritis, systemic features before joint problems are apparent, and an acute onset of widespread arthritis, especially in the elderly.

General features of the disease may precede joint involvement and include general malaise and fatigue. Signs affecting the joints are described in Ch. 19. The metacarpophalangeal joints, proximal interphalangeal (PIP) joints and wrists are most commonly affected (Fig. 36.1). Initially there is joint swelling, which may progress to subluxation of joints and deformities. There is wasting of small muscles resulting from disuse, vasculitis and peripheral neuropathy. There may be tenosynovitis and bursitis; rheumatoid nodules are present in approximately 20% of patients. The feet are similarly affected.

Atlantoaxial subluxation may give rise to neurological signs and spinal cord compression. Extra-articular manifestations are summarized in Fig. 36.2.

Investigations

The diagnosis of rheumatoid arthritis is made on a combination of clinical and laboratory findings. Investigations are discussed in Ch. 19. They should include:

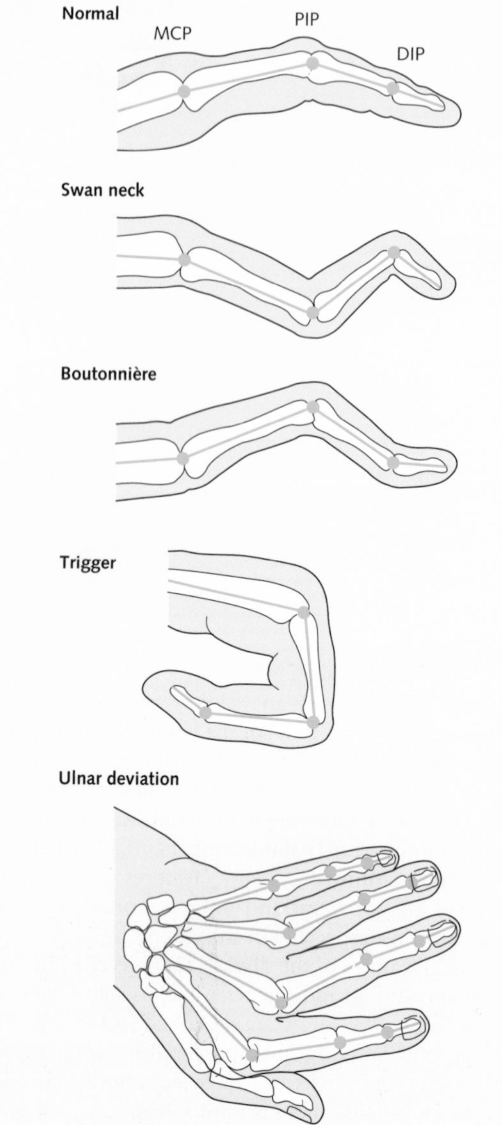

Fig. 36.1 Finger and hand abnormalities in rheumatoid arthritis. DIP, distal interphalangeal joint; MCP, metacarpophalangeal joint; PIP, proximal interphalangeal joint.

- Full blood count (anaemia of chronic disease, thrombocytosis or thrombocytopenia, leucopenia). Renal and liver function tests may help exclude other causes and will help with drug dosing. Potential causes of anaemia in rheumatoid arthritis are outlined in Fig. 36.3.
- Erythrocyte sedimentation rate (ESR).
- Rheumatoid factor, antinuclear antibodies and other autoantibodies including anticyclic citrullinated peptide (anti-CCP).
- Joint X-rays, especially of hands, wrists and feet: to aid in diagnosis and to monitor baseline at presentation.
- Aspiration of synovial fluid, if appropriate.

Management

The aims of treatment are to control symptoms, to maintain a normal life and to modify the underlying disease process and inflammation. Physiotherapy will help to keep joints mobile, strengthen muscles and prevent deformities. Surgery may be required to correct deformities (e.g. the repair of tendons, joint prostheses and arthrodesis). Resting the joints will relieve pain, and splints can help prevent deformities.

Drug treatment

While the initial measures should include analgesia with paracetamol or preferably a non-steroidal anti-inflammatory drug (NSAID), the early use of disease-modifying antirheumatic drugs (DMARDs) is considered best practice. The aim is to slow disease progression, slow joint destruction and maintain function. Several drugs that modify inflammatory cytokines are now available. Corticosteroids remain useful and effective but have numerous long-term side effects.

Non-steroidal anti-inflammatory drugs

These drugs have both analgesic and anti-inflammatory effects but do not alter disease progression. They inhibit the cyclo-oxygenase (COX) enzymes, of which there are two main isoforms: COX-2 is the inducible isoform responsible for inflammation, whereas COX-1 is constitutive and thought to produce the beneficial effects of prostaglandins. There are two categories of NSAID; drugs in the first, such as ibuprofen and diclofenac, inhibit both COX enzymes, reducing the production of prostaglandins in all tissues. They can have side effects, commonly gastrointestinal (including peptic ulceration, gastritis and haemorrhage), renal impairment and fluid retention. They should be used with caution in the elderly, during pregnancy and breastfeeding, and in coagulation defects. To reduce side effects they should be taken with food and combined with a proton pump inhibitor.

The second category is the selective COX-2 inhibitors (celecoxib). They are effective anti-inflammatory agents with a better side-effect profile in reducing gastrointestinal complications. However, their use has been associated with increased cardiovascular mortality and they should only be used when regular NSAIDs cannot be given.

Fig. 36.2 Organ systems affected by rheumatoid arthritis.

Organ system	Effects
Eyes	Sjögren's syndrome occurs in 15% of patients Scleritis causes a painful red eye, and may lead to uveitis and glaucoma Scleromalacia perforans is an uncommon complication where a rheumatoid nodule in the sclera perforates
Nervous system	Carpal tunnel syndrome (most common) Peripheral neuropathy causing glove and stocking sensory loss and occasionally motor weakness Mononeuritis multiplex due to vasculitis of vessels supplying nerves Atlantoaxial subluxation resulting in spinal cord compression
Lymphoreticular system	Generalized lymphadenopathy and splenomegaly may be present Felty's syndrome (seropositive arthritis, neutropenia and splenomegaly)
Blood	Normochromic normocytic anaemia or iron-deficiency anaemia (see Ch. 26) Raised ESR; CRP may be modestly raised or normal Reactive thrombocytosis
Respiratory system	Pleural effusions (more common in men) Rheumatoid nodules Diffuse fibrosing alveolitis Caplan's syndrome (the presence of large rheumatoid nodules and fibrosis in patients with RA exposed to various industrial dusts)
Cardiac	Pericarditis and pericardial effusions may occur
Skin	Vasculitis may produce nail-fold infarcts, ulcers and digital gangrene Peripheral oedema may be present and is due to increased vascular permeability
Kidneys	Secondary amyloidosis may affect the kidneys, leading to proteinuria, nephrotic syndrome and renal failure

CRP, C-reactive protein; ESR, erythrocyte sedimentation rate; RA, rheumatoid arthritis.

Fig. 36.3 Causes of anaemia in rheumatoid arthritis.

Anaemia of chronic disease
Hypersplenism due to splenomegaly (Felty's syndrome if also neutropenic)
Chronic blood loss from peptic ulceration due to steroid and NSAID administration
Bone marrow suppression by disease-modifying drugs such as gold and penicillamine
Folate deficiency (increased utilization of folate)

NSAID, non-steroidal anti-inflammatory drug.

Conventional disease-modifying anti-rheumatic drugs

DMARDs should now be considered early after the diagnosis of RA is made; the aim is to slow the disease process, maintaining structure and function. The most common drugs are methotrexate, sulfasalazine and ciclosporin. Current guidance suggests starting treatment with a combination of DMARDs where possible, which should include methotrexate unless it is contraindicated.

Methotrexate is a folate antagonist used in cancer chemotherapy. When taken once weekly, it has a powerful disease-modifying effect on RA, often seen within 4 weeks. Its side effects include gastrointestinal, hepatic, bone marrow and pulmonary toxicity; hence, a regular full blood count and liver function tests are needed. It is contraindicated in pregnancy.

Sulfasalazine is an effective DMARD but can be limited by side effects, including rashes, gastrointestinal intolerance, bone marrow suppression and hepatitis.

Ciclosporin is a calcineurin inhibitor. Leflunomide is a further immunomodulating drug acting through inhibition of pyrimidine synthesis.

The antimalarial drugs hydroxychloroquine and chloroquine can be used as DMARDs and are better tolerated. However, they are less effective against more severe RA. Retinopathy is a rare side effect. Gold and penicillamine are now rarely used.

Corticosteroids

The short-term use of corticosteroids for rapid symptomatic control in new-onset RA or flares of disease is well established. They are given alongside DMARDs, but the dose is tapered as soon as possible to avoid adverse effects. In a small percentage of patients, withdrawing steroids completely will cause a flare of disease, and these patients may be reliant on long-term low-dose steroids. Low-dose prednisolone may reduce the rate of joint destruction in moderate-to-severe RA of less than 2 years' duration, and possibly has a small disease-modifying effect in established disease. Corticosteroids may also be given intra-articularly to relieve pain, increase mobility and reduce deformity in one or a few joints.

Biological agents

In recent years there has been a huge increase in the number of agents targeted at specific molecules involved in the inflammatory response. The first to become widely used were tumour necrosis factor alpha (TNF-α) inhibitors, but agents against a wide array of cytokines have been developed. They are added to treatment when conventional DMARDs do not adequately control disease. Side effects are mainly due to suppression of the immune response and hypersensitivity.

- TNF-α inhibitors: TNF-α is a potent proinflammatory cytokine thought to be important in RA. Etanercept is a recombinant TNF-receptor protein which binds TNF-α. Infliximab, adalimumab, certolizumab and golimumab are monoclonal antibodies against TNF-α. They often produce marked improvement in patients with poorly controlled disease. The main concern is infection, especially reactivation of TB. They are expensive and current UK practice is to use them in patients with active RA not responding to at least two DMARDs, including methotrexate.
- B-cell inhibition: rituximab is a monoclonal antibody that selectively depletes CD20-positive B cells and is used in lymphomas. It is used with methotrexate in severe RA when treatment with other agents, including at least one TNF-α inhibitor, is unsuccessful.
- Other agents: tocilizumab, a monoclonal antibody targeting interleukin-6 (IL-6), is licensed for treatment when other agents have failed. Anakinra, an IL-1 receptor antagonist, and abatacept, a T-cell modulator, are not currently used outside clinical trials.

Surgery

Joint replacement may be indicated for severe pain or functional limitation despite maximal medical therapy. The timing of the decision to proceed with surgery is often difficult; if there is significant muscle atrophy, the patient may not benefit from the joint replacement.

Prognosis

RA is not just a joint disease limiting quality of life. It is a systemic disease that in its most severe form causes multi-organ dysfunction and shortens life. The life expectancy of patients whose joint disease does not remit with therapy is on average 15 years less than similar patients without RA.

OSTEOARTHRITIS

Osteoarthritis (OA) is the most common joint condition and affects approximately half the population by the age of 60 years. OA is a degenerative disorder affecting mainly the weight-bearing joints (e.g. the hips and knees). It is predominantly a disease of cartilage, which becomes eroded and progressively thinned as the disease proceeds. Risk factors include age, family history, obesity and female gender. People in certain occupations or sports players may be predisposed to OA in specific joints. It may also be secondary to other joint conditions and trauma.

Clinical features

Clinical signs and symptoms are described in Ch. 19. Joints commonly affected by OA include the hips, knees, distal interphalangeal (DIP) joints, first metacarpophalangeal (MCP) and metatarsophalangeal (MTP) joints, and lumbar and cervical spine. There is pain in affected joints, which is worse with movement and towards the end of the day, superimposed on a background of pain at rest. Morning stiffness may occur but usually lasts less than 30 min. The joints are stiff, immobile and deformed.

On examination, there may be swelling due to bony protuberances or joint effusions, crepitus on movement, limited joint movement and deformities. In some patients there will be a degree of inflammation. The pattern of joint involvement tends to be asymmetrical. In the hands, the most commonly affected joints are the DIP joints (Heberden's nodes), PIP joints (Bouchard's nodes) and first carpometacarpal joints, giving an appearance of 'square hands'. Unlike RA, there are no extra-articular manifestations of the disease.

Investigations

There are no biochemical abnormalities. Diagnosis is based on clinical findings and radiological changes of loss of joint space, subchondral sclerosis, subchondral cysts and marginal osteophytes (Fig. 36.4).

Management

Treatment options include combinations of drugs, physical treatments (e.g. weight reduction and heat application), electrotherapy (TENS), exercises, aids (e.g. walking sticks, special footwear, joint supports) and surgery (e.g. arthrodesis, arthroplasty, joint replacement).

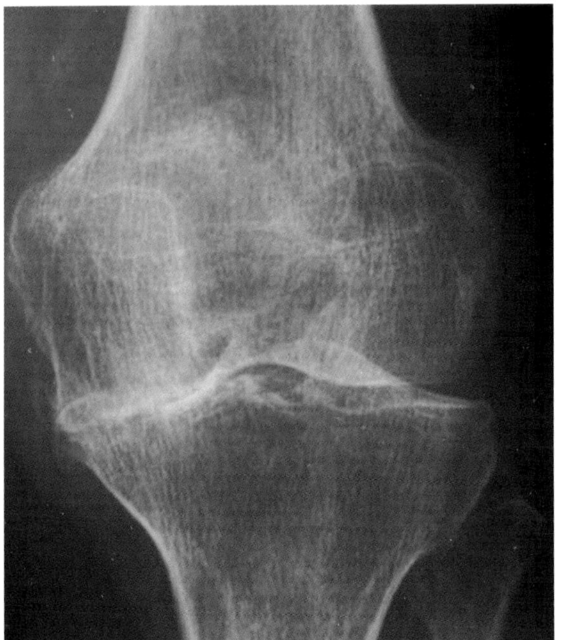

Fig. 36.4 Knee X-ray showing severe osteoarthritis with joint space narrowing and osteophyte formation in the medial site. Reprinted from Ko-Jen Li, Song-Chou Hsieh. Clinical Application of Musculoskeletal Ultrasound in Rheumatic Diseases. Journal of Medical Ultrasound. 2011 19(3):73–80, with permission from Elsevier.

Initially, simple analgesia (e.g. paracetamol) and topical NSAIDs should be prescribed for the pain. Oral NSAIDs are given if simple analgesia is not effective, and sometimes opioid analgesia is required. Intra-articular corticosteroids can be used for inflammatory exacerbations. Glucosamine, chondroitin and intra-articular hyaluronan are not currently recommended for the treatment of OA. Joint replacement is helpful in severe cases where pain is debilitating and unresponsive to other measures.

SPONDYLOARTHROPATHIES

This term (often replaced with 'seronegative arthritis') describes a group of related diseases with some common features including inflammation of joints of the axial skeleton, asymmetrical oligoarthritis and enthesitis. There is an association with HLA-B27 with familial clustering of cases. The following diseases are included:

- Ankylosing spondylitis.
- Reactive arthritis.
- Enteropathic arthritis.
- Psoriatic arthritis.
- Juvenile chronic arthritis.
- Undifferentiated spondyloarthropathy.

Ankylosing spondylitis

This most commonly affects young men (sex ratio 2:1) with a prevalence of approximately 1 in 2000. HLA-B27 is present in over 90% of patients.

Clinical features

The onset is insidious, with lumbar spinal involvement causing low back pain, and sacroiliitis causing pain in the buttocks or thighs, which may radiate down the back of the legs. The pain is typical for inflammatory pain with associated morning stiffness and improvement on exercise. Progressive spinal fusion and loss of movement occurs; eventually the patient has a fixed kyphotic spine, hyperextended neck, spinocranial ankylosis and a reduction in chest expansion, leading to a 'question mark' posture (Fig. 36.5). The hips are commonly affected, and other large joints may be involved in an asymmetrical distribution. Peripheral joints may also be affected, and dactylitis (causing 'sausage digits') is sometimes a feature. Enthesitis (inflammation of tendon insertions) often occurs at the Achilles, the supraspinatus tendon and the costochondral junctions. Extra-articular features include:

- General malaise.
- Uveitis: in approximately a third of cases.
- Bowel mucosal ulceration (in around 50%, usually asymptomatic) and inflammatory bowel disease.
- Aortic regurgitation: due to aortitis.
- Respiratory failure: secondary to kyphoscoliosis, rigidity and apical fibrosis.
- Neurological involvement such as cauda equina syndrome (in long-standing ankylosis), spinal cord compression (with atlantoaxial subluxation) or nerve root compression.

Investigations

The diagnosis of AS is made largely on features of the history and examination. The following investigations are useful and should be performed:

- ESR and C-reactive protein (CRP): often raised and may be useful for monitoring.
- HLA-B27: provides useful supporting evidence but it is also present in the healthy population.
- X-rays: sacroiliitis is indicated by irregular margins and sclerosis of adjacent bone; in long-standing disease, the classic finding is 'bamboo' spine with squaring of the vertebrae and calcification and ossification of intervertebral ligaments. In early disease these changes may not be present and MRI/CT may be useful if the diagnosis is not clear.

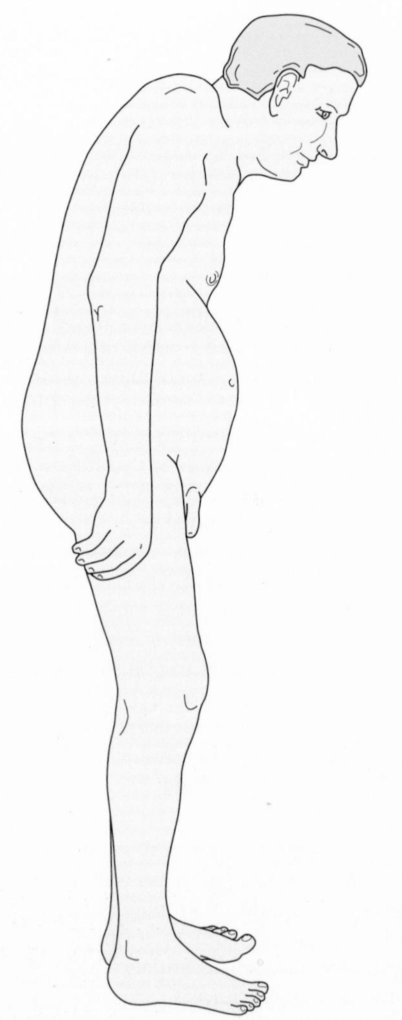

Fig. 36.5 Advancing ankylosing spondylitis. Eventually the trunk may become fixed in a fully flexed position, so that the patient cannot see directly ahead – the classic 'question mark' posture.

HINTS AND TIPS

Remember the extra-articular 'A's complicating ankylosing spondylitis:

- Apical fibrosis.
- Aortic regurgitation.
- Aortitis.
- Anterior uveitis.
- Achilles tendonitis and other enthesitides.
- Amyloidosis.

Management

Treatment includes analgesia with NSAIDs. Patients should be encouraged to exercise to prevent deformity, maintain movement and relieve symptoms. Sulfasalazine improves symptoms due to peripheral arthritis and morning stiffness; methotrexate is not effective in AS. TNF inhibitors have been shown to be effective and are used in severe disease. Although the majority of patients will be able to maintain a normal lifestyle, the prognosis is variable. The disease may be progressive, it may remit, or there may be recurrent episodes. In extreme cases, respiratory function may be impaired because of immobility of the spine and ribcage.

Reactive arthritis

Reactive arthritis occurs several days to weeks after enteritis or urethritis due to particular causative organisms, mainly *Salmonella, Yersinia, Campylobacter, Shigella* or *Chlamydia trachomatis*. When it occurs with non-specific urethritis (NSU) and conjunctivitis, and was formerly referred to as Reiter's syndrome. It usually affects young adults and is around 10 times more common in men than women, though this may be partly due to underdiagnosis.

Clinical features

The arthritis is often of acute onset, oligoarticular and asymmetrical, particularly affecting the lower limbs. It may be associated with non-articular inflammatory lesions, including plantar fasciitis and Achilles tendinitis. Other clinical features include:

- Urethritis: associated with penile discharge and dysuria. There may be circinate balanitis (an erythematous circular lesion on the glans with a pale centre).
- Conjunctivitis: usually mild and bilateral; iritis and anterior uveitis may also occur.
- Mouth ulcers.
- Keratoderma blennorrhagica: a pustular hyperkeratotic lesion on the soles of the feet.
- Nail dystrophy and subungual keratosis.
- General malaise and low-grade fever.
- Cardiovascular, respiratory and neurological complications are rare.

Investigations

The diagnosis is clinical and common autoantibodies are negative. Joint aspiration may help exclude septic and crystal arthritis. Evidence of the triggering infection should be sought with urine and faecal culture and urethral swabs, although these are often negative. HLA-B27 is positive in 60% of patients. X-rays do not aid the diagnosis of reactive arthritis.

Management

Treatment is symptomatic with analgesia (e.g. NSAIDs) and rest of affected joints. Painful effusions can be aspirated. Intra-articular or systemic steroids can be used in the acute phase, but if sustained treatment is needed sulfasalazine or methotrexate may be helpful. In most cases, the acute arthritis settles within 1–2 months; mild symptoms may persist for 6–12 months, but less than 10% develop chronic disease.

Psoriatic arthritis

This is a seronegative arthritis occurring in 10–15% of patients with psoriasis; in a minority of patients it precedes the skin condition. There are 5 clinical subtypes: distal arthritis alone, symmetrical polyarthritis (RA-like), axial arthritis (AS-like), asymmetrical oligoarthritis and arthritis mutilans. Distal arthritis is often considered the most specific feature and is probably the most common presenting pattern. However, the subtypes are not clear-cut, and over time the pattern may change in the same patient. There is nail pitting and onycholysis. Pitting oedema is sometimes present, and as with other seronegative arthritides enthesitis, dactylitis and eye signs may occur.

Radiology shows marginal erosions with new bone formation. Treatment is with analgesia and anti-inflammatory drugs. DMARDs and anti-TNF therapies may be effective and are used in severe cases.

Enteropathic arthropathies

These occur in patients with inflammatory bowel disease and usually affect the knees and ankles as a monoarthritis or asymmetrical oligoarthritis. Spondylitis and socroiliitis may occur. The aetiology is unknown, but the breakdown of mucosal integrity and subsequent exposure to multiple enteric bacteria may cause expansion of self-directed lymphocytes. Management should be aimed at the underlying bowel disease, which will usually improve the arthritis. NSAIDs and joint aspiration will provide symptomatic relief. In severe cases immunomodulatory treatment is sometimes required.

CRYSTAL ARTHROPATHY

Gout

Gout is a result of the deposition of sodium urate crystals in joints and soft tissues due to an abnormality of uric acid metabolism, affecting approximately 1 in 500 people in the UK. The risk is greater in men, those with high alcohol intake, hypertensives and the overweight. About a third have a positive family history. The underlying biochemical abnormality is an overproduction or underexcretion of uric acid resulting in hyperuricaemia. The main causes are given in Fig. 36.6.

Clinical features

Acute gout

The initial attack is typically in the first metatarsophalangeal joint with an acute onset of a red, hot, swollen, extremely painful big toe. It may be precipitated by alcohol, diet, starvation, diuretics or after surgery. A minority of patients have a polyarticular initial attack. In recurrent episodes other commonly affected areas include the ankle, wrist, knees and bursae. The patient may have high blood pressure, renal impairment or peripheral vascular disease. The renal disease may be secondary to uric acid stones.

COMMUNICATION

Patients with acute gout will often graphically describe the severity of their discomfort. It is a very painful condition.

Chronic tophaceous gout

In this stage of disease, which is now less frequent with effective treatment, there are deposits of urate in connective tissues, often visible on the helix of the ear or around joints (particularly hands and elbows). This causes joint erosion and disruption, leading to chronic arthritis and disability.

Fig. 36.6 Causes of gout.

Idiopathic
Drugs: diuretics, low-dose aspirin
Chronic renal impairment
Hypertension
Primary hyperparathyroidism
Hypothyroidism
Alcohol
Glucose-6-phosphate deficiency
Rapid cell turnover or destruction:
- Myeloproliferative disorders, e.g. polycythaemia rubra vera
- Lymphoproliferative disorders, e.g. leukaemia
- Severe psoriasis
- Tumour lysis syndrome, e.g. with initiation of chemotherapy

Investigations

The following investigations are important in patients with gout:

- Joint aspiration is the definitive test and helps exclude septic arthritis in the single hot swollen joint. Synovial fluid examined under polarized light microscopy shows needle-shaped, negatively birefringent crystals.
- X-rays may be normal in acute gout but show punched-out erosions and joint disruption in chronic gout.
- Serum uric acid may be high but there are a large number of false-positive and false-negative results. It is more useful for monitoring treatment.
- White cell count, CRP and ESR may be mildly raised in an acute attack.

Management

Acute attacks

These are normally treated with high doses of non-steroidal anti-inflammatory drugs (NSAIDs) such as naproxen 500 mg b.d. or ibuprofen 400 mg t.d.s. They should be used with care in patients with peptic ulcer disease, heart failure, hypertension and renal impairment.

When NSAIDs are contraindicated, colchicine can be used and is probably as effective, but often causes diarrhoea. If neither colchicine nor NSAIDs can be tolerated, steroids may be used. Intra-articular injection of steroid into an affected joint often provides symptomatic relief.

Prophylactic treatment

The patient should be advised on weight reduction, reducing alcohol consumption, avoiding precipitating foods such as red meat and avoiding precipitating drugs if possible.

If the patient has recurrent attacks, tophi, a documented state of uric acid overproduction (e.g. myeloproliferative disease) or renal disease, uric-acid-lowering drug therapy is indicated. The initiation of treatment may precipitate an acute attack; therefore, colchicine or NSAIDs should be used prophylactically for at least 1 month after the hyperuricaemia has been corrected. Uric acid lowering drugs should not be started during an acute attack.

Allopurinol and febuxostat inhibit xanthine oxidase, which catalyses the conversion of hypoxanthine to xanthine and of xanthine to uric acid. Allupurinol is the first-line treatment for prevention of gout, and is usually given once daily (initially 100 mg after food) and gradually increased to a maintenance dose of about 300 mg daily. Lower doses are given in patients with renal impairment. It may cause skin rashes.

Uricosuric drugs include probenecid and sulphinpyrazone. They may be used in patients with normal renal function when allopurinol is not tolerated. Aspirin antagonizes the effect of uricosuric drugs. They may lead to crystallization of urate in the urine and formation of urate stones, particularly in patients with disease of urate overproduction.

Rasburicase, a synthetic uricase which converts urate to allantoin, is used for prevention of gout and urate nephropathy in patients at risk of tumour lysis syndrome during chemotherapy.

Pseudogout

This is also known as calcium pyrophosphate dihydrate arthropathy and risk factors include old age, hyperparathyroidism, haemochromatosis, hypothyroidism and low phosphate or magnesium levels.

Acute attacks present with a monoarthritis or oligoarthritis, usually affecting the knees, hips or wrists, in contrast to gout. It is usually self-limiting and can be precipitated by an intercurrent illness. Chronic disease causes joint changes similar to osteoarthritis (but more severe) and may cause a polyarthritis.

Joint aspiration demonstrates the presence of crystals that are weakly positively birefringent in polarized light, and X-rays may reveal chondrocalcinosis in affected joints. Management is symptomatic with NSAIDs or colchicine and therapeutic joint aspiration. Intra-articular steroid injections are often helpful, and in chronic disease hydroxychloroquine can be considered. Any predisposing underlying conditions should be treated.

SYSTEMIC LUPUS ERYTHEMATOSUS

Systemic lupus erythematosus (SLE) is a multisystem, autoimmune connective tissue disorder. The prevalence in the UK is approximately 1 in 1000. It is around nine times more common in women and also more common in Asians and Afro-Caribbean people. Median age at onset in white women is between 30 and 50. The aetiology is unknown but is probably multifactorial; there is evidence of a genetic predisposition and environmental triggers (e.g. drugs such as hydralazine, ultraviolet light and viral infections) may have a role.

Clinical features

Common early features include fever, arthralgia, malaise, tiredness and weight loss. There is a huge spectrum of disease and any of the following systems may be involved.

Musculoskeletal system

This is involved in over 90% of cases. Arthralgia is usually symmetrical and migratory. Morning stiffness is milder than in RA, and examination findings may be mild compared to the symptoms. Erosive arthritis is rare. Myalgia and myositis can occur, and rarely there is a deforming arthropathy due to capsular laxity (Jaccoud's arthropathy). Aseptic necrosis affecting the hip or knee may rarely occur.

Skin

This is involved in approximately 80% of cases. Classically there is a 'butterfly' rash over the bridge of the nose and spreading over both cheeks (Fig. 36.7). Other features include photosensitivity, alopecia, livedo reticularis, Raynaud's phenomenon, nail-fold infarcts, purpura, urticaria and oral ulceration.

Subacute cutaneous lupus erythematosus (SCLE) is a subtype in which cutaneous symptoms predominate, although in around 50% of patients other organs are affected.

Discoid lesions may develop in SLE or may exist alone as discoid lupus erythematosus (DLE). There are discoid erythematous plaques on the face that progress to scarring and pigmentation; 5–10% of these patients develop mild systemic disease.

Nervous system

The central nervous system (CNS) is involved in 60% of cases. Psychiatric disturbances include depression and occasionally psychosis. Other features include:

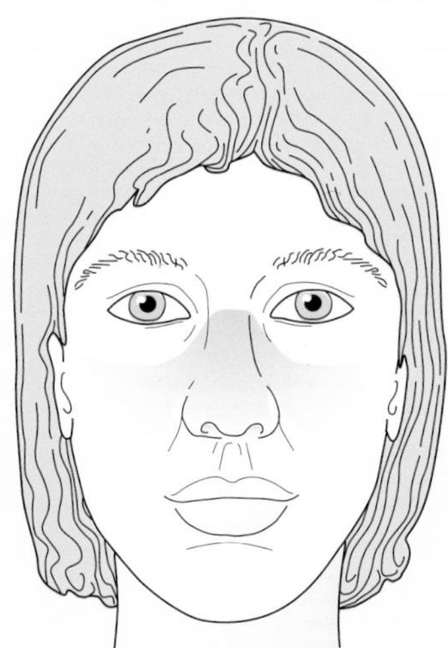

Fig. 36.7 Systemic lupus erythematosus showing the classic 'bat' or 'butterfly wing' rash.

- Seizures.
- Strokes.
- Peripheral neuropathies.
- Headache.
- Cognitive dysfunction.

Less common features include cranial nerve lesions and aseptic meningitis. Neurological involvement is likely due to vasculopathy, causing ischaemia, or autoantibody-mediated disease.

Respiratory system

The respiratory system is involved in approximately 50% of cases. Pulmonary manifestations include:

- Pleurisy with pleural effusions.
- Pneumonitis.
- Interstitial lung disease and 'shrinking lung syndrome' (reduced lung volumes but normal imaging).

Renal system

The renal system is involved in approximately 50% of cases and is associated with a poor prognosis. The patient may present with nephrotic or nephritic syndrome, hypertension or chronic renal failure. Proteinuria and haematuria are common. There are six main patterns of glomerular disease associated with immune complex deposition. Tubulointerstitial nephritis and renovascular disease may also occur.

Cardiovascular system

The cardiovascular system is involved in 40% of cases. There may be:

- Pericarditis with pericardial effusion.
- Myocarditis with consequent heart failure.
- Aortic valve lesions.
- Non-bacterial endocarditis of the mitral valve (Libman–Sacks endocarditis).

Blood and lymphatic systems

The ESR is markedly raised. There may be:

- Normochromic normocytic anaemia.
- Leucopenia.
- Thrombocytopenia.
- Haemolytic anaemia (rare).
- Generalized lymphadenopathy
- Splenomegaly ± hepatomegaly.
- Arterial and venous thrombosis. This may be part of the antiphospholipid syndrome.

Investigations

Diagnosis is often made using the American College of Rheumatology criteria (see Fig. 36.8). The following investigations are important in patients with SLE:

- Inflammatory markers: ESR is raised. CRP is usually normal.
- There may be anaemia, leukopenia or thrombocytopenia.
- Renal function, liver function, simple urinalysis and urine protein/creatinine ratio.
- Antinuclear antibody: positive in almost all cases (classically a homogeneous pattern) but not specific. Anti-double-stranded DNA (present in 75%) and anti-Sm (present in 25%) are more specific. The titres of anti-dsDNA rise in active disease.
- Serum complement levels are often reduced in active disease. Total immunoglobulins are raised.
- Renal biopsy: if there is involvement of the kidneys, renal biopsy shows characteristic histological changes, which can predict prognosis and guide treatment.

Treatment

General advice should be to quit smoking, which may increase active disease, and avoid sun exposure or use sunblock. Joint pain, headache or mild serositis can be managed with NSAIDs in patients with less severe disease. If necessary, anaemia can be corrected with transfusion. For acute exacerbations, steroids are given in high doses and gradually reduced depending on symptoms, signs and changes in ESR.

Immunosuppressive drugs are used for patients with more serious disease, such as with renal or CNS involvement, as they have a steroid-sparing effect. Drugs used include azathioprine, chlorambucil and cyclophosphamide, and there may be a role for the anti-CD20 molecule rituximab.

In some patients in whom NSAIDs are ineffective in controlling joint pain, or in whom skin manifestations predominate, the antimalarial drug hydroxychloroquine may be useful. It can cause retinal degeneration, so vision should be formally assessed at regular intervals.

Fig. 36.8 SOAPBRAIN MD. The ACR diagnostic criteria for SLE.

Serositis	Pleuritis or pericarditis
Oral ulceration	Oral or nasopharyngeal
Arthralgia	Involving more than 1 joint
Photosensitivity	Rash in reaction to sunlight
Blood abnormalities	Anaemia, leucopenia or thrombocytopenia
Renal involvemement	Proteinuria or casts
Antinuclear antibodies	Abnormal ANA titre
Immunological abnormalities	Antiphospholipid antibodies, anti-dsDNA or anti-Sm
Neurological involvement	Seizures or psychosis
Malar rash	Typical rash over bridge of nose and malar eminences
Discoid lesions	Raised patches with scaling

Four or more features are required.

Drug-induced lupus

Drug-induced lupus may occur with hydralazine in people who are genetically 'slow acetylators', and with procainamide, isoniazid, chlorpromazine and anticonvulsants. It remits when the drug is stopped. Renal and CNS involvement is rare. Anti-histone antibodies are present in over 95% of cases.

ANTIPHOSPHOLIPID SYNDROME

This condition manifests as an increased risk of arterial and venous thromboses and miscarriage in the presence of antibodies against phospholipid, particularly anticardiolipin antibody and lupus anticoagulant. Lupus anticoagulant causes a prolonged activated partial thromboplastin time, hence its name, but in vivo it is procoagulant. The raised APTT does not correct when the sample is mixed with normal plasma, but will normalize when phospholipid is added.

The condition may be primary, when pathogenesis is thought to be related to prior infection, but is also frequently described in the context of rheumatic disease, particularly SLE; around 50% of patients with lupus anticoagulant have SLE. Treatment is specialist and often requires high levels of anticoagulation.

POLYMYALGIA RHEUMATICA AND GIANT CELL ARTERITIS

These inflammatory conditions frequently occur together; around half of patients with giant cell arteritis (GCA) have polymyalgia. The underlying pathogenic mechanisms are incompletely understood and may be common to both conditions.

Polymyalgia rheumatica (PMR)

PMR is about three times more common than GCA. It is a clinical syndrome characterized by proximal muscle pain and stiffness. The incidence increases with age, with those under 50 rarely affected, and the prevalence is as high as 2% in patients aged over 60 years. It is two to three times more common in women than in men, more common in northern Europe than in southern Europe, and is rare in non-whites.

Clinical features

- Pain affecting shoulders (usually the first to be affected), hips and neck, predominantly of muscles.
- Severe morning stiffness that often persists for more than 1 h.
- Muscle tenderness.
- Acute illness of less than a month's duration.
- Anorexia and weight loss may be severe.

The distribution tends to be symmetrical, and systemic features such as sweating, malaise and depression are common. True weakness does not occur, although power and range of movement may be limited by pain. Synovitis may be present though it is usually overshadowed by the muscular symptoms.

Differential diagnosis

The differential diagnosis of PMR includes:

- Late-onset RA or spondyloarthropathy.
- Musculoskeletal: OA, rotator cuff disease, non-specific back pain, trochanteric bursitis.
- Other neuromuscular conditions, polymyositis and proximal myopathy.
- Occult malignancy if systemic features are marked.
- Hypothyroidism: due to myalgia and malaise.

Investigations

The following investigations are important in patients with PMR:

- ESR: usually over 40 mm/h; very high values can occur.
- Acute phase proteins: increased (e.g. CRP).
- Alkaline phosphatase: raised in approximately 30% of patients.
- A mild normochromic normocytic anaemia is common and platelets tend to be increased.
- Tests to exclude conditions capable of mimicking PMR: rheumatoid factor, thyroid function tests, creatine kinase if muscle weakness is suspected and autoantibodies if there are features suggesting connective tissue disease.

A temporal artery biopsy is not indicated unless features of GCA coexist.

Treatment

Symptoms almost always improve within a few days with corticosteroids. The ESR falls to normal within 2–3 weeks and the CRP becomes normal within 1 week. An initial daily dose of 15–20 mg of prednisolone is usually adequate to control symptoms. The dose should be continued for around a month before slowly reducing it while monitoring with follow-up appointments.

There is no indication for prophylactic high-dose steroids to prevent blindness as with giant cell arteritis. However, patients should be warned to look out for additional symptoms such as headache or blurred vision.

Approximately 50% of patients manage to discontinue steroids within 2 years. Management should be based on the clinical response, although a rise in ESR should prompt review. Relapses are most common in the first year but the incidence falls thereafter, and they are often associated with a reduction in steroid dose. Adding an NSAID to cover ache and stiffness may be of symptomatic help.

In patients who are developing the side effects of steroids, a 'steroid-sparing' immunosuppressant (e.g. methotrexate) should be considered under expert supervision. Prophylaxis against osteoporosis is usually indicated. In a few patients, it is impossible to withdraw steroids altogether and it is acceptable to maintain them indefinitely on prednisolone 2–3 mg/day.

Prognosis

The prognosis is good provided the steroid dosage is not excessive. Most patients can be reassured that treatment can usually be discontinued after 2–4 years with a low rate of recurrence thereafter.

Giant cell arteritis

This disease usually occurs in patients over 60 years old and is very rare before the age of 50. The classical symptoms are of temporal arteritis, causing temporal headache with tender, reddened non-pulsatile arteries. The headache may be severe and is often worse at night. Involvement of other cranial arteries may cause a tender scalp, pain in the jaw during eating (jaw claudication), skin necrosis or tongue ischaemia. Involvement of the vertebral arteries may lead to TIA or stroke, and disease of the ophthalmic arteries may lead to retinal ischaemia or infarction causing amaurosis fugax, blurred vision or irreversible blindness. Features of polymyalgia rheumatica (see above) may be present, including systemic features.

Investigations

The ESR is usually raised, up to 100 mm/h, although a normal ESR does not exclude the diagnosis. C-reactive protein, platelets and alkaline phosphatase levels are commonly raised. Temporal artery biopsy is required to make a definitive diagnosis. 'Skip lesions' may lead to false negatives, and a long biopsy specimen should be obtained.

Treatment

Treatment is with high doses of prednisolone (60 mg daily). This relieves the headache within 24 h and averts the risk of blindness, which occurs in up to 50% of patients if untreated. The prednisolone is gradually reduced to a maintenance level, and the dose is monitored by symptoms and serial ESRs. Treatment may have to be continued for many years, and itself carries a significant morbidity from side effects.

HINTS AND TIPS

Steroids should never be delayed if GCA is suspected. Temporal artery biopsy may remain positive for several weeks after steroids are started.

VASCULITIS

Classification

Vasculitis is a term referring to many different conditions all causing inflammation of blood vessels. Vasculitis may be a primary condition or it may occur in the context of other inflammatory conditions such as rheumatoid arthritis, SLE or infection. The primary vasculitides may be classified according to the size of the vessels affected (Fig. 36.9).

Aetiology and pathology

The common feature of the vasculitides is the presence of leucocytes in the vessel wall causing inflammation and ultimately necrosis. This may lead to obstruction of the vessel and ischaemia, or the vessel may rupture causing bleeding.

The precise trigger of inflammation remains obscure. In several of these conditions autoantibodies are present, particularly anti-neutrophil cytoplasmic antibodies (ANCA), and it is likely that they play a pathogenic role.

Fig. 36.9 Chapel Hill classification of vasculitis by size of vessel affected.

Large arteries	Takayasu arteritis (affects branches of aorta) Giant cell arteritis (see above)
Medium-sized arteries	Polyarteritis nodosa (PAN) Kawasaki disease (children, often affects coronary arteries) Primary CNS vasculitis
Small arteries	Wegener's granulomatosis* Microscopic polyangiitis (MPA)† Churg–Strauss syndrome† Henoch–Schönlein purpura

**, Associated with c-ANCA; †, associated with p-ANCA.*

Clinical features

The clinical features of vasculitis vary widely and they are often difficult to diagnose. They may affect blood vessels anywhere in the body, often causing systemic symptoms such as fatigue, weakness and fever, as well as single or multi-organ failure. Features include the following:

- Skin: purpuric or petechial rash, livedo reticularis.
- Upper airway symptoms (rhinitis, congestion) in Wegener's granulomatosis.
- Pulmonary symptoms: cough, haemoptysis, wheeze.
- Myalgia.
- Neurological signs: mononeuritis multiplex, seizures, focal signs.
- Renal involvement: the main cause of death. Patients may present with hypertension, proteinuria, an acute nephritic syndrome, nephrotic syndrome or renal failure.
- Cardiac involvement (PAN or Kawasaki disease): Coronary arteritis may cause angina and myocardial infarction. There may be pericarditis.

The combination of renal impairment and pulmonary haemorrhage suggests ANCA-associated vasculitis (Wegener's, MPA) or Goodpasture's disease.

Investigations

The following tests should be carried out:

- Full blood count, renal and liver function, ESR, creatine kinase.
- Urinalysis ± protein–creatinine ratio.
- Autoantibody screen including ANA and complement (lupus) ANCA.
- Chest X-ray and ECG.

A biopsy will often be required to make a definitive diagnosis. Other tests may be necessary depending on the organs involved.

Treatment

In some cases of mild vasculitis, for instance when it is limited to skin involvement or arthralgia, symptomatic treatment with NSAIDs may be sufficient. This is particularly true of Henoch–Schönlein purpura, of which the majority of cases are self-limiting. However, a significant minority of patients develop renal involvement and monitoring is extremely important.

In other vasculitides, some form of immunomodulatory treatment is usually required due to the risk of progression and irreversible organ damage. This is usually in the form of high-dose corticosteroids at first, though resistant disease may require additional immunosuppression in the form of cyclophosphamide. In the ANCA-associated vasculitides both therapies are started simultaneously to obtain rapid control of the disease. Kawasaki disease is treated with IV immunoglobulin.

Prognosis varies according to the form of vasculitis. Aggressive ANCA-associated vasculitis or PAN carries a 5-year mortality of up to 90% if untreated. Most patients respond well to therapy, but 5-year mortality may still be as high as 30%.

Behçet's disease

This is a recurrent progressive multisystem disease of unknown aetiology. It is thought that most features are due to vasculitis, and all sizes of blood vessel are involved. Painful ulceration of the oral and genital regions is common. Other features of Behçet's disease may include:

- Skin lesions: nodules, pustules, erythema nodosum.
- Eyes: uveitis, hypopyon, retinal vasculitis.
- Vessels: aneurysms and venous thrombosis in large vessels.
- Joints: seronegative arthritis.
- CNS complications: brainstem syndromes, meningoencephalitis.
- GI tract: pain, nausea, diarrhoea mimicking inflammatory bowel disease.

Treatment is with steroids for ulcers and systemic features. In resistant cases colchicine or cytotoxic drugs (e.g. azathioprine) may be needed.

OTHER CONNECTIVE TISSUE DISORDERS

Systemic sclerosis

Systemic sclerosis is a multisystem disease that mainly occurs in middle-aged women. It presents with Raynaud's phenomenon in more than 75% of cases. The aetiology is unknown. There may be an association with certain HLA types. There are abnormalities of both humoral and cellular immunity. Early in the disease, the skin is oedematous and the blood vessels show arteritis and thickening. There is an increase in collagen and progressive fibrosis of viscera. The condition may be divided into diffuse cutaneous (DSSc) or limited cutaneous (LSSc) types, depending on the degree of skin involvement. Very rarely it may occur without skin involvement, when it is termed 'systemic sclerosis sine scleroderma'. LSSc may show the characteristic features of CREST syndrome (Fig. 36.10).

Clinical features

There is general malaise, lassitude, fever and weight loss. The following systems may be involved.

Skin

The previous term for systemic sclerosis was scleroderma, reflecting the thickening and hardening of the skin associated with increased collagen content. In LSSc skin involvement is limited to the hands, forearms, face and neck; involvement of other areas is indicative of DSSc. Patients classically have a beaked nose, facial telangiectasia and tight skin around the mouth causing difficulty in opening the mouth wide (Fig. 36.11). The skin becomes smooth, waxy and atrophic with pigmentation or depigmentation. There may be digital

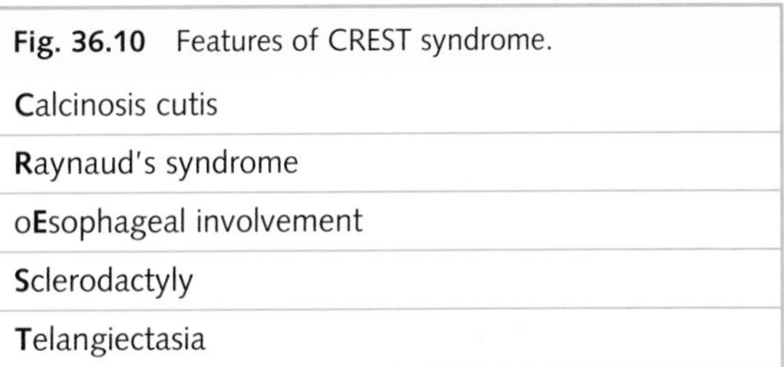

Fig. 36.10 Features of CREST syndrome.

Calcinosis cutis
Raynaud's syndrome
o**E**sophageal involvement
Sclerodactyly
Telangiectasia

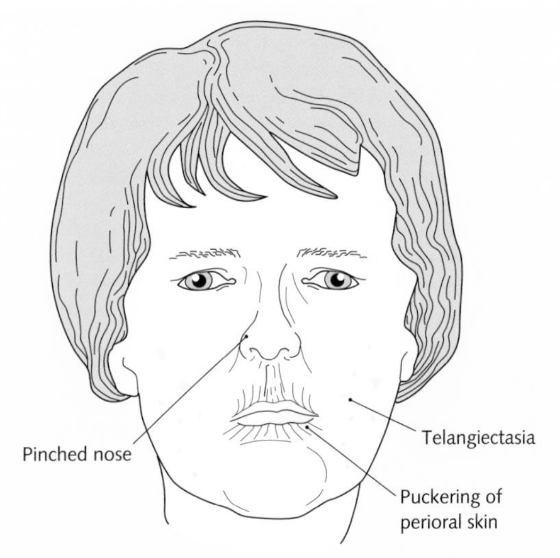

Fig. 36.11 Systemic sclerosis, showing pinched nose, multiple telangiectasia, and tightening of the skin around the mouth. The skin may also be waxy and shiny.

oedema ('sausage-shaped' fingers), with subsequent sclerodactyly. Raynaud's phenomenon is common and there may be subcutaneous calcification. Itch may be prominent.

Morphoea or localized scleroderma is a relatively benign condition affecting only the skin, especially on the trunk and limbs. Plaques evolve to produce waxy, thickened skin and induration. These may enlarge or new lesions may appear over time. Resolution is associated with hyperpigmentation. Only rarely does morphoea proceed to systemic sclerosis.

Gastrointestinal system

Oesophageal involvement is very common. Reduced peristalsis, dilatation and oesophageal sphincter dysfunction may cause dysphagia or heartburn in about half of affected patients. Reflux may lead to strictures. Dilatation and atony of the small bowel can cause bacterial overgrowth with malabsorption and steatorrhoea.

Respiratory system

There is interstitial fibrosis in around 70% of patients, which predominantly affects the lower lobes of the lungs but can be diffuse. A restrictive lung defect is seen, which may progress to respiratory failure. There may be aspiration pneumonia (due to oesophageal dysmotility) and pulmonary hypertension in advanced disease.

Musculoskeletal system

Polyarthralgia and flexion deformities develop due to fibrosis of tendons. Myopathy and polymyositis can occur.

Cardiovascular system

Myocardial fibrosis can cause arrhythmias and conduction defects. Pericardial effusions and pericarditis can occur, and right heart failure secondary to pulmonary hypertension is seen.

Renal system

Subclinical renal involvement is present in up to 80% of patients. Chronic kidney disease in scleroderma appears to have a benign prognosis. However, scleroderma renal crisis occurs in up to 15% due to an obliterative endarteritis of renal vessels, leading to progressive renal failure and hypertension, which may be fatal.

Eyes

Eyelid and conjunctival abnormalities can occur, and tear secretion may be reduced.

Investigations

The following investigations may help diagnose systemic sclerosis:

- Antinuclear antibodies: these are present in 80% of patients (nucleolar pattern in scleroderma; rheumatoid factor is positive in 30%). Anti-centromere antibodies are associated with LSSc, whereas anti-DNA topoisomerase-1 (anti-Scl70) antibodies are associated with DSSc.
- ESR: often raised.
- FBC: may show a normochromic normocytic anaemia or a haemolytic anaemia.
- Hand X-rays: may show calcinosis.

CXR, ECG and urinalysis should be performed, as should baseline renal function. Further investigation should be guided by symptoms and initial findings, for instance barium swallow or oesophageal manometry for reflux.

Management

Treatment is symptomatic (e.g. nifedipine or electrically heated gloves may help with Raynaud's phenomenon). Antacids, proton pump inhibitors or histamine H_2 antagonists will help relieve heartburn. Physiotherapy may help when joints are affected, and NSAIDs can be given for joint pain. Hypertensive renal crises are emergencies and should be treated aggressively with angiotensin-converting enzyme (ACE) inhibitors and optimal supportive care. There is little evidence that immunomodulatory therapy or antifibrotic therapy is of significant benefit for most patients. However, patients with widespread skin disease or lung fibrosis may benefit from steroids or other immunosuppressants.

Prognosis

The course of the disease is variable but is usually slowly progressive. Death usually occurs from lung, renal or cardiac complications. The overall mean 5-year survival is approximately 90%. The prognosis may be better for LSSc.

Polymyositis and dermatomyositis

These are inflammatory disorders of muscle, of which the precise aetiology is unknown. The two conditions share the histological features of muscle fibre necrosis with regeneration and inflammatory cell infiltrate. However, there are important differences: dermatomyositis involves the skin, has a greater association with cancer (up to 15% of cases are associated with an underlying malignancy), and both the distribution and composition of the inflammatory infiltrate are different. They can occur at any age, with a peak incidence at around 50 years old, with women twice as likely to be affected as men. The incidence of associated malignancy increases with age.

Clinical features

The clinical features of polymyositis and dermatomyositis include the following:

- Progressive symmetrical and proximal muscle weakness, usually gradual in onset but occasionally acute. Muscle wasting in advanced cases.

- Muscle pain and tenderness: about 50% of patients.
- Fibrosis: flexion deformities of the limbs.
- Arthralgia and arthritis: about 50% of patients.
- Skin involvement in dermatomyositis: purple 'heliotrope' colour around the eyes, and sometimes the rest of the face, with periorbital oedema; violaceous, oedematous lesions over the knuckles (Gottron's papules); telangiectasia, nail-fold infarcts.
- Muscle weakness can affect the oesophagus, leading to dysphagia.
- Raynaud's phenomenon.
- Lung fibrosis or respiratory muscle weakness, which may require ventilatory support.
- Myocarditis: usually mild.
- Features of other rheumatic diseases such as Sjögren's syndrome and SLE.

Investigations

- Creatine kinase is almost always raised and can be used to monitor the disease. A raised CK-MB or troponin can be seen in myocarditis.
- Muscle biopsy: necrosis of muscle fibres with swelling and disruption of muscle cells; fibrosis, thickening of blood vessels and inflammatory changes.
- ESR: usually raised and there may be a normochromic normocytic anaemia.
- Autoantibodies: myositis-specific antibodies, such as anti Jo-1, may be positive. Antinuclear antibodies are also often present.
- Investigations for underlying malignancy.

The major differential diagnosis is inclusion body myositis, which is usually asymmetric and distal. A muscle biopsy will usually distinguish the two.

Management

High-dose steroids should be prescribed in the acute phase. The dose can be gradually tapered. Immunosuppressive drugs (e.g. methotrexate or azathioprine) may be required if there is a poor response to steroids. Physiotherapy may help to restore muscle power.

Prognosis

The 5-year survival is approximately 80%, but a significant number of those will experience considerable disability. Lung or heart involvement, high autoantibody titres and underlying malignancy are associated with a poorer outcome.

Sjögren's syndrome

This is a chronic autoimmune disease leading to destruction of epithelial exocrine glands resulting in keratoconjunctivitis sicca (dry eyes) and/or xerostomia (dry mouth). It can be primary or secondary if associated with a connective tissue disorder (commonly RA). There is an association with certain HLA class II types. Other exocrine glands may be involved. Systemic manifestations include:

- Arthralgia, polyarthritis, myalgia.
- Raynaud's phenomenon, vasculitis and other skin involvement.
- Renal involvement in 20% of patients.
- Pulmonary: fibrotic lung disease, usually mild.
- Parotid gland enlargement in one-third.
- Peripheral neuropathy and focal CNS lesions.

It is associated with other organ-specific autoimmune diseases (e.g. thyroid disease, vitiligo, pernicious anaemia, primary biliary cirrhosis and chronic active hepatitis). There is an increased risk of lymphoma.

Investigations

The following investigations are important in patients with Sjögren's syndrome:

- Anti-Ro and anti-La antibody titres raised. ANA often present.
- Immunoglobulins: raised.
- Rheumatoid factor: present.
- Schirmer's test: this is a method of quantifying conjunctival dryness. A strip of filter paper is put under the lower eyelid and the distance along the paper that tears are absorbed is measured. This should be more than 10 mm in 5 min.
- Biopsy of secretory glands shows a lymphocytic and plasma cell infiltrate of the secretor.

Treatment

The mainstay of therapy is conservative treatment to protect the eye and relieve the oral symptoms with artificial saliva and tears. Attempts to modify the progression of the disease have shown little reward, although newer trials suggest there is a role for anti-B-cell therapies such as rituximab.

Mixed connective tissue disease

This is a term used for a condition that combines features of SLE, scleroderma and polymyositis but the symptoms and signs do not fit neatly into one of the well-defined syndromes. The features may occur sequentially, and patients may therefore be given another diagnosis before it is clear that they have MCTD. It affects women more than men and presents in young adults. It is associated with high titres of antinuclear antibodies (ANA), often positive in a speckled pattern, and high titres of antibody to an extractable nuclear antigen such as ribonucleoprotein. The condition may respond

Fig. 36.12 Immunological tests.

Test	Associated disorder
Antinuclear factor (ANA)	SLE: rheumatoid arthritis Sjögren's syndrome: MCTD, systemic sclerosis
Anti-double-stranded-DNA antibodies	SLE
Rheumatoid factor	Rheumatoid arthritis: SLE, MCTD, Sjögren's syndrome
Anti-Ro (SSA), anti-La (SSB) antibodies	Sjögren's syndrome
Antiphospholipid antibodies (e.g. anticardiolipin)	Antiphospholipid syndrome
Antiribonucleoprotein antibodies	MCTD
Jo-1 antibodies	Polymyositis, dermatomyositis
Antineutrophil cytoplasmic antibodies (ANCA)	p-ANCA (peripheral): polyarteritis nodosa c-ANCA (classical): Wegener's granulomatosis
Antiacetylcholine receptor antibodies	Myasthenia gravis
Anti-GM1 antibodies	Multifocal motor neuropathy, Guillain–Barré syndrome
Anti-GAD antibodies	Stiff person syndrome

ANA, antinuclear antibody; GAD, glutamate decarboxylase; MCTD, mixed connective tissue disease; SLE, systemic lupus erythematosus.

to steroids. Immunological tests for this disorder and others are summarized in Fig. 36.12.

Relapsing polychondritis

This is a disorder in which there is inflammation of cartilage and other tissues of unknown aetiology. The ears and eyes are commonly affected, but the airways, heart valves, joints and kidneys may also become involved. In around a third of patients it is associated with vasculitis or other rheumatic disease. There is a very small evidence base for treatment; steroids or dapsone are often used before immunosuppressive drugs are tried. Airway and heart valve involvement may cause early mortality.

SKIN DISEASE

Psoriasis

Psoriasis is a chronic inflammatory skin disease that affects roughly 2% of the population. Psoriasis may present at any age, with a peak incidence in the late 20s, and affects the sexes equally. It may be triggered by stress, trauma, infection and drugs (e.g. lithium, chloroquine and beta-blockers), but may also arise in the absence of these.

Evidence suggests that it is an immune-mediated disease with associated hyperproliferation of keratinocytes. Pathologically, an immune cell infiltrate containing cells of both the adaptive and innate immune system can be seen in the epidermis, and there is epidermal thickening with increased numbers of epidermal cells.

Clinical features

The lesions in psoriasis are typically clearly marginated, salmon-pink plaques topped by a silvery scale, most frequently found over the extensor surfaces of the limbs (e.g. elbows and knees). They may be severely itchy. Involvement of the scalp with a thickened hyperkeratotic scale is also common. Plaques may vary in size and shape and can be discoid, serpiginous or circinate (ring-like). In extreme cases, erythroderma may occur. Removal of the scales leaves pinpoint bleeding sites (Auspitz's sign), and Köbner's phenomenon is seen (i.e. it lesions arise at sites of trauma). Various less common forms have been described as follows:

- Guttate psoriasis: an eruption of small psoriatic lesions over the entire body; it typically occurs after streptococcal pharyngitis.
- Flexural psoriasis: lesions have a pinkish, glazed appearance, are clearly demarcated and are non-scaly. The commonest sites of involvement are the groin, perianal and genital regions and inframammary folds.
- Pustular psoriasis: affects the palms or soles, with well-demarcated scaling and erythema. The pustules are white, yellow, green or brown when dried.

Extradermal manifestations include nail involvement (pitting and onycholysis) in 25% and some form of arthropathy in 10% of patients with psoriasis. The condition is usually chronic but flares and remission may be seen.

Management

For mild conditions, treatment other than reassurance and an emollient may be unnecessary. In more troublesome cases topical therapy can be highly effective; different therapies may need to be tried to see what suits the patient. Systemic therapy is used only if topical treatments are inadequate.

Topical therapy

Corticosteroids applied topically are rapidly effective, and are often used as first-line treatment, but rarely induce long-term remission and lead to skin atrophy with chronic use. Salicylic acid is useful as an adjunct to remove surface scale. Side effects include irritation or toxicity when large areas are treated. Coal tar has both anti-inflammatory and antiproliferative properties but use is limited by its unpleasant appearance and odour, and it should not be used on the face due to irritation. However, when the lesions are extensive, coal tar baths are useful. Dithranol is very effective in psoriasis but can cause severe skin irritation and should therefore be started at low concentrations and gradually built up. Topical vitamin D derivatives such as calcipotriol are effective for mild-to-moderate psoriasis and do not have an unpleasant odour; hypercalcaemia is a rare complication. Tazarotene is a topical retinoid which is useful as an adjunct to other agents in mild-to-moderate plaque psoriasis. Many of these drugs are formulated as shampoos for scalp psoriasis.

Systemic therapy

Ultraviolet B radiation therapy alone is helpful in mild-to-moderate, guttate or chronic plaque psoriasis. If unsuccessful, photochemotherapy using psoralens with long-wave ultraviolet A irradiation (PUVA) is effective in some patients. Special lamps are required and short-term side effects include burning; in the long term there may be cataract formation, accelerated ageing of the skin (solar elastosis) and increased risk of skin cancer. Acitretin is a retinoid (vitamin A derivative) given orally for severe resistant or complicated psoriasis. It is valuable combined with UV therapy. Side effects can include cracked lips, hair thinning, pruritus, paronychia and nose bleeds, and it is teratogenic. Cytotoxic drugs (e.g. methotrexate and ciclosporin) can be used for severe resistant psoriasis. They are for use only by specialists. If disease does not respond to these, biological agents including anti-TNF (etanercept, infliximab) and anti-IL-12/IL-23 (ustekinumab) therapies can be used. Fumaric acid has been used in Germany for many years and may be as effective as methotrexate; further trials are awaited.

Eczema/dermatitis

The terms eczema and dermatitis are often used interchangeably, and refer to non-specific inflammation of the skin. It can be broadly separated into cases occurring due to an external factor (e.g. contact dermatitis) and those occurring endogenously (e.g. atopic, seborrhoeic). Clinically, lesions are often vesicular, rupturing to leave a raw, weeping surface. They may be diffuse, irritating and sometimes painful. Itch is common and often severe, and secondary infection may occur. With chronicity, lesions become scaly, thickened and pigment is lost.

Classification

Atopic eczema

This affects around 10% of the population. It usually starts in infancy, and although the majority experience significant improvement or clearing of the condition by adulthood, the skin may remain sensitive to irritants throughout life. It is thought that the barrier function of the skin is impaired, allowing irritant substances to penetrate and activate immune cells. In infants there are exudative, crusted, itchy areas over extensor surfaces and cheeks. By childhood and adulthood the lesions are more localized and seen on the antecubital and popliteal fossae, face, neck, wrists and ankles. There is pruritus, with skin thickening and increased markings. Investigations include prick tests to common allergens, and raised serum immunoglobulin E (IgE). It may be associated with asthma and hay fever.

Contact dermatitis

Irritant contact dermatitis: the hands are the most common affected site. There is erythema, vesiculation and fissuring. Irritants include detergents, bleaches and soaps. Risk is increased in certain occupations (e.g. hairdressers and engineers).

Allergic contact dermatitis: this is a delayed hypersensitivity reaction which requires previous sensitization, which may occur after one episode of contact or slowly over years. Patch testing produces a marked, prolonged response even to dilute quantities of the allergen. The pattern of eczema depends on the site of contact and there is often a sharp cut-off where contact ends, although spread to other sites may occur. Thin, moist skin is the most vulnerable. Common allergens include:

- Dyes.
- Nickel: buttons and zips.
- Chromates: cement and leather.
- Cosmetics: fragrances, preservatives.
- Rubber.
- Resins: glues.
- Plants.
- Topical antibiotics.

Seborrhoeic dermatitis

Seborrhoeic dermatitis in adults manifests as a scaly, crusty, red, itchy eruption with yellowish scales, appearing on oily areas of the skin (e.g. the face, flexures and scalp (dandruff)).

Other subtypes

- Discoid eczema: in this form there are itchy, vesicular, round lesions distributed over the body.
- Dyshidrotic eczema: also known as pompholyx, this is an extremely itchy, vesicular dermatitis affecting palms, soles and fingers.

Management

Where possible, the cause should be established and removed, although in practice this may be very difficult. A patient with suspected contact dermatitis should be patch-tested to establish the diagnosis. Atopic eczema usually requires the regular application of an emollient with short courses of a mild-to-moderate topical corticosteroid, the least potent that is effective. In more severe eczema, more potent steroids may be needed, and if itching is a major problem consideration should be given to the administration of antihistamines. Secondary infection is common and should be promptly treated. In severe, resistant atopic dermatitis, systemic steroids may be used, or ciclosporin if steroid therapy fails.

For dry, fissured, scaly lesions, treatment is with emollients and emulsifying ointment as soap substitutes. For weeping eczema, treatment is with topical corticosteroids, wet dressings of potassium permanganate, and topical antibacterials. Coal tar is used occasionally in chronic atopic eczema. Seborrhoeic dermatitis is treated with medicated shampoo, antifungals and topical steroids.

Acne vulgaris

This is a papulopustular inflammatory condition, usually affecting the face and trunk, which affects approximately 90% of adolescents. Whilst usually mild and short-lived, it can persist into adulthood and may be severely disfiguring and psychologically damaging. There is increased keratinization of the sebaceous duct leading to blockage, increased production of sebum, and colonization by *Propionibacterium acnes*. These events cause the primary lesion, the comedo, which may be open (blackhead) or closed (whitehead). They often become inflamed, forming papules, pustules or cysts. Healing can leave residual scarring.

Management

A sympathetic approach is needed; dispel myths that the patient is dirty or that acne is caused by eating chocolate or greasy food. Advise on washing the face with soap and water frequently to degrease the skin, but to avoid rubbing the skin roughly. Topical treatments include benzoyl peroxide, retinoids, azelaic acid or salicylic acid, all of which will reduce comedones. Benzoyl peroxide also has antibacterial action and is useful for inflamed lesions. In mild-to-moderate acne with inflammation, topical or oral antibiotics (courses up to 6 months) such as erythromycin or tetracyclines are effective.

COMMUNICATION

Even mild acne can be a distressing condition for young people and requires a sympathetic approach often involving other family members.

Isotretinoin is a retinoid used for severe acne unresponsive to systemic antibiotics, and acts primarily by reducing sebum secretion. It is teratogenic and has other side effects including dry mouth and myalgia. In females, hormone manipulation with antiandrogens and ethinylestradiol can be highly effective and an alternative to isotretinoin.

Herpes simplex

More than 80% of adults have serological evidence of prior herpes simplex virus type 1 (HSV-1) infection, usually from childhood. It is the cause of the cold sore, herpes labialis. HSV-2 is more commonly associated with genital herpes. Primary infection is usually asymptomatic; following this the virus survives latent in cell bodies of nerve ganglia. Reactivation, which may occur in times of stress, causes a burning, stinging neuralgia, which precedes or accompanies the development of lesions. These take the form of small groups of vesicles with an erythematous base in orolabial and genital areas. Diagnosis is clinical but vesicular fluid or scrapings can show HSV. Treatment is with topical, oral or IV aciclovir or oral valaciclovir. Herpes simplex may cause an encephalitis (see Ch. 34), and in immunocompromised patients disseminated HSV infection may occur.

Herpes (varicella) zoster

Primary infection with HZV causes chickenpox (varicella), usually in childhood; if occurring in adulthood it may be severe. There is fever and a widespread vesiculopapular rash. Following recovery the virus lies dormant in the dorsal root ganglia until immunosuppression or illness causes reactivation, termed shingles. Typically, dermatomal pain and paraesthesia precede the appearance of maculopapular then vesicular lesions restricted to that dermatome. Shingles is usually thoracic or in the ophthalmic division of the trigeminal nerve. Disseminated herpes can cause shingles in a non-dermatomal distribution. Diagnosis is clinical, although analysis of vesicular fluid or scrapings can demonstrate herpes zoster. If ophthalmic, or in an immunosuppressed host, then treatment with IV aciclovir is indicated. Oral antivirals, if started within 72 h of symptoms, will aid healing and reduce post-herpetic neuralgia. Corticosteroids may help acute pain but do not prevent post-herpetic neuralgia, which is best treated with amitritpyline, gabapentin or carbamazepine. It may prove difficult to control and specialist advice should be sought. The patient may be isolated until non-infectious (when the lesions crust after 7–10 days), and certain groups such as the immunocompromised, pregnant women or healthcare workers without previous infection should avoid contact.

Lichen planus

This mainly affects middle-aged adults. The cause is unknown but may be related to disturbances of immune function. Lichen-planus-like reactions occur with certain drugs, such as sulphonamides, sulphonylureas, methyldopa, thiazides, beta-blockers and drugs that alter immune function (e.g. antimalarials, gold salts, penicillamine).

The lesions are purple, polygonal and planar or flat-topped papules, with a largely peripheral and symmetrical distribution. Scarring occurs with chronic disease. Linear lesions may follow trauma or scratching (Köbner's phenomenon). Lesions may occur on the buccal mucosa or in the nails. The presence of Wickham's striae (fine white lacy lines coursing over the papule) helps to distinguish the disease. Post-inflammatory hyperpigmentation is also a useful diagnostic sign.

The lesions usually last for 12–18 months if untreated. Systemic steroids may be required to suppress intractable itching. Less acute disease can be managed with topical corticosteroids with an antihistamine at night to control the itching.

Erythema multiforme

This can present in a variety of ways but the classic lesion is circular with central intensity or blistering giving a 'target' appearance. They usually occur on the limbs in a symmetrical distribution. The lesions may be preceded by a prodrome of fever, sore throat, headache, arthralgia and gastroenteritis. When severe, the mucosae may be involved, and it is termed erythema multiforme major. Despite significant overlap, there is a move to distinguish this from Stevens–Johnson syndrome (see below).

Causes of erythema multiforme

- Systemic infections, especially viruses and mycoplasma, account for 90% of cases. Herpes simplex virus is most commonly implicated.
- Drugs (e.g. barbiturates, sulphonamides, penicillin, salicylates).
- Malignancy.
- Autoimmune rheumatic disease (e.g. RA, SLE).

Stevens–Johnson syndrome and toxic epidermal necrolysis

These related conditions are severe reactions, usually to a medication (e.g. allopurinol, antibiotics, antiepileptics) but also to infection or a rarer cause such as vaccination. They are characterized by the acute onset of fever, skin and mucosal lesions, and skin sloughing. TEN is the more severe form in which at least 30% of the skin is sloughed. The mainstay of management is optimal supportive treatment with attention to nutrition, fluid balance and prevention of infection. The offending medication should be stopped and any causative infection treated. Steroids are usually given and IV immunoglobulin may have a role. Mortality in TEN is up to 35%.

Pemphigus vulgaris and bullous pemphigoid

These are autoimmune, bullous conditions affecting mainly people aged over 60. In pemphigus antibodies are directed against an epidermal cell adhesion molecule, causing flaccid, fragile blisters to develop within the epidermis. It affects mucosa and skin, with denuded areas remaining after the blisters rupture. Treatment is with steroids and immunosuppressive agents.

In pemphigoid, the antibodies affect the basement membrane, leading to blisters between the dermis and epidermis. It may occur spontaneously or in response to medication. The blisters are tense and widespread, occurring particularly in flexures.

Erythema nodosum

This manifests as painful nodular lesions, usually on the anterior shins, that go through similar colour changes to a bruise. New crops of lesions emerge while earlier lesions are fading, and it may become necrotic. It is five times more common in women, with a peak incidence between 20 and 50 years. The most common causes are infections, sarcoidosis or drugs, but in a significant proportion of cases no cause is found.

Causes of erythema nodosum

- Bacterial infections, esp. *Streptococcus* spp., tuberculosis, leprosy.
- Sarcoidosis.
- Drugs (e.g. sulphonamides, oral contraceptive pill, dapsone).
- Crohn's disease and ulcerative colitis.
- Behçet's disease.
- Viral (e.g. EBV) and fungal (e.g. cocciomycosis) infections.

Vitiligo

Vitiligo is characteristically well-demarcated, roughly symmetrical areas of depigmentation. There is loss of melanocytes, thought to be due to an autoimmune process. Around 30% of cases are associated with organ-specific autoimmune disease (e.g. Addison's, pernicious anaemia, alopecia, Hashimoto's thyroiditis).

Pyoderma gangrenosum

This presents with violaceous nodules, which then undergo necrosis to produce an ulcer with an overhanging edge. They heal leaving a scar. There is a clear underlying cause in around half of cases, such as inflammatory bowel disease, neoplasia, Wegener's granulomatosis and myeloma. Systemic steroids and ciclosporin are the first-line treatment. Treatment of the underlying disease, if present, often results in healing of the ulcers.

SKIN MANIFESTATIONS OF SYSTEMIC DISEASE

Systemic disease often involves the skin, ranging from the life-threatening purpuric rash of meningococcal septicaemia, which must not be missed, to rare lesions providing clues to a diagnosis. The following is a small selection; many other diseases (e.g. chronic liver disease) have skin signs, which have been highlighted in the relevant chapters.

Inflammatory bowel disease

Both ulcerative colitis and Crohn's disease are causes of erythema nodosum and pyoderma gangrenosum. Crohn's is associated with aphthous ulceration and perianal skin tags, fistulae or abscesses.

Diabetes mellitus

Skin manifestations include recurrent infections, ulcers, necrobiosis lipoidica diabeticorum (shiny areas on the shins with a yellowish colour and telangiectasia), granuloma annulare (purplish annular lesions with the skin surface remaining intact) and fat necrosis at the site of injections.

Coeliac disease

Coeliac disease is associated with dermatitis herpetiformis. There are symmetrical clusters of pruritic urticarial lesions, particularly in the gluteal region and extensor aspects of the elbows and knees. They progress to vesicles and bullae. Direct immunofluorescence shows granular deposits of IgA along the dermal papillae. Treatment is with dapsone.

Hyperthyroidism

Pretibial myxoedema is seen in Graves' disease. There is skin thickening over the shins due to glycosaminoglycan deposition.

Neoplasia

There are many skin manifestations of internal malignancy, including the following:

- Acanthosis nigricans (especially with gastric carcinoma): areas of pigmented rough thickening of the skin in the axillae or groin with warty lesions.
- Dermatomyositis.
- Erythema gyratum repens: a rare 'wood grain' erythema associated with lung cancer.
- Secondary skin metastases.
- Acquired ichthyosis: dry, scaly skin, associated with lymphoma.
- Thrombophlebitis migrans (especially with pancreatic carcinoma): successive crops of tender nodules affecting superficial veins throughout the body.

Sarcoidosis

Erythema nodosum may occur. Granulomatous inflammation of the skin (cutaneous sarcoid) may manifest as papules, nodules, plaques or lupus pernio (a diffuse bluish plaque with small papules affecting the nose).

Rheumatic fever

This may cause erythema marginatum, round erythematous lesions with central clearing. They may come and go over hours.

Neurofibromatosis

This condition is autosomal dominant and may include the following features:

- Café au lait spots (light brown macules).
- Axillary freckling.

- Violaceous dermal neurofibromata.
- Subcutaneous nodules.

Lyme disease (borreliosis)

The classical rash is erythema chronicum migrans, which starts off as a small red papule before slowly enlarging to form a ring with a raised border. It lasts for 2 days to 3 months. Lyme disease is caused by *Borrelia burgdorferi*, a spirochaete spread by ticks from deer. Within the UK, it is most common in the New Forest. Other features include malaise, arthralgia, lymphadenopathy, CNS abnormalities (e.g. meningitis and peripheral neuropathies) and cardiac disease including conduction disturbances and myocarditis. Treatment is with doxycycline, penicillin or a third-generation cephalosporin (e.g. cefotaxime).

Hyperlipidaemia

Tendon xanthomata are associated with familial hypercholesterolaemia. Eruptive xanthomata occur with greatly elevated serum lipid concentrations. Xanthelasmata are yellow plaques commonly found on the eyelids which may indicate hyperlipidaemia.

SKIN TUMOURS

Basal cell carcinoma

This is the most common skin tumour and is frequently seen in elderly, fair-skinned people. Lesions mainly occur on the face, especially at the side of the nose or in the periorbital skin. There are several subtypes. Nodular BCC is the most common, and is flesh-coloured with a pearly, rolled edge. Dilated blood vessels can be seen over the surface, and central ulceration often occurs (causing a 'rodent ulcer'). Superficial BCC occurs mainly on the trunk, and is a mildly erythematous lesion with scale and 'micropapules' at the border. Other forms, which may be more aggressive, are less common. Any type of BCC may produce pigment. They tend to be locally invasive, but metastases are very rare. Treatment is by surgical excision, cryotherapy or radiotherapy.

Squamous cell carcinoma

This tumour arises from the epidermis or skin appendages and is most commonly seen on damaged or chronically irritated skin, especially areas of sun exposure. It is invasive and can metastasize, although this is rare (less than 1%). Long-term sun exposure is the most important aetiological factor. Azathioprine therapy is also strongly linked to SCC development. Tumours are often hyperkeratotic, crusted and indurated, and may ulcerate. Other variants include SCC in situ (Bowen's disease), a slow-growing, scaly patch with a well-defined border. Carcinoma may develop in long-standing venous ulceration; when this occurs it is termed a Marjolin's ulcer. Keratoacanthoma is a rapidly growing differentiated tumour with a central core of keratin; although they usually resolve spontaneously with scarring, they are histologically similar to SCC and around 6% progress to SCC.

Treatment of SCC is by excision or radiotherapy.

Malignant melanoma

HINTS AND TIPS

Sites of malignant melanoma with a poor prognosis are BANS: Back of the Arm, Neck and Scalp.

This tumour is increasing in incidence and occurs particularly in fair-skinned people with exposure to sunlight. It is a major cause of cancer in young people. Some melanomas arise in pre-existing moles. There are four types: superficial spreading, nodular, lentigo maligna and acral lentiginous. Properties that help identify malignant melanoma are as follows:

- Rapid enlargement.
- Diameter >7 mm.
- Bleeding or crusting.
- Increasing variegated pigmentation, particularly blue–black or grey.
- An indistinct border or irregular border.
- Sensory change.
- Small 'satellite' lesions around the principal lesion.

The prognosis is related to the depth of the tumour assessed histologically (Breslow thickness). The 5-year survival for patients with a tumour <1 mm thick is more than 90%. If the thickness is >3 mm, the 5-year survival rate is around 60%. Metastasis is common, particularly to lung, liver and brain. The prognosis is worst for lesions on the scalp or neck.

Management

Prevention is important, with avoidance of exposure to direct sunlight and use of effective sunscreen lotions. Self-examination should be practised, and people should be aware of the warning signs and symptoms listed above. Treatment is by excision with skin grafting if necessary. Chemotherapy and radiotherapy are used for palliation.

SKIN INFECTION

Cellulitis

This is skin infection involving the dermis and subcutaneous fat, manifesting as erythematous, warm, oedematous areas. The lower limb is the most common site but it may occur anywhere. Systemic features of infection, such as fever, tachycardia and hypotension, may occur in more severe, rapidly progressing cellulitis. Predisposing factors include breaks in the skin (e.g. due to trauma, ulcers or drug use), fungal foot infection, oedema, diabetes and immunosuppression. The most common causative organisms are *Staphylococcus aureus* and beta-haemolytic streptococcus species. Treatment is with antibiotics according to local sensitivities; in severe cases they may need to be given intravenously.

Erysipelas is infection of the upper dermis; the infected areas are raised and clearly demarcated. The face is involved more often, and systemic features are common.

Impetigo

This is superficial skin infection with *S. aureus* or beta-haemolytic streptococcus, usually seen in children. Lesions begin as papules before progressing to vesicles. These may form bullae, or may break down to form a thick golden crust. Treatment is with antibiotics.

Necrotizing fasciitis

This invasive infection of the subcutaneous tissues is often caused by group A streptococci, though anaerobic bacteria may be involved. The skin is often affected but may be spared. Progression is rapid and unremitting; mortality is around 25%. Treatment is with antibiotics and surgical debridement.

Further reading

Berden, A., Goceroglu, A., Jayne, D., et al., 2012. Diagnosis and management of ANCA associated vasculitis. BMJ 344, e26.

British Association of Dermatologists: publishes guidelines and reviews of many aspects of skin disease in the 'clinical standards' section of its website. Available online at: http://www.bad.org.uk.

British Society for Rheumatology: publishes guidelines and reviews of all aspects of rheumatology. Available online at: http://www.rheumatology.org.uk.

D'Cruz, D., Khamashta, M., Hughes, G., 2007. Systemic lupus erythematosus. Lancet 369, 587–596.

Graham-Brown, R.A.C., Bourke, J.F., 2007. Mosby's colour atlas and text of dermatology, second ed. Mosby Elsevier, Edinburgh.

Griffiths, C., Barker, J., 2007. Pathogenesis and clinical features of psoriasis. Lancet 307, 263–271.

Hassan, N., Dasgupta, B., 2011. Giant cell arteritis. BMJ 342, d3019.

Marsland, D., Kapoor, S., 2008. Crash Course: Rheumatology and Orthopaedics. Elsevier Mosby, Edinburgh.

National Institute for Health and Clinical Excellence (NICE), 2008. Prostate cancer. Clinical guideline CG58. Available online at: http://www.nice.org.uk/CG58.

National Institute for Health Clinical Excellence (NICE), 2009. Rheumatoid arthritis. Clinical guideline CG79. Available online at: http://www.nice.org.uk/CG79.

Haematological disorders

Objectives

The key learning points for this chapter:

- What is meant by 'haematinics'.
- The different types of sickle cell crisis.
- The classification and causes of anaemia.
- The difference between acute and chronic leukaemia.
- What is meant by the Philadelphia chromosome.
- The diagnosis and treatment of multiple myeloma.
- The meaning and importance of 'B symptoms'.
- The different patterns of bleeding seen in haemophilia and von Willebrand's disease.
- Inherited conditions associated with an increased risk of venous thromboembolism.

ANAEMIA

Anaemia is a common clinical problem as it may result from many different pathological processes. The aetiology, clinical evaluation, complications and investigation policy have been considered in Ch. 29. The general approach to management is outlined first, and then specific conditions are discussed in detail. Anaemia can be classified by the size of the red cells seen on microscopy or by the underlying cause (e.g. iron deficiency, haemolysis).

General approach to management

Discover the underlying cause

Remember that there may be more than one cause of anaemia in any one patient – this can catch out the unwary! For example, folate deficiency and iron deficiency may both be present in coeliac disease. In some diseases, such as rheumatoid arthritis, there are several potential causes of anaemia (see Ch. 36).

Treat the underlying cause

The anaemia will recur if the underlying problem persists (e.g. peptic ulceration, colonic neoplasm).

Correct the anaemia

The method of correction will depend on the type of anaemia and presence of complications. In general, iron, vitamin B_{12} and folate should only be prescribed when the patient has been appropriately investigated and shown to have a deficiency.

Iron replacement

Oral iron replacement therapy (e.g. ferrous sulphate) should be continued for 3 months after the haemoglobin returns to normal to replace iron stores. However, in patients who have deficiency due to chronic bleeding this may mask further blood loss. Side effects include nausea, diarrhoea or constipation, and abdominal pain. The stools usually become very dark or black. If side effects occur, the dose can be reduced or the preparation changed, for instance to ferrous gluconate. IM or IV iron can be given but only if there is poor patient compliance with oral therapy, severe gastrointestinal disturbance with oral therapy, malabsorption or in specific situations such as patients on dialysis and some cancer patients.

Vitamin B_{12} replacement

Most causes of vitamin B_{12} deficiency are due to malabsorption and so vitamin B_{12} is given by IM injection in the form of hydroxocobalamin. Initially it is given every other day for 2 weeks to replace stores. Maintenance dosing is every 3 months and is usually lifelong.

Folate replacement

Oral folic acid corrects anaemia and replaces stores (a higher dose may be needed in malabsorption states). Lower-dose oral folic acid should be given as prophylaxis against neural tube defects to women prior to conception and throughout the first 12 weeks of pregnancy.

There is a complex relationship with cancer; trials have raised the possibility of a slightly increased risk of cancer with long-term treatment, and some rare tumours are folate dependent. It should be given only when there is a definite indication. It should not be given alone in megaloblastic anaemia unless vitamin B_{12} status has been shown to be normal, as although it will partially normalize the anaemia of vitamin B_{12} deficiency, the neurological sequelae will continue to worsen and may be precipitated.

COMMUNICATION

Make sure patients are clear that over-the-counter preparations do not contain sufficient iron for replacement and that replacement must continue for at least 3 months to replace iron stores.

Blood transfusion

Blood is given as packed red blood cells (red cell concentrate, RCC) which have been separated from whole blood. In an emergency, where time does not allow cross-matching, O RhD-negative blood can be given safely. Most labs can provide group-matched blood within about 30 min; fully cross-matched blood takes longer. Regular blood transfusion may be necessary in chronic anaemia which is not corrected by supplements. Fig. 37.1 summarizes the complications of transfusion.

Splenectomy

Splenectomy is useful in hereditary spherocytosis and refractory autoimmune haemolytic anaemia. Other indications for splenectomy include trauma, refractory idiopathic thrombocytopenic purpura, and symptomatic splenomegaly (e.g. myelofibrosis, lymphoma and leukaemia). Complications of splenectomy include thrombocytosis and increased susceptibility to infection with encapsulated bacteria (mainly pneumococcus, meningococcus, *Haemophilus influenzae* type B). Patients should be immunized with vaccines against these organisms. Lifelong daily penicillin for prophylaxis is often started post-splenectomy, but this practice may decrease with increasingly resistant bacteria; patients can also be given antibiotics to have on standby in case of fever.

Erythropoietin

Recombinant erythropoietin (EPO) has revolutionized the management of the anaemia associated with chronic renal failure. It is given up to three times a week as subcutaneous or IV injections. Adequate iron stores are needed and it is less effective in inflammatory states. It is also approved for treatment of chemotherapy-induced anaemia in certain situations.

Complications include hypertension and a rare pure red cell aplasia associated with anti-EPO antibodies. Incidence has decreased with newer agents.

Fig. 37.1 Complications of blood transfusion.

Complication	Cause
Haemolytic reaction	ABO incompatibility (acute, severe), extravascular haemolysis (delayed by 3 days to 3 weeks, mild/clinically silent)
Anaphylaxis	Hypersensitivity to plasma proteins
Febrile reaction	Antibodies to white cells
Volume overload	Particularly the elderly and in megaloblastic anaemia
Coagulopathies	Platelets and clotting factors are reduced by a dilutional effect in massive transfusion
Infection	Virus (HIV, hepatitis B and C, EBV, CMV), Gram-negative bacteria (uncommon)
Haemosiderosis	With repeated transfusions
Alloimmunization	Antibodies may develop to red cells, leucocytes, platelets and plasma proteins despite receiving compatible blood; this may cause problems the next time the patient receives a transfusion
Graft-versus-host disease	Uncommon: preventable by using irradiated blood (important in transplant recipients)
Air embolism	Particularly if given via central lines
Thrombophlebitis	At cannula site
TRALI (transfusion-associated lung injury)	Unpredictable, non-cardiogenic pulmonary oedema

CMV, cytomegalovirus; EBV, Epstein–Barr virus; HIV, human immunodeficiency virus.

Causes of anaemia

Some specific causes of anaemia are outlined below. For an approach to the diagnosis of anaemia and a more extensive list of causes, see Ch. 29.

Anaemia of chronic disease

Aetiology and pathology

Many chronic diseases, particularly infective, inflammatory or malignant processes, are associated with anaemia. The pathology is multifactorial, with inappropriate utilization of adequate iron stores, reduced erythropoietin production, reduced response to erythropoietin and reduced RBC survival. It has a different pathogenesis and treatment to anaemia seen in chronic renal failure.

Presentation and complications

Presentation is with the typical symptoms and signs of anaemia, and complications may occur. Signs of the underlying disease may also be present.

Investigations

Characteristic findings are:

- Normochromic normocytic anaemia (may be hypochromic, microcytic).
- Low serum iron but normal/high serum ferritin.
- Increased iron stores in bone marrow.
- Total iron-binding capacity (TIBC) is low. This helps differentiate from iron deficiency anaemia (IDA) when TIBC is raised.
- A raised erythrocyte sedimentation rate (ESR), neutrophilia and thrombocytosis, in addition to the anaemia, constitutes a 'reactive' blood picture reflecting the primary pathology.

HINTS AND TIPS

Remember that ferritin is an acute phase protein and may be misleading in acute illness.

Treatment

- Treat the underlying disease.
- If mild and asymptomatic, no treatment is necessary.
- If symptomatic, consider transfusion. EPO is used in rare cases.

Haemolytic anaemia

There are many different types of haemolytic anaemia, which may be classified according to whether the disorder is inherited or acquired, and whether the red cell lysis occurs in the peripheral circulation ('intravascular') or in the monocyte-macrophage system – the liver, spleen and lymph nodes ('extravascular'). Abnormalities common to all haemolytic anaemias are as follows:

- Jaundice due to raised unconjugated bilirubin.
- Raised reticulocyte count.
- Raised lactate dehydrogenase.
- Reduced haptoglobin levels.

Abnormalities specific to certain causes of haemolytic anaemia are outlined in the sections below. Chronic haemolytic anaemia leads to increased folate requirements, which may not be met, causing a coexistent folate deficiency picture.

Glucose-6-phosphate dehydrogenase (G6PD) deficiency

This X-linked recessive condition occurs in around 200 million people worldwide; the most severe form occurs in Mediterraneans. G6PD deficient erythrocytes are susceptible to oxidative stress, which causes haemoglobin to precipitate (Heinz bodies) and haemolysis to occur. In the most common forms the patient is normally asymptomatic, with episodes of acute intravascular and extravascular haemolysis precipitated by infection, drugs or eating fava beans.

- There is reduced G6PD concentration and activity. The blood film in an acute episode shows bite cells, blister cells, Heinz bodies and red cell fragments.
- Treatment is primarily by avoiding precipitants and treating underlying causes. Transfusion may be required in acute episodes.

Pyruvate kinase deficiency

This recessively inherited enzyme deficiency causes a chronic extravascular haemolysis of variable severity, which may be apparent at birth. There is reduced ATP production. In mild disease, the anaemia is often well tolerated due to right shift of the oxygen dissociation curve. Patients may develop complications of chronic haemolysis such as gallstones, hepatosplenomegaly and problems associated with iron overload.

- The blood film is often non-specific. Pyruvate kinase activity is usually low with raised levels of 2,3-diphosphoglycerate.
- Treatment is with transfusion when required; splenectomy is usually reserved for severe cases.

Hereditary spherocytosis

This encompasses a number of inherited defects of membrane proteins, most of which are autosomal dominant, causing reduced deformability of RBCs, membrane loss and extravascular destruction. The severity is variable, and around 25% of patients have no anaemia and are not diagnosed until adulthood. However, most patients present in childhood with a mild-to-moderate anaemia, jaundice and splenomegaly. Aplastic crisis can occur in association with viral illness, most commonly parvovirus B19. Complications of long-term haemolysis may develop:

- The blood film shows spherocytes and reticulocytes, and bone marrow examination reveals a compensatory erythroid hyperplasia. The spherocytes show increased osmotic fragility on testing.
- Splenectomy should be considered on an individual patient basis taking into account the severity of the anaemia and complications. Folate supplementation may be required.
- Hereditary elliptocytosis is an autosomal dominant condition with a similar but milder presentation to that of hereditary spherocytosis. Blood film shows elliptical RBCs. Most cases require no treatment but the severity is variable, and severe forms may also require splenectomy and folate supplementation.

Sickle cell disease

This is covered below.

Autoimmune haemolytic anaemia (AIHA)

In these acquired conditions haemolysis occurs when antibodies bind to the cell surface, either inducing complement-mediated intravascular haemolysis or extravascular destruction. It can be classified according to the temperature at which the antibodies bind: warm AIHA, cold agglutinin disease, or mixed.

- Warm AIHA is usually idiopathic but may occur with infection, other autoimmune disease or malignancy. There is anaemia and jaundice ± splenomegaly. In addition to the non-specific findings, the direct antigen test is positive. Blood film shows anisocytosis, reticulocytes and spherocytes. Treatment is with steroids; splenectomy or immunosuppressants are considered if steroids do not control the haemolysis.
- Cold agglutinin disease is usually due to IgM antibodies, occurring following infection with *Mycoplasma pneumoniae* or infectious mononucleosis, or in association with haematological malignancy. Complement-mediated haemolysis occurs in the periphery where the temperature is lower, causing a variable degree of anaemia and peripheral discoloration. Treatment is by avoiding cold, transfusion, and treating any underlying condition. When severe, rituximab and plasma exchange may be effective.

Mechanical haemolytic anaemia

Mechanical destruction ('shearing') of red blood cells can occur in certain diseases or iatrogenically. The most common iatrogenic cause is poorly functioning heart valves; high velocity flow and turbulence across a valve can cause fragmentation of red cells.

Microangiopathic haemolytic anaemia occurs when widespread activation of the coagulation cascade leads to fibrin strand formation in small vessels, causing shearing of RBCs. This occurs in disseminated intravascular coagulation (DIC), thrombotic thrombocytopenic purpura (TTP), haemolytic uraemic syndrome (HUS) and HELLP syndrome. These are covered later in the chapter.

Paroxysmal nocturnal haemoglobinuria (PNH)

PNH is an acquired disorder of a haematopoietic precursor cell. An acquired abnormality of a membrane protein renders a proportion of the patient's RBCs vulnerable to lysis by complement. Other cell lines are involved, and the classical triad is of pancytopenia, haemolysis and hypercoagulability.

Sickle cell anaemia

HINTS AND TIPS

Do not deny sickle cell patients adequate analgesia during a crisis through a misplaced fear of drug dependency.

Sickle cell anaemia is an inherited (autosomal recessive) condition that most commonly affects Afro-Caribbeans but is also found in the Middle East and Mediterranean. The condition provides advantage in infection with falciparum malaria. It is one cause of sickle cell disease, a term that also encompasses other inherited causes of sickling.

Pathology

A single base mutation in the DNA on chromosome 11 causes substitution of glutamic acid for valine at position 6 in the haemoglobin beta chain (HbS). When HbS becomes deoxygenated it aggregates in an organized fashion, forming polymers within the RBCs that are less soluble and less deformable. As a result the erythrocyte shape becomes distorted and changes from a biconcave disc to a 'sickle' shape; the sickle cells cannot readily pass through the microcirculation and become trapped in small vessels (causing infarction) and in the spleen, where they are destroyed.

Clinical features

In the homozygote, severity is variable and dependent on factors such as the level of fetal haemoglobin (HbF) and the co-inheritance of alpha-thalassaemia trait. It may present from the third month onwards when levels of HbF start to fall. There is chronic haemolysis, with intermittent crises and complications. There are four types of sickle cell anaemia crisis:

- Aplastic: usually due to parvovirus B19 infection. Profound anaemia and reticulocytopenia occurs – usually self-limiting but transfusion may be required.

- Sequestration: sequestration may occur in the spleen or liver. The haemoglobin drops rapidly, with a compensatory increase in reticulocytes. The involved organs enlarge rapidly. Splenic sequestration is seen only in children as the spleen is usually infarcted by the age of 6 years. Exchange transfusion may be required.
- Painful: due to vascular occlusion. Can be precipitated by dehydration, hypoxia, infections and cold exposure. Almost any organ can be affected. Small bones of the hands and feet are most often affected in childhood ('hand–foot syndrome'). In older patients, the lungs, hips, shoulders and spine are more commonly involved. Vascular occlusion is the cause of serious complications as detailed below.
- Haemolytic: this is rare and may be associated with coexistent G6PD deficiency. The haemoglobin drops rapidly, with a compensatory increase in reticulocytes. Increased haemolysis is also seen in association with other crises.

Complications

- Anaemia, usually well tolerated.
- Infection: mainly susceptibility to infection with encapsulated organisms due to hyposplenism (see Splenectomy section), but also infection of infarcted bone causing osteomyelitis (*Salmonella* spp.).
- Vessel occlusion: splenic infarction, TIA and stroke, renal papillary necrosis, priapism, aseptic necrosis of the femoral head, placental infarction and spontaneous abortion.
- Gallstones.
- Leg ulceration.
- Acute chest crisis: due to vascular occlusion, infection and bone marrow embolism. New infiltrates can be seen on X-ray. Mortality is around 3%.

Investigations

- Normochromic normocytic anaemia, with reticulocytosis, raised LDH and low haptoglobin.
- Sickle cells, target cells and nucleated RBCs on blood film (features of hyposplenism may also be present following splenic infarction; see Fig. 29.6).
- Haemoglobin electrophoresis or chromatography demonstrates HbS. HbF levels may be raised.
- Leucocyte and platelet counts may also be raised.
- Prenatal diagnosis can be made using polymerase chain reaction (PCR) techniques on chorionic villous samples.

The findings are often more severe in episodes of crisis. Other tests may reveal organ-specific complications.

Treatment

Immunization against encapsulated bacteria and prompt treatment of infection is extremely important. During episodes of crisis, supportive care must include effective analgesia as well as optimization of hydration and oxygenation. Blood transfusion is often necessary. Other treatments include the following:

- Hydroxycarbamide (hydroxyurea): this cytotoxic drug is indicated in patients with painful crises, significant anaemia or other complications. It increases fetal haemoglobin levels and reduces the frequency of crises. It causes a macrocytosis and myelosuppression in a dose-dependent manner, and there may be a risk of leukaemia with long-term treatment.
- Long-term folate (increased folate utilization because of haemolysis).
- Prophylactic penicillin in children.
- Exchange transfusions if recurrent crises or significant organ damage.
- Management by a multidisciplinary sickle cell team reduces admissions and improves patients' quality of life.

The only curative treatment is haematopoietic cell transplantation, which is only carried out in patients with severe disease who have an HLA-matched sibling. There is ongoing research into gene therapy to increase the expression of HbF.

Prognosis

There is 5% mortality in the first 10 years of life. Median life expectancy is estimated to be in the mid 50s, with death most commonly due to infection.

Note that in the sickle cell trait (a heterozygous carrier state) the disease is much milder, with little or no anaemia and a normal blood film. It also provides significant protection against malaria. Crises may be caused in extreme conditions. The most common complication is renal disease.

Thalassaemia

Thalassaemia is an inherited disease of defective haemoglobin production; normal haemoglobin synthesis is summarized in Fig. 37.2. The prevalence of thalassaemia is 2.5–15% in affected areas. Alpha-thalassaemia affects those in the Mediterranean, Africa, the Middle East and south-east Asia, whereas beta-thalassaemia is found in China, the Mediterranean, the Middle East and India. It is an inherited condition. The alpha globin gene is on chromosome 16 and the beta gene on chromosome 11.

Pathophysiology

- Reduced production of one or more of the haemoglobin chains (most importantly alpha or beta) results in a relative excess and accumulation of the other chain ('imbalanced globin chain synthesis'). There are many known mutations which result in varying degrees of reduced globin synthesis.
- The unstable haemoglobin precipitates, causing ineffective erythropoiesis and haemolysis.

Fig. 37.2 Normal haemoglobin synthesis.

Normal haemoglobin is composed of four polypeptide chains (tetramer)
At various stages of development, different polypeptide chains are produced (ζ, ε, α, γ, δ and β)
In the embryo (first 8 weeks' gestation), three different haemoglobins are produced by the yolk sac, Hb Gower-1 (ζ_2, ε_2), Hb Gower-2 (α_2, ε_2) and Hb Portland (ζ_2, γ_2)
Fetal haemoglobin (HbF) is composed of two α chains and two γ chains (α_2, γ_2) and is the major haemoglobin of intrauterine life. It declines rapidly around birth and constitutes less than 1% haemoglobin by 6 months of age. HbF is produced predominantly by the liver until 30 weeks, after which the bone marrow takes over. It has an avid affinity for oxygen
Production of β chains increases rapidly at 36 weeks' gestation; 96% adult haemoglobin is HbA (α_2, β_2), 3.5% is HbA_2 (α_2, δ_2) with the remainder being HbF
The genes for the globin chains α and ζ are found clustered on chromosome 16. The genes for the remaining chains are located in a cluster on chromosome 11
Each person has four α genes (two on each chromosome 16) and two β genes (one on each chromosome 11)

- There is deficiency of alpha chains in alpha-thalassaemia and of beta chains in beta-thalassaemia.

Clinical features

- The clinical presentation is dependent on the underlying abnormality, as described in Figs 37.3 and 37.4. Note that carriers with only one defective copy of the gene (or two in alpha-thalassaemia) are usually asymptomatic.
- Skeletal change occurs due to expansion of erythropoietic bone marrow.
- Thalassaemia provides an advantage in infection with falciparum malaria.
- Aplastic crises may occur with parvovirus B19 infection.

Microcytic anaemia is the abnormality on a blood film in beta-thalassaemia minor. Differentiation from iron deficiency is possible on the basis of ferritin levels, red cell distribution width (RDW, a measure of homogeneity of red cell size) and clinical suspicion. MCV is usually lower in thalassaemia than IDA.

Management

- Transfusion to maintain an adequate haemoglobin (>10 g/dL) initiated during childhood to ensure normal growth and development.

Fig. 37.3 Characteristic features of the alpha-thalassaemias.

Subtype	Silent carrier	Alpha-thalassaemia trait	HbH disease	Hydrops fetalis
Genetic abnormality	One alpha gene deleted	Two alpha genes deleted	Three alpha genes deleted	Four alpha genes deleted
Clinical features	Asymptomatic	Usually asymptomatic	Haemolytic anaemia Splenomegaly Bone changes May be symptomatic at birth	Hepatosplenomegaly Gross oedema Hypoalbuminaemia Extramedullary haematopoiesis
Haematological findings	Usually no abnormality	Hypochromia Microcytosis	Hypochromia Microcytosis Reticulocytosis HbH (β_4) on electrophoresis Inclusion bodies with cresyl blue	Hypochromia Microcytosis Reticulocytosis Target cells Nucleated red cells Hb Bart's (γ_4) on electrophoresis
Survival	Normal	Normal	Variable	Stillborn or death shortly after birth

HbH, haemoglobin H.

Fig. 37.4 Characteristic features of the beta-thalassaemias.

Subtype	Beta-thalassaemia minor	Beta-thalassaemia intermedia	Beta-thalassaemia major
Genetic abnormality	Heterozygous abnormality in beta globin gene	Homozygous or mixed heterozygous abnormality in beta globin gene	Homozygous abnormality in beta globin gene
Clinical features	Usually asymptomatic Splenomegaly on imaging	Variable – possible features: Extramedullary haematopoiesis Hepatosplenomegaly Skeletal deformity Gallstones Leg ulcers Thrombosis Pulmonary hypertension	Failure to thrive (3–6 months) Jaundice Extramedullary haematopoiesis Hepatosplenomegaly Skeletal deformity Haemosiderosis Recurrent infections Cardiac failure Gallstones Leg ulcers
Haematological findings	Mild anaemia Microcytosis with normal RDW Hypochromia Target cells Poikilocytosis HbA_2 high HbF may be raised	Moderate anaemia but usually not transfusion-dependent Microcytosis Hypochromia Target cells Poikilocytosis	Transfusion-dependent severe anaemia Microcytosis Hypochromia Target cells Anisopoikilocytosis Reticulocytosis Nucleated RBCs Basophilic stippling Inclusion bodies on supravital staining with methyl violet HbA absent or very low HbF high
Survival	Normal	Variable. Usually survive to adulthood even without treatment	Death in childhood without treatment; bone marrow transplantation may be curative

Hb, haemoglobin; RBC, red blood cell; RDW, red cell distribution width.

- Iron chelation to prevent haemosiderosis using desferrioxamine.
- Splenectomy can reduce transfusion requirements but should be avoided where possible because of the increased susceptibility to infection.
- Long-term folate supplementation in severe disease (beta-thalassaemia major).
- Vitamin D and calcium for skeletal abnormalities.
- Haematopoietic stem cell transplant is an effective treatment for patients with beta-thalassaemia major, particularly children. However, HLA-matched cells are not always available.
- Current research emphasis is on the prospect of using gene therapy techniques.
- Prenatal diagnosis and genetic counselling should be available.

Pernicious anaemia

This is an autoimmune condition and has an incidence of roughly 2 per 10 000. However, it is suspected that pernicious anaemia is underdiagnosed and true rates may be much higher, especially in the elderly. There is a strong association with other autoimmune diseases.

Pathology

- Immunoglobulin G (IgG) autoantibodies are produced against gastric parietal cells and intrinsic factor.
- This causes gastric mucosal atrophy with loss of parietal cells and achlorhydria.
- Production of intrinsic factor, necessary for vitamin B_{12} absorption, is reduced.
- Binding of vitamin B_{12} to intrinsic factor is impaired.

Clinical features

- The onset is usually insidious and is more common after the age of 50 years.
- Symptoms include those of anaemia and the neurological complications of vitamin B_{12} deficiency.
- Examination may reveal anaemia, glossitis, mild jaundice due to haemolysis, low-grade pyrexia, mild splenomegaly and neurological signs.

- Complications of anaemia (see Ch. 29).
- Neurological abnormalities from vitamin B_{12} deficiency (peripheral neuropathy, subacute combined degeneration of the cord, dementia, optic atrophy).
- Increased risk of gastric carcinoma.

Investigations

- Macrocytic anaemia with typical blood film (see Fig. 29.6).
- White cell and platelet counts: may be low.
- Serum vitamin B_{12}: low, with abnormal Schilling test (now rarely performed).
- Megaloblastic bone marrow: large erythrocytes, large hypersegmented neutrophils.
- Bilirubin and LDH increased (due to breakdown of abnormal RBCs).
- Parietal cell antibody in 90% (seen in up to 50% of healthy elderly).
- Intrinsic factor antibody in 50%.
- Gastroscopy should be considered to exclude gastric carcinoma.

Treatment

- Lifelong vitamin B_{12} replacement.
- Initial response to treatment can be demonstrated by an increase in reticulocyte count.

Blood transfusion may be required if the patient is haemodynamically compromised or demonstrating ischaemic stress. However, as the patient is often elderly with comorbidities, and the circulation may be hyperdynamic, the risk of precipitating heart failure must be considered. Response to vitamin B_{12} is often rapid and transfusion can often be avoided.

Aplastic anaemia

This refers to a condition of pancytopenia, i.e. deficiency of all three marrow cell lines, due to a lack of precursor cells in the bone marrow. It may be congenital or acquired, and is one cause of 'bone marrow failure'. In Caucasians, incidence is around 3 per million per year.

Aetiology

Most cases of aplastic anaemia are idiopathic, and it is thought that an autoimmune process is the most likely reason for precursor cell destruction. In a minority of cases of acquired aplastic anaemia there may be a clear link to exposure to viruses, drugs or radiation. The most common form of congenital aplastic anaemia is Fanconi anaemia, a polygenic autosomal recessive or X-linked condition.

Clinical features

- Symptoms of anaemia.
- Excess bleeding due to thrombocytopenia.
- Susceptibility to infection due to leucopenia.

Investigations

- Pancytopenia.
- Absence of compensatory reticulocytosis.
- Bone marrow biopsy shows reduced haematopoietic cells and replacement with fat cells.

Management

- Supportive measures: platelet and blood transfusion, prompt treatment of infection.
- Stem cell transplant in younger patients with severe aplastic anaemia.
- Immune suppression alone in older patients: antithymocyte globulin and ciclosporin are commonly used.

Sideroblastic anaemia

Sideroblastic anaemia refers to conditions where anaemia is associated with an excess of abnormal sideroblasts: nucleated erythrocyte precursors containing iron granules. There is a defect of haem synthesis, leading to disordered erythropoiesis and excess iron in the marrow.

Aetiology

Sideroblastic anaemia can be congenital or acquired:

- Congenital: X-linked.
- Acquired: in myelodysplastic syndrome (see below) or secondary to drugs (e.g. isoniazid, pyrazinamide), alcohol, lead poisoning, myeloproliferative disease, connective tissue disease.

The patient presents with symptoms of anaemia.

Management

MCV may be low, normal or raised depending on the underlying cause. Ferritin is raised. Bone marrow examination reveals ring sideroblasts, where haem has accumulated into granules that are situated in a perinuclear ring. Treatment is supportive, with blood transfusion, withdrawal of causative agents and iron chelation.

Bone marrow infiltration

Any cause of bone marrow infiltration, if extensive enough, can cause bone marrow failure and anaemia. The causes include proliferative syndromes with fibrosis, amyloid, sarcoidosis lymphoma/leukaemia and metastatic malignancy.

Lead poisoning

This is now rare in developed countries but may occur in adults due to industrial exposure, and in children from inhalation or ingestion of lead-containing products. Presentation may be with gastrointestinal upset, irritability and reduced consciousness, foot drop or wrist drop, and the Burton line on the gums.

Complications include peripheral neuropathy, encephalopathy, anaemia and nephropathy.

Management

- Blood lead levels.
- Full blood count: hypochromic anaemia with basophilic stippling of RBCs.
- Discuss with poisons information services.
- Treat with disodium calcium edetate (drug of choice), succimer, dimercaprol or penicillamine.

MYELODYSPLASTIC SYNDROMES

These chronic myeloid conditions are classified as neoplastic disorders. They arise from acquired mutations in a haematopoietic stem cell, which then develops and proliferates abnormally, resulting in an abnormal population of cells in the bone marrow that interferes with normal haematopoiesis. There is a risk of transformation into acute leukaemia. They are more common in men and in the elderly.

Classification

MDS is classified according to how many of the cell lines are affected, the proportion of blast cells (early precursor cells) in the marrow, and whether specific chromosomal deletions are present. Sideroblastic anaemia is seen in refractory anaemia with ring sideroblasts (RARS). Risk of leukaemic transformation is highest in refractory anaemia with excess blasts (RAEB). For more information, see Further reading.

Clinical features

The symptoms are non-specific and reflect the underlying deficiency. Patients may present with symptoms due to one or a combination of anaemia, leucopenia and thrombocytopenia.

Investigations

- Full blood count: anaemia with low reticulocytes. Thrombocytopenia and leucopenia may be present.
- Blood film: poikilocytes (abnormally shaped red cells) and anisocytosis (unequal size).
- Bone marrow exam: hypercellular with abnormal precursors. Ring sideroblasts in RARS. Increased blast cells in RAEB.
- Cytogenetics on bone marrow samples may detect underlying chromosomal abnormalities in the clone, which have prognostic implications.

Management

A prognostic score should be calculated to help guide treatment. Other factors which are taken into account are the wishes of patients, and their ability to withstand different treatment regimens. Approaches are as follows:

- Supportive care, including transfusions or red cells and platelets, and prompt treatment of infection.
- Low-intensity chemotherapeutic drugs such as azacytadine. These may prolong life but do not offer a cure.
- High-intensity chemotherapy and stem cell transplant: reserved for younger patients with high-risk disease.

There are many clinical trials underway investigating the efficacy of different regimens.

LEUKAEMIA

The leukaemias are a group of conditions characterized by the malignant proliferation of leucocytes in the bone marrow. The cells spill out into the bloodstream and may infiltrate other organs.

In the acute leukaemias, there is a proliferation of early lymphoid and myeloid precursors (blasts), which do not mature. The clinical course is very aggressive and they are rapidly fatal without treatment.

The chronic leukaemias have a more indolent course and are characterized by the proliferation of lymphoid and myeloid cells that reach maturity (lymphocytes and neutrophils, respectively).

All leukaemias are best managed by specialists and chemotherapy is a rapidly changing field. Most patients are in clinical trials and only the principles need be understood by students and junior doctors.

COMMUNICATION

Leukaemia is a frightening diagnosis for most patients. Make sure they understand the particular form they have and the outlook with modern therapy.

Acute lymphoblastic leukaemia

Epidemiology and aetiology

Acute lymphoblastic leukaemia (ALL) is the most common malignancy in children under 15 years. Only 15% of ALL cases occur in adults. Its aetiology is unknown but is probably multifactorial. A genetic predisposition is suggested by concordance in twins, and the incidence is increased in Down's syndrome and ataxia telangiectasia. The classification of ALL was previously according to the FAB system, but the WHO has recommended moving to classification by underlying cell type (B or T cell) and cytogenetic abnormality.

Pathology

- Lymphoblasts proliferate uncontrollably in the bone marrow and cause bone marrow failure.
- Lymphoblasts circulate in the bloodstream and can infiltrate the lymph nodes, liver, spleen, kidneys, testicles and central nervous system (CNS), causing organ failure.
- The pathological cell is a B-cell precursor in 80% of ALL and a T cell in the remainder.

Clinical features

- Peaks of incidence are at age 5 years and over 65 years.
- The history is usually short, as the disease is so aggressive (days to a few weeks).
- Rapidly proliferating tumour cells in the bone marrow cause bone pain or symptoms of bone marrow failure (Fig. 37.5).
- There may be fever, lymphadenopathy and hepatosplenomegaly on examination.
- Symptoms or signs due to other organ involvement may be present: for instance meningism or cranial neuropathies with CNS involvement.

Investigations

- Normochromic normocytic anaemia with low reticulocyte count.
- High white cell count due to lymphoblasts; neutropenia may be present.
- Thrombocytopenia.
- Bone marrow is hypercellular and dominated by lymphoblasts (usually >50%).
- Cytogenetic abnormalities may be present (e.g. hyperdiploidy or the Philadelphia chromosome).
- Urate and LDH high.

Fig. 37.5 General features of bone marrow failure.

Cells affected	Result	Manifestation
Red cell precursors	Anaemia	Lethargy, dyspnoea, pallor
White cell precursors	Neutropenia	Recurrent infections, fever
Platelet precursors	Thrombocytopenia	Bleeding, bruising, purpura

- Mediastinal mass on chest X-ray in T-cell ALL.
- Cerebrospinal fluid examination may show lymphoblasts, increased pressure and increased protein.

Treatment

All chemotherapy requires careful supportive care with hydration, prophylactic antibiotics, antiviral and antifungal drugs, septic surveillance, blood products to support pancytopenia, bone marrow colony-stimulating factors such as granulocyte colony-stimulating factor, monitoring of coagulation, and allopurinol to prevent tumour lysis syndrome and gout from the increased purine metabolism.

Treatment should be managed in a specialized unit and include:

- Cytotoxic chemotherapy in three phases: induction of remission, consolidation and maintenance. The regimen may be tailored to the cytogenetic profile: for instance using a tyrosine kinase inhibitor in Philadelphia chromosome-positive ALL.
- CNS prophylaxis: intrathecal methotrexate, cranial irradiation if high risk.
- Monitoring for relapse followed by prompt treatment with salvage chemotherapy.
- Allogeneic bone marrow transplantation often improves outcomes and can be curative. It is usually reserved for patients with high-risk ALL.

Prognosis

Prognosis is poor in infants and adults with a 5-year event-free survival of 30–40%. In children the 5-year-event-free survival is 70–80%. However, prognosis is very variable and depends upon other factors, including white cell count at presentation, null-cell or T-cell phenotype, male sex and the type of cytogenetic abnormalities.

Acute myeloid leukaemia

AML accounts for 20% of all leukaemias and 80% of adult acute leukaemias. It is much less common in children.

Aetiology

Most cases arise with no clear cause, though many risks are recognized:

- Ionizing radiation: survivors of Hiroshima.
- Chemical exposure: leather and rubber workers (benzene).
- Previous chemotherapy: alkylating agents.
- Predisposing diseases: myeloproliferative diseases, aplastic anaemia and myelodysplasia, which can transform to acute leukaemia.

Fig. 37.6 French–American–British (FAB) classification of AML.

FAB subtype	Name (predominant cell type)	Specific clinical features
M1	Undifferentiated myeloblastic	–
M2	Myeloblastic	Most common
M3	Promyelocytic	DIC may cause fatal bleeding
M4	Myelomonocytic	Gingival, skin and meningeal infiltration
M5	Monocytic	Gingival, skin and meningeal infiltration Lymphadenopathy and DIC may occur
M6	Erythroleukaemia	Particularly older patients
M7	Megakaryocytic	–

AML, acute myeloid leukaemia; DIC, disseminated intravascular coagulation.

Pathology

- Accumulation of immature haematopoietic blast cells in the bone marrow, which can cause bone marrow failure.
- Blasts can infiltrate the gums, liver, spleen, skin and, less commonly, the CNS.
- AML is traditionally classified as shown in Fig. 37.6. The more recent WHO classification is shown in Fig. 37.7.
- Disseminated intravascular coagulation (DIC) has a recognized association with promyelocytic leukaemia, which carries the t(15:17) translocation (previously M3).
- Gingival hypertrophy and skin lesions are features of monocytic subtypes M4 and M5.
- When the circulating white cell count is very high, leukostasis may occur, resulting in hyperviscosity symptoms.

Presentation

- More frequent with increasing age (median age at presentation is 65 years).
- Symptoms are due to marrow failure (Fig. 37.5) or organ infiltration by leukaemic cells.
- Eye involvement is relatively common.
- Bone pain, joint pain and malaise may be prominent symptoms.
- Significant hepatomegaly and splenomegaly may occur. Lymphadenopathy is rare.

Fig. 37.7 WHO classification of AML.

AML with recurrent genetic abnormalities	Generally better prognosis. Includes: t(8:21): Auer rods seen t(15:17): promyelocytic leukaemia. DIC may occur
AML with multilineage dysplasia	With or without preceding myeloproliferative disorder or myelodysplasia
AML/MDS related to therapy	Following alkyating agents or radiation
AML not otherwise categorized	

AML, acute myeloid leukaemia; DIC, disseminated intravascular coagulation; MDS, myelodysplastic syndrome.

Investigations

- Normochromic normocytic anaemia with low reticulocyte count.
- High white cell count due to circulating blasts; neutropenia may be present.
- Thrombocytopenia.
- Blasts may contain Auer rods (diagnostic of AML).
- Bone marrow is hypercellular with blasts constituting at least 20%. Flow cytometry on the marrow aspirate will help identify the specific cell type.
- Cytogenetic abnormalities may be present in around 50% of patients. For example, an 8:21 translocation is associated with a favourable outcome, whereas monosomy of chromosome 5 is a poor marker.
- Urate and LDH high.
- Calcium and phosphate may also be raised.
- Abnormal renal or liver function may reflect organ failure due to infiltration.

Treatment

Treatment should be managed in a specialized unit. Broad principles are as follows:

- Supportive care as for all leukaemias (see ALL).
- Intensive cytotoxic chemotherapy: induction of remission and post-remission (consolidation) therapy. The exact regimen is determined by the

subtype and the risk group, and most patients are in a clinical trial.
- Bone marrow transplantation following remission may improve outcome in high-risk patients.
- Salvage chemotherapy is required when remission is not achieved or relapse occurs early.
- There are many new agents under investigation, including enzyme inhibitors and immunotherapeutics such as gemtuzumab.
- Monitoring of residual disease is performed with bone marrow inspection, cytogenetics and molecular techniques such as PCR.

Treatment of elderly patients is often difficult due to the adverse effects of chemotherapy, and lower-intensity regimens are required.

Prognosis

- In most patients, cure/complete remission should be the aim; up to 75% of patients enter remission. Long-term survival is very variable and dependent on patient-specific factors.
- Poor prognostic factors include increasing age, very high white cell count, secondary leukaemia (e.g. previous myelodysplasia), certain cytogenetic abnormalities and the presence of DIC.

Chronic lymphocytic leukaemia

Epidemiology and aetiology

Chronic lymphocytic leukaemia (CLL) is the most common leukaemia in the developed world (30% of all leukaemias). The incidence increases with age and it is twice as common in males. B-cell CLL and small lymphocytic lymphoma are thought to be part of a spectrum of disease. The aetiology is unknown. Other leukaemias of mature lymphocytes not covered here include hairy cell leukaemia and pro-lymphocytic leukaemias.

Pathology

- Proliferation of small lymphocytes in bone marrow, blood and lymphoid tissues.
- These are morphologically mature but functionally abnormal.
- 95–98% of CLL patients have B-cell phenotype (remainder are T cells).

Clinical features

- Some patients are asymptomatic; others may describe malaise, weight loss, night sweats, recurrent infections, bleeding or symptoms of anaemia.
- Lymphadenopathy is usually found (60%).
- Hepatosplenomegaly may also be present.
- Skin involvement is common.

Investigations

- Monoclonal lymphocytosis with 'smear' or 'smudge' cells seen on film.
- Anaemia may be due to marrow infiltration or autoimmune haemolysis (DAT-positive).
- Thrombocytopenia may be due to marrow infiltration or autoimmune destruction.
- Bone marrow shows accumulation of mature lymphocytes constituting over 30% of cells.
- Cytogenetic and immunological analysis will offer diagnostic and prognostic information.
- Hypogammaglobulinaemia occurs in 50% and predisposes to infection.

Treatment

CLL usually follows an indolent course. Staging the disease will help guide treatment. The only potential cure is with stem cell transplant, which carries a high risk of treatment-related mortality. Initially the disease is often asymptomatic, and monitoring is sufficient. When disease becomes symptomatic or rapidly progressive, treatment is indicated. There are ongoing clinical trials.

- Chlorambucil (an alkylating agent) is an older, established treatment.
- Combination therapy involving fludarabine, cyclophosphamide and rituximab has shown good results in clinical trials. Other potential agents are bendamustine and alemtuzumab.
- Autoimmune phenomena are responsive to oral prednisolone.
- Radiotherapy may be beneficial in symptomatic, localized disease.
- Splenectomy is sometimes used in refractory hypersplenism.

Prognosis

- Dependent on extent of disease (survival ranges from 1.5 years to over 12 years).
- In around 10% of CLL, Richter transformation to high-grade lymphoma occurs as a terminal event.

Chronic myeloid leukaemia

CML accounts for 20% of all leukaemias. It can be considered as a myeloproliferative disease. It occurs mainly in middle age, most commonly between 40 and 60 years, with a male preponderance.

Pathology

CML is a malignant proliferation of myeloid cells of unknown aetiology. There is a characteristic chromosome 9:22 reciprocal translocation – the 'Philadelphia chromosome'. The resulting fusion gene *bcr/abl* possesses elevated tyrosine kinase activity and is believed to be pathogenic in CML.

Clinical features

- Symptoms include lethargy, weight loss, sweats and left hypochondrial discomfort (enlarging spleen).
- Symptoms of anaemia or thrombocytopenia may be present.
- On examination there is splenomegaly, which may be massive.
- Hepatomegaly is present in 50% of cases but lymphadenopathy is uncommon.
- The natural history is characterized by a chronic phase lasting several years, followed by an acute, aggressive phase similar to acute leukaemia.
- Leukostasis may occur with very high leukocyte counts.

Investigations

- Raised white cell count (often very high) with full range of immature and mature myeloid cells.
- Anaemia may be due to marrow infiltration or hypersplenism.
- Thrombocytosis is common.
- Bone marrow demonstrates accumulation of myeloid cells.
- 95% of patients have the Philadelphia chromosome on light microscopy. The other 5% demonstrate the fusion protein through molecular studies.
- Neutrophil alkaline phosphatase is low.
- Urate and LDH are high.
- Serum vitamin B_{12} is high.

Treatment

- Good supportive therapy as needed.
- Imatinib, a specific tyrosine kinase inhibitor (TKI) targeting the *bcr/abl* fusion protein, revolutionized treatment of CML. It is well tolerated and produces clinical and cytogenetic response in the vast majority of cases. Newer TKIs have been developed and clinical trials are ongoing.
- Alpha-interferon and hydroxycarbamide are rarely used and only if there is intolerance to TKIs.
- Allogeneic bone marrow transplantation may be curative and should be considered in young patients with an HLA-matched sibling and those with blast crisis.
- Leucopheresis will reduce the white count quickly in leukostasis.
- Frequent monitoring of response to treatment is extremely important.

Prognosis

- Chronic phase: median time 2–6 years. With TKIs 93% are progression-free at 6 years.
- Acute phase: median survival 3 months without treatment.
- Transformation is to AML in two-thirds of patients and to ALL in the remainder.

MULTIPLE MYELOMA

The incidence of multiple myeloma is 5 per 100 000 (1% of all malignancies, 10–15% of all haematological malignancies), occurring mainly in the elderly. An abnormal proliferation of plasma cells causes features such as a paraprotein, skeletal lesions, bone marrow failure, renal impairment and hypercalcaemia.

It is one of a number of diseases associated with abnormal proliferation of a clone of plasma cells (terminally differentiated B cells), also including:

- Monoclonal gammopathy of uncertain significance (MGUS): presence of a paraprotein but <5% plasma cells in marrow and no end-organ damage. 1% per year progress to myeloma.
- Smouldering multiple myeloma: greater than 10% plasma cells in the bone marrow but no end-organ damage (anaemia, hypercalcaemia, renal impairment, bone lesions).
- Waldenström's macroglobulinaemia: production of large amounts of IgM.
- Primary systemic amyloidosis: production of light-chain fibrils which are deposited in organs.

Pathology

- Neoplastic proliferation of a single clone of plasma cells.
- The malignant cells secrete a monoclonal immunoglobulin or light chain and normal immunoglobulin production is suppressed. The plasma cells can form tumours called plasmacytomas.
- Osteoclast activity is increased, resulting in bone reabsorption.
- AL (systemic) amyloidosis affects 10% of cases.

Clinical features

- Symptoms of anaemia may be present.
- Bone pain due to osteolytic lesions and pathological fractures affect two-thirds of patients.
- Hypercalcaemia is often present, causing typical symptoms (see Ch. 35).
- Renal impairment: often due to light-chain deposition or hypercalcaemia.
- Recurrent infections result from impaired antibody response and hypogammaglobulinaemia.
- Examination usually reveals pallor alone.
- Spinal cord compression and radiculopathy can result from compression by tumour or vertebral collapse.

- Polymerization of the monoclonal antibody occasionally results in hyperviscosity syndrome.

Investigations

- Normochromic normocytic anaemia.
- Rouleaux (RBCs sticking together) and background immunoglobulin staining may be seen on the blood film.
- Plasma viscosity and ESR: usually high.
- Serum protein electrophoresis demonstrates a monoclonal paraprotein. In 60% it is IgG, 25% IgA. Free light chains are not usually detected with this method. Quantification and serial measurement of the paraprotein enables effective monitoring.
- Free light chains may be detected in the urine ('Bence Jones protein') with urine electrophoresis, or in the serum with a serum free light-chain assay. The majority of paraprotein-negative myeloma secrete free light chains; a small number are truly non-secretory.
- Skeletal survey with X-rays reveals generalized osteopenia, 'punched-out' lytic lesions ('pepperpot skull') and pathological fractures. Bone scans are not helpful.
- Bone marrow aspirate shows that over 10% of bone marrow cells are plasma cells. Cytogenetic analysis is increasingly helpful for prognosis.
- Calcium high; alkaline phosphatase usually normal.
- Renal failure may result from a number of factors (Fig. 37.8).
- Beta-2-microglobulin level usually high.

HINTS AND TIPS

Psychological care of very sick or terminally ill patients is an important part of their management, and referral to a clinical psychologist may help patients cope with their illness.

Treatment

- Monitoring only in MGUS and smouldering myeloma.
- Supportive treatment with antibiotics, blood products, analgesics and correction of hypercalcaemia where necessary.
- Autologous stem cell transplant (ASCT) improves event-free survival (though is not curative) and is performed when the patient is healthy enough to undergo the high-dose chemotherapy required.
- Prior to ASCT, chemotherapy is required to induce remission. There are several potential regimens, such as CTD (cyclophosphamide, thalidomide, dexamethasone). Newer agents such as bortezomib are effective.
- In patients not eligible for ASCT, induction chemotherapy regimens may be modified to minimize toxicity.
- There may be a role for maintenance therapy after ASCT or induction chemotherapy.
- Following relapse, the treatment depends on the individual case. Further induction chemotherapy may be used, and there may be a role for a second ASCT. In those not able to tolerate the above, lenalidomide offers improved survival.
- Allogeneic transplantation may be curative but has a high mortality. It is an option for younger patients, after proper discussion of the risks.
- Radiotherapy may be useful where there is localized disease causing bony pain.

Please see Further reading for more details.

Fig. 37.8 Causes of renal failure in multiple myeloma.

Hypercalcaemia
Hyperuricaemia
Precipitated light chains
Amyloidosis
NSAIDs prescribed for bone pain

NSAIDs, non-steroidal anti-inflammatory drugs.

Prognosis

- The prognosis is very variable. Median survival is roughly 4 years.
- Poor prognostic factors include certain cytogenetic profiles, high beta-2-microglobulin levels (most accurate), high paraprotein levels, high urea, low haemoglobin, increasing age and low albumin.

LYMPHOMA

Lymphomas are neoplastic proliferations of lymphocytes that form solid tumours within lymphoid tissue. They are split into two broad categories on the basis of histological findings: Hodgkin's disease (Reed–Sternberg (RS) cells present) and non-Hodgkin's lymphoma (all others).

Hodgkin's disease

Incidence and aetiology

The incidence of Hodgkin's disease is 5 in 100 000; it is one of the most common malignancies in young adults and accounts for around 10–15% of all lymphomas. There is a bimodal age distribution with peaks at 20–30 years and above 50 years with a male

Fig. 37.9 Rye classification of Hodgkin's disease.

Subtype	Percentage	Prognosis
Lymphocyte-rich classical HD	5	Excellent
Nodular lymphocyte-predominant HD	5	Excellent
Mixed cellularity	30	Intermediate
Lymphocyte depleted	<5	Poor
Nodular sclerosing	60	Variable

preponderance in childhood Hodgkin's disease. Its aetiology is unknown but there is a link with Epstein–Barr virus (EBV) and an increased risk in immunodeficient states (e.g. HIV, immunosuppressant therapy). It mainly affects Caucasian populations and is more common in higher socioeconomic groups.

Pathology

- Characteristic RS cells in a background of inflammatory infiltrate.
- RS cells are large bi- or multinuclear cells with prominent 'owl-eyed' nucleoli.
- Hodgkin's disease is divided, using the Rye classification, into five histological subgroups (Fig. 37.9).
- The pathological cell in nodular lymphocyte-predominant Hodgkin's disease is a variant of the RS cell, sometimes termed the 'popcorn cell'.

Clinical features

- Symptoms are due to painless lymph node enlargement (particularly cervical, axillary and mediastinal) and/or 'B symptoms' (Fig. 37.10).
- Lymphadenopathy is supradiaphragmatic in 90% of patients and mediastinal disease may cause dry cough and exertional dyspnoea.
- Affected lymph nodes feel rubbery and are non-tender.
- Some patients describe pruritus and alcohol-induced lymph node pain.
- Pallor and hepatosplenomegaly may also be found on examination.

Fig. 37.10 'B symptoms' of lymphoma.

Weight loss >10% of initial weight over previous 6 months
Drenching night sweats
Fever >38°C

Investigations

- Diagnosis requires lymph node biopsy, and excision of a whole node is performed if possible to provide adequate structural information. Needle aspiration is insufficient.
- Staging of disease is then performed with whole-body CT or PET-CT (Fig. 37.11).
- Bone marrow examination is usually required for staging, especially if B symptoms are prominent. Reed–Sternberg cells in the bone marrow indicates stage IV disease.
- Normochromic normocytic anaemia, neutrophilia, eosinophilia and thrombocytosis.
- Alkaline phosphatase may be raised.

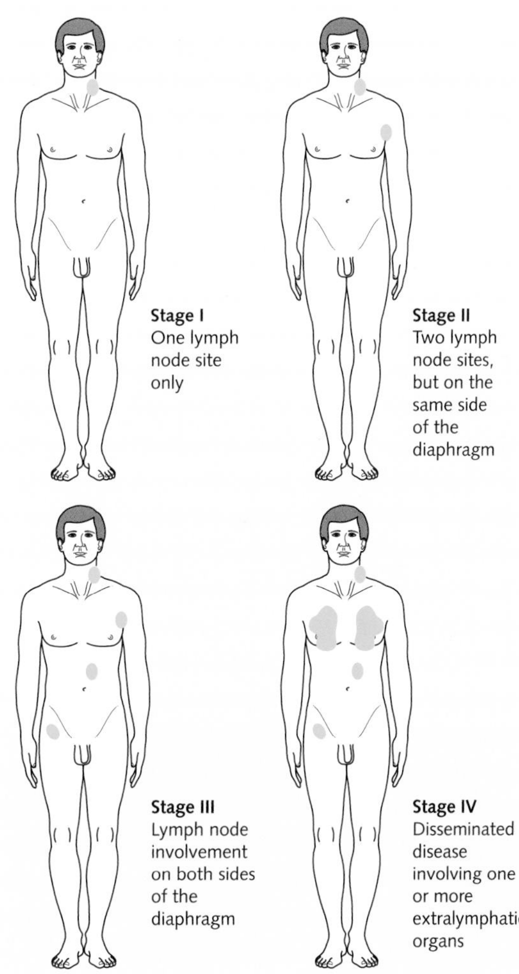
Stage I
One lymph node site only
Stage II
Two lymph node sites, but on the same side of the diaphragm
Stage III
Lymph node involvement on both sides of the diaphragm
Stage IV
Disseminated disease involving one or more extralymphatic organs

Fig. 37.11 Ann Arbor staging of malignant lymphomas. Diagram shows stages I–IV. When you stage a patient you give a number (I–IV) and a letter (A or B). The letter A denotes the absence of B symptoms and B denotes the presence of B symptoms. For example, patients at stage IIA have stage II lymphoma without B symptoms.

- LDH raised in bulky disease (prognostic indicator and marker of disease activity).
- Urate high in bulky disease.
- ESR and CRP often raised.
- Chest X-ray: mediastinal lymphadenopathy
- Staging laparotomy or splenic biopsy is very rarely performed when the diagnosis is suspected but there is no other accessible pathological tissue.

Treatment

- Early disease (stages I–II) without adverse prognostic factors (see below) is treated with up to four cycles of ABVD (Adriamycin (doxorubicin), bleomycin, vinblastine, dacarbazine) chemotherapy and radiotherapy.
- Early disease with adverse prognostic factors is treated with longer courses of chemotherapy (tailored to response as measured by PET scan) and radiotherapy.
- Extensive disease (stage III–IV) is treated with chemotherapy alone. ABVD is the accepted standard. Other regimens are BEACOPP and Stanford V.
- Relapse is treated with alternative chemotherapy regimen or high-dose chemotherapy followed by autologous haematopoietic stem cell transplant.

Prognosis

The outlook for the predominantly young patients is good and a positive outcome should be expected.

- Prognosis is greatly affected by histological type and stage of disease at presentation. With treatment, early disease without adverse factors has 10-year survival of up to 97%. Even advanced disease has 5-year survival rates of over 50%.
- Poor prognostic indicators include B symptoms, high-stage, lymphocyte-depleted histology, increasing age, bulky mediastinal disease, high ESR and low albumin.

Non-Hodgkin's lymphoma

Incidence and aetiology

Non-Hodgkin's lymphoma (NHL) accounts for over 3% of all cancer-related deaths. Incidence increases with age and the condition is more common in males. The aetiology is multifactorial, including:

- Genetic predisposition.
- Immunosuppression (particularly human immunodeficiency virus (HIV) infection, also transplant recipients).
- Viruses (e.g. EBV, particularly Burkitt's lymphoma).
- A possible link with exposure to ionizing radiation.

Pathology

- Highly heterogeneous group of conditions in terms of pathological cell type and clinical course.
- Neoplastic proliferation of B (usually) or T lymphocytes within the lymphoid system forming solid tumours which do not have RS cells.
- The most commonly used classification is the WHO classification, which was updated in 2008, and classifies neoplasms by the cell of origin.
- In practical terms it is often useful to classify lymphomas as indolent/low grade or aggressive/high grade although disease behaviour varies greatly between individuals, and transformation frequently occurs.

Clinical features

- Indolent lymphoma (such as most follicular lymphomas) usually presents with slowly enlarging lymphadenopathy and less commonly with B symptoms.
- Aggressive lymphoma (such as lymphoblastic, diffuse large B-cell or Burkitt's lymphoma) may present with a rapidly growing mass and commonly with B symptoms.
- A great number of symptoms and signs may be present due to involvement of extranodal sites including skin, lung, bowel, CNS and bone.
- Low-grade NHL progresses slowly but cure is unlikely; high-grade NHL causes death within months if untreated, but may be cured in up to 40% of patients.
- Lymphadenopathy, hepatosplenomegaly, pallor and involvement of extranodal sites should be looked for on examination.

Investigations

- Lymph node biopsy for histology, immunohistochemistry and cytogenetics.
- Staging should then be performed to determine the extent of disease using the Ann Arbor system (Fig. 37.11). This usually comprises CT or PET scan and bone marrow biopsy.
- Circulating lymphoma cells are sometimes seen on the peripheral film.
- Full blood count may show evidence of bone marrow failure if extensively infiltrated.
- LDH and urate may be high in bulky disease.
- Paraproteinaemia and immune paresis (reduction in normal immunoglobulins) may be found.
- Lumbar puncture if there is any suspicion of CNS involvement. The CSF should be sent for cytology or flow cytometry.

Treatment

Indolent NHL

Follicular lymphoma is the most common subtype.

- Stage I or II disease: radiotherapy offers a small chance of cure. Observation is reasonable if radiotherapy would cause significant morbidity.

- Stage III or IV: observation if asymptomatic. In symptomatic disease, rituximab is given with combination chemotherapy. After successful induction therapy, rituximab is given as maintenance treatment.
- Combination chemotherapy ± rituximab can be given in refractory disease. There is also a role for autologous stem cell transplant.

Aggressive NHL

Diffuse large B-cell lymphoma is the most common subtype.

- Limited stage I or II disease: radiotherapy, rituximab (monoclonal anti-CD20) and short-course chemotherapy. CHOP (cyclophosphamide, hydroxydaunorubicin (doxorubicin), Oncovin (vincristine), prednisolone) is the gold standard.
- In stage III and IV disease, or bulky early-stage disease, treatment is rituximab and longer courses of chemotherapy(usually 6–8 cycles).
- Relapsed or refractory disease is treated with alternative chemotherapy with the aim of proceeding to stem cell transplant in eligible patients.

Rituximab is not used in T-cell lymphoma.

Prognosis

- Low-grade NHL: median survival is around 8–10 years.
- High-grade NHL: 40% 5-year disease-free survival.
- Poor prognostic factors include increasing age, high LDH, extensive disease, T-cell phenotype, certain extranodal sites, poor performance status and low-grade NHL that has transformed into high-grade NHL.

MYELOPROLIFERATIVE DISEASE

These conditions, like myelodysplastic syndromes (MDS), are chronic myeloid neoplasms caused by proliferation of a myeloid precursor cell. The abnormal cells differentiate into mature cells and, in contrast to MDS, evidence of this is seen in the peripheral blood. There are four classical syndromes: chronic myeloid leukaemia (associated with the Philadelphia chromosome and covered above), essential thrombocythaemia (ET), polycythaemia vera (PV) and primary myelofibrosis (PMF). An acquired mutation of *JAK2* is present in around 95% of patients with PV and up to 60% of patients with ET or PMF.

Polycythaemia vera

In PV there is an increased number of circulating erythrocytes (raised haematocrit) which cannot be ascribed to other causes (e.g. chronic hypoxia). There is a risk of developing myelofibrosis or transformation to acute leukaemia.

Clinical features

- Symptoms of raised haematocrit include headache, weakness, sweating and dizziness.
- Arthralgia and pruritus are commonly experienced.
- Thrombosis may cause visual disturbance.
- The patient looks plethoric (red complexion) and splenomegaly is present.

Investigations

- Full blood count: raised haematocrit. Thrombocytosis and leucocytosis in 50%.
- Arterial blood gas and erythropoietin level help exclude secondary polycythaemia.
- *JAK2* mutation analysis on peripheral blood.
- Bone marrow examination may be required if there is doubt about the diagnosis or concern about transformation. There is hypercellularity with reduced iron stores.

Treatment

- In simple erythrocytosis: venesection to lower the haematocrit.
- If coexistent thrombocytosis or thrombotic events: hydroxyurea.

Essential thrombocythaemia

In essential thrombocythaemia (ET), the platelet count is markedly elevated and the platelets are functionally abnormal. Life expectancy is usually normal with treatment.

Clinical features

- The majority of patients are asymptomatic at the time of diagnosis.
- Patients may report headache, lightheadedness or syncope.
- Episodes of thrombosis and/or bleeding may occur.
- Transformation to PV, acute leukaemia or myelofibrosis may occur. Most commonly the condition evolves to myelofibrosis (5–10% at 10 years).

Investigations

- Causes of a reactive thrombocytosis must be excluded.
- Full blood count shows elevated platelets >600 on two separate occasions.
- Blood film may show bizarre-looking platelets and platelet aggregates.
- Bone marrow examination: hypercellularity, abundant megakaryocytes without significant fibrosis.
- *JAK2* mutation present in around 60%.

Treatment

- Observation alone is sufficient in young patients at low risk of thrombosis.
- Aspirin is useful for mild symptoms in low-risk patients.
- Platelet-lowering therapy is required for patients at high risk of thrombosis; hydroxyurea and anagrelide are both effective.

Primary myelofibrosis

In primary myelofibrosis (PMF), there is proliferation of abnormal cells in all three cell lines, accompanied by release of growth factors which cause bone marrow fibrosis.

Clinical features

- Systemic symptoms: fatigue, weight loss, night sweats.
- Extramedullary haematopoiesis leads to massive splenomegaly, which may cause discomfort or early satiety. Hepatomegaly is often present.
- There is an increased risk of thrombotic events.

Investigations

- Full blood count: anaemia. Platelet and white cell counts are often abnormal but may be elevated or lowered.
- Blood film shows anisocytosis, teardrop erythrocytes and immature neutrophils.
- Bone marrow: often very difficult to obtain aspirate ('dry tap'). Biopsy shows extensive fibrosis.
- Cytogenetics: may help estimate prognosis.

Treatment

- Allogeneic stem cell transplant is the only curative treatment.
- Hydroxyurea is often effective at improving symptoms and reducing splenomegaly. Splenectomy may be required.

Survival is very variable. In high-risk patients it may be as little as 1–2 years from diagnosis, but in low-risk patients may be as long as 20 years. The decision of whether to proceed with stem cell transplant, taking into account the high mortality associated with the treatment, is often very difficult.

BLEEDING DISORDERS

An increased tendency to bleeding can result from abnormalities of platelets, the coagulation pathway or blood vessels. The differential diagnosis, clinical findings and investigation of these disorders are discussed in detail in Ch. 28. Specific conditions and their management are considered here.

Haemophilia A

Haemophilia A affects 1 in 8000 males. As an X-linked recessive inherited condition it affects only males, although heterozygous females may experience mild symptoms.

Pathology

There are many mutations to the factor VIII gene that may cause haemophilia. The abnormal forms have reduced factor VIII activity. The condition is classified as mild, moderate and severe depending on factor activity relative to normal (i.e. <1%, 1–5% or >5%, respectively).

Presentation

- Severity of bleeding correlates with level of factor VIII activity (lower levels correspond to more severe symptoms).
- Bleeding into joints (haemarthrosis) and muscles is common, and may be spontaneous or secondary to trauma.
- Recurrent haemarthroses and intramuscular haematomas cause long-term disability due to arthropathy and contractures.
- Haematuria and intracranial bleeding may occur.
- Bleeding from small cuts is usually minor due to normal platelet function.
- After trauma, bleeding is out of proportion and often delayed.

Investigations

- APTT (activated partial thromboplastin time): prolonged; normalizes with addition of 50% normal plasma.
- PT (prothrombin time): normal.
- Bleeding time: normal.
- Factor VIII assay: low.

Treatment

- Usually managed in specialized haemophilia centres.
- When there is bleeding or the patient requires surgery, factor VIII levels can be increased in two ways – mild haemophilia with desmopressin (DDAVP); moderate or severe haemophilia with recombinant factor VIII concentrates.
- Other aspects of management include analgesia (avoiding aspirin), joint replacement, synovectomy for arthropathy, regular dental care, and psychosocial and genetic support.

Prognosis and complications

Life expectancy should be normal with current therapies. Previously the complications of receiving factor VIII concentrates included exposure to HIV, hepatitis B and C as it was derived from donated blood. This is much reduced with recombinant factor VIII. The development of inhibitors to infused factor VIII results in a much worse prognosis.

Haemophilia B (Christmas disease)

Incidence is 1 per 30 000. It is also an X-linked recessive inherited condition. There is decreased plasma factor IX activity. The clinical features are identical to haemophilia A.

Investigations

- APTT: prolonged.
- PT: normal.
- Bleeding time: normal.
- Factor IX assay: low.

Treatment

Treatment is with recombinant factor IX. Desmopressin has no effect on factor IX levels. Otherwise, treatment is the same as for haemophilia A. With current therapies life expectancy should be normal.

Von Willebrand's disease

Von Willebrand's disease (vWD) occurs in 1% of the general population. It is an inherited (autosomal dominant) condition.

Pathology

- Deficiency of von Willebrand factor (vWF).
- vWF is a plasma protein that mediates platelet adherence to the subendothelium and platelet aggregation. It also binds and stabilizes factor VIII.

Presentation

- Both sexes are equally affected.
- Severity of disease is variable.
- Most patients present with bleeding similar to platelet disorders: bruising, bleeding into the skin, mucosal bleeding (epistaxis, bleeding gums, gastrointestinal bleeding).
- Menorrhagia and bleeding following surgery, dental extractions, trauma and delivery are common.
- In some patients binding to factor VIII is affected, resulting in low factor VIII levels and a clinical picture similar to haemophilia.

Investigations

- Platelets: normal in number and structure.
- APTT: prolonged (may be normal).
- PTT: normal.
- Prolonged bleeding time and elevated platelet function analyser result.
- vWF assays: low.

Treatment

Aspirin should be avoided. Treatment is with desmopressin, tranexamic acid or plasma-derived factor VIII concentrates (which contain large amounts of vWf) in haemorrhage or perioperatively. Life expectancy is usually normal.

Immune thrombocytopenia (ITP)

In ITP, thrombocytopenia results from antibody-mediated destruction of platelets in the spleen and liver. It affects both adults and children, with an incidence in adults of around 40 cases per million. The cause is often unclear, but it may occur following viral illnesses, in the context of other autoimmune disease (such as SLE) or lymphoproliferative disease, or following administration of certain drugs. When there is an underlying cause it is termed 'secondary' ITP.

Clinical features

- Easy bruising, petechial or purpuric rash.
- Mucosal bleeding and menorrhagia.
- Haematuria and gastrointestinal bleeding is uncommon.
- Splenomegaly is rarely present in isolated ITP and should prompt consideration of an underlying diagnosis.

Investigations

- Full blood count: isolated thrombocytopenia, or anaemia if significant bleeding.
- Blood film: platelet clumps in pseudothrombocytopenia due to EDTA-mediated aggregation. The sample should be repeated in a citrate or heparin tube.
- Bone marrow examination: required in older patients, when systemic symptoms are present, or if there are other cytopenias that are not easily explained.

Treatment

It may be difficult to know when to start treatment. Generally, if patients are symptomatic and platelets are below 30×10^9/L, treatment is required. Otherwise, careful monitoring and advice may be sufficient.

- Transfused platelets are rapidly destroyed and should only be given in significant acute bleeding.

- IV immunoglobulin will rapidly (but temporarily) raise the platelet count.
- High-dose oral prednisolone achieves a response in up to 75%. Steroids should be withdrawn slowly.
- Splenectomy or other immunosuppressive therapy may be required if relapse occurs.

DISSEMINATED INTRAVASCULAR COAGULATION

This is a syndrome characterized by a specific haematological response to a wide range of insults.

Aetiology

DIC may be caused by:

- Malignancy: mucus-secreting adenocarcinomas, prostate, pancreatic carcinoma, acute promyelocytic leukaemia (AML–M3).
- Infection: Gram-negative (most commonly) or Gram-positive sepsis.
- Obstetric: amniotic fluid embolism, placental abruption, pre-eclampsia, HELLP syndrome, septic abortion.
- Tissue damage: rhabdomyolysis, fat embolism, severe trauma, burns.
- Immunological: incompatible blood transfusion, drug reaction, anaphylaxis.
- Liver disease: acute fatty liver of pregnancy, fulminant liver failure.
- Others: snake bites, acute pancreatitis.

Pathology

- Initially, intravascular coagulation is precipitated by release of tissue factor or procoagulant substances into the circulation from injured cells, malignant cells, or damaged endothelium.
- Microthrombi form throughout the microcirculation causing ischaemia and infarction.
- Platelets, fibrin and clotting factors are consumed by the thrombotic process and the fibrinolytic system becomes activated; these two processes result in a tendency to bleed, and haemorrhage may be significant.

Presentation

- DIC is often severe and life-threatening, but may be chronic and compensated when due to malignancy.
- Thrombosis can cause widespread ischaemia or infarction leading to renal failure, liver failure and CNS involvement.
- Bleeding is often into the skin or from recent venepuncture sites.
- Gastrointestinal and pulmonary haemorrhage may also occur.

Investigations

- Platelet count: low.
- PT and APTT: prolonged.
- Fibrinogen: usually low (may be normal as acute phase reactant).
- D-dimers/fibrin degradation products: high.
- Blood film: fragmented RBCs due to microangiopathic haemolysis.

Treatment

- Treatment of the underlying disease is the first priority and may resolve the DIC.
- Meticulous supportive care (e.g. fluids, antibiotics, debridement of gangrene).
- Replacement of platelets and clotting factors (using fresh frozen plasma or cryoprecipitate) may be used if there is haemorrhage or risk of haemorrhage (e.g. in surgery).
- Pharmacological inhibitors of coagulation or fibrinolysis (e.g. heparin or tranexamic acid) may be beneficial in certain circumstances but their use is controversial.

Prognosis

Mortality is up to 80% in severe DIC and is usually due to the underlying disease.

> **COMMUNICATION**
>
> Raised total protein with a normal albumin level should raise suspicion of the presence of a paraprotein.

THROMBOTIC DISORDERS AND THROMBOEMBOLISM

> **HINTS AND TIPS**
>
> The causes of thromboembolism can be broken down by Virchow's triad:
> - Changes in the vessel wall.
> - Changes in the blood flow.
> - Changes in the composition of the blood.

Thromboembolism is common, and the increased incidence of deep vein thrombosis following long journeys (so-called 'economy class syndrome') has made it a well-known area among the public.

Fig. 37.12 Risk factors for venous thromboembolism.

Aetiology	Risk factor	
Inherited (decreasing order of thrombotic risk)	Antithrombin III deficiency Protein C deficiency Protein S deficiency Factor V Leiden mutation (activated protein C resistance) Prothrombin 20210A mutation Hyperhomocysteinaemia Dysfibrinogenaemia (10% have thrombophilia, 90% coagulopathy)	
Acquired	Physiological	Pregnancy Obesity Increasing age
	Initiating events (immobilization)	Surgery Trauma Long distance travel
	Pathological	Malignancy Venous trauma Oestrogens Nephrotic syndrome Antiphospholipid syndrome Hyperviscosity syndromes Paroxysmal nocturnal haemoglobinuria Inflammatory bowel disease

Aetiology

Risk factors for venous thromboembolism are outlined in Fig. 37.12.

Pathology

- Venous thrombosis can be caused by abnormal vessel walls, venous stasis or hypercoagulable blood.
- Thrombosis may be precipitated by a specific provoking event such as surgery or a physiological state such as pregnancy.
- The lower limbs are the most common site of thrombosis.
- Small clots may break off and cause pulmonary embolus or, very rarely, cerebral infarction by paradoxical embolus in patients with a patent foramen ovale.

Presentation

- Deep vein thrombosis (DVT) causes local pain, swelling, redness and oedema.
- The diagnosis can be difficult to make on clinical grounds.
- Pulmonary embolus (PE) causes sudden onset of pleuritic chest pain, dyspnoea and haemoptysis.
- Patients with inherited hypercoagulable states may present with venous thromboses without obvious precipitants, in unusual places (e.g. Budd–Chiari syndrome), at an early age or with spontaneous abortions.
- Antiphospholipid syndrome and hyperhomocysteinaemia increase the risk of arterial as well as venous thromboses.

Investigations

- Careful clinical examination should be performed to look for an underlying cause such as malignancy, and investigations requested appropriately.
- The pre-test probability of VTE should be evaluated with an accepted scoring system.
- In cases where the risk score is low or equivocal, D-dimer measurement may be helpful. It is a sensitive but non-specific test, and helps to exclude DVT.
- The final step is to perform the appropriate imaging test on the at-risk patients. This may be ultrasound, ventilation–perfusion scanning or CT pulmonary angiography (CTPA).
- A baseline platelet count and clotting screen should always be performed.
- If the patient is young, ask if there have been recurrent episodes, recurrent spontaneous abortions or a family history of thromboembolism, and consider hereditary thrombophilia. Assays are available to detect these abnormalities.

Treatment if thrombosis is proven

- Anticoagulation with low-molecular-weight heparin should be started. It is licensed for both DVT and PE. The lack of need for monitoring has allowed the treatment of DVT as an outpatient. The indications for unfractionated heparin are decreasing; among them are renal failure or mechanical heart valves.
- Oral warfarin should be given simultaneously and monitored using the international normalized ratio (INR), which should be maintained between 2 and 3.
- Heparin should be continued until the INR is therapeutic.
- If heparin is contraindicated, agents such as the hirudins or fondaparinux can be used.
- Newer oral anticoagulants, such as dabigatran and rivaroxaban, are being introduced in certain contexts and may eventually replace warfarin completely.

HINTS AND TIPS

Warfarin alone is initially PROcoagulant due to its more rapid inhibition of PROtein C and S.

Treatment period

The length of time a patient should be anticoagulated is controversial and always under review, but as a general rule is 3–6 months depending on the extent and the existence of a precipitating factor such as a period of immobilization.

Above-knee DVTs are at increased risk of propagating along the venous system and embolizing to the lungs. Two or more thromboses, whether provoked or unprovoked, indicate that lifelong anticoagulation is required.

THROMBOTIC THROMBOCYTOPENIC PURPURA AND HAEMOLYTIC URAEMIC SYNDROME

These two conditions are characterized by thrombosis and microangiopathic haemolytic anaemia. They share several features and are often considered together. Mortality is up to 80% without treatment.

Haemolytic uraemic syndrome (HUS)

HUS is most common in children, and 90% of cases occur following a diarrhoeal illness, particularly with pathogenic *Escherichia coli*. The remaining 10% can be due to a variety of causes including viruses, drugs and cancer. Complement abnormalities may underpin the pathogenesis.

Clinical features

The cardinal features of HUS are acute kidney injury, thrombocytopenia and haemolytic anaemia. Involvement of other organs, particularly the liver and CNS, occurs in up to 20%.

Investigations

- Haematology: anaemia, thrombocytopenia DAT negative.
- Biochemistry: renal impairment, raised LDH, raised bilirubin.
- Blood film: red cell fragments, reticulocytes.
- Coagulation studies: normal (as opposed to DIC).

Treatment

- Typical HUS (following diarrhoea) is usually self-resolving with supportive care. Dialysis is sometimes required.
- Plasma exchange or immunosuppression may be required.
- Eculizumab (anti-complement) may be effective.

Thrombotic thrombocytopenic purpura

Thrombotic thrombocytopenic purpura (TTP) is a rare disease, most common in young adults. It is a combination of signs, symptoms and characteristic blood film appearance. Reduced ADAMTS-13 (a metalloproteinase) activity allows large von Willebrand factor multimers to enter the circulation, causing platelet aggregation and microthrombi.

Clinical features

The classical 'pentad' consists of:

- Haemolytic anaemia: typical symptoms.
- Thrombocytopenia: bleeding.
- Acute kidney injury.
- Prominent neurological features such as lethargy, headache, confusion and seizures.
- Pyrexia that is not caused by infection.

These features may not all be present and clinical suspicion is necessary.

Investigations

- Blood film: anaemia, reticulocytosis, thrombocytopenia and fragmented red cells (schistocytes).
- Bilirubin and LDH: increased due to haemolysis.

- Coagulation: usually normal.
- ADAMTS-13 assays are available but take too long to help with diagnosis.

Treatment

Plasma exchange has vastly improved the prognosis and most people achieve a lasting response. Immunosuppression is also used.

Further reading

Bird, J., Owen, R., D'Sa, S., et al., 2011. Guidelines for the diagnosis and management of multiple myeloma. Br. J. Haematol. 154, 32–75.

British Society for Haematology: publishes guidelines and reviews of all aspects of haematology. Available online at: http://www.b-s-h.org.uk.

Campbell, P., Green, A., 2006. The myeloproliferative disorders. N. Engl. J. Med. 355, 2452–2466.

Campo, E., Swerdlow, S., Harris, N., et al., 2011. The 2008 WHO classification of lymphoid neoplasms and beyond: evolving concepts and practical applications. Blood 117, 5019–5032.

National Institute for Health and Clinical Excellence (NICE), 2011. Anaemia management in people with chronic kidney disease. Clinical guideline CG114. Available online at: http://www.nice.org.uk/CG114.

Noris, M., Remuzzi, G., 2009. Atypical haemolytic uraemic syndrome. N. Engl. J. Med. 361, 1676–1687.

Reed, D., Williams, T., Gladwin, M., 2010. Sickle-cell disease. Lancet 376, 2019–2031.

Tefferi, A., Vardiman, J., 2009. Myelodysplastic syndromes. N. Engl. J. Med. 361, 1872–1885.

Infectious diseases

Objectives

The key learning points for this chapter:

- How the human immunodeficiency virus causes disease in humans.
- The definition and use of highly active antiretroviral therapy.
- The findings in the full blood count and blood film in malaria.
- The methods of prevention you should advise in a malarial area.
- The problems posed by resistant bacteria and strategies to combat them.

INTRODUCTION

Infections affecting specific systems have been discussed in the appropriate chapters. This chapter considers three important and very different infections – human immunodeficiency virus (HIV), malaria and drug-resistant bacteria, in particular methicillin-resistant *Staphylococcus aureus* (MRSA).

HIV AND AIDS

Epidemiology

The Department of Health estimates that around 90 000 adults in the UK are living with HIV, of whom a quarter are unaware of the diagnosis. The World Health Organization estimates that around 35 million people worldwide are infected with HIV, more than three-quarters of whom live in sub-Saharan Africa. In some countries, such as Botswana, the adult prevalence of HIV is up to 25%, and it is threatening the stability of society. There has been a huge drive to increase the provision of antiretroviral therapies to these countries, but the development of effective strategies remains difficult.

Aetiology

HIV-1 was first identified in 1983; it is found throughout the world and is the main cause of disease in humans.

HIV-2 is endemic in west Africa and less common outside this region. It accounts for around 5% of worldwide HIV cases. Its similarity to the simian immunodeficiency virus led to the theory of cross-species transfer gaining widespread acceptance as its origin in humans.

HIV can be transmitted by sexual, parenteral and vertical routes (Fig. 38.1).

Pathology

HIV is a lentivirus, which is a subgroup of the human retroviruses. Its genetic information is stored in a single strand of ribonucleic acid (RNA). Three specific genes produce proteins essential for HIV survival (Fig. 38.2). The virus can infect any cells expressing CD4 (notably T-helper cells which are central to the immune response) as well as macrophages, monocytes and microglia. CD4 acts as a receptor for glycoprotein (gp120) on the virus envelope, allowing the virus to enter the cell. Co-receptors such as CXCR4 and CCR5 are recognized as important and potential therapeutic targets.

The enzyme reverse transcriptase makes DNA copies of the virus RNA, which become integrated into the host cell's genome, resulting in production of more virus particles. The normal function of the infected cells is disrupted and the host cells are eventually destroyed.

Because the principal cells affected are those of the immune system, HIV infection is characterized by diseases resulting from immunodeficiency (e.g. infections and malignancies).

Presentation

Staging of HIV/AIDS was initially developed in 1985, and there are currently two main systems in use. The American CDC staging system uses the CD4 count and the presence of certain HIV-related illness to classify the clinical stage as A, B or C (see Fig. 38.3). The WHO system is designed for use when access to a CD4 count is not always available and describes four stages outlined below. Fifty per cent of untreated patients will develop the acquired immune deficiency syndrome (AIDS) after 10 years. A minority remain asymptomatic for many

Fig. 38.1 Routes of HIV transmission.

Route	Examples
Sexual	Vaginal intercourse, anal intercourse
Parenteral	IV drug abuse, blood transfusion, needlestick injury
Vertical (i.e. from mother to fetus)	During gestation or delivery, via breast milk

Fig. 38.2 HIV genes and the proteins they encode.

Gene	Protein
pol	Reverse transcriptase (makes DNA copies of the viral RNA) and integrase (for insertion into host DNA)
gag	Core protein p24
env	Encodes gp41, a transmembrane protein, and gp120, an external glycoprotein (for fusion with host cell)

Fig. 38.3 CDC staging of HIV infection.

$CD4^+$ count (cells/ μL)	A: Asymptomatic, acute HIV or PGL	B: Symptomatic conditions, not AIDS defining	C: AIDS indicator illness
>500	A1	B1	C1
200–499	A2	B2	C2
<200	A3	B3	C3

PGL, persistent generalized lymphadenopathy.

years without treatment. Depending on the level of persistent viraemia, they are classified as 'long-term non-progressors' or 'elite controllers'.

Primary HIV infection

In the majority of patients this results in a 'seroconversion illness' occurring around 4 weeks after infection. Symptoms are similar to those seen with other viral infections, including fever, arthralgia, headaches, rash, generalized lymphadenopathy and occasional neurological abnormalities. The illness is self-limiting and usually resolves within 8 weeks.

Clinical stage 1

During this early stage of HIV infection the patient is either asymptomatic or has persistent generalized lymphadenopathy: rubbery, mobile, enlarged lymph nodes at multiple sites. Biopsy shows non-specific reactive histiocytosis.

Clinical stage 2

During this stage (which broadly corresponds to CDC stage B) the illness is symptomatic, and conditions occur that are due to immune deficiency or HIV infection itself. Although many of these may occur in other clinical situations, they are more severe in the context of HIV. However, these are not 'AIDS-indicator' illnesses. Constitutional symptoms are common. See Fig. 38.4.

Clinical stages 3 and 4

In stages 3 and 4 constitutional symptoms may be more severe, and the conditions that occur indicate that the immunosuppression is more profound. The appearance of these conditions, detailed in Fig. 38.4, are a guide to initiating or changing treatment. Any system can be affected. Malignancies are seen with increased frequency and may be associated with specific viral infections (see Fig. 38.5). These stages broadly correspond to CDC stage C, although there are some minor discrepancies.

Investigations

All investigations for HIV infection should be performed under the strictest confidentiality. The condition is far more treatable than in the past, but the diagnosis still has social, financial, health and psychological implications. Education and counselling are important. In the USA, the CDC advocates HIV screening for adults as part of routine medical care. This practice has not yet become widespread in the UK.

The presence of HIV infection can be assessed by the measurement of viral antigens, HIV RNA detection, the immune response to the infection (anti-HIV antibodies) or the effects of the infection ($CD4^+$ count). Fig. 38.6 summarizes the findings at the different stages.

In practice, the diagnosis is usually made using HIV antibody tests. The screening test is repeated if positive or borderline. If repeatedly positive, another assay such as Western blotting is used to confirm the diagnosis. This combination of tests gives high sensitivity and specificity.

HIV antibodies may be undetectable for up to 3 months after infection and this is a window for false-negative results; if clinical suspicion is high, testing needs to be repeated or a different method used.

Once the diagnosis is reached the disease activity should be assessed. This is done by quantifying both HIV RNA viral load and $CD4^+$ cell count. The prognosis is worse with a higher viral load and lower CD4 count, as these indicate a more rapid progression from early to

Fig. 38.4 Features of symptomatic HIV infection.

Organ/system	WHO stage	Example
Mouth	2	Angular stomatitis, recurrent oral ulceration, parotid enlargement
	3	Oral hairy leucoplakia, oral candidiasis, necrotizing gingivitis/periodontitis
	4	**Chronic oral herpes simplex infection**
Gastrointestinal	2	Hepatosplenomegaly
	3	Persistent diarrhoea or malnutrition
	4	**HIV wasting syndrome**, HIV rectal fistula, oesophagitis **(HSV, CMV, *Candida*)**
	Not in WHO staging	Hepatobiliary disease (***Mycobacteria***, hepatitis B, **CMV**, microsporidia), colitis (*Campylobacter, Salmonella, Shigella,* ***Cryptosporidium***, *Giardia,* **CMV**), anal carcinoma
Cardiovascular	4	HIV-associated cardiomyopathy
	Not in WHO staging	Pericardial effusions, conduction abnormalities, dilated cardiomyopathy, pulmonary hypertension, non-infectious endocarditis
Respiratory	2	Recurrent upper respiratory infection (e.g. tonsillitis, sinusitis)
	3	Pulmonary TB, **severe recurrent bacterial pneumonia**, lymphoid interstitial pneumonitis, chronic HIV-associated lung disease (e.g. bronchiectasis)
	4	**Lower respiratory candidiasis, *Pneumocystis jirovecii* pneumonia**
	Not in WHO staging	Fungal pneumonia
Neurological	4	**CNS toxoplasmosis, cryptococcal meningitis, HIV encephalopathy, progressive multifocal leucoencephalopathy, CNS lymphoma**
	Not in WHO staging	Myelopathy, peripheral neuropathy, inflammatory demyelinating polyneuropathy, retinitis (e.g. **CMV**)
Renal	4	HIV-associated nephropathy (HIVAN) Severe nephrotic syndrome with characteristic FSGS
Haematological	3	Unexplained anaemia, neutropenia or thrombocytopenia
	4	B-cell non-Hodgkin's lymphoma
	Not in WHO staging	**Burkitt's lymphoma, immunoblastic lymphoma**
Dermatological	2	Herpes zoster, fungal nail infections (*Candida,* tinea), seborrhoeic dermatitis, itchy papular eruptions, extensive molluscum contagiosum
	4	**Kaposi's sarcoma, genital herpes simplex**
	Not in WHO staging	Squamous cell carcinoma, crusted scabies
Reproductive	Not in WHO staging	**Invasive cervical carcinoma**
Other/systemic	2	Weight loss <10%
	3	Persistent fever
	4	**Disseminated TB, disseminated non-TB mycobacterial infection**, recurrent severe bacterial infection (not pneumonia), disseminated fungal infection (e.g. **histoplasmosis**), **cryptosporidiosis**, visceral herpes simplex, **CMV infection other than liver/spleen/lymph nodes, Kaposi's sarcoma**

AIDS-indicator illnesses (CDC 1993, Stage C) are shown in bold; FSGS, focal segmental glomerulosclerosis.

Fig. 38.5 Malignancies seen with increased frequency and associated viruses.

Tumour	Associated virus
Kaposi's sarcoma	Human herpes virus 8
Cerebral lymphoma	Epstein–Barr virus
Non-Hodgkin's lymphoma	Epstein–Barr virus
Hodgkin's disease	Not determined
Cervical carcinoma	Human papillomavirus
Anal carcinoma	Human papillomavirus

late stages of infection. Viral load and CD4 count are also used to follow the response to drug therapy.

Drug resistance is problematic in a small proportion of patients, and testing for resistant strains at diagnosis is recommended.

COMMUNICATION

Do not be afraid to perform an HIV test. It is important to discuss your intention with the patient, but counselling is no longer considered essential.

Treatment

The treatment of HIV has changed hugely in the last 10 years. HIV is not curable, but the advent of highly active antiretroviral therapy (HAART) has greatly improved disease control and life expectancy. The aim is to reduce viral load to as low as possible and raise CD4$^+$counts. HAART involves the use of several drugs from different classes in order to reduce the development of resistant viral strains and to maximize the treatment response. In contrast to the pre-HAART era, drug therapy is begun early in the disease process, and is advised for patients with a CD4 count below 350 cells/μL or those with AIDS-indicator illnesses. The role of HAART in primary infection is not yet established. The three common classes are:

- Nucleoside analogue reverse transcriptase inhibitors (e.g. zidovudine, lamivudine and didanosine).
- Non-nucleoside analogue reverse transcriptase inhibitors (e.g. efavirenz and nevirapine).
- Protease inhibitors (e.g. ritonavir, indinavir and saquinavir).

Newer drugs include integrase inhibitors (e.g.raltegravir), fusion inhibitors and CCR5 receptor antagonists (e.g. maraviroc). Fig. 38.7 shows the sites of action. Treatment should be under HIV specialists and the exact regimen varies from person to person. The legion of potential side effects and interactions from these drugs provides another reason for specialist care.

As HIV treatment has improved, the incidence of HIV-associated infection and malignancy has changed and in many cases diminished. Opportunistic infections commonly seen in HIV are shown in Fig. 38.8. Tuberculosis, particularly following the emergence of drug-resistant strains, is problematic in parts of the world where HIV incidence is high. Kaposi's sarcoma (KS) and non-Hodgkin's lymphoma are frequently seen in HIV infection. Treatment of KS includes HAART, local treatments (radiotherapy or intralesional chemotherapy) or systemic chemotherapy.

Prevention

Despite HAART, there is no 'cure' for HIV infection; preventative measures must remain the highest priority. Such measures include education, the provision of clean needles for IV drug abusers, the use of condoms, the screening of blood products and organs donated for transplantation, and avoidance of breastfeeding in HIV-positive mothers. Research continues into new treatments and the possibility of a vaccine. Post-exposure prophylaxis (PEP) reduces transmission rates in healthcare workers following needlestick injury.

Fig. 38.6 Investigation at different stages of HIV infection.

Phase	Viral replication	p24	HIV antibodies	CD4$^+$ count
Primary infection	High	Detectable until HIV antibodies appear	Detectable 3 weeks to 3 months after exposure	Transient fall due to high viral load, but returns to normal when HIV antibodies appear
Stage 1 (WHO)/ A (CDC) (Asymptomatic/ PGL)	Low	Undetectable as antibody in excess to antigen	Detectable	Normal
Advanced, symptomatic stages	High	Detectable	Detectable	Falls; when <200 cells/μL risk of infection is very high and development of AIDS is likely

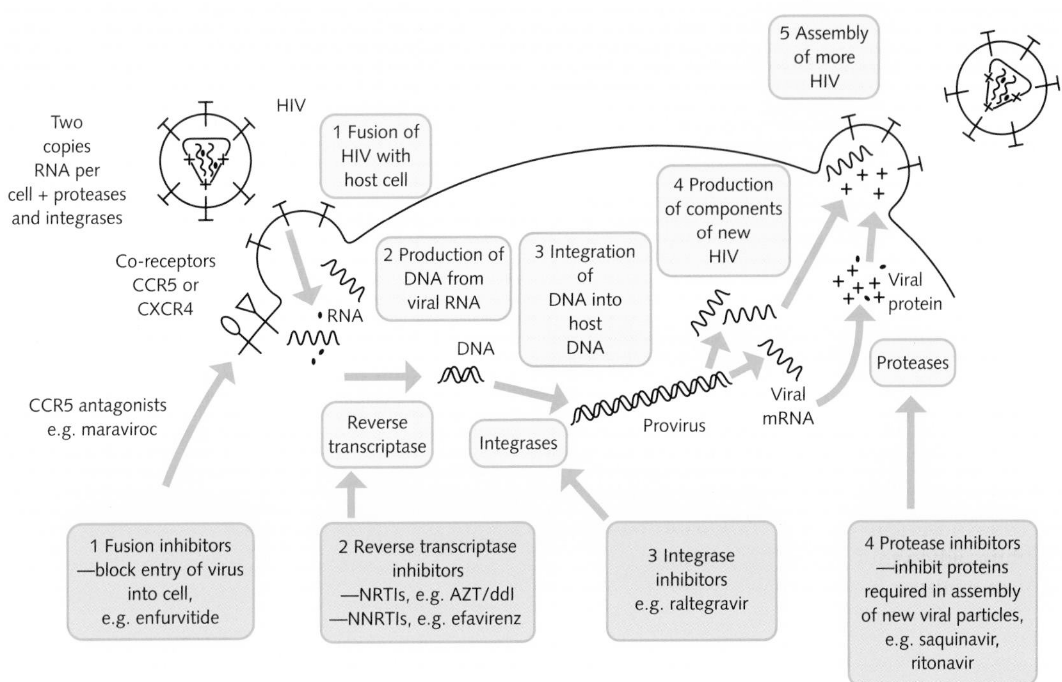

Fig. 38.7 Site of action of HIV drugs. AZT, zidovudine; ddI, didanosine; NNRTIs, non-nucleoside reverse transcriptase inhibitors; NRTIs, nucleoside reverse transcriptase inhibitors.

Fig. 38.8 Treatment and prophylaxis of opportunistic infections.

Infection	Treatment	Treatment alternatives	Indication for prophylaxis	Prophylactic drug regimes
Pneumocystis jirovecii	Oral or IV co-trimoxazole Steroids may be beneficial	IV pentamidine, or clindamycin + primaquine, or dapsone + trimethoprim	Secondary prevention or $CD4^+$ <200 cells/μL	Oral co-trimoxazole, or nebulized pentamidine, or dapsone + pyrimethamine
Toxoplasmosis	Sulfadiazine + pyrimethamine + folate	Clindamycin replacing sulfadiazine	Secondary prevention or $CD4^+$ <200 cells/μL positive serology	Pyrimethamine + sulfadiazine, or clindamycin, or co-trimoxazole, or dapsone
Cytomegalovirus	Ganciclovir or foscarnet		Secondary prevention	Ganciclovir or foscarnet
Herpes simplex	Aciclovir	Valaciclovir or foscarnet	Secondary prevention	Aciclovir
Herpes zoster	Aciclovir	Valaciclovir or foscarnet or famciclovir		
Cryptococcal meningitis	Amphotericin B ± flucytosine, or fluconazole		Secondary prevention	Fluconazole
Mycobacterium avium complex	Rifampicin + ethambutol + clarithromycin	Rifabutin replacing rifampicin	Secondary prevention	Azithromycin or clarithromycin
Candida	Fluconazole	Ketoconazole or itraconazole	Secondary prevention	Fluconazole

Prognosis

This is strongly related to viral load and $CD4^+$ count. Untreated patients with a $CD4^+$ count <50 cells/μL have a 90% 3-year mortality rate while it is only 25% if the count is >250 cells/μL. The long-term prognosis in people who respond well to HAART with high $CD4^+$ counts and unrecordable viral load is not known, but many are asymptomatic and living normal lives more than 10–15 years post diagnosis.

MALARIA

Epidemiology

Worldwide, malaria affects over 200 million people and causes around 1 million deaths each year. It is endemic in the tropics and subtropics. It is seen in temperate zones when imported by people who have visited or come from endemic areas. In the UK, approximately 2000 cases are notified each year.

Aetiology

The disease is caused by protozoal infection with one of the species of the genus *Plasmodium* (*P. vivax, P. ovale, P. malariae* or *P. falciparum*).

Pathology

Malaria is spread from an infected person to a non-infected person by sporozoites from the bite of a female *Anopheles* mosquito. The sporozoites multiply in hepatocytes, leading to thousands of merozoites, which then invade red blood cells. In addition, *P. vivax* and *P. ovale* organisms persist in the liver as hypnozoites which may lie dormant for months or years. Schizogony (asexual reproduction) then occurs in red blood cells; eventually cells rupture, releasing malaria parasites, malaria antigen, haemoglobin, cytokines (especially tumour necrosis factor) and other constituents of the red blood cells into the bloodstream, causing the typical clinical picture.

This occurs every 72 h in *P. malariae* (quartan malaria), every 48–72 h in *P. vivax* and *P. ovale* (tertian malaria) and every 48 h in *P. falciparum* (subtertian malaria). *P. vivax, P. ovale,* and *P. malariae* invade up to 2% of the circulating red blood cells. *P. falciparum* may affect over 10% of cells, producing a potentially life-threatening illness.

Fig. 38.9 demonstrates the life cycle of malaria.

Presentation

Malaria is characterized by periodic high fever, sweating and rigors, which coincide with release of merozoites from erythrocytes. Nausea and vomiting, abdominal pain, diarrhoea, headache, cough and arthralgia/myalgia may also be present. Splenomegaly is commonly found but mild icterus and massive hepatomegaly may also be present. Fig. 38.10 summarizes the complications of *P. falciparum* malaria.

Investigations

- Thin and thick blood films: thick films allow parasites to be identified; thin films are useful in species identification. The degree of parasitaemia is important. Repeat films may be needed.
- Antigen detection kits are useful for rapid diagnosis. PCR may be more sensitive than microscopy, but takes much longer. It is useful for species or strain identification.
- Anaemia and leucocytosis may occur. Thrombocytopenia is common.
- Urea and electrolytes: renal failure.
- C-reactive protein: normally raised.
- Coagulopathy: may be a feature of *P. falciparum* infection.
- Liver function tests: often become abnormal. Raised bilirubin due to haemolysis.
- Hyponatraemia: *P. falciparum.*
- Hypoglycaemia may be seen.

Treatment

The treatment of malaria is under constant review as resistant strains develop. Up-to-date information regarding prophylaxis and treatment of malaria should be obtained from local infectious disease centres.

> **COMMUNICATION**
>
> Travellers, including those returning to visit their home countries, need careful instruction about the need for malaria prophylaxis, both medication and precautions against mosquito bites.

The acute episode

Management of the acute episode includes:

- Supportive care as appropriate; severe cases should be managed in a critical care setting.
- Oral chloroquine for *P. vivax, P. ovale* and *P. malariae.*
- *P. falciparum* is commonly resistant to chloroquine. There are three common regimens used: quinine (IV if severe) with doxycycline or clindamycin; Co-artem (artemether–lumefantrine); and atovaquone–proguanil.

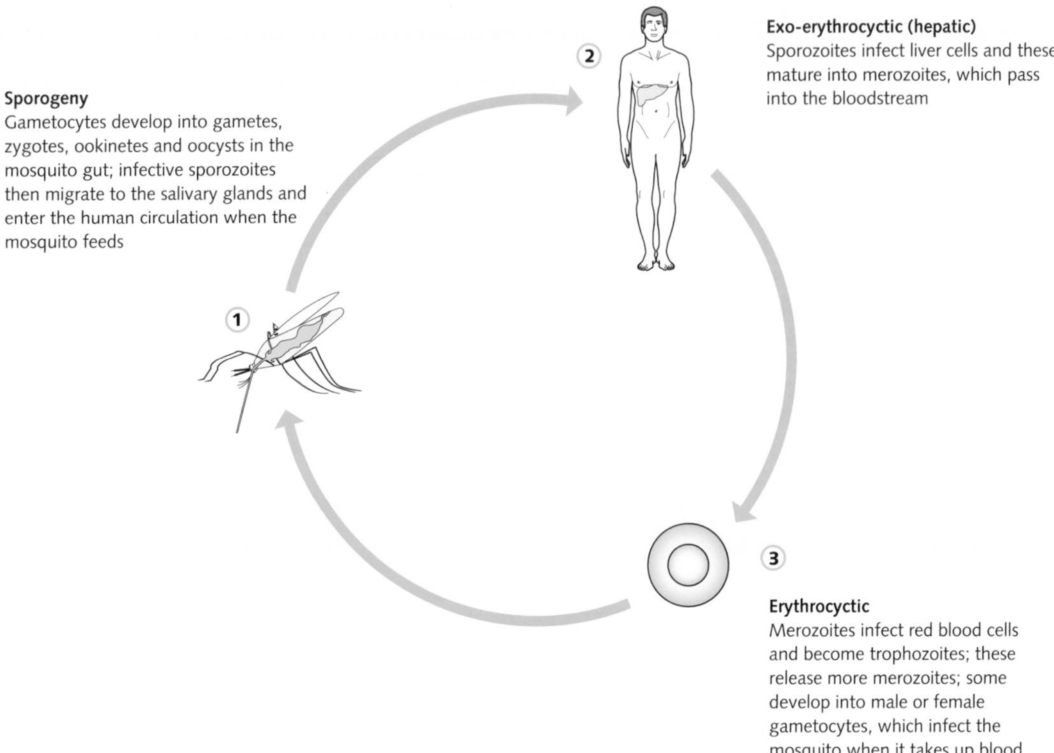

Sporogeny
Gametocytes develop into gametes, zygotes, ookinetes and oocysts in the mosquito gut; infective sporozoites then migrate to the salivary glands and enter the human circulation when the mosquito feeds
1
2
Exo-erythrocyctic (hepatic)
Sporozoites infect liver cells and these mature into merozoites, which pass into the bloodstream
3
Erythrocyctic
Merozoites infect red blood cells and become trophozoites; these release more merozoites; some develop into male or female gametocytes, which infect the mosquito when it takes up blood

Fig. 38.9 The malaria transmission cycle.

Fig. 38.10 Complications of infection by *Plasmodium falciparum.*

Cerebral malaria (hyperpyrexia, coma, death)
Hypoglycaemia
Acute respiratory distress syndrome
Seizures
Severe intravascular haemolysis with haemoglobinuria ('blackwater fever')
Acute renal failure
Hepatic necrosis
Jaundice
Haemolytic anaemia
Lactic acidosis
Coagulopathy (including DIC)

DIC, disseminated intravascular coagulation.

- IV artesunate may offer a survival advantage over IV quinine in severe complicated malaria.
- Exchange transfusion may be useful when there is a high level of parasitaemia.

Eradication therapy

The eradication of liver parasites to prevent future relapse:

- Necessary in *P. ovale* and *P. vivax*.
- Primaquine is used. Consider testing for glucose-6-phosphate dehydrogenase deficiency prior to commencing treatment as severe haemolysis may occur in these patients.

Prevention

With the emergence of resistant organisms, the avoidance of mosquito bites and mosquito control take on greater importance.

Chemoprophylaxis

For chemoprophylaxis, refer to up-to-date information (e.g. the *British National Formulary* or the London School of Hygiene and Tropical Medicine). It should be started 1 week prior to travel and continued for at least 4 weeks after return.

Medications used include chloroquine, proguanil–atovaquone, mefloquine and doxycycline. All have side effects and the risks and benefits should be made available to patients.

Avoidance of mosquito bites

Mosquito nets and repellents are vital. Appropriate clothing should be worn: i.e. long sleeves and trousers around dawn and dusk, which is when the female *Anopheles* mosquito is most active.

Spray bedroom with insecticide last thing in the evening.

Prognosis

Prognosis is excellent with *P. vivax, P. ovale* and *P. malariae* infection. *P. falciparum* is still a life-threatening condition, and cerebral malaria is of particular concern, with mortality of up to 20%.

DRUG-RESISTANT BACTERIA

The last decade has seen an increase in the emergence of drug-resistant strains of bacteria, commonly ascribed to the overuse of low-dose antibiotics which exert an environmental pressure on the pathogens. Drug resistance may be acquired via mutation or bacterial plasmid transfer.

Drug-resistant bacteria are important in terms of mortality, morbidity and increased cost. The subject is frequently politicized, often driven by sensationalist reporting of the latest 'superbug' or 'killer bacteria'. Patients may be worried about these infections when they come to hospital.

As a medical student and doctor, the single biggest contribution to be made to limiting spread is effective hand hygiene with hand washing or alcohol gel. Most hospitals have a 'bare below the elbow' policy: shirts should be short-sleeved or have the sleeves rolled up. Ties are less commonly worn, and should be tucked in or clipped to shirts. Remember to clean your stethoscope regularly as well!

Methicillin-resistant *Staphylococcus aureus*

MRSA results in the same range of presentations as other *S. aureus* infections but is highly resistant to antibiotic therapy. It is not untreatable. MRSA is resistant to most beta-lactam antibiotics, but often sensitive to vancomycin, teicoplanin and linezolid, as well as other antibiotics in individual cases.

In hospital, patients are routinely screened (nose/axilla/groin) for MRSA. Patients are often admitted with MRSA colonization, especially those from long-term care facilities. Those positive have eradication therapy, barrier nursing if needed and special precautions are taken in certain situations (e.g. they may be last on a theatre list, so it can be cleaned post operation to prevent contamination of other patients).

Other resistant bacteria

- Vancomycin-resistant enterococci (VRE) may have emerged due to the increased use of vancomycin treatment for MRSA and *C. difficile*. Enterococci are common gut flora but in at-risk patients may cause UTI, wound infections and bacteraemia.
- Resistant Gram-negative bacteria such as *Pseudomonas* are a common problem in chronic suppurative respiratory conditions, such as bronchiectasis and cystic fibrosis, as well as intensive care units where they may cause ventilator-associated pneumonia.

Further reading

British HIV Association: publishes guidelines and reviews on HIV. Available online at: http://www.bhiva.org.

British Society for Antimicrobial Chemotherapy: has information about MRSA and other bacterial infections encountered. Available online at: http://www.bsac.org.uk.

Interim WHO Clinical Staging of HIV/AIDS and HIV/AIDS case definitions for surveillance 2005. Available online at: http://www.who.int/hiv/pub/guidelines/clinicalstaging.pdf.

Lalloo, D., Shinegadia, D., Pasvol, G., et al., 2007. UK malaria treatment guidelines. J. Infect. 54, 111–121.

London School of Hygiene and Tropical Medicine: provides information on tropical medicine. Available online at: http://www.lshtm.ac.uk.

Drug overdose and abuse

Objectives

The key learning points for this chapter:

- How to assess a patient with suspected drug overdose.
- The general approach to management of patients with possible drug overdose.
- The management of specific common drug overdoses.

EPIDEMIOLOGY

Drug overdose results in a significant proportion of all acute hospital admissions and has an overall incidence of around 2 per 1000 population. Around 25% of suicides are due to deliberate drug overdose. Admission following the use of illegal drugs is also frequently seen – common substances are covered in Figs 39.1 and 39.2.

AETIOLOGY

Overdose may be due to the following:

- Accidental: particularly in children.
- Deliberate: in suicide, attempted suicide or deliberate self-harm, homicide or child abuse (e.g. Münchhausen's syndrome by proxy).
- Iatrogenic: e.g. drug interactions, reduced metabolism/excretion (renal failure, liver failure).

PRESENTATION

History

Drug overdose in many patients results in a mild illness requiring little intervention. However, some patients take many tablets or cocktails of drugs, causing a life-threatening state requiring intensive care. Around 80% of patients are conscious and able to provide a history. In all patients, particularly the unconscious, further history from family, friends and the ambulance staff is likely to be very helpful and should be actively sought. Always consider overdose in any unconscious patient. Where possible, try to establish the following facts.

What drugs were taken and when?

It is very common for more than one drug to be taken, and alcohol is often also used. Try to establish which tablets were taken, how many and how long ago to establish the likely ongoing risk and to help plan investigation and treatment. However, it is good policy to treat the patient and not the history, as this may be unreliable.

Try to assess the suicide risk

Features conferring higher suicide risk are detailed in Fig. 39.3. It is important to cover the events leading to the overdose – did the patient intend suicide at the time or was it an impulsive reaction to an acute stressor such as an argument? Evidence that the act was premeditated should be sought (e.g. collecting tablets over a period of time, a suicide note, taking tablets when the patient expected to be alone). The actions after taking the overdose, and the course of events leading to hospital admission are also important – did the patient themselves ring for help? Ask about ongoing suicidal ideation and low mood.

COMMUNICATION

Patients presenting with deliberate self-harm or attempted suicide are often challenging and difficult to engage. If the patient is happy for friends or family to be present, ensure they are involved. Input from psychiatry is also very important.

Examination

The examination should be in three stages: assess how ill the patient is; look for evidence to suggest the likely drug(s) involved; and look for complications of overdose.

How ill is the patient?

The first priority is ABC – check the Airway, Breathing and Circulation. Assessment of conscious level, pulse, blood pressure, temperature and blood glucose should then be made.

Fig. 39.1 Specific measures in the management of drug overdose with certain of the more common drugs.

Drug	Toxic side effects	Specific management
Opiates	Respiratory depression, drowsiness or coma, pinpoint pupils, hypotension, bradycardia, hypothermia, pulmonary oedema	Naloxone 0.8–2 mg IV (may need to be repeated every 2–3 min to a maximum of 10 mg because of its short half-life); can be administered by continuous IV infusion
Benzodiazepines	Drowsiness, dysarthria, nystagmus, ataxia, coma, respiratory depression; fairly safe if taken alone but potentiate the effects of other sedative drugs, which are often taken at the same time	Flumazenil 200 μg over 15 s, then 100 μg every 60 s until response (maximum dose 1 mg); should be used cautiously
Paracetamol	Nausea and vomiting in the first 24 h; acute hepatocellular necrosis may develop after 3 days with as few as 20 tablets causing jaundice, encephalopathy, hypoglycaemia and abdominal pain; renal tubular necrosis may also occur	Monitor blood pressure, prothrombin time, glucose, creatinine, pH, and for signs of encephalopathy: these parameters determine the need for specialist referral; check paracetamol levels from 4 h onwards (treatment may begin before result is available if significant overdose suspected); use nomogram to determine whether antidote should be given if less than 24 h since tablets were taken Give acetylcysteine (Parvolex) by IV infusion Oral methionine may be given instead if overdose less than 12 h before
Aspirin	Nausea, vomiting, tinnitus, deafness, sweating, hyperventilation, tachycardia, delirium, seizures, coma, impaired clotting, hypokalaemia, hypoglycaemia, metabolic acidosis (respiratory alkalosis initially)	Correct dehydration, hypokalaemia and hypoglycaemia If plasma salicylate levels >500 mg/L (3.6 mmol/L), urinary alkalinization with sodium bicarbonate under close supervision In severe poisoning (>700 mg/L or 5.1 mmol/L), haemodialysis may be life-saving
Iron	Usually accidental affecting children Causes haemorrhagic enteritis (corrosion) with nausea, vomiting, abdominal pain, haematemesis, bloody diarrhoea, acute hepatocellular necrosis, metabolic acidosis, peritonitis, hypotension, coma	Desferrioxamine by IV or IM injection
Digoxin	Nausea, vomiting, diarrhoea, hyperkalaemia, bradyarrhythmias, tachyarrhythmias, altered colour vision, delirium	Correct electrolyte disturbance Temporary ventricular pacing in atrioventricular block Digoxin-specific antibody fragments (Digibind) in severe overdose
Beta-blockers	Bradycardia, hypotension, cardiac failure, convulsions, coma, asystole	Atropine IV for bradycardia Glucagon IV in severe overdose
Heparin	Haemorrhage	IV protamine sulphate
Warfarin	Haemorrhage	IV vitamin K, IV infusion of concentrates of factors II, VII, IX and X, or fresh frozen plasma
Tricyclic antidepressants	Tachycardia, dry mouth, drowsiness, mydriasis, increased reflexes, seizures, coma Prolonged QT interval may cause VT/SVT	Supportive measures; special attention to acidosis Sodium bicarbonate if significant overdose Lidocaine for arrhythmia

Is there any evidence to suggest an underlying cause?

Relatives or ambulance staff may have brought bottles from the scene. Look for evidence on the patient such as diabetic cards or hospital appointment cards (e.g. insulin overdose). The hospital's electronic system may alert you to their last prescription and if they have taken overdoses previously. Also look for:

- Pinpoint pupils: opiates, organophosphates.
- Dilated pupils: tricyclic antidepressants, amphetamines, cocaine.
- Nystagmus: phenytoin, alcohol.

Fig. 39.2 Features and management of common illegal drug overdose.

Substance	Clinical features	Management
Heroin and other opioids (smack, junk, gear, horse)	See Fig. 39.1	See Fig. 39.1
Cocaine/crack cocaine (coke, charlie, snow)	Euphoria, tachycardia, agitation, hyperthermia, coronary artery spasm, seizures, acidosis	Sedation, active cooling, GTN. Beta-blockers are contraindicated
Ketamine (K, special K)	Dissociation, hypertension, arrhythmia, respiratory depression	Supportive measures
Mephedrone (miaow miaow, M-cat)	Agitation, tachycardia, hypertension, seizures	Supportive measures
Gammahydroxybutyrate (GHB)	Euphoria, dizziness, hypotonia, bradycardia, respiratory depression	Supportive measures. GHB is rapidly metabolized and cleared
MDMA/amphetamines (ecstasy, speed, pills)	Agitation, tachycardia, psychosis, hyperthermia, rhabdomyolysis	Supportive measures, sedation, beta-blockers

Fig. 39.3 Features indicating a high suicide risk.

Elderly
Male
Previous suicide attempts
Unemployed
Socially isolated (single, living alone)
Chronic debilitating illness (psychiatric or physical)
Drug or alcohol abuse

- Burns around the mouth: corrosives.
- Hyperventilation: aspirin.
- Needle marks: opiates, benzodiazepines, stimulants.

Have any complications occurred?

Fig. 39.4 summarizes complications of drug overdose. Note that a low-reading thermometer can be used to detect hypothermia.

Fig. 39.4 Complications of drug overdose.

Coma
Respiratory depression
Hypotension or hypertension
Arrhythmias
Seizures
Head injury
Hypothermia or hyperthermia
Aspiration pneumonia
Rhabdomyolysis (can cause renal failure)
Organ failure
Gastric stress ulceration

INVESTIGATIONS

- Paracetamol and salicylate levels should be measured in all patients.
- Urea and electrolytes (including magnesium), blood glucose, serum osmolarity, creatine kinase.
- Baseline clotting and liver function tests in paracetamol overdose.
- Drug levels can be measured in the blood, gastric contents and urine. The timing may be important (e.g. paracetamol overdose).
- Arterial blood gas to assess respiratory depression or stimulation (opiates, salicylate) and acid-base status.
- ECG is advisable in all patients, as many drugs can cause arrhythmia in overdose.
- Chest X-ray: if evidence of aspiration.
- If unconscious, consider further imaging to rule out an intracranial event.

MANAGEMENT

The management of drug overdose can be divided into three parts: general measures for all patients; specific measures according to the drug taken; and psychiatric assessment and social input when the patient recovers physically.

General approach

Supportive care

- If unconscious, assess airway and give oxygen via a face-mask.
- If not maintaining airway, call anaesthetist as the patient may need intubation.

- Some patients may require assisted ventilation.
- Maintain blood pressure with IV fluid as required.
- Measure observations regularly – patients who seem well may deteriorate rapidly.
- Attach cardiac monitor if arrhythmia is suspected or the patient is known to have taken tricyclic antidepressants or cardiac medications, e.g. beta-blockers, digoxin.
- In arrhythmia, correct hypoxia, acidosis or electrolyte imbalance; antiarrhythmic agents should be used with caution as they can exacerbate the arrhythmia.
- Convulsions should be treated with IV benzodiazepines.

Preventing absorption in the bowel

Gastrointestinal absorption may be decreased with activated charcoal. Induced emesis is not recommended. Gastric lavage is very infrequently used, and only if the patient presents very shortly after ingestion and if recommended by the National Poisons Information Service (NPIS).

- Activated charcoal binds poisons in the stomach preventing absorption.
- It is more effective the sooner it is given, and is usually used within 1 h of ingestion.
- Repeated doses are very infrequently used.
- It is contraindicated in drowsy patients (risk of aspiration).
- It is ineffective for iron, lithium, potassium, alcohol and cyanide.
- Whole bowel irrigation is not routinely recommended but can be considered in iron overdose or in enteric-coated drugs.

Increase elimination of drug

Elimination of drugs can be increased using urinary alkalinization or dialysis.

Urinary alkalinization

- Increases renal excretion of mildly acidic drugs.
- Used in severe salicylate, phenobarbital and amphetamine overdose.
- A good urinary output is required. Fluid balance, electrolytes and acid–base status should be monitored very carefully.

Dialysis

Dialysis is used in severe overdose when other methods are contraindicated, unsuccessful or likely to be unsuccessful. Haemodialysis is especially useful for overdose of salicylate, lithium, alcohols and polyethylene glycol. Haemoperfusion is useful for protein-bound drugs but is very rarely performed.

Specific antidotes

Advice for overdose of any drug or ingestion of any poisons can be obtained 24 h a day from a number of poisons information centres run by the NPIS. Each A&E department and hospital switchboard will have a list of national numbers, as well as access to the NPIS online database, Toxbase, which provides a vast amount of detailed information.

Fig. 39.1 summarizes the features and management of overdose of some of the more common drugs.

HINTS AND TIPS

Some people are at higher risk of serious harm from paracetamol overdose and require treatment at lower serum levels. Risk factors include malnourishment, liver disease, long-term alcohol excess and taking liver enzyme inducing drugs (e.g. phenytoin, carbamazepine).

Psychiatric and social assessment

Once the acute event and medical management is completed, an assessment of the patient's psychiatric state (ongoing suicidal risk) and social circumstances should be made, however trivial the overdose may have appeared. Where appropriate, psychiatrists and social care workers should be involved.

ILLEGAL DRUGS

Due to their nature there is often less information available on the treatment of adverse effects associated with illegal drugs. In addition, new drugs emerge and quickly become widely used – such as mephedrone in the recent past. Toxbase is very useful in this regard. Fig. 39.2 details some of the features seen with commonly used illegal drugs.

ALCOHOL MISUSE AND WITHDRAWAL

Alcohol is widely used throughout the world. Lifetime incidence of alcohol dependence is between 5 and 15% in Europe; although this represents only a minority of those who drink alcohol, the problem is huge in terms of morbidity, mortality and healthcare costs. The 'CAGE' questionnaire is commonly used as a screening tool for alcohol problems (Fig. 39.5).

Fig. 39.5 The CAGE questionnaire.

Have you ever felt you needed to **C**ut down on your drinking?
Has anyone ever **A**nnoyed you by criticizing your drinking?
Have you ever felt **G**uilty about your drinking?
Have you ever needed a drink in the morning – an '**E**ye-opener' – to make yourself feel better?
A positive answer to any of these questions is indicative of possible alcohol dependence.

Alcohol-related health problems

- Acute intoxication: alcohol causes euphoria and reduced inhibition. In greater quantities it may cause reduced conscious level, respiratory depression, atrial fibrillation, hypoglycaemia and hypotension.
- Alcohol withdrawal: tremor, sweating, tachycardia, irritability, agitation, hallucinations, delusions, seizures. Symptoms usually start within 24 h of last alcohol intake.
- Gastrointestinal: gastritis, oesophagitis, varices, alcoholic liver disease (see Ch. 32).
- Cardiovascular: arrhythmia, cardiomyopathy, hypertension.
- Respiratory: increased incidence of pneumonia and TB due to reduced clearance of pathogens.
- Neurological: cortical atrophy, cerebellar degeneration, peripheral neuropathy, Wernicke's encephalopathy/Korsakoff's syndrome.
- Endocrine: gynaecomastia, testicular atrophy, osteoporosis.
- Increased risk of cancer particularly oesophageal and head and neck cancers.

Management of alcohol dependence

Alcohol withdrawal

Patients experiencing alcohol withdrawal are difficult to treat and, despite initial willingness, often self-discharge. It is important to see the patient and assess their symptoms rather than give instructions over the telephone. The standard treatment is a course of benzodiazepines, usually chlordiazepoxide, which is slowly reduced over several days; most hospitals have a dosing protocol. Seizures should be treated with IV benzodiazepines if necessary, and occasionally antipsychotics such as haloperidol are required for severe withdrawal psychosis.

Patients also require thiamine (IV in the form of Pabrinex) and investigation of any alcohol-related conditions. Fluid replacement may be difficult; dextrose may be the most suitable IV fluid but should not be given before the first dose of Pabrinex due to the risk of precipitating Wernicke's encephalopathy.

Long-term treatment

Regular psychosocial input is essential. Longer-term managed withdrawal regimens may be needed for extremely heavy drinkers who have struggled in the past. Once withdrawal has been completed there are three currently recommended pharmacological aids:

- Naltrexone: a partial agonist at opioid receptors. It reduces cravings, and is usually continued for 6 months to 1 year.
- Acamprosate: its mechanism of action is not completely known. It reduces cravings and is continued for 6 months to 1 year if initially successful.
- Disulfiram: this causes an unpleasant reaction on ingestion of any alcohol. The patient has to be suitable and willing to undergo treatment. Cravings are not reduced and compliance is often poor.

Further reading

Battista, E., 2012. Crash Course: Pharmacology, fourth ed. Mosby Elsevier, Edinburgh.

National Institute for Health and Clinical Excellence (NICE), 2004. Self-harm. Clinical guideline CG16. Available online at: http://www.nice.org.uk/CG16.

National Institute for Health and Clinical Excellence (NICE), 2011. Alcohol dependence and harmful alcohol use. Clinical guideline CG115. Available online at: http://www.nice.org.uk/CG115.

Vale, J.A., Bradberry, S.M., Bateman, D.N., 2010. Poisoning by drugs and chemicals. In: Warrell, D.A., Cox, T.M., Firth, J.D. (Eds.), Oxford Textbook of Medicine, fifth ed. Oxford University Press, Oxford, pp. 873–922.

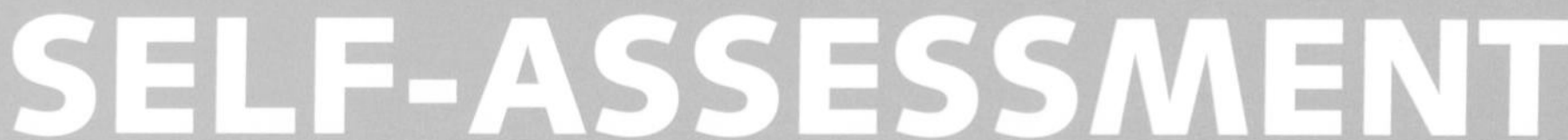

SELF-ASSESSMENT

Single best answer questions (SBAs) 407

Extended-matching questions (EMQs) 419

SBA answers 429

EMQ answers 439

Single best answer questions (SBAs)

Indicate which one of the five options is the correct answer.

History taking

1. Which one of the following is not important in the patient with a chronic cough?
   A. Nocturnal symptoms.
   B. Taking angiotensin II receptor blockers.
   C. Change in voice character.
   D. Nasal problems (chronic cough if no pre-existing lung disease is present).
   E. Occupation.

2. Which one of the following drugs and side effects are incorrectly linked?
   A. Nitrofurantoin and pulmonary fibrosis.
   B. Angiotensin-converting-enzyme inhibitors and angio-oedema.
   C. Digoxin and visual field defects.
   D. Amiodarone and photosensitive rash.
   E. Ethambutol and disturbance of colour vision.

3. Which one of the following is incorrect?
   A. 20 cigarettes per day for 20 years equals 20 pack years.
   B. 30 cigarettes per day for 25 years equals 32.5 pack years.
   C. A 750-mL bottle of 12% wine contains 9 units.
   D. A pint of bitter contains roughly 2 units.
   E. Alcohol problems can be initially assessed with the 'CAGE' questions.

Examination

1. Which one of the following statements regarding hand signs is correct?
   A. Clubbing may be caused by uncomplicated chronic bronchitis.
   B. Koilonychia usually indicates liver disease.
   C. Osler's nodes and Bouchard's nodes both occur in osteoarthritis.
   D. Asterixis is specific for hepatic encephalopathy.
   E. Leuconychia is consistent with hypoalbuminaemia.

2. Which one of following would suggest a lower rather than an upper motor neurone lesion?
   A. Fasciculation.
   B. Increased tone.
   C. Extensor plantar response.
   D. Clonus.
   E. Relatively little wasting.

3. Which one of the following is not true of pulsus paradoxus?
   A. The volume of the pulse decreases in inspiration.
   B. Can be confirmed by detecting >10 mmHg difference in systolic pressure during the breathing cycle.
   C. Is a sign of severe asthma.
   D. Is called pulsus paradoxus because it is the opposite of what normally happens to the pulse.
   E. Can occur in cardiac tamponade.

4. Which of the following would not help distinguish between a kidney and the spleen on abdominal examination?
   A. Dullness to percussion.
   B. A notch on the medial border.
   C. Ability to 'get above' the mass.
   D. Ability to ballot the mass.
   E. Absence of bowel sounds in the left upper quadrant.

5. Which one of the following is not characteristic of a jugular venous, as opposed to carotid, pulsation?
   A. Palpable pulse.
   B. Movement with respiration.
   C. A double waveform.
   D. Movement with posture.
   E. A rise when pressure is applied below the right costal margin.

6. Which one of the following is a true sign of a large uncomplicated pneumothorax?
   A. Tracheal deviation away from the pneumothorax.
   B. A clicking sound synchronous with the heart sounds.
   C. Symmetrical expansion of the chest.
   D. Increased breath sounds over pneumothorax.
   E. Reduced percussion note over pneumothorax.

The clerking

1. Which one of the following is not true of a medical clerking?
   A. It is a legal document.
   B. It is essential to follow a particular order.
   C. The time and date are essential.
   D. It should incorporate a problem list.
   E. It should be completed with a name, signature and bleep number.

ations

1. en investigating suspected pulmonary embolus, which one of the following is true?
   A. The D-dimer is useful to exclude pulmonary embolus but not to diagnose it.
   B. The diagnosis is confirmed by the presence of right bundle branch block.
   C. A perfusion scan is better than CTPA if the patient has chronic obstructive pulmonary disease.
   D. The troponin level will be unrecordable.
   E. If the CT pulmonary angiogram is negative for pulmonary embolism then a formal angiogram should be performed to confirm the diagnosis.

2. Regarding arterial blood gas monitoring, which one of the following is incorrect?
   A. $P\text{CO}_2$ can be considered an 'acid' gas.
   B. If the $P\text{CO}_2$ is low or normal in type I respiratory failure, ventilation is adequate.
   C. Metabolic compensation involves the retention of bicarbonate ions by the liver.
   D. A raised anion gap is compatible with the presence of exogenous acid in the blood.
   E. An increased base excess accompanies a rise in bicarbonate levels.

3. Regarding the ECG, which one of the following is correct?
   A. The PR interval is measured from the end of the P wave to the start of the QRS complex.
   B. Normal electrical axis is from -90° to $+90^\circ$.
   C. P mitrale is suggested by a peaked P wave taller than 2.5 mm in lead II.
   D. Q waves in leads II, III and aVF indicate a previous transmural anterior myocardial infarction.
   E. The normal QRS duration is ≤ 0.12 s.

4. Which one of the following causes a reduced mean corpuscular volume?
   A. Hypothyroidism.
   B. Alcohol.
   C. Pernicious anaemia.
   D. Beta-thalassaemia trait.
   E. Chronic renal failure.

5. Which one of the following does not cause raised ESR?
   A. Multiple myeloma.
   B. Anaemia.
   C. Polycythaemia.
   D. Increasing age.
   E. Giant cell arteritis.

6. Which one of the following causes hypocalcaemia?
   A. Renal cell carcinoma.
   B. Milk-alkali syndrome.
   C. Renal impairment.
   D. Sarcoidosis.
   E. Pseudopseudohypoparathyroidism.

7. Which one of the following is an incorrect pair?
   A. Increased urea-to-creatinine ratio with gastrointestinal bleeding.
   B. High alkaline phosphatase and gamma-glutamyltranspeptidase with hepatitis.
   C. High D-dimer and venous thromboembolism.
   D. High creatine kinase and polymyositis.
   E. High HbA1c and poor diabetic control.

8. When performing a short synacthen test, which one of the following is correct?
   A. You are testing for excess cortisol production.
   B. A flat response is a normal response.
   C. It is performed overnight.
   D. Synacthen is synthetic adrenocorticotrophic hormone.
   E. It can separate adrenal and pituitary causes of cortisol deficiency.

9. Regarding the chest X-ray, which one of the following is incorrect?
   A. Loss of the right heart border indicates consolidation in the right middle lobe.
   B. Cardiomegaly is defined as a cardiothoracic ratio of >0.5 in a posteroanterior film.
   C. Airspace (alveolar) shadowing could be caused by pulmonary infection.
   D. Sarcoidosis may cause bilateral hilar lymphadenopathy.
   E. Kerley B lines are perihilar in distribution.

Cardiovascular disorders

1. A 49-year-old lady is found to have a heart murmur during a routine preoperative assessment clinic. Which one statement regarding heart murmurs is correct?
   A. A pansystolic murmur loudest at the apex radiating to the axilla is most likely mitral regurgitation.
   B. Mitral stenosis with atrial fibrillation (AF) would give a diastolic murmur with presystolic accentuation.
   C. Left-sided heart murmurs are best heard in inspiration.
   D. Aortic regurgitation is best heard in the left lateral position.
   E. An opening snap is heard in aortic stenosis just after the first heart sound.

2. A 50-year-old diabetic man is found to have a persistent blood pressure of 164/92 mmHg. Which one of the following would be the most appropriate initial management?
   A. Atenolol.
   B. Bendroflumethiazide.
   C. Better diabetic control.
   D. Enalapril.
   E. Low salt diet.

3. Which one of the following findings suggests that aortic stenosis is clinically significant?
   A. The apex beat is not displaced.
   B. The blood pressure is 160/94 mmHg.
   C. The murmur is heard all over the praecordium.
   D. The murmur radiates to the carotids.
   E. There is left ventricular hypertrophy on the ECG.

4. A 63-year-old man is admitted with an episode of severe, central chest pain and dyspnoea. An ECG is performed in the emergency department which shows anterior ST elevation of >2 mm. The patient receives primary percutaneous coronary intervention. He recovers well and on discharge his renal function is normal, cholesterol 4.5 mmol/L and triglycerides 3.4 mmol/L. Which of the following medications should be prescribed on discharge?
   A. Ramipril, simvastatin, warfarin and atenolol.
   B. Ramipril, simvastatin, aspirin and atenolol.
   C. Losartan, bezafibrate, aspirin and diltiazem.
   D. Losartan, simvastatin, clopidogrel and atenolol.
   E. Ramipril, bezafibrate, aspirin and atenolol.

5. Which one statement regarding chronic left ventricular failure is false?
   A. Can be classified by the New York Heart Association scale.
   B. Diuretics improve symptoms.
   C. Digoxin has no role unless in atrial fibrillation.
   D. May predispose to ventricular arrhythmias.
   E. All patients should try angiotensin-converting-enzyme inhibitors unless contraindicated.

6. Which one of the following statements is false with regards to atrial fibrillation (AF)?
   A. Can cause heart failure in previously well-controlled heart disease.
   B. Results in an increased risk of stroke.
   C. Is usually caused by rheumatic fever.
   D. Results in absent P waves on the ECG.
   E. May be a finding in acute pulmonary embolus.

7. A 23-year-old human resource manager attends the emergency department with palpitations. She described the sensation as very fast and regular. An ECG is performed and shows a regular, narrow QRS complex with a rate of 200. Shortly after admission the symptoms spontaneously resolve and a repeat ECG shows a normal PR interval with a positive delta wave in V_1. Which one of the following is the most likely diagnosis?
   A. Atrial flutter.
   B. Ventricular fibrillation.
   C. Ventricular re-entry tachycardia.
   D. Atrioventricular nodal re-entry tachycardia.
   E. Atrioventricular re-entry tachycardia.

8. Which one statement regarding the jugular venous pressure is false?
   A. Is measured from the suprasternal notch with the patient sitting at 45°.
   B. Reflects right ventricular preload.
   C. Cannon waves indicate complete heart block.
   D. An elevated non-collapsing JVP may indicate superior vena caval obstruction.
   E. Tricuspid regurgitation results in large 'v' waves.

9. A 65-year-old diabetic lady with known hypertension presents to the emergency department with retrosternal chest tightness. An ECG reveals T-wave inversion in V_2–V_4. Her 12-h serum troponin level comes back as 10 times the upper limit of normal. Which single investigation will provide the most diagnostic information?
   A. Cardiac catheterization.
   B. Exercise tolerance test (ETT).
   C. Echocardiography.
   D. 24-h ECG monitor.
   E. Radionuclide cardiac perfusion scanning.

10. Which one of the following is a cause of essential hypertension?
    A. Conn's syndrome.
    B. Phaeochromocytoma.
    C. Coarctation of the aorta.
    D. Renal artery stenosis.
    E. Idiopathic.

11. Which statement regarding the assessment of the pulse is false?
    A. The character should be assessed centrally.
    B. A slow rising pulse indicates mitral stenosis.
    C. Pulsus alternans indicates poor left ventricular function.
    D. Rate, rhythm, volume and character should be assessed.
    E. The heart rate will increase during inspiration in sinus rhythm.

Respiratory disease

1. A 51-year-old builder was involved in a high-speed road traffic incident. Basic first aid was provided at the scene according to ATLS principles and he was subsequently transferred to hospital. Whilst being formally assessed, one of the FY2 doctors in the emergency department noticed the patient's oxygen saturations had dropped to 85%. He is concerned the patient may have a tension pneumothorax. Which one of the following is not a feature of a tension pneumothorax?
   A. The trachea is deviated towards the affected side.
   B. Increased percussion note over the pneumothorax.
   C. Asymmetrical expansion of the chest.
   D. Absent breath sounds over the pneumothorax.
   E. A raised JVP.

2. A 51-year-old Pilates instructor suffered a bimalleolar fracture of her ankle which required open reduction and internal fixation (ORIF). The operation was a

success and she was discharged with a 3-week course of low-molecular-weight heparin (LMWH). Four weeks post-op she developed progressive shortness of breath and a dry cough. She attended the emergency department where a CT pulmonary angiogram revealed large bilateral pulmonary embolisms. Which one of the following statements would be correct regarding pulmonary embolus?

A. The S_1 Q_3 T_3 pattern is the most common ECG abnormality.
B. This case is unusual since haemoptysis is the most common symptom.
C. Is rarely associated with undiagnosed malignancy.
D. One of the earliest signs is a resting tachycardia.
E. Requires 1 year of warfarin therapy.

3. A 17-year-old girl is admitted to hospital with a wheeze and severe dyspnoea. Which one of the following statements is true with regards to the assessment and management of an acute asthma attack?

A. The peak flow measure is unhelpful.
B. A normal $P\text{CO}_2$ is reassuring.
C. IV magnesium may be indicated.
D. Death is extremely rare.
E. IV bronchodilator is much better than nebulized therapy.

4. An 67-year-old gardener presents to his GP with a 3-day history of productive cough, fevers and anorexia. On examination the patient has coarse crackles at the right base with bronchial breathing. The GP suspects this is pneumonia and refers the patient to be seen in hospital for a chest X-ray and blood cultures. Which one of the following does not score a point in the severity assessment for community-acquired pneumonia?

A. Blood urea $>$7 mmol/L.
B. Systolic blood pressure $>$90 mmHg.
C. Respiratory rate $>$30 per min.
D. Confusion.
E. Age $>$65 years.

5. A 72-year-old retired car mechanic presents with a 6-month period of weight loss, cough and occasional haemoptysis. A chest X-ray reveals a mass in the right hemithorax with associated hilar shadowing. A CT is performed and subsequent bronchoscopy and biopsy makes the diagnosis of squamous cell carcinoma of the lung. Which one of the following statements is true regarding squamous cell carcinoma of the lung?

A. Is associated with the syndrome of inappropriate antidiuretic hormone secretion.
B. Is associated with hypercalcaemia.
C. Is the most common cause of Eaton–Lambert myasthenic syndrome.
D. Chemotherapy is the mainstay of treatment.
E. Rarely metastasizes to bone.

6. Which of these drugs is most likely to be associated with interstitial lung disease?

A. Amiodarone.
B. Amoxicillin.
C. Doxycycline.
D. Enalapril.
E. Sotalol.

7. A 46-year-old woman with a known diagnosis of sarcoidosis presents to the emergency department with worsening dyspnoea. A chest X-ray is performed and subsequently reported as stage 3 pulmonary sarcoidosis. Which one of the following is the X-ray most likely to show?

A. A pleural effusion.
B. Bilateral hilar lymphadenopathy.
C. Bilateral hilar lymphadenopathy with reticunodular shadowing.
D. Fibrocystic sarcoidosis typically with upward hilar retraction, cystic and bullous change.
E. Bilateral pulmonary infiltrates.

8. A 19-year-old student is brought in by ambulance to the emergency department with severe dyspnoea. His peak flow is 100 L/min (normally 650 L/min). His respiratory rate is 40/min and auscultation of his chest reveals barely audible breath sounds. His mother tells you that he had been hyperventilating for approximately 30 min prior to admission. What would you expect the arterial blood gas result to be?

A. pH 7.29, $P\text{CO}_2$ 6.3 kP, $P\text{O}_2$ 9.2 kP, bicarbonate 45 mmol/L.
B. pH 7.51, $P\text{CO}_2$ 7.9 kP, $P\text{O}_2$ 9.6 kP, bicarbonate 37 mmol/L.
C. pH 7.39, $P\text{CO}_2$ 5.3 kP, $P\text{O}_2$ 7.1 kP, bicarbonate 30 mmol/L.
D. pH 7.51, $P\text{CO}_2$ 2.0 kP, $P\text{O}_2$ 9.6 kP, bicarbonate 14 mmol/L.
E. pH 7.57, $P\text{CO}_2$ 3.2 kP, $P\text{O}_2$ 10.2 kP, bicarbonate 27 mmol/L.

9. A 56-year-old publican is admitted to the emergency department with dyspnoea. Whilst he is waiting to be seen by the doctor, the nurse administers oxygen through nasal cannula at 2 L/min as his oxygen saturations were 89%. Which one of the following most accurately reflects the fraction of oxygen inspired ($F\text{iO}_2$)?

A. 98%.
B. 50%.
C. 35%.
D. 28%.
E. 24%.

10. Which one of the following has not shown proven benefit in chronic obstructive pulmonary disease?

A. Smoking cessation.
B. Long-term home oxygen therapy (LTOT).
C. Routine use of inhaled corticosteroids.

D. Non-invasive ventilation.
E. Pulmonary rehabilitation.

11. Which one statement regarding malignant mesothelioma is true?
A. Is a tumour of the lung parenchyma.
B. Usually accompanies pulmonary asbestosis.
C. Is diagnosed by pleural plaques on chest X-ray or CT.
D. Has a good prognosis.
E. May result in compensation for patient and/or family.

12. Which one statement is false regarding obstructive sleep apnoea?
A. Exclusively occurs in overweight people.
B. Is occasionally treated with surgery.
C. Causes excessive daytime sleepiness.
D. Is associated with non-respiratory disorders.
E. Can be central or secondary to collapsing airways.

Gastroenterology

1. A 67-year-old man underwent an oesophagogastroduodenoscopy (OGD) for reflux symptoms. Barrett's oesophagus was diagnosed. Which one of the following statements regarding this condition is true?
A. Approximately 25% will progress to adenocarcinoma.
B. The condition predominantly affects the middle third of the oesophagus.
C. The condition is asymptomatic in most cases.
D. Is treated surgically in the first instance.
E. The condition is characterized by dysplasia from squamous cell epithelium to columnar cell epithelium.

2. A 43-year-old midwife presents with constant, epigastric pain radiating to the back. She had been suffering with intermittent episodes of right upper quadrant (RUQ) pain for the previous 6 months. Serum amylase is 1400 U/mL. A diagnosis of suspected pancreatitis is made. Which one of the following statements is true?
A. A serum amylase of >2500 U/mL indicates severe pancreatitis.
B. The most likely aetiology is gallstones.
C. The Rockall score is used to assess severity.
D. A recognized early complication of pancreatitis is pseudocyst formation.
E. Pancreatitis is the only possible diagnosis.

3. A 58-year-old alcoholic with known liver cirrhosis presents with copious amounts of haematemesis. A variceal bleed is suspected. Which one of the following statements is true for the management of a large upper gastrointestinal (GI) haemorrhage?
A. A detailed history and examination is a priority.
B. A large bleed causes an immediate decrease in haemoglobin concentration.
C. Causes a decrease in urea concentration.
D. The investigation of choice is a CT scan.
E. Re-bleeding carries a higher mortality.

4. A 24-year-old primary school teacher presents with abdominal pain and bloody diarrhoea. He has a colonoscopy which shows features of ulcerative colitis (UC). Which one of the following features is associated with UC?
A. Transmural inflammation.
B. Pseudopolyps.
C. Perianal lesions.
D. Skip lesions.
E. More common in smokers.

5. A 76-year-old retired accountant presents with a change in bowel habit, tenesmus and weight loss. A colonoscopy is done and shows a carcinoma of the colon. Which one of the following statements is true about colorectal cancer?
A. The majority occur in patients with a strong family history.
B. The cancer is likely to be in the ascending colon.
C. Right-sided tumours usually present earlier.
D. May present with an iron-deficiency anaemia alone.
E. Only a minority of tumours can be resected surgically.

6. An 87-year-old lady was admitted for severe pneumonia and treated with a broad-spectrum beta-lactamase. On the 10th day of her admission she develops perfuse diarrhoea with cramping abdominal pain. A diagnosis of pseudomembranous colitis is made after further investigation. Which one of the following statements is true?
A. Is caused by *Clostridium difficile* itself.
B. Can be prevented by using alcohol hand gel after each patient contact.
C. Is diagnosed by demonstrating an erythematous, ulcerated mucosa covered by a membrane on sigmoidoscopy.
D. May be complicated by toxic dilatation of the colon.
E. Is treated with IV metronidazole in first instance.

7. A 22-year-old female medical student registers with a new GP. On her health questionnaire she states that she has been diagnosed with irritable bowel syndrome (IBS). Which one statement about IBS is true?
A. The condition is rare.
B. The condition is more common in males.
C. IBS may present with rectal bleeding.
D. It is a diagnosis of exclusion.
E. It is usually treated with 100% success.

8. A 49-year-old mother of two presents to the emergency department (ED) with right upper quadrant (RUQ) pain and fever. On examination she is tender in the RUQ but not jaundiced. The ED doctor suspects she has cholecystitis secondary to gallstones. Which one of the following statements about gallstone disease is true?
   A. Most are radio-opaque.
   B. They are often asymptomatic.
   C. Their incidence decreases with age.
   D. They cannot cause bowel obstruction.
   E. Charcot's triad is diagnostic of cholecystitis.

9. Which one of the following may be said of viral hepatitis?
   A. Hepatitis A may cause chronic hepatitis.
   B. Hepatitis B is transmitted via the faecal–oral route.
   C. Chronic hepatitis B infection may be complicated by hepatocellular carcinoma.
   D. Hepatitis C causes acute hepatic failure.
   E. Hepatitis E is not transmitted via the faecal–oral route.

10. Which of the following is the classic appearance of the stool in intussusception?
   A. Fatty stool.
   B. Melaena.
   C. Putty-coloured stool.
   D. Redcurrant jelly stool.
   E. Watery stool.

11. A 53-year-old woman with a previous diagnosis of autoimmune hepatitis and cirrhosis is seen in the acute medical assessment unit after being referred by her GP for increasing abdominal distension. On examination her body weight is 110 kg and she has bilateral pitting oedema up to her knees. She is not jaundiced. Shifting dullness is elicited on examination of the abdomen. Which one of the following is the greatest contributing mechanism to the fluid retention in this patient?
   A. Increased sodium absorption in the renal tubules.
   B. Inferior vena cava (IVC) obstruction.
   C. Lymphatic obstruction.
   D. Portal hypertension.
   E. Hypoalbuminaemia.

Genitourinary disorders

1. Which one of the following conditions is not an indication for emergency haemodialysis/ haemofiltration in acute kidney injury (AKI)?
   A. Pulmonary oedema.
   B. Serum creatinine >500 μmol/L.
   C. Severe acidosis.
   D. Resistant hyperkalaemia.
   E. Uraemic pericarditis.

2. A 62-year-old diabetic man is admitted with urinary sepsis. On routine blood tests he is found to have a serum potassium level of 6.8 mmol/L. An ECG is performed immediately. Which one of the following changes would you not expect to see?
   A. Tented T waves.
   B. Absent P waves.
   C. Broad QRS complexes.
   D. U waves.
   E. Sinusoidal waveform.

3. A 5-year-old boy presents with a pale puffy face and swollen legs. There is generalized oedema on clinical examination. Which one of the following is least in keeping with nephrotic syndrome?
   A. Low serum albumin.
   B. Haematuria.
   C. High serum cholesterol.
   D. >3 g protein in a 24-h urine collection.
   E. Oval fat bodies in the urine.

4. A 59-year-old lady is being investigated for haematuria. A diagnosis of glomerulonephritis is suspected. Which one of the following tests is not indicated?
   A. X-ray kidney, ureter, bladder (KUB).
   B. Urine microscopy.
   C. Serum and urine immunoelectrophoresis.
   D. Complement levels.
   E. Antineutrophil cytoplasmic (ANCA) and antiglomerular basement membrane (anti-GM) antibodies.

5. Which one of the following statements does not apply to acute kidney injury?
   A. Oliguria always occurs.
   B. Hypovolaemia is a common cause.
   C. Mortality may be high, especially in the context of multi-organ distress syndrome (MODS).
   D. The majority of patients regain normal renal function.
   E. An early ultrasound scan is important.

6. Which one of the following statements is correct with respect to chronic kidney disease (CKD)?
   A. Hypertension is a rare cause.
   B. Patients with proteinuria do better.
   C. Lowering the blood pressure is dangerous.
   D. Microcytic anaemia is a feature.
   E. Dietary phosphate must be decreased.

7. An 18-year-old girl present with rigors, lower abdominal pain and urinary frequency. Which of the following tests is not indicated?
   A. DMSA scan.
   B. Urine microscopy and culture.
   C. Urine beta-HCG (pregnancy test).
   D. Abdominal X-ray.
   E. Full blood count.

8. Which one statement regarding urinary tract infections (UTI) is true?
   A. Are more common in females.
   B. Affect 5% of the female population at least once.
   C. Are always symptomatic.
   D. Are less common in catheterized patients.
   E. Never ascend to involve the kidneys.

9. A 32-year-old man has a rotator cuff repair under general anaesthetic as a day case. Routine blood tests and urine dip had been unremarkable during preoperative assessment. He is discharged after an uncomplicated operation with paracetamol and indometacin for pain. He presents 2 weeks later to his GP with significant bilateral ankle oedema. On examination his blood pressure is 125/72 mmHg. Urine dipstick reveals 3+ protein, but no haematuria. Plasma creatinine is 65 mmol/L (normal). What is the most likely diagnosis?
   A. Membranous nephropathy.
   B. Acute tubular necrosis.
   C. Interstitial nephritis.
   D. Lupus nephritis.
   E. Minimal change nephropathy.

Neurology

1. A 63-year-old woman presents 2 h after sudden-onset right-sided weakness. She takes warfarin for atrial fibrillation. Which one of the following statements is correct?
   A. Imaging of the brain should be done within the next 24 h but is not urgent.
   B. If the CT scan shows haemorrhage, warfarin should be reversed with cryoprecipitate.
   C. Because she takes warfarin, the stroke is definitely haemorrhagic.
   D. Haemorrhage is the most common cause of stroke.
   E. Facial weakness in stroke usually spares the forehead.

2. A 26-year-old man presents with a severe, throbbing, unilateral headache preceded by odd visual symptoms. It is worsened by loud noises, bright light or moving around. He is afebrile. Which one of the following statements is correct?
   A. The most likely diagnosis is meningitis.
   B. Subarachnoid haemorrhage commonly has visual warning symptoms.
   C. A triptan is a suitable treatment in this case
   D. Acute migraine headache can be treated with beta blockers
   E. Patients with cluster headache typically avoid movement.

3. You see a 55-year-old man in clinic who has noticed a gradually worsening, low-frequency tremor in his right hand over the last 6 months. Which one of the following statements is true?
   A. Parkinson's disease is usually symmetrical in onset.
   B. The tremor of Parkinson's disease is more noticeable at rest.
   C. Levodopa is definitely the best treatment for this patient.
   D. A radio-iodine scan is necessary to make the diagnosis in this case.
   E. Rigidity is an uncommon feature.

4. You see a 23-year-old woman in clinic. She experienced an episode of visual blurring in her right eye, associated with pain on movement, which came on over hours and has improved over the last month. Which one of the following statements is correct?
   A. This is definitely MS.
   B. It is unusual to get MS at this age.
   C. Night vision is likely to be most affected.
   D. If there are lesions on MRI, her risk of developing MS is higher.
   E. Vision only improves in a minority of patients.

5. A 19-year-old male student is admitted with confusion, fever, photophobia and a purpuric rash. His friends say he was complaining of a severe headache and has vomited. Which one of the following is correct?
   A. *Streptococcus* is the most likely causative organism.
   B. The diagnosis should be confirmed with blood cultures before treatment.
   C. *Listeria* is a common cause in young adults.
   D. Lumbar puncture should be performed immediately.
   E. He should be treated urgently with IV antibiotics.

6. Which one of the following statements is correct regarding raised intracranial pressure?
   A. The headache is worse at the end of the day.
   B. Tachycardia is part of the Cushing reflex.
   C. Papilloedema is not caused by raised ICP.
   D. 6th nerve palsy is a feature.
   E. Abdominal pain is a feature.

7. A 64-year-old woman presents with progressive weakness that started in her legs. She has noticed 'flickering' of her muscles. Which one of the following is correct regarding motor neurone disease?
   A. It is more common in women.
   B. Commonly causes sensory problems as well as motor problems.
   C. May present with diplopia.
   D. The 5-year survival is almost 75%.
   E. May cause a mixture of upper and lower motor neurone symptoms.

8. A 45-year-old man presents following a severe sudden-onset headache that occurred during exercise. CT scan shows blood in the subarachnoid space. Which

one of the following statements is correct regarding this condition?
A. Mortality is low.
B. The majority are preceded by a 'sentinel headache'.
C. Reduced consciousness following initial improvement may be due to hydrocephalus.
D. He should be given beta-blockers.
E. Fluid intake should be restricted.

9. A 44-year-old woman presents with symptoms of raised intracranial pressure. MRI scan reveals a solitary lesion. Which one of the following statements is correct regarding intracerebral tumours?
A. Primary tumours are more common than secondary tumours.
B. If primary tumour is suspected, MRI is sufficient to determine the type of tumour.
C. Meningiomas may be cured with surgical resection.
D. Glioblastomas are indolent tumours with a good prognosis.
E. Breast cancer rarely metastasizes to the brain.

10. A 64-year-old man present following a 'blackout'. Which one of the following statements is correct regarding the cause?
A. Seizure is probable if urinary incontinence occurred.
B. Jerking or twitching is never seen in vasovagal syncope.
C. An ECG is unlikely to be helpful in determining the cause.
D. Biting the tip of the tongue suggests a seizure.
E. Syncope on exertion suggests a cardiac cause.

Endocrinology

1. Which one of the following allows a diagnosis of diabetes to be made?
A. Fasting plasma glucose of 6.0.
B. Random glucose of 10.9.
C. Random glucose of 11.2 and polyuria.
D. Fasting glucose of 6.9 and 2-h glucose of 10.4.
E. Fasting glucose of 6.6 and 2-h glucose of 7.5.

2. A 17-year-old woman with diabetes is found unconscious by her mother following a chest infection. Which one of the following is correct regarding DKA?
A. Insulin replacement should be the first treatment.
B. In young patients there is no need to worry about fluid overload.
C. Hypoventilation is typical.
D. Antibiotics are often required.
E. Raised blood sugar and clinical signs are sufficient for the diagnosis.

3. Which one of the following is correct regarding the long-term treatment of diabetes?
A. Type 1 diabetes can often be managed with oral medication.
B. The aim should be an HbA1c below 10%.
C. Sulphonylureas are first choice in overweight patients.
D. Metformin is contraindicated in renal failure.
E. Once-daily subcutaneous insulin is the treatment of choice for type 1 diabetes.

4. A 66-year-old woman who takes long-term low-dose steroids for rheumatoid arthritis sustains a Colles' fracture. Which one of the following statements is correct regarding osteoporosis?
A. It is frequently painful.
B. It is less common in women.
C. Hypocalcaemia is seen on testing.
D. A T-score of −2.0 is diagnostic.
E. The prevalence is around 25% in Caucasian women aged 80 or over.

5. A 58-year-old man presents with polyuria, dehydration and abdominal pain. Blood tests reveal a calcium level of 3.2. Which one of the following is correct?
A. Sarcoidosis is a cause of hypercalcaemia.
B. Treatment with bisphosphonates is urgently required.
C. If the calcium returns to normal with treatment, no further investigation is needed on this occasion.
D. Protein-bound calcium is the relevant value.
E. Malignancy is a rare cause.

6. A 42-year-old man comes to see you because his family are concerned his appearance has changed. He has experienced headaches over the last year. Which one of the following is a feature of acromegaly?
A. Increased interdental spacing.
B. Homonymous hemianopia.
C. Retrognathism.
D. Hypergonadism.
E. Hypoglycaemia.

7. A 36-year-old woman complains of constipation, weight gain and constantly feeling cold. Which one of the following is incorrect regarding hypothyroidism?
A. Viral thyroiditis is a cause of hypothyroidism.
B. A microcytic anaemia is common.
C. Hypercholesterolaemia may occur.
D. If hyponatraemia is present, it is prudent to rule out hypoadrenalism before treating.
E. Myxoedema coma is a rare but life-threatening complication.

8. Which one of the following statements is correct regarding Addison's disease?
A. The majority of cases in the developed world are due to infection.

B. U&Es in crisis show hyponatraemia and hyperkalaemia.
C. Diagnosis is usually made with a random cortisol measurement.
D. Aldosterone replacement with fludrocortisone is the most important treatment in addisonian crisis.
E. Hypopigmentation is common.

9. A 37-year-old woman presents with tremor, palpitations and loose stools. Which one of the following may be seen in thyrotoxicosis of any aetiology?
A. Atrial fibrillation.
B. Pretibial myxoedema.
C. Finger clubbing.
D. Menorrhagia.
E. Bilateral proptosis.

10. Which one of the following hormones is secreted by the posterior pituitary?
A. Thyroid-stimulating hormone.
B. Adrenocorticotrophic hormone.
C. Growth hormone.
D. Anti-diuretic hormone.
E. Prolactin.

Rheumatology and skin

1. Which one of the following is not a complication of rheumatoid arthritis?
A. Diffuse fibrosing alveolitis.
B. Obstructive lung disease.
C. Pleural effusion.
D. Anaemia of chronic disease.
E. Pericardial effusion.

2. Which one of the following is a typical feature of rheumatoid arthritis?
A. Bamboo spine.
B. Bouchard's nodes.
C. Boutonnière deformity.
D. Heberden's nodes.
E. Telescoping of the digits.

3. Which one of the following X-ray findings is not a typical feature of osteoarthritis?
A. Soft tissue thickening.
B. Loss of joint space.
C. Subchondral sclerosis.
D. Osteophytes.
E. Subchondral cysts.

4. An obese 52-year-old man comes to see you with pain in his left knee that is worse on weight bearing and at the end of the day. It is now limiting his daily activity. X-ray shows features of osteoarthritis. Which one of the following statements is incorrect?
A. He should be advised to lose weight.
B. He may benefit from non-steroidal anti-inflammatory drugs.
C. When other treatments are ineffective, joint replacement may well be indicated.
D. Anti-TNF alpha drugs are a reasonable treatment.
E. He may benefit from physiotherapy.

5. A 56-year-old man who recently started an additional drug for hypertension presents with a hot, swollen first MTP joint. Which one of the following is unlikely to have precipitated his condition?
A. Diuretics.
B. High alcohol intake.
C. Starvation.
D. Trauma.
E. Excess intake of dairy products.

6. A 19-year-old man complains of lower back pain and stiffness, which is worse in the morning and improves after about 45 min. There is no history of trauma. Which one of the following investigations will not help reach the diagnosis?
A. Erythrocyte sedimentation rate.
B. HLA serotyping.
C. Anti-neutrophil cytoplasmic antibodies (ANCA).
D. Plain X-rays.
E. MRI scan of the lumbar/sacral spine.

7. Which one of the following is not a feature of idiopathic SLE?
A. Raised ANA.
B. Anti-smooth muscle antibodies.
C. Photosensitive rash.
D. Abnormal full blood count.
E. Seizures.

8. Which one of the following is not a feature of CREST syndrome?
A. Conjunctivitis.
B. Raynaud's phenomenon.
C. Oesophageal involvement.
D. Sclerodactyly.
E. Telangiectasia.

9. An 18-year-old man comes to see you with erythematous plaques over his elbows and knees, which have progressed over the last 2 months. He is concerned about his appearance. The lesions have a fine, silvery scale. Which one of the following treatments is not used for this condition?
A. Corticosteroids.
B. Benzoyl peroxide.
C. Vitamin D derivatives.
D. UVB radiation therapy.
E. Anti-TNF therapy.

10. Which one of the following features is not true regarding melanoma?
    A. Small satellite lesions help identify malignant melanoma.
    B. Metastasis to the brain is common.
    C. The prognosis is worse for lesions on the legs.
    D. Chemotherapy is a palliative measure.
    E. Five-year survival for lesions less than 1-mm thick is greater than 90%.

Haematology

1. A 68-year-old man complains of tiredness and grumbling epigastric symptoms over the last 2–3 months. He has a history of peptic ulcer disease. Full blood count reveals haemoglobin of 8.2 and microcytosis. Which one of the following is true regarding his condition?
    A. Ferritin is likely to be raised.
    B. Total iron binding capacity will be reduced.
    C. Bone marrow iron stores are likely to be normal.
    D. The reticulocyte count is likely to be significantly raised.
    E. The platelet count is often raised.

2. A 19-year-old Afro-Caribbean woman is admitted with severe pain in her back and legs. She is known to have sickle cell anaemia. Her haemoglobin is 8.0. Which one of the following statements is correct?
    A. Underlying infection must be sought.
    B. Opiate analgesia should be withheld due to the risk of dependence.
    C. She should be given an urgent blood transfusion.
    D. Painful crises are due to increased haematopoiesis.
    E. Sequestration crises are often seen in adults.

3. A Mediterranean man presents with jaundice, nausea and vomiting 24 h after a meal of lamb and broad beans. His haemoglobin is 8.3. Which one of the following statements is correct?
    A. The diagnosis is pyruvate kinase deficiency.
    B. The blood film will show Howell–Jolly bodies.
    C. LDH is likely to be low.
    D. Infection is a common precipitant of this condition
    E. The reticulocyte count is likely to be low.

4. Which one of the following is incorrect regarding DIC?
    A. It may be associated with the M3 form of AML.
    B. The D-dimer level is elevated.
    C. It may be chronic and compensated.
    D. It is more common with Gram-negative than Gram-positive infection.
    E. Inhibitors of fibrinolysis are the mainstay of treatment.

5. Which one of the following is true regarding bleeding disorders?
    A. Haemophilia A is an autosomal recessive condition.
    B. Treatment of bleeding in haemophilia A and B is with recombinant clotting factors.
    C. Most patients with Von Willebrand's disease present with haemarthrosis.
    D. Von Willebrand's disease can be treated with recombinant factor VIII.
    E. Haemophilia B affects the sexes equally.

6. Which of the following investigations is the best to confirm a suspected diagnosis of lymphoma?
    A. Excision biopsy.
    B. Fine needle aspiration biopsy.
    C. Bone marrow aspiration and trephine biopsy.
    D. PET scan.
    E. CT scan of neck, chest, abdomen and pelvis.

7. Which one of the following blood film findings is incorrectly linked to the condition?
    A. Heinz bodies: G6PD deficiency.
    B. Auer rods: acute lymphoblastic leukaemia.
    C. Smudge cells: CLL.
    D. Tear drop erythrocytes: myelofibrosis.
    E. Basophilic stippling: lead poisoning.

8. A 63-year-old man presents with back pain, which came on after jarring his back getting off a bus. X-ray of the spine shows a compression fracture, and blood tests show hypercalcaemia and renal impairment. You are worried about myeloma. Which one of the following investigations will not help?
    A. Serum free light-chain assay (SFLCA).
    B. Urine electrophoresis.
    C. Survey of skeleton with plain X-rays.
    D. Bone marrow examination and trephine biopsy.
    E. Isotope bone scan.

9. Which of the following statements is true regarding myeloproliferative disease?
    A. Polycythaemia is always caused by malignant proliferation.
    B. The *JAK2* mutation in present in 95% of patients with myeloproliferative disease.
    C. Myelofibrosis carries the best prognosis of these disorders.
    D. In ET the platelet count is elevated but the platelets function abnormally.
    E. First-line treatment of CML is with alpha-interferon.

10. A 24-year-old woman presents with her second spontaneous deep vein thrombosis. Which one of the following tests will not help identify an underlying thrombophilia?
    A. Protein C.
    B. Protein S.
    C. Antithrombin III.
    D. ADAMTS-13 antibodies.
    E. Lupus anticoagulant.

Infectious diseases

1. Which one of the following should not be used to treat MRSA?
   A. Vancomycin.
   B. Linezolid.
   C. Teicoplanin.
   D. Piperacillin/tazobactam.
   E. Tigecyline.

2. A 37-year-old man returns from Asia where he was treated for acute malaria infection. Four months later he presents with fever, sweating and nausea. Malaria caused by *P. vivax* is diagnosed. After acute treatment, which one of the following treatments does he need?
   A. Atovaquone.
   B. Primaquine.
   C. Artemether.
   D. IV quinine.
   E. Chloroquine.

3. Which one of the following is true regarding HIV infection?
   A. It is a DNA retrovirus.
   B. It cannot be transmitted from mother to child.
   C. Seroconversion may be asymptomatic.
   D. It commonly presents with Kaposi's sarcoma.
   E. It is best treated with single-agent therapy.

4. Which one of the following is not a common cause of urinary tract infection?
   A. *Pseudomonas*.
   B. *Klebsiella*.
   C. *Proteus*.
   D. *Streptococcus pyogenes*.
   E. *Escherichia coli*.

5. Which one of the following is true of HIV infection?
   A. HIV-2 is the most common type worldwide.
   B. It predominantly depletes CD8 T cells.
   C. The risk of HIV transmission from a needlestick injury is lower than that of hepatitis B transmission.
   D. Persistent generalized lymphadenopathy is an AIDS indicator illness.
   E. Drug therapy is only started when the CD4 count falls below 200 cells/μL.

Toxicology

1. Which one of the following is incorrect regarding examination findings in overdose?
   A. In aspirin overdose the respiratory rate is frequently raised.
   B. Cocaine overdose causes dilated pupils.
   C. Pinpoint pupils are seen in opiate overdose.
   D. Beta-blockers usually cause paradoxical tachycardia in overdose.
   E. Tricyclic antidepressant overdose causes dry mouth.

2. Which of the following is correct regarding general treatment of overdose?
   A. Gastric lavage should always be tried if the equipment is available.
   B. Activated charcoal is useful in drowsy patients who can't tell you what they have taken.
   C. Urinary alkalinization is useful for acidic drugs.
   D. Dialysis is ineffective for salicylate overdose.
   E. Whole bowel irrigation is routinely recommended when the drug has passed through the stomach.

3. Which of the following is incorrect regarding specific treatment of overdose?
   A. Naloxone for opiate overdose is often given as an infusion due to its short half-life.
   B. Flumazenil can be given for benzodiazepine overdose.
   C. *N*-acetylcysteine for paracetamol overdose can only be given intravenously.
   D. Oral methionine is effective in aspirin overdose.
   E. 'Digibind' is a fragment of digoxin-specific antibody given in severe overdose.

4. Which of the following is not a feature of alcohol withdrawal?
   A. Tremor.
   B. Hallucinations.
   C. Bradycardia.
   D. Seizures.
   E. Sweating.

5. Which of the following features do not indicate an elevated suicide risk?
   A. Unemployment.
   B. Chronic illness.
   C. Female gender.
   D. Social isolation.
   E. A history of substance abuse.

General

1. Paroxysmal supraventricular tachycardia in Wolff–Parkinson–White syndrome is best treated by:
   A. Digoxin.
   B. IV adenosine.
   C. Open cardiac surgery.
   D. Radiofrequency ablation.
   E. Sotalol.

2. A 30-year-old IV drug user is admitted with multiple lower lobe lung abscesses. The most likely diagnosis is:
   A. Aspergillosis.
   B. Aspiration pneumonia.
   C. HIV infection.
   D. Right-sided infective endocarditis.
   E. Tuberculosis.

3. Purple plaques with white striae on wrists and mucous membranes suggest a diagnosis of:
   A. Erythema multiforme.
   B. Lichen planus.
   C. Molluscum contagiosum.
   D. Porphyria cutanea tarda.
   E. Psoriasis.

Extended-matching questions (EMQs)

1. Chest pain

A. Aortic stenosis.
B. Angina pectoralis.
C. Inferior non-ST elevation myocardial infarction.
D. Anteroseptal non-ST elevation myocardial infarction.
E. Asthma.
F. Costochondritis.
G. Pulmonary embolus.
H. Mitral valve prolapse.
I. Hypertrophic obstructive cardiomyopathy.
J. Dressler's syndrome.

For each of the following patients, select the most likely diagnosis from the list of options.

1. A 56-year-old man with hypertension and known angina presents with central tight chest pain similar to his normal angina but increasing in frequency and now present at rest. ECG shows ST depression and T-wave inversion in leads V_1–V_4.
2. A 45-year-old man presents with pleuritic chest pain 6 weeks after a myocardial infarction. A friction rub can be heard on auscultation and the ECG shows ST elevation in all leads.
3. A 64-year-old woman smoker with hypertension and hypercholesterolaemia reports 4 weeks of reproducible retrosternal 'band-like' chest tightness on exertion. It is relieved by rest. ECG is normal.
4. A previously well 45-year-old woman smoker presents with left-sided pleuritic chest pain and dyspnoea on exertion. ECG shows right-axis deviation and T-wave inversion in leads V_1–V_3. Resting oxygen saturations are 93% on air.
5. A 25-year-old rower presents with chest pain and dizziness on exertion. He has a pansystolic murmur at the apex and fourth heart sound on examination. ECG shows left ventricular hypertrophy. His uncle died aged 32 years from an unknown cause.

2. Haematuria

A. Benign prostatic hypertrophy.
B. Goodpasture's syndrome.
C. Acute pyelonephritis.
D. Acute cystitis.
E. Prostatic carcinoma.
F. Ureteric calculi.
G. Bladder carcinoma.
H. Renal cell carcinoma.
I. Wegener's granulomatosis.
J. IgA nephropathy.

For each of the following patients, select the most likely diagnosis from the list of options.

1. A 23-year-old woman presents with fever, tachycardia and tenderness in the left loin. The white cell count is raised and the urine is cloudy.
2. A 70-year-old man describes intermittent colicky left loin pain, weight loss and night sweats. He has noted testicular changes, which, on examination, are a varicocele. The haematuria is macroscopic.
3. A 36-year-old woman presents with malaise, recurrent epistaxis, haemoptysis and microscopic haematuria. Examination reveals septal perforation and nodules on the chest X-ray. The serum creatinine is elevated at 307 μmol/L.
4. A 39-year-old man presents to the emergency department in high summer with severe colicky right loin pain radiating down into the scrotum. Examination is unremarkable and the dipstick shows haematuria.
5. A 78-year-old man with long-standing nocturia, poor urinary stream and terminal dribbling notices macroscopic haematuria towards the end of the urine stream. He has become more lethargic and is troubled by lower back pain.

3. Dyspnoea

A. Pulmonary tuberculosis.
B. Aspergilloma.
C. Diaphragmatic palsy.
D. Interstitial lung disease.
E. Bronchopneumonia.
F. Pneumoconiosis.
G. Mesothelioma.
H. Left ventricular systolic dysfunction.
I. Sarcoidosis.
J. Diastolic cardiac dysfunction.

For each of the following patients, select the most likely diagnosis from the list of options.

1. A 45-year-old man with two previous anterior myocardial infarctions, hypertension and diabetes describes increasing dyspnoea, especially orthopnoea. Cardiomegaly is noted on chest X-ray.
2. The above patient undergoes coronary artery bypass graft surgery involving a prolonged intensive care admission. He remains dyspnoeic but his orthopnoea is more pronounced. Chest X-ray appears to show more elevated hemidiaphragms.

3. A 51-year-old patient with dyspnoea has marked bibasal crackles on auscultation. The dyspnoea does not improve with diuretics and subsequent echocardiography is normal.
4. A 60-year-old ex-builder presents with dyspnoea and cough. Chest X-ray shows extensive pleural thickening and calcification plus a pleural effusion. This is blood-stained at aspiration.
5. A 40-year-old homeless patient presents with dyspnoea, weight loss, cough and haemoptysis. The chest X-ray shows left upper lobe consolidation with cavitation. Heaf testing is strongly positive.

4. Abnormal full blood counts

A. Pernicious anaemia.
B. Acute lymphoblastic leukaemia.
C. Sarcoidosis.
D. Folate deficiency anaemia.
E. Acute myeloid leukaemia.
F. Hodgkin's lymphoma.
G. Disseminated intravascular coagulation.
H. Multiple myeloma.
I. Haemolytic uraemic syndrome.

For each of the following patients, select the most likely diagnosis from the list of options.

1. A 63-year-old woman presents with lethargy, malaise and bone pain. Investigations show a normocytic anaemia, elevated serum urea, creatinine and calcium levels. The total protein is raised, although the albumin is within the normal range.
2. A 40-year-old man presents with lethargy, malaise and several recent chest infections. A full blood count result is all within the normal ranges but the blood film comments on the presence of Auer rods.
3. A 64-year-old woman with vitiligo has a full blood count measured for investigation of lethargy. She is anaemic and has a mean corpuscular volume of 120 fL. She has antigastric parietal cell antibodies in her serum.
4. A 34-year-old man undergoing mechanical ventilation for severe pneumonia begins to bleed from previous venepuncture sites and mucosal surfaces. The platelet count and haemoglobin, which had been normal, begin to fall and his clotting tests, including D-dimers, become deranged.
5. A 24-year-old woman with lethargy, malaise and night sweats notices enlarged lymph glands in her neck. A full blood count is carried out before biopsy. An eosinophilia is the only abnormality.

5. Rheumatological

A. Rheumatoid arthritis.
B. Osteoarthritis.
C. Reactive arthritis.
D. CREST syndrome.
E. Polymyalgia rheumatica.
F. Dermatomyositis.
G. Ankylosing spondylitis.
H. Systemic lupus erythematosus.
I. Antiphospholipid syndrome.
J. Mixed connective tissue disorder.

For each of the following patients, select the most likely diagnosis from the list of options.

1. A 57-year-old female smoker has noticed weakness over the last month, especially when getting up from a chair. The thigh muscles are tender and creatine kinase is raised. She has purplish lesions over her knuckles. Chest X-ray shows a lesion consistent with lung cancer.
2. A 25-year-old Afro-Caribbean woman is referred for investigation of three miscarriages. She is concerned by how her skin reacts to sunlight and the development of alopecia. Her musculoskeletal symptoms are of a small joint arthralgia. Proteinuria is present on urine testing.
3. A 55-year-old man with a body mass index of 35 is troubled by pain in the left hip. This is predominantly present on weight bearing and is worsened by exercise. X-ray reports loss of the joint space.
4. A 31-year-old woman reports pain on urinating, right knee and left ankle pain. She is normally fit and well, although she was off work for 10 days before presentation with diarrhoea.
5. A 74-year-old man has had trouble with muscle pain in his thighs and shoulders over the last 3 weeks. The pain is worse getting out of a chair, going up stairs and lifting his arm to comb his hair. He says he is very stiff in the mornings. The ESR is 64.

6. Signs on chest examination

A. Bronchial breathing.
B. Expiratory wheeze.
C. Trachea deviated to left.
D. Trachea deviated to right.
E. Stridor.
F. Increased percussion note.
G. Whispering pectoriloquy.
H. Inspiratory crackles.
I. Intercostal muscle recession.
J. Stony dullness.

For each of the following patients, select the physical signs that best fit the clinical scenario from the list of options.

1. A patient with a large retrosternal goitre.
2. A right tension pneumothorax.
3. A patient with right upper lobe fibrosis due to sarcoidosis.
4. A patient with poorly controlled asthma.
5. A patient with a large pleural effusion.

7. Abdominal swellings

A. Aortic aneurysm.
B. Ascites.
C. Fibroid uterus.
D. Polycystic kidneys.
E. Ventral hernia.
F. Transplanted kidney.
G. Ovarian cyst.
H. Hepatomegaly.
I. Splenomegaly.
J. Enlarged bladder.

For each of the following patients with a palpable abdominal mass, suggest the most likely cause from the list of options.

1. A 34-year-old male with Cushingoid features has a smooth mass palpable in the right iliac fossa.
2. An 81-year-old with urinary incontinence following a hernia repair and a suprapubic smooth tender mass.
3. A 35-year-old lady is admitted with a thunderclap headache and has masses in both hypochondria.
4. A 79-year-old lady complains of a swelling in the centre of her abdomen that appears when she sits up and disappears when she lies down.
5. A 38-year-old lady is admitted smelling of alcohol. She is confused, with multiple spider naevi, asterixis and a tense, swollen abdomen.

8. Headache

A. Meningitis.
B. Encephalitis.
C. Subarachnoid haemorrhage.
D. Tension headache.
E. Migraine.
F. Cluster headache.
G. Glaucoma.
H. Giant cell arteritis.
I. Trigeminal neuralgia.
J. Raised intracranial pressure.

For each of the following patients, select the most likely diagnosis from the list of options.

1. A 21-year-old university student presents with a severe headache of gradual onset. He cannot tolerate the opthalmoscope and is febrile.
2. A 56-year-old woman has recently been experiencing severe shooting pain over one side of her face, lasting a few seconds and occurring many times per day. She has noticed that eating seems to bring it on.
3. A 39-year-old businessman presents with a rapid onset of severe pain around his right eye that is associated with lacrimation, lasts 1–2 h and has been occurring nightly for 2 weeks.
4. A 69-year-old lady describes a worsening headache and pain in her jaw when she chews. Her vision is normal. Her erythrocyte sedimentation rate is 88 mm/h.
5. A 28-year-old male with a family history of kidney disease presents with a sudden-onset severe occipital headache. He has neck stiffness.

9. Altered level of consciousness

A. Brainstem infarction.
B. Drug overdose.
C. Hepatic encephalopathy.
D. Hypoglycaemia.
E. Hyponatraemia.
F. Hypothermia.
G. Meningitis.
H. Renal failure.
I. Schizophrenia.
J. Subarachnoid haemorrhage.

For each of the following patients, select the most likely diagnosis from the list of options.

1. A 93-year-old lady is brought in following a sudden loss of consciousness. Two days later, she remains deeply unconscious with pinpoint pupils.
2. A 42-year-old man is brought in after a sudden collapse. Subhyaloid haemorrhages are seen on fundoscopy.
3. A dishevelled 22-year-old woman is brought in having been found in the street. She responds to painful stimuli and has pinpoint pupils.
4. A 56-year-old man is brought in by ambulance. He is extremely drowsy and jaundiced. His wife says he has been 'battling the drink' for years and has been coughing up dark sputum recently.
5. An elderly, hypertensive lady is admitted in a postictal state after a witnessed tonic–clonic seizure. She has recently been commenced on a diuretic for her hypertension.

10. Endocrine tests

A. 2-h oral glucose tolerance test.
B. Dexamethasone suppression test.
C. Domperidone test.
D. Insulin-like growth factor 1 measurement.
E. Insulin stress test.
F. Prolonged fast.
G. Prolonged glucose tolerance test.
H. Short synacthen test.
I. Thyrotrophin-releasing hormone test.
J. Water deprivation test and response to desmopressin.

For each of the following clinical scenarios, select the most appropriate investigation from the list of options.

1. A patient presents with headaches. You notice interdental spacing, large hands and feet, hypertension and prominent supraorbital ridge.
2. A 39-year-old woman complains of episodic fainting, which is most likely to occur if she misses a meal.
3. A 28-year-old women with vitiligo complains of lethargy. She is noted to have pigmented palmar creases and oral mucosa.
4. A 29-year-old man has recently been discharged following a significant head injury. He now presents with polyuria, polydipsia and hypernatraemia.
5. A 50-year-old woman is referred to clinic with hirsutism, weight gain, diabetes and hypertension.

11. Diarrhoea

A. HIV.
B. Traveller's diarrhoea.
C. Colorectal carcinoma.
D. Crohn's disease.
E. Thyrotoxicosis.
F. Irritable bowel syndrome.
G. Villous adenoma of the rectum.
H. Diverticulitis.
I. Systemic sclerosis.
J. Chronic pancreatitis.

For each of the following patients, select the most likely diagnosis from the list of options.

1. A 75-year-old man with a history of chronic constipation presents with acute left iliac fossa pain and loose motion mixed with blood.
2. An 82-year-old lady presents to her GP with episodic diarrhoea and constipation, vague lower abdominal pain and increasing tiredness.
3. A 35-year-old office manager presents with a 3-month history of episodic diarrhoea, bloating and abdominal cramps. He reports no weight loss but says his symptoms seem only to occur during his working day.
4. A 38-year-old man with a long-term history of alcohol excess and multiple hospitalizations presents to his GP with weight loss and loose, offensive stools.
5. A returning 19-year-old gap year student presents with a 1-month history of diarrhoea, sweating and palpitations.

12. Dysphagia

A. Systemic sclerosis.
B. Candidiasis.
C. Plummer–Vinson syndrome.
D. Oesophageal cancer.
E. Pharyngeal pouch.
F. Achalasia.
G. Hiatus hernia.
H. Coeliac disease.
I. Ischaemic heart disease.
J. Gastro-oesophageal reflux disease.

For each of the following patients, select the most likely diagnosis from the list of options.

1. A 40-year-old man with a long-term history of intermittent dysphagia to both solids and liquids presents with severe retrosternal chest pain.
2. A 32-year-old lady recently diagnosed with renal impairment gives a history of heartburn and dysphagia associated with exertional dyspnoea.
3. A 60-year-old lifelong smoker presents with a history with painful difficulty in swallowing that started with solids but has now progressed to liquids.
4. A 55-year-old obese lady presents with painful difficulty in swallowing and disturbed sleep due to bouts of coughing.
5. A 41-year-old lady presents with painless difficulty in swallowing associated with a dry rash at the corners of her mouth.

13. Cranial nerves

A. Horner's syndrome.
B. Argyll Robertson pupil.
C. Bell's palsy.
D. 6th nerve palsy.
E. Ramsay Hunt syndrome.
F. 3rd nerve palsy.
G. Pituitary adenoma.
H. Senile miosis.
I. 4th nerve palsy.
J. Holmes–Adie pupil.

For each of the following patients, select the most likely diagnosis from the list of options.

1. A 56-year-old man presents to his GP complaining of loss of peripheral vision bilaterally. On examination it is noted that he has an enlarged lower jaw and is hypertensive.
2. On review at the endocrine clinic, a 64-year-old woman is noted to have a unilateral drooping eyelid and a fixed and dilated pupil with the eye looking downwards and outwards.
3. A 49-year-old man with a hard, irregular, palpable, right-sided thyroid swelling presents with a drooping eyelid on the same side. On examination you also notice that his right pupil is constricted.

4. A 28-year-old woman presents with left-sided facial weakness associated with a vesicular rash in the external auditory meatus.
5. A 79-year-old diabetic man has a fall walking down the stairs – on questioning he reports that he has had double vision on looking downwards for some months.

14. Clinical features in endocrine disease

A. Phaeochromocytoma.
B. Acromegaly.
C. Hypothyroidism.
D. Diabetes mellitus.
E. Addison's disease.
F. Conn's syndrome.
G. Digoxin.
H. Cushing's syndrome.
I. Hyperthyroidism.
J. Prolactinoma.

For each of the following patients, select the most likely diagnosis from the list of options.

1. A 34-year-old man presents with a history of abdominal pain and weight loss. On examination he has pigmented buccal mucosa and a systolic blood pressure of 92 mmHg.
2. A 48-year-old with a long-term history of severe asthma presents complaining of weight gain and bruising easily.
3. A 44-year-old man presents with headaches, sweating, tremor, weight loss and palpitations. He is hypertensive. Blood tests reveal a raised calcium.
4. A 48-year-old man reports muscle cramps, weakness and headaches. He is hypertensive. U&Es show hypokalaemia and mild hypernatraemia.
5. A 68-year-old man who was recently diagnosed with atrial fibrillation presents with new-onset gynaecomastia. On examination he has normal testicles and no signs of liver disease.

15. Renal impairment

A. Myeloma.
B. Contrast nephropathy.
C. Churg–Strauss syndrome.
D. Wegener's granulomatosis.
E. Diabetes mellitus.
F. Leukaemia.
G. Amyloidosis.
H. ACE inhibitors.
I. Polycystic kidney disease.
J. Systemic lupus erythematosus.

For each of the following patients with renal impairment, select the most likely diagnosis from the list of options.

1. A 24-year-old lady with a history of recurrent urinary tract infections presents with loin pain and haematuria. On examination she is noted to have hypertension. Her mother is on dialysis.
2. A 32-year-old man presents with a history of haemoptysis, epistaxis, mouth ulcers, lethargy and arthralgia. He is found to have renal impairment.
3. A 65-year-old lady with a long history of bronchiectasis presents with loose stools. She is found to have renal impairment and proteinuria.
4. A 52-year-old with poorly controlled diabetes is admitted with suspected acute renal colic and investigated with ultrasound and IV pyelography. His renal function subsequently worsens 3 days after admission.
5. A 72-year-old man with recurrent infections and bony pain. A full blood count shows an Hb of 9.6.

16. Hepatobiliary disease

A. Sclerosing cholangitis.
B. Wilson's disease.
C. Acute cholecystitis.
D. Biliary colic.
E. Haemochromatosis.
F. Primary biliary cirrhosis.
G. Hepatitis C.
H. Pancreatic cancer.
I. Alcoholic hepatitis.
J. Chronic pancreatitis.

For each of the following patients, select the most likely diagnosis from the list of options.

1. A 55-year-old man is found to have elevated fasting glucose. On examination he has grey-appearing skin and an enlarged liver.
2. A 40-year-old lady with a history of Addison's disease presents with lethargy and pruritus. Blood tests show an elevated serum bilirubin and ultrasound shows no evidence of obstruction.
3. An overweight 52-year-old lady presents with vomiting and right upper quadrant pain that radiates to the back. On examination she has rebound tenderness over the right upper quadrant and a full blood count shows raised white cells.
4. A 45-year-old man under investigation for abnormal liver function tests develops a tremor and has several fits.
5. A 60-year-old alcoholic with a history of alcohol-induced pancreatitis presents with jaundice and back pain. An ultrasound of his liver shows a dilated common bile duct at 11 mm.

17. Seizures

A. Febrile convulsion.
B. Glioma.
C. Alcohol withdrawal.
D. Meningitis.
E. Absence seizure.
F. Encephalitis.
G. Temporal lobe epilepsy.
H. Alcohol toxicity.
I. Hypocalcaemia.

For each of the following patients, select the most likely diagnosis from the list of options.

1. A 15-year-old girl is brought in by her parents after several episodes where she says she has a feeling of 'deja-vu' and then becomes unresponsive, but appears awake and picks at her clothes. She can't remember the episodes, which last around 2 min.
2. A 10-year-old boy is admitted to hospital with a non-blanching rash and decreased level of consciousness. In A&E he begins to have a generalized seizure.
3. A 36-year-old pub landlord is admitted to hospital with a fractured tibia. At 36 h after admission he starts hallucinating and has a seizure.
4. A 38-year-old previously fit and well man presents to his GP feeling depressed with a history of two witnessed generalized seizures and early-morning headaches.
5. A 5-year-old boy is noticed by his mother to have episodes of unresponsiveness. On EEG a pattern of three spike-and-wave discharges per second is seen.

18. Miscellaneous neurological disorders

A. Skeletal muscle.
B. Sciatic nerve.
C. Peripheral nerves.
D. Cavernous sinus.
E. Substantia nigra.
F. Neuromuscular junction.
G. Frontal lobe.
H. Common peroneal nerve.
I. Dorsal columns.
J. Middle cerebral artery.

For each of the following symptoms and signs, select the most likely location of the lesion from the list of options.

1. Painless muscle weakness that worsens on repetitive contraction.
2. Progressive paraparesis or tetraparesis with lower motor neurone signs and sensory symptoms following a diarrhoeal illness.
3. Painful proximal muscle weakness manifested by difficulty getting up from chair or climbing stairs.
4. Unilateral footdrop and weakness of ankle eversion associated with numbness over the dorsum of the foot.
5. Loss of vibration sense and reduced proprioception, with preservation of pain and temperature sensation.

19. The hands

A. Koilonychia.
B. Leukonychia.
C. Onycholysis.
D. Splinter haemorrhage.
E. Janeway's lesions.
F. Half-and-half nails.
G. Dupuytren's contracture.
H. Beau's lines.
I. Quincke's sign.
J. Osler's nodes.

For each of the following patients, select the most likely diagnosis from the list of options.

1. A patient with coeliac disease has a microcytic anaemia. You notice an unusual appearance of their nails.
2. A 40-year-old lady recently discharged from the ITU with urinary septicaemia has horizontal grooves in her nails.
3. A 63-year-old lady with joint pain and a rash over her elbows finds that part of her nail is coming away from the nail bed on her ring finger.
4. A 55-year-old with a history of rheumatic heart disease has a pulsation of the nail bed.
5. A 31-year-old IV drug user is admitted generally unwell. On examination, a pansystolic murmur is noted as well as non-tender macules on his palm.

20. Dermatological manifestations of disease

A. Thrombophlebitis migrans.
B. Lyme disease.
C. Acanthosis nigricans.
D. Pyoderma gangrenosum.
E. Behçet's disease.
F. Erythema ab igne.
G. Erythema multiforme.
H. Xanthelasmata.
I. Herpes zoster.
J. Erythema nodosum.

For each of the following patients, select the most likely diagnosis from the list of options.

1. A 52-year-old man who recently started a course of antibiotics for a chest infection presents with circular lesions with central blistering that are distributed symmetrically on his limbs.
2. A 67-year-old lady with gastric cancer develops areas of pigmented rough, thickened skin in her groin and axillae.
3. A 35-year-old with inflammatory bowel disease develops painful lesions on the anterior shin.
4. A 40-year-old Turkish lady with joint pain develops painful ulceration of her mouth, followed by her genitalia.
5. A 45-year-old male presents to his GP with exertional chest pain. On examination it is noted that he has yellow plaques over the eyelids.

21. Chest pain

A. Acute myocardial infarction.
B. Angina.
C. Costochondritis.
D. Dissecting aortic aneurysm.
E. Herpes zoster.
F. Oesophageal spasm.
G. Pericarditis.
H. Pulmonary embolism.
I. Reflux oesophagitis.
J. Thoracic vertebral collapse.

For each of the following patients, select the most likely diagnosis from the list of options.

1. Acute onset of chest pain radiating round from the back in a band on both sides of the chest.
2. Central chest pain precipitated by bending forward or lying flat.
3. Central chest pain relieved by sitting forward.
4. Central chest pain with local tenderness along the sides of the sternum.
5. Right-sided chest pain exacerbated by coughing.

22. Haemoptysis

A. Acute bronchitis.
B. Bronchiectasis.
C. Carcinoma of the lung.
D. Exacerbation of chronic obstructive pulmonary disease.
E. Goodpasture's syndrome.
F. Hereditary haemorrhagic telangiectasia.
G. Mitral stenosis.
H. Pneumonia.
I. Pulmonary embolism.
J. Tuberculosis.

For each of the following patients, select the most likely diagnosis from the list of options.

1. A 25-year-old man with fever and rusty-coloured sputum.
2. A 35-year-old woman with a history or recurrent nose bleeds and a family history of haemoptysis.
3. A 45-year-old woman with copious purulent sputum and brisk haemoptysis.
4. A 45-year-old woman with shortness of breath and pink, frothy sputum.
5. A 50-year-old man with haematuria and haemoptysis.

23. Jaundice

A. Acute alcoholic hepatitis.
B. Acute viral hepatitis.
C. Gilbert's syndrome.
D. Carcinoma of the head of the pancreas.
E. Cholangitis.
F. Chronic biliary cirrhosis.
G. Gallstones.
H. Haemolysis.
I. Leptospirosis.
J. Paracetamol toxicity.

For each of the following patients with jaundice, select the most likely diagnosis from the list of options.

1. A 50-year-old woman with central abdominal pain and a history of weight loss over 4 months.
2. A 50-year-old woman with a history of ulcerative colitis and a recent onset of fever, rigors and jaundice.
3. A 60-year-old woman with recurrent episodes of right hypochondrial pain.
4. A 25-year-old woman with a 2-week history of muscle pains and fever.
5. A 35-year-old farm worker with fever, red eyes and abdominal pain.

24. Disturbance of micturition

A. Chronic kidney disease.
B. Diabetes insipidus.
C. Diabetes mellitus.
D. Glomerulonephritis.
E. Hypercalcaemia.
F. Hypokalaemia.
G. Inappropriate secretion of antidiuretic hormone.
H. Nephrotic syndrome.

I. Overhydration.
J. Pyelonephritis.

For each of the following patients, select the most likely diagnosis from the list of options.

1. A 20-year-old man with shortness of breath, a pH of 7.25 and a P_{aCO_2} of 2.5 kPa.
2. A 35-year-old man with polyuria whose chest X-ray shows bilateral hilar lymphadenopathy.
3. A 50-year-old woman treated with lithium for depression.
4. A 65-year-old man with polyuria, bone pain and Bence Jones protein in the urine.
5. A 75-year-old woman with loin pain, frequency and dysuria.

25. Joint problems

A. Ankylosing spondylitis.
B. Gout.
C. Neuropathic arthropathy (Charcot's joint).
D. Osteoarthritis.
E. Polymyalgia rheumatica.
F. Pseudogout.
G. Psoriatic arthropathy.
H. Reactive arthritis.
I. Rheumatoid arthritis.
J. Septic arthritis.

For each of the following patients, select the most likely diagnosis from the list of options.

1. A 70-year-old man complains of symmetrical swelling and pain of both wrists and elbows.
2. A 24-year-old heroin user presents with an acutely painful, swollen, red left knee. He is febrile and cannot weight bear.
3. A 76-year-old man with long-standing diabetes presents with a distorted, swollen left ankle that is not very painful.
4. A 70-year-old woman complains of pain on walking with limited range of movement of the left hip.
5. An 86-year-old woman complains of pain and swelling in her left wrist. Aspirated fluid reveals weakly positively birefringent crystals.

26. Renal disease

A. Amyloidosis.
B. Antiglomerular basement membrane disease (Goodpasture's syndrome).
C. HIV-associated nephropathy.
D. IgA nephropathy.
E. Lupus nephritis.
F. Minimal change nephropathy.
G. Multiple myeloma.
H. Pyelonephritis.
I. Sarcoidosis.
J. Wegener's granulomatosis.

For each of the following patients, select the most likely diagnosis from the list of options.

1. A 12-year-old boy with hypoalbuminaemia, oedema and frothy urine.
2. A 25-year-old man who feels well but has macroscopic haematuria 2 days after an upper respiratory tract infection.
3. A 30-year-old man with weight loss and renal impairment showing focal segmental glomerulosclerosis on renal biopsy.
4. A 45-year-old man with acute kidney injury associated with fever, sinusitis, nose bleeds and haemoptysis.
5. A 65-year-old woman with anaemia associated with lytic bone lesions.

27. Calcium problems

A. Bony metastases.
B. Familial hypocalciuric hypercalcaemia.
C. Hyperthyroidism.
D. Hypoparathyroidism.
E. Multiple myeloma.
F. Primary hyperparathyroidism.
G. Sarcoidosis.
H. Secondary hyperparathyroidism.
I. Squamous carcinoma of the lung.
J. Tertiary hyperparathyroidism.

For each of the following patients, select the most likely diagnosis from the list of options.

1. A 30-year-old man with bilateral hilar lymphadenopathy.
2. A 35-year-old woman with muscle cramps and perioral tingling following a recent neck operation.
3. A 45-year-old woman with an incidental finding of raised calcium and low phosphate.
4. A 50-year-old man with renal impairment, normal calcium and high phosphate.
5. A 65-year-old man with weight loss and sclerotic lesions in ribs on chest X-ray.

28. Nerve lesions

A. Carpal tunnel syndrome.
B. Diabetic neuropathy.
C. Guillain–Barré syndrome.
D. Lead poisoning.
E. Mononeuritis multiplex.

F. Multiple sclerosis.
G. Pancoast tumour.
H. Spinal cord infarction.
I. Subacute combined degeneration of the cord.
J. Syringomyelia.

For each of the following patients, select the most likely diagnosis from the list of options.

1. A 60-year-old man with abdominal pain and weakness in both feet.
2. A 65-year-old woman with loss of vibration and joint position sense in the feet with extensor plantars.
3. A 70-year-old man with pain in the right shoulder and weakness of the small muscles of the right hand.
4. A 70-year-old man with weakness of the small muscles of both hands with loss of pain and temperature sensation in the hands.
5. A 70-year-old woman with pain in the right forearm at night and weakness of the right thumb.

29. Investigations in gastrointestinal disease

A. Anti-tissue transglutaminase antibodies.
B. Low blood caeruloplasmin.
C. Positive antimitochondrial antibody.
D. Raised 24-h urine 5-HIAA.
E. Raised alpha-fetoprotein.
F. Raised CA125 level.
G. Raised serum amylase.
H. Raised serum ferritin.
I. Raised serum glucagon.
J. Raised unconjugated bilirubin.

For each of the following patients, select the most likely diagnosis from the list of options.

1. A 30-year-old woman with weight loss, steatorrhoea and a blood film suggesting hyposplenism.
2. A 50-year-old man with a mass in the right hypochondrium and episodes of flushing and diarrhoea.
3. A 50-year-old woman with pruritus and obstructive jaundice.
4. A 55-year-old man with acute abdominal pain radiating to the back.
5. A 55-year-old man with darkening skin, arthralgia, impotence and abnormal liver function.

30. Headache

A. Cluster headache.
B. Giant cell arteritis.
C. Meningitis.
D. Migraine.
E. Post-herpetic neuralgia.
F. Sinusitis.
G. Subarachnoid haemorrhage.
H. Temporomandibular joint problems.
I. Tension headache.
J. Trigeminal neuralgia.

For each of the following patients, select the most likely diagnosis from the list of options.

1. A 30-year-old man with severe pain around the right eye lasting about an hour and occurring daily for the last 2 weeks.
2. A 30-year-old woman with a constant headache described as a band around the head for 3 weeks.
3. A 50-year-old woman with hypertension and acute onset of severe pain around the back of the head.
4. A 55-year-old woman with headache worse on bending over and tenderness over the forehead.
5. A 70-year-old woman with headache and tenderness over her forehead and scalp.

SBA answers

History taking

1. B – ACE inhibitors, not AIIRBs, are implicated in chronic cough. Nocturnal symptoms may indicate asthma or gastro-oesophageal reflux disease. Voice change may indicate malignancy. Nasal problems are a common cause. Occupational exposure to irritants may cause cough.
2. C – Digoxin may affect colour vision. Nitrofurantoin, amiodarone, cytotoxics and methotrexate may cause lung fibrosis. Amiodarone may cause a slate-grey skin change. The patient should be told to report any colour vision change after starting ethambutol.
3. B – 30 = 1.5 packs per day multiplied by 25 years = 37.5 pack years.

Examination

1. E – Clubbing may occur in lung cancer or with chronic suppurative lung disease, e.g. bronchiectasis. Koilonychia is a sign of iron deficiency. Osler's nodes are a feature of endocarditis. Asterixis also occurs in other forms of encephalopathy, e.g. carbon dioxide retention.
2. A – Fasciculation would suggest an LMN lesion. Wasting may occur with UMN lesions due to disuse but it is predominantly an LMN sign.
3. D – Pulsus paradoxus is an exaggeration of the normal change in pulse volume with the respiratory cycle.
4. E – The presence or absence of bowel sounds does not help. Dullness to percussion and a palpable notch are characteristic of the spleen. If the mass is a kidney you should be able to palpate between the mass and costal margin. Kidneys are ballotable.
5. A – A venous pulsation cannot be felt. JVP normally falls with inspiration; Kussmaul's sign in cardiac tamponade is a paradoxical rise of the JVP in inspiration. The normal JVP has an 'a' and a 'v' wave. As the patient reclines the JVP moves higher in the neck. 'e' describes the hepatojugular reflex.
6. B – This is Hamman's sign and occurs occasionally with left-sided pneumothoraces and also in pneumomediastinum. Tracheal deviation suggests a tension pneumothorax requiring emergency management. Expansion and breath sounds are reduced on the side of the pneumothorax. The percussion note is increased: 'hyper-resonance'.

The clerking

1. B – In certain cases it is better to change the order to emphasize more relevant features.

Investigations

1. A – D-dimer is a sensitive but non-specific test. With a low-risk score it can be used to exclude PE. RBBB supports the diagnosis, indicating right heart strain, but does not confirm it. Underlying lung disease makes perfusion scans difficult to interpret. Troponin level may rise slightly as the right ventricle is stressed. Under normal circumstances, after a negative CTPA no other tests are needed and an alternative diagnosis should be considered.
2. C – Bicarbonate is retained by the kidney in metabolic compensation. Rising CO_2 levels lower the pH. Normal CO_2 indicates that oxygenation is the problem but ventilation is adequate. Raised anion gap occurs for instance with lactic acidosis.
3. E – Increased QRS duration suggests ventricular conduction delay. PR interval is measured from the beginning of the P wave. Normal axis is from $-30°$ to $+90°$C suggests P pulmonale. Q waves in II, III and a VF suggest previous inferior infarction.
4. D – Beta-thalassaemia trait causes reduced MCV. Pernicious anaemia causes vitamin B_{12} deficiency and megaloblastic anaemia. Chronic renal failure causes anaemia with normal MCV.
5. C – Polycythaemia does not increase the ESR and may lower it.
6. C – Renal impairment causes hypocalcaemia. RCC may cause hypercalcaemia, mainly by metastasis to bone. Other causes of lytic lesions in bone are lung, breast, thyroid and prostatic malignancy. In milk-alkali syndrome there is increased calcium intake. In pseudopseudohypoparathyroidism biochemistry is normal.

7. B – High alkaline phosphatase and GGT traditionally indicate obstructive biliary disease. Urea-to-creatinine ratio is also increased in simple dehydration. D-dimer will be elevated in VTE, but remember that many things elevate the D-dimer and a negative result is more useful. Creatine kinase is released when skeletal muscle is damaged. HbA1c is used to monitor therapy.

8. D – The short synacthen test looks for cortisol deficiency. Cortisol should rise with synacthen in normal individuals. The dexamethasone suppression test is performed overnight. A long synacthen test or ACTH level is needed to determine the cause.

9. E – Kerley B lines are visible at the periphery in pulmonary oedema.

Cardiovascular disorders

1. A – Mitral regurgitation is commonly loudest at the apex and radiates to the axilla. There is no presystolic accentuation in the context of AF due to the absence of atrial contraction. Left-sided heart murmurs are best heard in expiration, right-sided best in inspiration (due to decreased venous return). Aortic regurgitation is best heard at the left sternal edge in expiration with the patient sitting up. An opening snap is a feature of mitral stenosis.

2. D – Patients aged under 55 should be started on an ACE inhibitor. Although lifestyle changes should be advised, if the blood pressure is persistently over 160 mmHg systolic medical therapy is indicated, especially in the context of diabetes. If mono-therapy is unsuccessful, a calcium channel blocker should be added. If the blood pressure remains high on this a diuretic, such as bendroflumethiazide, would be the third agent. Beta-blockers, such as atenolol, are now only used if the blood pressure remains raised despite the use of the above agents. Diabetic control is crucial, but does not reduce the blood pressure.

3. E – Although aortic stenosis can cause a narrow pulse pressure, the absolute value is unhelpful in assessing degree of stenosis. The murmur may help in the initial diagnosis, either its severity or radiation are an indicator of clinical significance (as a matter of fact in critical aortic stenosis there may be no murmur due to the severe impairment of flow). Left ventricular hypertrophy on ECG indicates functionally important aortic stenosis.

4. B – All acute coronary syndrome (ACS) patients should be on secondary prevention for atherosclerotic disease. The evidence shows an ACE inhibitor (e.g. ramipril), a beta-blocker (e.g. atenolol), a statin (e.g. simvastatin) and aspirin all individually reduce mortality. Although fibrates are effective in reducing both LDL cholesterol and triglycerides, there is insufficient mortality data for these agents. An angiotensin receptor blocker (e.g. losartan) is only indicated if the patient does not tolerate an ACE inhibitor. Warfarin is not indicated in isolated ACS.

5. C – Digoxin is indicated in sinus rhythm as it improves symptoms (RADIANCE trial). The New York Heart Association classification is used to classify the degree of failure on the basis of symptoms. Diuretics improve symptoms, but have no mortality benefit, whereas ACE inhibitors improve both morbidity and mortality. Left ventricular failure predisposes to arrhythmias, especially if the ventricle is dilated.

6. C – Although rheumatic fever may indeed result in atrial fibrillation, in the UK ischaemic heart disease and hypertension are far more common causes of AF. Atrial contraction contributes 10–30% of ventricular filling and AF may therefore cause heart failure on the background of existing heart disease. Anticoagulation with either aspirin or warfarin should be instigated in any patient with AF unless contraindications exist. The ECG changes associated with AF are absent P waves and irregular, narrow QRS complexes. Pulmonary embolism is a cause of AF.

7. E – The delta wave described in this clinical scenario is pathognomonic for Wolff–Parkinson–White syndrome (WPW). WPW is a form of atrioventricular re-entry tachycardia since the re-entry circuit is not through the AV node. The rate described is unlikely to be atrial flutter as this tends to be multiples of 75 depending on the degree of block. Ventricular fibrillation is not compatible with life.

8. A – It is measured from the sternal angle (the angle of Louis – the angle formed between the manubrium and sternum). Answers B–E are all true.

9. A – This lady has suffered an NSTEMI. She will be at high risk of subsequent MI and death (GRACE score) in light of her age, co-morbidities and troponin elevation. Cardiac catheterization is thus indicated as an inpatient. This investigation will be able to show the culprit lesion, but also allows for revascularization at the same time. Investigations that stress the myocardium (e.g. ETT or radionuclide perfusion scanning) in patients that have been admitted with an NSTEMI are contraindicated. Echocardiography may show the extent of the damage by the ischaemic event, but offers no treatment potential. 24-h ECH monitoring has no role in this clinical setting.

10. E – Essential hypertension is the same as primary hypertension. This idiopathic condition is responsible for 95% of cases of hypertension. Conn's syndrome (hyperaldosteronism), phaeochromocytoma (catecholamine-producing tumour), coarctation of the aorta and renal artery stenosis are all causes of secondary hypertension.

11. B – A slow rising pulse is a feature of aortic stenosis. The character of the pulse should be assessed centrally (e.g. carotid – ensure to check one side at a time!). Pulsus alternans is the physical finding of a variable pulse waveform of strong and weak beats – a feature of ventricular impairment. Venous return is decreased during inspiration which causes reduced vagal tone and results in an increased heart rate.

Respiratory disease

1. A – A tension pneumothorax is a medical emergency that requires immediate decompression (large-bore cannula in the second intercostal space, mid-clavicular line). It is a clinical diagnosis based on the following features on examination. The trachea is deviated away from the affected side. There will be no breath sounds and a hyperresonant percussion note on the affected side. When the tension pneumothorax becomes sufficiently large to compromise cardiovascular function, venous return to the heart will be impaired, resulting in a raised JVP.

2. D – Tachycardia is a common finding in pulmonary embolism and the most common ECG abnormality. Although the S_1 Q_3 T_3 pattern is often mentioned in textbooks, it is encountered in <20% of pulmonary embolism cases. Haemoptysis may well be a feature; the most common symptom is pleuritic chest pain. Treatment depends on the cause and ranges from 6 months of LMWH (as would be the case here) to lifelong warfarin.

3. C – In severe asthma, IV magnesium may be beneficial. Peak flow is a helpful tool, especially when compared to the patient's normal performance, in predicting severity. Peak flow values of <33% of normal indicate a life-threatening asthma attack. Blood gases are a particularly important tool in the assessment of severe asthma. A normal $P\text{CO}_2$ is suggestive the patient is getting tired (it should be low due to hyperventilation) and is not reassuring at all. Death is not uncommon. There is no evidence to support the use of IV bronchodilators over nebulized equivalents.

4. B – The CURB65 score is used to assess severity for community-acquired pneumonia. Confusion, defined as an abbreviated mini mental test score of <8, scores 1 point. A serum urea of >7 mmol/L scores 1 point. A systolic blood pressure of <90 mmHg scores 1 point. A respiratory rate of >30 scores 1 point. Age >65 scores 1 point. A score of 0–1 is mild pneumonia, 2 is moderate and 3–5 is severe. Typically, mild pneumonia is treated in the community, moderate potentially in hospital and severe definitely in hospital commonly with IV antibiotics.

5. B – Syndrome of inappropriate antidiuretic hormone secretion and Eaton–Lambert myasthenia syndrome are both associated with small-cell lung cancer. Squamous cell carcinoma may produce parathyroid-related peptide causing hypercalcaemia. The mainstay of treatment is surgery, although patients often present with metastases which commonly occur in bone, the adrenal glands, brain and liver.

6. A – Amiodarone may cause lower zone pulmonary fibrosis, particularly in the context of pre-existing lung disease. Other causes of lower zone fibrosis are rheumatoid arthritis, asbestosis, idiopathic and drugs such as methotrexate and nitrofurantoin.

7. E – There are 4 stages of chest X-ray changes associated with pulmonary sarcoidosis. Answer B is stage 1, answer C is stage 2, answer E is stage 3 and answer D is stage 4. Pleural effusions are not a feature in this classification.

8. C – The scenario described above is one of a life-threatening asthma attack. The most important features here are the considerable length of the attack and the apparent lack of effective ventilation. In the acute setting the CO_2 would be low, with an associated respiratory alkalosis, (answers D and E) due to hyperventilation. Once the patient gets tired the $P\text{CO}_2$ will be in the normal range (**this is a bad sign**) and the pH will subsequently normalize. If ICU/HDU input is sought at this point, the patient will deteriorate and develop type II respiratory failure.

9. E – Although the fraction of inspired oxygen is highly dependent on respiratory rate and oxygen flow rate through the delivery system, it is useful to have some rough idea of the concentrations of oxygen given. Inspired room air has $F\text{iO}_2$ of 21%, whereas a non-rebreath mask at 15 L/min is as close to an $F\text{iO}_2$ of 100% as possible. Venturi masks have special valves that closely regulate the $F\text{iO}_2$ and are commonly available at concentrations of 28%, 35% and 40%. A simple facemask delivering oxygen at 5 L/min roughly delivers $F\text{iO}_2$ of 50%.

10. C – Routine use of inhaled corticosteroids is only indicated if FEV_1 <50% with 2 exacerbations per year. All the other answers have proven benefit in COPD.

11. E – The condition is usually caused by industrial asbestos exposure and may therefore result in compensation for the patient and/or family. It is a tumour of the pleura rather than the lung parenchyma. Associated pulmonary asbestosis is only found in approximately 15% of cases. The prognosis is poor.

12. A – Although a raised body mass index (BMI) is a risk factor for obstructive sleep apnoea, the condition is seen in patients with a normal BMI. Management is conservative in first instance (sleep hygiene, weight loss, alcohol avoidance, etc.) and positive pressure airway support, although surgery may be indicated if these fail. The condition causes excessive daytime sleepiness, which can be assessed by the Epworth sleepiness score. Hypertension and possibly coronary artery disease are associated with obstructive sleep apnoea. The condition can be central (i.e. a reduced respiratory drive), due to collapse of the airway (e.g. the soft palate), or a combination of both.

Gastroenterology

1. C – Barrett's oesophagus is usually asymptomatic. Less than 1% progress to adenocarcinoma per year. It is characterized by metaplasia from squamous to columnar epithelium in the distal part of the oesophagus. The underlying cause is gastro-oesophageal reflux disease (GORD) which is typically managed medically with lifestyle changes, and proton pump inhibitors.

2. B – Pancreatitis is an inflammatory condition of the pancreas most commonly caused by alcohol or gallstones. The history of intermittent RUQ pain is suggestive of biliary colic in a female in her forties. The likelihood is thus that this is gallstone pancreatitis. Severity can be assessed using the modified Glasgow or APACHE-II scoring systems. The Rockall score is used to predict mortality in gastrointestinal bleeding. Pseudocyst formation is not an early complication – it tends to occur after 2–6 weeks. Although a serum amylase of 1400 U/mL is high, occasionally a perforated viscus may present in a similar manner with serum amylase concentrations >1000 U/mL.

3. E – A large upper GI bleed is a medical emergency and should be initially managed according to advanced life support principles of Airway, Breathing and Circulation. Fluid resuscitation is a priority. Blood results may show a raised urea (secondary to red cell ingestion) and may initially show a normal haemoglobin concentration as there has been no chance for haemodilution in the very acute setting. The investigation of choice is an oesophagogastroduodenoscopy. Re-bleeding carries an immediate mortality of 40%.

4. B – Transmural inflammation, perianal lesions and skip lesions are all features of Crohn's disease. UC is less common in smokers, the converse of which is true for Crohn's disease. Pseudopolyps are associated with UC.

5. D – The symptoms described here are suggestive of a left-sided tumour. The more distal the disease the more likely it is to cause a change in bowel habit. Tenesmus is suggestive of rectal disease. Right-sided tumours typically present late and may present as iron-deficiency anaemia. More than 90% of tumours can be resected surgically.

6. D – Pseudomembranous colitis is a serious infection, commonly hospital acquired. It is caused by the toxins produced by *Clostridium difficile*. As is the case for all forms of colitis, toxic dilatation of the colon is a complication. Diagnosis of *C. difficile* infection is made by toxin-positive stool culture, pseudomembranous colitis is diagnosed endoscopically. Prevention is predominantly through hand washing using soap and water (to eliminate the bacterial spores) and careful use of antibiotics. Initial treatment is with oral metronidazole or oral vancomycin.

7. D – IBS is a diagnosis of exclusion that can only be made once organic causes have been excluded (such as coeliac disease, inflammatory bowel disease, etc.). The condition is more common in females between the ages of 20 and 40. Symptoms are central or lower abdominal pain, commonly relieved by defecation, abdominal bloating and altered bowel habit. Rectal bleeding is not a feature. Treatment may require input from dieticians, surgeons, psychiatrists or gynaecologists and is not always successful.

8. B – Gallstones are commonly asymptomatic. Their incidence increases with age, parity, raised BMI and they are more common in females. Occasionally, a large gallstone can erode through the gallbladder into the adjacent duodenum, causing a gallstone ileus. A minority of gallstones are radio-opaque owing to their composition: they commonly contain cholesterol and/or bile salts. Charcot's triad (RUQ pain, jaundice and rigors) is suggestive of cholangitis.

9. C – Hepatitis A may relapse, but does not cause chronic hepatitis. Hepatitis B transmission is parenteral and infection may be complicated by hepatocellular carcinoma. Hepatitis C is usually asymptomatic in the acute phase. Hepatitis E is transmitted via the faecal-oral route.

10. D – Intussusception affects children more commonly than adults. In 20% of cases there may be redcurrant jelly stool, although this is a late sign. Melaena is stool containing metabolized blood (indicating an upper gastrointestinal bleed). Fatty stool (or steatorrhoea) or putty-coloured stool is a feature of obstructive jaundice or chronic pancreatitis. Watery stool is common in gastroenteritis.

11. A – Although portal hypertension and hypoalbuminaemia have some effect on fluid retention, renal sodium handling has the greatest effect. It is thought that aldosterone plays an important role in the mechanism and it may be that renal sensitivity to aldosterone is enhanced in liver cirrhosis. There is no suggestion of IVC or lymphatic obstruction in this clinical scenario.

Genitourinary disorders

1. B – Pulmonary oedema, severe acidosis, resistant hyperkalaemia and symptomatic uraemia are all indications for emergency haemodialysis/haemofiltration in the context of AKI. Serum creatinine is used as a marker of renal function, but raised levels are not an indication for haemodialysis/haemofiltration.

2. D – ECG changes associated with hyperkalaemia are tented T waves, small or absent P waves, broad QRS complexes and, eventually, sinusoidal waveform (this is commonly followed by ventricular fibrillation and needs IMMEDIATE senior input and management). U waves are seen on an ECG in association with hypokalaemia (as well as depressed ST segments).

3. B – Haematuria is not a feature of nephrotic syndrome (it is a feature of nephritic syndrome). High serum cholesterol, low albumin, significant proteinuria and oval fat bodies in the urine are all features of nephrotic syndrome.

4. A – A KUB X-ray is not indicated in this case. The preferred initial imaging modality would be ultrasound scan (potentially with a renal biopsy). Urine microscopy would be used to look for red cell casts which are pathognomonic for glomerular bleeding. Immunoelectrophoresis is used to exclude myeloma. Hypocomplementaemia occurs in lupus nephritis, membranoproliferative glomerulonephritis, cryoglobulinaemia and infective-endocarditis-associated glomerulonephritis. ANCA and anti-GM antibodies are associated with glomerulonephritis and is a treatable cause.

5. A – Non-oliguric AKI occurs, but is less common. Pre-renal renal impairment is the most common cause for AKI, particularly in the hospital setting. Hypovolaemia is a cause of pre-renal renal impairment. AKI has a significant mortality, particularly when associated with other organ impairment (>50 %). Approximately two-thirds of patients regain normal renal function. An early ultrasound scan is important in excluding post-renal (obstructive) causes.

6. E – CKD is commonly caused by hypertension; of course it may also be a result of CKD. Proteinuria is a poor indicator of disease progression as patients tend to experience a faster decline in renal function. Blood pressure should be maintained at 130/80 mmHg to reduce the rate of glomerular damage. Decreased production or erythropoietin combined with impaired iron utilization results in normochromic normocytic anaemia. Impaired renal excretion of potassium and phosphate must be balanced by decreased oral intake.

7. D – This is the classical presentation of pyelonephritis. Midstream urine (MSU) should be dipsticked and subsequently sent for microscopy culture and sensitivities. Any female of childbearing age presenting with abdominal pain must have a pregnancy scan to rule out an ectopic pregnancy. The preferred imaging modalities would be a DMSA scan or an ultrasound scan – an abdominal X-ray would not be indicated in this scenario. A full blood count would be likely to show a raised white cell count in keeping with infection.

8. A – Females are at increased risk of UTI as a result of a shorter urethra with its meatus closer to the anus. The condition will affect 25–35% of women at least once. UTIs are commonly asymptomatic, the management of which is controversial. Infection is a frequent and dangerous complication of urinary catheterization. A simple UTI may ascend the ureters and cause pyelonephritis.

9. C – The most likely diagnosis is indometacin-induced interstitial nephritis. The diagnosis would be confirmed by renal biopsy. Indometacin should be stopped, and the patient might benefit from oral steroids. Membranous nephropathy may present like this, but is not normally associated with surgical procedures. Acute tubular necrosis is often due to prolonged hypotension, of which there is no suggestion in this clinical scenario. There is nothing in the history to suggest lupus nephritis. Minimal-change nephropathy is unlikely to be caused by a relatively minor orthopaedic procedure and indometacin.

Neurology

1. E – Facial weakness is usually due to an UMN lesion which spares the forehead. As this patient is on warfarin, CT scan is required urgently to rule out haemorrhage. If haemorrhage is present and the INR is raised, warfarin should be reversed with prothrombin complex concentrate. Ischaemic strokes can occur in patients on warfarin if the INR is subtherapeutic for a prolonged period of time, or occasionally if the INR is therapeutic. Haemorrhage accounts for around 20% of strokes.
2. C – Meningitis is not as likely as migraine – the patient is afebrile and the visual symptoms would be atypical. A minority of subarachnoid haemorrhages are preceded by a 'sentinel bleed' but visual warning symptoms are not typical. Beta-blockers are sometimes used for migraine prophylaxis. Patients with cluster headache are typically restless, as opposed to those with migraine. Triptans are effective for acute migraine.
3. B – Symptoms are asymmetrical in onset; symmetrical onset implies an alternative diagnosis such as the Parkinson's plus syndromes. He is young, and a dopamine agonist is often preferred as first line in younger patients. A radio-iodine scan may be helpful if the diagnosis is in doubt, but is not required. Rigidity is one of the cardinal features of parkinsonism, the others being tremor, bradykinesia and postural instability.
4. D – Optic neuritis is commonly due to MS, but it can occur in isolation or be due to other pathologies such as infection or vasculitis. Colour vision is usually affected more. In 90% of patients the vision gradually improves over weeks to months following the initial event. The risk of developing MS following an episode of optic neuritis is higher if white matter lesions are present on MRI. MS typically occurs between the ages of 20 and 40.
5. E – The purpuric rash is most likely to occur in meningococcal infection. *Streptococcus pneumoniae* is a common cause but does not usually cause a purpuric rash. *Listeria* is more common in the elderly, alcoholics and the newborn. Lumbar puncture is required but not immediately, and the presence of severe headache, confusion and vomiting should warn you of raised ICP. Treatment with IV ceftriaxone or benzylpenicillin is urgently required along with supportive measures and notification of ITU.
6. D – It is commonly referred to as a 'false localizing sign'. The headache is typically worse in the morning. The Cushing reflex is a late sign consisting of hypertension and bradycardia. Fundoscopy should be performed to look for papilloedema if raised ICP is suspected. Nausea and vomiting may occur; abdominal pain is not a feature.
7. E – MND is slightly more common in men. It does not affect the sensory nerves or the extraocular muscles. Prognosis is poor; survival beyond 5 years is very rare. It usually causes a mixture of upper and motor neurone signs.
8. C – Mortality of subarachnoid haemorrhage is 50%. Only 30% are preceded by a sentinel headache. As well as hydrocephalus, other causes of worsening GCS are vasospasm and re-bleeding. Treatment is with good fluid intake, analgesia and nimodipine. Neurosurgery may be required.
9. C – Metastases are more common than primary tumours. If primary tumour is suspected, stereotactic biopsy is required. Meningiomas, when small, can be simply observed. Surgery is often successful. Glioblastomas are aggressive tumours with a poor prognosis. Breast cancer, as well as lung and skin cancer, commonly metastasizes to the brain.
10. E – Syncope on exertion should prompt investigations to look for aortic stenosis or hypertrophic cardiomyopathy. Urinary incontinence and a few jerks/twitches are commonly seen during syncope. ECG is mandatory and may reveal arrhythmia. Biting the side of the tongue is suggestive of a seizure.

Endocrinology

1. C – A, normal; B, further testing required; C, diabetes; D, impaired glucose tolerance; E, impaired fasting glucose.
2. D – Antibiotics are often required for underlying infection, which is a common cause of DKA. Patients are usually very dehydrated and correcting the fluid balance is the priority. In young patients, particularly, overzealous fluid replacement can precipitate cerebral oedema. Compensatory hyperventilation (Kussmaul respiration) to 'blow off' carbon dioxide is commonly seen. The diagnosis requires demonstration of acidosis, ketosis and diabetes.

3. D – Type 1 diabetes requires treatment with subcutaneous insulin and is usually treated with a basal-bolus regimen of four injections per day. The aim is an HbA1c between 6.5 and 7.5%. Type 2 diabetes can initially be managed with oral medication. Metformin is first line but contraindicated in renal failure. Sulphonylureas often cause weight gain.

4. E – Osteoporosis is not painful until a fracture is sustained. It is more common in women. Calcium, phosphate and alkaline phosphatase should be normal. A T-score of less than −2.5 is diagnostic.

5. A – Sarcoidosis is one cause of hypercalcaemia. Malignancy, including myeloma, is a common cause. Even if the calcium quickly returns to normal with treatment, it is important to find the underlying cause. Ionized calcium is the relevant value, and correction for the albumin level should be done. Hydration alone may normalize the calcium level; bisphosphonates are required if rehydration is insufficient.

6. A – If present, the visual field defect is a bitemporal hemianopia in acromegaly. Prognathism is common. Hypogonadism and hyperglycaemia are common.

7. B – A mildly macrocytic anaemia is often seen. Viral thyroiditis can cause transient hyperthyroidism followed by hypothyroidism. Treating a patient with concurrent hypoadrenalism with thyroxine can precipitate an Addisonian crisis. Myxoedema coma is rare but mortality is up to 20%.

8. B – Autoimmune destruction is most common in the developed world; worldwide, infection, especially TB, is more common. Diagnosis is made with the short synacthen test. Rehydration, correction of electrolyte abnormalities and replacement of cortisol with hydrocortisone are most important in crisis. In the long term, most patients also require fludrocortisone. Hyperpigmentation is seen in Addison's, but there is an association with vitiligo.

9. A – Sinus tachycardia is also common. Menhorrhagia occurs in hypothyroidism; thyrotoxicosis causes amenorrhoea. Pretibial myxoedema, proptosis and clubbing (thyroid acropachy) are all specific to Graves' disease.

10. D – ADH (also called arginine vasopressin) is synthesized predominantly in the hypothalamus and released by the posterior pituitary. The main hormones secreted by the anterior pituitary are TSH, ACTH, GH, LH and FSH.

Rheumatology and skin

1. B – Obstructive lung disease is not caused by rheumatoid arthritis; all the other options are potential complications. In lung fibrosis, spirometry shows a restrictive pattern.

2. C – Bamboo spine is seen in advanced ankylosing spondylitis. Heberden's nodes and Bouchard's nodes are osteophytic outgrowth in osteoarthritis over the distal and proximal interphalangeal joints, respectively. Telescoping of the digits is seen in psoriatic arthritis mutilans.

3. A – Soft tissue thickening is sometimes seen as a feature of rheumatoid arthritis, but soft tissue is poorly visualized on plain X-ray. The others are classical findings of OA on plain X-ray.

4. D – Anti-TNF therapy is used for autoimmune conditions such as rheumatoid arthritis. Weight loss, physiotherapy and NSAIDs may give symptomatic benefit. The condition is likely to progress and he may require joint replacement.

5. E – Dairy products do not precipitate gout and may protect against it. The other four factors are recognized precipitants.

6. C – The symptoms should make you think of ankylosing spondylitis, and ANCA is unlikely to be helpful here – it is used when a vasculitis is suspected. HLA-B27 is present in over 90% of patients with AS and provides useful further evidence. Plain X-rays may show characteristic changes; if not, MRI can detect early sacroiliitis. ESR is usually raised in inflammatory conditions but will be normal in mechanical back pain.

7. B – Anti-smooth muscle antibodies are seen in autoimmune hepatitis. Anti-Sm (Smith) and anti-dsDNA antibodies are highly specific for SLE. ANA is present at a raised titre in almost all cases. Photosensitive rash is typical. Abnormalities on the full blood count include leukopenia, anaemia and thrompcytopenia. Seizures and psychosis may occur.

8. A – The 'C' in CREST syndrome stands for calcinosis cutis, when calcium is deposited in the skin.

9. B – Erythematous plaques over extensor surfaces with a silvery scale are typical of psoriasis. Benzoyl peroxide is used to treat acne. Anti-TNF therapy is used for severe psoriasis when other treatments fail.

10. C – Along with rapid enlargement, bleeding/crusting, sensory change, diameter >7 mm and indistinct border, satellite lesions help identify malignancy. Metastasis to lungs, liver and brain is

common. The prognosis is worse for scalp or neck lesions. Excision is the only curative treatment and cure rates are good for early lesions.

Haematology

1. E – The picture is of iron deficiency anaemia. Ferritin is usually low, though it may be normal as it is an acute phase reactant. TIBC is raised. Iron deficiency anaemia only occurs once bone marrow stores of iron have been exhausted. The reticulocyte count is usually normal in IDA. Platelet count is often raised due to ongoing bleeding.
2. A – Painful crises are caused by vaso-occlusion and can be precipitated by infection, cold, hypoxia and dehydration. Adequate analgesia should be given, including opiates. Haemoglobin of 8 may well be normal in this patient; transfusion may be required at some point but does not need to be given urgently if the anaemia is well tolerated. Sequestration crisis is only seen in children as the spleen undergoes infarction in most patients by the time they are teenagers.
3. D – Haemolysis following ingestion of fava beans (broad beans) is typical of glucose-6-phosphate dehydrogenase deficiency. In haemolytic anaemia LDH is raised and the reticulocyte count increases. Howell–Jolly bodies are seen in hyposplenism. Infection and drugs are other common precipitants.
4. E – It is associated with promyelocytic leukaemia (AML-M3) as well as some other malignancies. When seen in malignancy it is occasionally more mild and chronic than in acute disease. D-dimer is elevated and fibrinogen is low due to consumption. Gram-negative sepsis and obstetric complications are other common causes. Supportive measures are the mainstay of treatment.
5. B – Haemophilia A and B are X-linked conditions and hence affect males almost exclusively. Von Willebrand's disease presents like platelet deficiency with mucosal and skin bleeding. It is treated with plasma-derived factor VIII. Bleeding in haemophilia A and B is treated with recombinant factor VIII and IX, respectively.
6. A – Excision of a whole lymph node gives information about the type of cells present and the lymph node architecture. FNA is often insufficient. Full-body CT scan and bone marrow examination are needed to stage the disease. PET scan is becoming more widely used for staging.
7. B – Auer rods are seen in acute myeloid leukaemia.
8. E – Isotope bone scan. This will not detect the lesions of myeloma, which appear as 'punched-out' holes on plain X-ray. SFLCA is more sensitive than urine electrophoresis but may not be universally available. Bone marrow examination will give an estimate of the proportion of plasma cells and will confirm the diagnosis.
9. D – Secondary polycythaemia is commonly caused by chronic hypoxia, such as in COPD. The *JAK2* mutation is present in 95% of patients with PV, but fewer of those with ET or MF. In CML the causative abnormality is the Philadelphia chromosome, a translocation. First-line treatment is with imatinib, a tyrosine kinase inhibitor. ET carries the best prognosis of these disorders.
10. D – ADAMTS-13 antibodies are present in thrombotic thrombocytopenic purpura and are not commonly tested for.

Infectious diseases

1. D – Piperacillin is a penicillin and is not effective against MRSA. The other antibiotics are commonly used against MRSA but resistance to some of them, such as vancomycin, is increasing.
2. B – Primaquine. He requires eradication therapy for hypnozoites that occur with *P. vivax* and *P. ovale*. The other agents are used in treatment of the acute illness.
3. C – HIV is an RNA retrovirus. Vertical transmission is common, but the risk can be lowered with antiretrovirals and avoiding breastfeeding. Seroconversion is asymptomatic in a minority of patients. Kaposi sarcoma is a late-stage complication. Combination therapy is used.
4. D – *Streptococcus pyogenes* is a group A streptococcus which often causes skin or soft tissue infection, sometimes invasive, and strep throat.
5. C – The risk of hepatitis B transmission following a needlestick injury is up to 60% compared with a 0.3% risk of HIV transmission. HIV-1 is most common. CD4 T-cells are mainly affected. PGL may exist in stage 1 illness. HAART is started when the CD4 count is less than 350.

Toxicology

1. D – Beta-blockers almost always cause bradycardia in overdose. Sotalol, an atypical beta-blocker which is occasionally used for arrhythmias, may give rise to polymorphic ventricular tachycardia.

2. C – Alkalinizing the urine increases the excretion of acidic drugs. Dialysis is especially useful for large salicylate overdoses. Gastric lavage and whole bowel irrigation are very infrequently used. Activated charcoal is contraindicated in drowsy patients.
3. D – Oral methionine is an alternative to *N*-acetylcysteine for mild paracetamol overdose. There is no specific treatment for aspirin overdose.
4. C – Alcohol withdrawal causes tachycardia.
5. C – Male gender is associated with a higher risk.

General

1. D – Radiofrequency ablation.
2. D – Right-sided infective endocarditis.
3. B – Lichen planus.

EMQ answers

1.

1. D The ECG changes indicate anteroseptal ischaemia.
2. J
3. B
4. G Not all chest pain and ECG changes are cardiac in origin. Remember to look for underlying causes of pulmonary embolism.
5. I This is of autosomal dominant inheritance.

2.

1. C
2. H The presence of a varicocele indicates possible tumour spread to the left renal vein. Remember the venous drainage of the left testicle.
3. I The presence of upper airway symptoms and signs implies this is Wegener's rather than other 'pulmonary–renal' syndromes.
4. F
5. E The back pain is worrying as it may indicate the presence of bony metastases.

3.

1. H
2. C Cardiac failure is not the only cause of orthopnoea. Cardiac surgery, internal jugular catheterization and prolonged ICU admission are all associated with phrenic nerve dysfunction.
3. D Not all crackles heard on auscultation are caused by cardiac failure.
4. G
5. A

4.

1. H The elevated total protein is due to the excess immunoglobulin produced. Plasma cells may be seen on the peripheral blood film.
2. E
3. A Vitamin B_{12} deficiency may be found with other autoimmune diseases. Schilling tests are rarely carried out now.
4. G
5. F Eosinophilia – 'Hodgkin's, histamine or helminths' (the three 'H's).

5.

1. F The lesions are Gottron's papules. Up to 15% of cases are associated with malignancy.
2. H The recurrent miscarriages indicate that the antiphospholipid syndrome may also be present.
3. B Compare the pattern of symptoms of osteoarthritis versus inflammatory arthritis.
4. C
5. E

6.

1. E Stridor is an inspiratory noise resulting from tracheal compression. A thyroid goitre may displace the trachea but as it is in the midline this may be either to the left or right.
2. C The trachea is pushed away by the increasing pressure in the right hemithorax.
3. D Scarred fibrotic tissue pulls the trachea towards itself.
4. B Airflow obstruction during expiration causes a polyphonic expiratory wheeze.
5. J The fluid causes a stony dull percussion note and reduced air entry. Expansion may also be reduced.

7.

1. F This is a common place to put a transplanted kidney. His Cushing's syndrome can be explained by steroid therapy to prevent organ rejection.
2. J Elderly men may have bladder outflow obstruction due to enlarged prostate glands. These may cause urinary retention with overflow incontinence, e.g. postoperatively.
3. D She has polycystic kidneys. These are associated with an increased risk of subarachnoid haemorrhage.
4. E Divarification of the recti is accentuated by sitting up.
5. B She has ascites due to decompensated alcoholic liver disease. The decompensation causes encephalopathy and may be precipitated by an alcohol binge.

8.

1. A This must be treated as suspected meningitis.
2. I Attacks of trigeminal neuralgia are often triggered by innocuous stimuli.

3. F Clusters last 4–12 weeks and are followed by pain-free periods of months.
4. H Prompt therapy with steroids is required to avoid permanent damage to her vision. A temporal artery biopsy may confirm the diagnosis but may be falsely negative because of 'skip lesions'.
5. C There is an increased incidence of subarachnoid haemorrhage in polycystic kidney disease.

9.

1. A The sudden onset suggests a vascular cause. Loss of consciousness is uncommon in strokes unless the brainstem is affected. This may occur in brainstem stroke or from the pressure effects of huge infarction or haemorrhage.
2. J The sudden onset again suggests a vascular cause and in this context the subhyaloid haemorrhages are pathognomonic of subarachnoid haemorrhage.
3. B The most likely explanation is an opiate overdose. This could be assessed by giving the patient naloxone (an opiate antagonist).
4. C Decompensated liver disease often causes encephalopathy. It is often precipitated by infection, constipation and gastrointestinal bleeding.
5. E Diuretic therapy is a common cause of hyponatraemia, which in turn can cause an altered mental state and seizures.

10.

1. D The suspected diagnosis is acromegaly. A useful screening test is IGF-1 levels. An isolated measurement of growth hormone level is not useful.
2. F Investigations directed at finding an endocrine cause for suspected hypoglycaemic episodes are usually negative. However, the only way to exclude an insulinoma is to conduct a prolonged fast and measure serum glucose and C-peptide levels if symptoms occur.
3. H Autoimmune Addison's disease is suspected. Administration of an exogenous adrenocorticotrophic hormone (Synacthen) will fail to produce an increase in serum cortisol.
4. J His cranial diabetes insipidus will be demonstrated by a failure to concentrate the urine during a water deprivation test as the serum osmolality rises. If desmopressin is administered the urine will concentrate within an hour as the renal tubules remain responsive to antidiuretic hormone.
5. B Cushing's syndrome is suspected and will be confirmed if the administration of exogenous steroids fails to suppress adrenal steroid synthesis.

11.

1. H Left iliac fossa pain and bloody diarrhoea is typical of diverticulitis.
2. C
3. F The absence of nocturnal symptoms points to a non-organic cause for the patient's symptoms.
4. J In alcoholic patients a common cause of hospitalization is acute pancreatitis – with repeated attacks and continued alcohol abuse the pancreas does not secrete sufficient enzymes and malabsorption ensues.
5. E Noticeable sweating and palpitations are suggestive of excessive thyroxine levels.

12.

1. F Achalasia is a condition of mostly unknown aetiology characterized by a lack of relaxation in the lower oesophageal sphincter due to degeneration of the myenteric plexus. Dysphagia, retrosternal cramps, regurgitation and weight loss are characteristic.
2. A Most patients with systemic sclerosis have oesophageal involvement.
3. D
4. J Obesity is a risk factor for GORD and the night-time bouts of coughing are due to aspiration of gastric fluid.
5. C Plummer–Vinson syndrome is a narrowing in the upper oesophagus associated with iron-deficiency anaemia, glossitis and angular stomatitis.

13.

1. G Peripheral visual field loss is suggestive of bitemporal hemianopia. This can be caused by a lesion at the optic chiasm such as pituitary adenoma, which in this case has also manifested itself with features of growth hormone excess.
2. F Third nerve palsy may be caused by vascular lesions in patients with diabetes. The pupil may be spared.
3. A The other two features of Horner's syndrome are enophthalmos and anhydrosis. In this case the cause is a preganglionic lesion – thyroid neoplasm.
4. E Shingles of the geniculate ganglion.
5. I Diabetes is a common cause.

14.

1. E
2. H Secondary to long-term steroid use in this case.

3. A Phaeochromocytoma. The raised calcium should make you think of coexisting parathyroid adenoma and multiple endocrine neoplasia.
4. F The hypokalaemia often causes muscle symptoms.
5. G A pharmacological cause of gynaecomastia. Examples of others are spironolactone, oestrogens and cimetidine. Prolactinoma would cause testicular atrophy.

15.

1. I This is an autosomal dominant inherited condition in which cysts develop in the teenage years, associated with berry aneurysms, mitral valve prolapse, liver cysts and malignant change.
2. D This vasculitis affects the respiratory system and kidneys most commonly. An early diagnosis is important, as it is treatable.
3. G Due to the chronic inflammation affecting her gastrointestinal tract and kidneys.
4. B The risk is greatest in those with diabetes mellitus and pre-existing renal disease.
5. A There are several possible causes of renal impairment in myeloma, including hypercalcaemia, NSAIDs, amyloidosis and light-chain deposition.

16.

1. E Iron deposition affects the joints, heart, liver, pancreas, skin and causes hypogonadism due to pituitary deposition.
2. F Associated with autoimmune conditions such as Addison's, Raynaud's, thyroid disease and systemic sclerosis. The lack of pain and lack of evidence of obstruction on ultrasonography make cancer less likely.
3. C Not simple biliary colic because of features of peritonism and a raised white cell count.
4. B A rare inherited disorder with copper accumulation particularly in the liver and basal ganglia.
5. H One of the causes of this is chronic pancreatitis.

17.

1. G This is a typical history of complex partial seizures seen in temporal lobe epilepsy. There is an association with febrile convulsions in childhood.
2. D
3. C Incidence of alcohol excess is known to be high in this social group.
4. B Early-morning headaches are suggestive of raised intracranial pressure.
5. E

18.

1. F Symptoms suggestive of myasthenia gravis.
2. C Guillain–Barré syndrome.
3. A Features are of an inflammatory myopathy, e.g. polymyositis.
4. H Common peroneal nerve palsy – the peroneal nerve is susceptible to entrapment and injury.
5. I Dorsal column pathology occurs in vitamin B_{12} deficiency and advanced syphilis.

19.

1. A Koilonychia (spoon-shaped nails) is associated with iron-deficiency anaemia.
2. H Beau's lines. Caused by arrest of nail growth after severe acute illness.
3. C In this case caused by psoriasis; other causes are trauma and fungal nail infection.
4. I A sign of aortic regurgitation.
5. E Found in infective endocarditis.

20.

1. G The cause in this case was an antibiotic (penicillin). Other causes are systemic infections, collagen disorders and vitamin deficiency.
2. C Classically associated with gastric malignancy.
3. J
4. E More common in Turkey, as well as in Iran and Japan.
5. H

21.

1. J Onset of pain is often acute, with vertebral collapse from tumour or osteoporosis and the pain radiates round in the dermatome from that level.
2. I Increased pressure in the abdomen from bending down can precipitate acid reflux, as can lying flat when an incompetent oesophageal sphincter allows reflux.
3. G Pericarditic chest pain is characteristically relieved by sitting up.
4. C In costochondritis the pain is usually bilateral down the costal cartilages as they attach to the sternum.
5. H Pleuritic chest pain of any cause will be exacerbated by coughing, respiration and movement.

22.

1. H In pneumonia, red cells released into the alveoli as part of consolidation may degenerate into browny haemosiderin pigment and be cleared by coughing as rusty sputum.

2. F Hereditary haemorrhagic telangiectasia (Osler–Weber–Rendu syndrome) is dominantly inherited and associated with arteriovenous malformations in the mucosa of the mouth, nose and gastrointestinal tract, and in the lungs and brain.
3. B All causes of bronchiectasis can produce brisk bleeding from dilated blood vessels in the walls of inflamed dilated bronchi.
4. G In pulmonary oedema the fluid may be just frothy and clear but it may be blood-stained when red cells are also released into the alveoli.
5. E Goodpasture's syndrome is associated with antiglomerular basement membrane antibody, which cross-reacts with basement membrane in the lung.

23.

1. D Carcinoma of the pancreas often presents with pain, which often radiates to the back.
2. E Ascending cholangitis is usually associated with ulcerative colitis and causes jaundice, fever, rigors and sepsis.
3. G Gallstones cause acute cholecystitis; the gallbladder is not usually palpable because of the recurrent inflammation.
4. B The jaundice of acute viral hepatitis is often preceded by less specific symptoms of fever, malaise, muscle and joint pains.
5. I Leptospirosis (Weil's disease) is caused by spirochaetes. An acute viral illness is followed by jaundice, bleeding and abdominal pain in around 10% of cases.

24.

1. C A metabolic acidosis suggests diabetic ketoacidosis; acute kidney injury might also, but such acidosis would not be expected in chronic kidney disease.
2. E Sarcoidosis is the most likely cause of bilateral hilar lymphadenopathy in a young man, and hypercalcaemia is a complication.
3. B Nephrogenic diabetes insipidus is a complication of lithium treatment.
4. E These would be the characteristic findings of multiple myeloma, which is often complicated by hypercalcaemia.
5. J It is important in the history to distinguish frequency from polyuria.

25.

1. I Symmetrical polyarticular inflammation could be rheumatoid arthritis or psoriatic arthropathy, but there is no mention of a rash.
2. J Septic arthritis is an emergency as the joint will rapidly be destroyed.
3. C Neuropathic joints become damaged because trauma can occur not limited by pain in the joint; however, they are often painful subsequently.
4. D Problems in a single, large, weight-bearing joint are most likely to be osteoarthritis, confirmed by X-ray.
5. F Old age is a risk factor for pseudogout.

26.

1. F
2. D
3. C
4. J
5. G

27.

1. G
2. D Hypoparathyroidism is a common complication of thyroid surgery.
3. F
4. H
5. A Metastatic lesions are sclerotic. Myeloma lesions are osteolytic.

28.

1. D
2. I
3. G
4. J
5. A

29.

1. A
2. D
3. C
4. G
5. H

30.

1. A
2. I
3. G
4. F Tenderness over the forehead may also be present in tension headache. In sinusitis there are usually nasal symptoms.
5. B

Index

Note: Page numbers followed by *b* indicate boxes, *f* indicate figures and *t* indicate tables.

A

abbreviated mental test score 139*f*
abdominal examination 18–22
  inspection 20, 20*f*
abdominal mass 21*f*
abdominal pain 5, 85–90
  differential diagnosis 85, 86*f*
  examination 87–88, 87*f*
  investigations 88–89, 88*f*
abdominal swelling 6
  questions 421
abducens nerve (VI) 24, 25
abscess
  central nervous system 302, 302*f*
  cerebral 109
  liver 272
absence attacks (petit mal) 303
acarbose 318
accessory nerve (XI) 26, 26*f*
ACE inhibitors 183, 186, 187, 190, 198, 202
achalasia 246
acidosis 277
acne rosacea 126
acne vulgaris 126, 362
acoustic neuroma 163*f*
acromegaly 336–338
  aetiology 336
  clinical features 336, 337*f*
  diagnosis 337
  management 337–338
  prognosis 338
actinic (solar) keratoses 125
action tremor 14
activated partial thromboplastin time (APTT) 168
acute coronary syndromes 183–184
  NSTEMI 186–190
  STEMI 184–186, 184*f*
acute kidney injury 273–275
  aetiology 273
  causes 274*f*
  clinical features 273
  investigations 273–274
  management 274–275
  prognosis 275
acute lymphoblastic leukaemia 375–376
acute myeloid leukaemia 376–378, 377*f*
acute respiratory distress syndrome *see* ARDS
adalimumab 348
Addisonian crisis 341
Addison's disease 341–342, 341*f*
adenosine 193, 194
adrenal gland disorders 339–343, 339*f*
  Addison's disease 341–342, 341*f*
  congenital adrenal hyperplasia 343
  Conn's syndrome 342
  Cushing's syndrome 339–341, 340*f*
  phaeochromocytoma 342–343
adrenocortical tumours 341
adult polycystic kidney disease 284
age
  and hypertension 200, 200*f*
  and ischaemic heart disease 179
air pollution 223
alcohol
  and hypertension 200
  units of 3*f*
alcohol abuse 402–403, 403*f*
  health problems 403
  management 403
alcoholic liver disease 268–269
alfacalcidol 331
allergic contact dermatitis 126
allergies 2–3
allopurinol 352
α-1 antitrypsin deficiency 223, 272
α-blockers 203
alteplase 185
amantadine 297
amaurosis fugax 110, 290*b*
amiloride 266
aminophylline 222*f*
amiodarone 195
amphetamines 401*f*
anaemia 66, 171–178, 367–375
  aplastic 374
  causes 369–375
    bone marrow infiltration 374
    chronic disease 175–176, 175*f*, 369
    chronic kidney disease 277
    lead poisoning 374–375
    paroxysmal nocturnal haemoglobinuria 370
    rheumatoid arthritis 117*b*, 347*f*
  differential diagnosis 171, 172*f*
  examination 173–174, 173*f*
    blood tests 174–176, 175*f*
  haemolytic 172*f*, 369–370
    autoimmune 370
    mechanical 370
  history 171–173
  investigations 174–177, 176*f*
  management 367
    blood transfusion 368, 368*f*
    erythropoietin 368
    folate replacement 367–368
    iron replacement 367
    splenectomy 368
    vitamin B_{12} replacement 367
  pernicious 373–374
  sickle cell 175*f*, 370–371
  sideroblastic 374
  thalassaemia 175*f*, 371–373, 372*f*, 373*f*
anakinra 348
anaplastic carcinoma 326
ANCA-positive vasculitis 280
angina 188*f*
angiography
  cerebral 114
  ischaemic heart disease 181, 182
angioplasty 183
angiotensin II receptor blockers 198, 202
anion-exchange resins 327
ankle swelling 4–5
ankylosing spondylitis 117–118, 349–350, 350*f*
anorexia 4
anosmia 7
anterior horn cell lesions 154*f*
anti-double-stranded-DNA antibodies 360*f*
anti-GAD antibodies 360*f*
anti-GM1 antibodies 360*f*
antiacetylcholine receptor antibodies 360*f*
antiarrhythmic drugs 194–196, 195*f*
antibiotics
  bronchiectasis 239
  infective endocarditis 211–212
  meningitis 114*b*, 301
  pneumonia 227–228, 228*f*
  urinary tract infection 282
  see also individual drugs

anticholinergics 297
antidiuretic hormone (ADH) 91, 92*f*
antiepileptic drugs 305–306
antiglomerular basement membrane disease 280
antineutrophil cytoplasmic antibodies (ANCA) 360*f*
antinuclear factor 360*f*
antiphospholipid antibodies 360*f*
antiphospholipid syndrome 354
antiplatelet drugs 182, 186, 187, 190, 290
antiretroviral therapy 394
antiribonucleoprotein antibodies 360*f*
antithyroid drugs 325
antoantibodies, neurological disease 159*f*
anuria 91
anxiety, palpitations 50
aortic coarctation 214
aortic regurgitation 207, 208*f*
aortic stenosis 206–207, 207*f*, 214
apex beat 15
aplastic anaemia 374
appetite 4
ARDS 242, 242*f*
arginine vasopressin *see* antidiuretic hormone
Argyll Robertson pupil 23
arms *see* upper limbs
arrhythmias 188*f*, 189–196
  antiarrhythmic drugs 194–196, 195*f*
  bradycardias 193–194
  clinical features 190
  investigations 190–191
  supraventricular 189, 191–193
  ventricular 189, 193, 193*f*
  see also palpitations; and specific arrhythmias
arterial blood gases 40, 217
arthritis 212
ascites 21*f*, 88, 265–266
aspartate aminotransferase 185
Aspergillus spp. 241
aspiration pneumonia 226
aspirin 182, 185, 186, 187
  overdose 400*f*
asterixis 14, 17, 20
asthma 219–221
  aetiology 219
  clinical features 219–220, 224*f*
  diagnosis 220
  differential diagnosis 220
  management 220–221
    chronic therapy 220–221, 221*f*
    emergency treatment 221, 222*f*
  pathophysiology 219
atenolol 182, 187
atherosclerosis *see* ischaemic heart disease
atonic/akinetic epilepsy 303
atopic dermatitis/eczema 125, 361
atrial fibrillation 52*b*, 191, 191*f*
atrial flutter 192, 192*f*
atrial myxoma 213
atrial septal defect (ASD) 213
atrioventricular block 189
atypical facial pain 295
auscultation 16, 16*f*, 18, 21–22, 22*f*
  dyspnoea 46
Auspitz's sign 360
autoimmune haemolytic anaemia 370
autoimmune hepatitis 271
autoimmune polyendocrine syndromes 343
azathioprine 255

B

Babinski response 29*f*
back pain 121–124
  causes 122*f*
  differential diagnosis 121
  examination 123
  history 121–123
  investigations 123
  red flags 122*f*
  yellow flags 122*f*
bacterial gastroenteritis 259
bacterial overgrowth 251
bacteriology, PUO 59
Bamford classification 142, 145*f*, 289–290
barium meal 63
Barrett's oesophagus 246
basal cell carcinoma 127, 365
Beau's lines 13
Becker muscular dystrophy 308–309
beclomethasone 221*f*
bedside manner 1
Behçet's disease 357
Bell's palsy 311, 312*f*
bendroflumethiazide 202
benign oesophageal stricture 246
benign positional vertigo 163*f*
benzhexol 297
benzodiazepine overdose 400*f*
Berger's disease 280
β-2 agonists 221*f*
β-blockers 182, 186, 187, 190, 195, 198, 203
  overdose 400*f*
biguanides 317
bile-acid sequestrants 327
biliary tract cancer 262
bilirubin
  metabolism 80*f*
  see also jaundice
biochemistry
  lymphadenopathy/splenomegaly 150
  osteomalacia 306
  see also specific conditions
bisoprolol 182
bisphosphonates
  osteoporosis 329
  Paget's disease 330
blackouts *see* syncope
bleeding *see* haemorrhage; and specific conditions
bleeding disorders 384–386
  haemophilia A 384–385
  haemophilia B (Christmas disease) 385
  immune thrombocytopaenia 385–386
  von Willebrand disease 385
blind spot 23*f*
blood lipids
  fasting 190
  and ischaemic heart disease 180
blood pressure 14, 17, 103
  abdominal pain 87
  see also hypertension
blood tests
  abdominal pain 89
  acute kidney injury 274
  acute pancreatitis 263
  anaemia 174–176, 175*f*
  back pain 123
  bowel habit changes 72
  bruising/bleeding 167–168
  cardiac failure 197
  chest pain 39
  colorectal cancer 257
  confusional states 140
  cough/haemoptysis 55
  dyspepsia 63
  glomerular disease 279
  haematemesis/melaena 67
  haematuria/proteinuria 101
  headache/facial pain 112
  jaundice 82*f*
  joint disease 118
  lung cancer 230
  lymphadenopathy/splenomegaly 150, 150*f*
  neurological deficit 159
  palpitations 52
  pneumonia 227
  pulmonary embolism 228
  PUO 58–59
  questions 420
  respiratory failure 217
  stroke 144–145
  urinary symptoms 94
  see also specific conditions
blood transfusion 368, 368*f*
blue bloaters 223
body habitus 12
bone disease 328–332
  osteomalacia 331
  osteoporosis 328–329
  Paget's disease 329–330, 330*f*
  renal osteodystrophy 277, 331–332

bone marrow
failure 376*f*
infiltration 176–177, 374–375
bone mineral density (BMD) 328, 329
bone pain 9*f*
Bouchard's nodes 13, 117, 348
boutonnière deformity 346*f*
bowel habits 6, 71–74
differential diagnosis 71
examination 71, 73*f*
history 71
investigations 72–74
see also constipation; diarrhoea
bowel sounds 88
Bowen's disease 125, 365
brachial artery 14–15
brachial plexus lesions 154*f*, 157*f*
bradycardias 193–194
see also specific types
bradykinesia 296
breast, examination 31
breathlessness *see* dyspnoea
bronchiectasis 19*f*, 239
bronchitis 221–223
bronchodilators 225
bronchoscopy 56, 227
bronchospasm, clinical findings 19*f*
Brudzinski's sign 111, 301
bruising/bleeding 165–170
complications 166–167
differential diagnosis 165–166
examination 167, 167*f*
history 166–167
investigations 167–170, 168*f*, 169*f*, 170*f*
Budd-Chiari syndrome 272
budesonide 221*f*
bulbar palsy 311
bullous pemphigoid 126, 363
buttock pain 5

C

cachexia 87
CAGE questionnaire 403*f*
calcitonin 329, 330
calcitriol 331
calcium
homeostasis 333*f*, 426
see also hypercalcaemia; hypocalcaemia
calcium channel blockers 183, 187, 190, 203
calf
pain 5
swelling 4–5
candidiasis 127
carbimazole 325
carcinoid syndrome 252
carcinoid tumours 252
cardiac enzymes 184–185, 185*f*, 186
cardiac failure 188–189, 196–200
aetiology 196
clinical features 196–197
congestive 197
investigations 197
Killip classification 189*f*
left heart 196–197
management 197–200
New York Heart Association classification 196*f*
right heart 197
cardiac rehabilitation 199
cardiac rupture 188*f*, 189
cardiac transplantation 199
cardiogenic shock 188–189, 189*f*
cardiomemo 52
cardiomyopathy 210–211, 210*f*
dilated 210
hypertrophic/obstructive 183
restrictive/infiltrative 211
cardiovascular disease 179–216
acute coronary syndromes 183–184
NSTEMI 186–190
STEMI 184–186, 184*f*
arrhythmias 188*f*, 189–196
cardiac failure 188–189, 196–200
examination 14–17
hypertension 103–108, 200–204
ischaemic heart disease 179–183
questions 408–409, 430–431
symptoms 4–5
systemic lupus erythematosus 353
systemic sclerosis 358
valvular heart disease 204–209
see also specific conditions
carditis 212
Carnett's sign 88
carotenaemia 12
carotid artery 14–15
carotid pulse 15*f*
carpal tunnel syndrome 309
carvedilol 187
catechol-O-methyltransferase inhibitors 297
cellulitis 127, 365–366
central nervous system 289–312
cerebrovascular disease 289–293
classification 303–304, 303*f*
epilepsy 132*f*, 141, 302–306
headache syndromes 7, 109–114, 293–295
infections 300–302
encephalitis 302
meningitis 109, 114*b*, 300–302
spinal cord 302
intracranial tumours 306–307, 307*f*
movement disorders 295–298
multiple sclerosis 298–300
spinal cord disorders 310
systemic lupus erythematosus 353
cerebellar lesions 154*f*
gait 159*f*
symptoms 157*f*
cerebellar tremor 298
cerebral abscess 109
cerebral angiography 114
cerebral hemispheres, lesions of 154*f*, 157*f*
cerebral tumours 110
cerebrospinal fluid, meningitis 302*f*
cerebrovascular accident/event *see* stroke
cerebrovascular disease 289–293
extra-axial haemorrhage 291–293
stroke 141–146, 289–290
certolizumab 348
CHADS score 191
CHADS2 score 141*b*, 291*f*
Charcot's joints 316
chest pain 4, 5, 37–42, 38*f*
associated symptoms 38
cause 38
central 37
differential diagnosis 37, 38*f*
dyspepsia 61
examination 38–39, 39*f*
history 37–38
nature of pain 38
onset and progression 37–38
site and radiation 38
investigations 39–41
arterial blood gases 40
blood tests 39
chest X-ray 40
ECG 40, 40*f*
echocardiogram 40
exercise test 41
percutaneous coronary intervention 40
upper gastrointestinal endoscopy 41
pleuritic 37
questions 419, 425
risk factors 38, 39
chest wall, tenderness 37
chest X-ray
chest pain 40
confusional states 140
infective endocarditis 211
pericarditis 209
PUO 59
tuberculosis 234
Cheyne-Stokes respiration 45
Chlamydia pneumoniae 181
cholecystitis
acute 261–262
chronic 262
cholestasis screen 83
chronic kidney disease 275–278
aetiology 276
classification 276*f*

chronic kidney disease (*Continued*)
clinical features 276
investigations 276–277
management 277–278
chronic lymphocytic leukaemia 378
chronic myeloid leukaemia 378–379
chronic obstructive pulmonary disease *see* COPD
Chvostek's sign 334
ciclosporin 347
cirrhosis 21*f*
clasp-knife phenomenon 27
claudication 5
clerking 33–36
questions 407, 429
sample 34
clopidogrel 182, 187
Clostridium difficile 258–259
clotting factor disorders 166
clubbing 13, 13*f*, 14, 45, 66
abdominal pain 87
cluster headache 110, 111, 294
coagulation abnormalities 165–166
acquired factor inhibitors 166
factor deficiency 166
vitamin K deficiency 165
coagulation pathway 168*f*
coagulation tests 168, 170*f*
cocaine 401*f*
coeliac disease 250–251
skin manifestations 364
collapsing pulse 14*f*
colonoscopy 73
anaemia 177
colorectal disease
C. difficile and pseudomembranous colitis 258–259
diverticular disease 258
ischaemic colitis 259
lower gastrointestinal bleeding 259, 259*f*
microscopic colitis 259
colorectal neoplasia 256–257
benign disease 256–257
colorectal cancer 257–258, 257*f*
coma 131
differential diagnosis 132*f*
examination 133–134, 134*f*
community-acquired pneumonia (CAP) 226
computed tomography *see* CT
confusional states 137–140
differential diagnosis 137
examination 139–140, 139*f*
history 137–139
investigations 140
congenital adrenal hyperplasia 343
congenital central hypoventilation syndrome 241–242
connective tissue disorders 357–360
mixed connective tissue disease 359–360
polymyositis/dermatomyositis 358–359
relapsing polychondritis 360
Sjögren's syndrome 359
systemic lupus erythematosus 352–354
systemic sclerosis 357–358, 357*f*
Conn's syndrome 342
consciousness, loss of *see* loss of consciousness
consolidation, clinical findings 19*f*
constipation, differential diagnosis 72*f*
contact dermatitis 361
coordination 27
COPD 221–226
acute exacerbation 224, 225
aetiology 223
clinical features 223–224
investigations 224, 224*f*
management 224
long term 224–225
surgery 225
pathophysiology 223
prognosis 225–226
coronary artery bypass graft (CABG) 183, 183*f*
Corrigan's sign 15, 207
corticosteroids *see* steroids
cortisol
deficiency 344
excess 344
cortisol releasing hormone test 344
cough 5, 43, 53–56
differential diagnosis 53
examination 54, 55*f*
history 53–54, 54*b*
investigations 54–56
Courvoisier's law 261*b*
COX-2 inhibitors 346
crackles 46
cranial diabetes insipidus 338–339, 339*f*
cranial nerves 22–27
questions 422
see also individual nerves
creatinine kinase 185
crepitations 46
CREST syndrome 357*f*
Creutzfeld-Jakob disease 138
Crohn's disease 251, 253*f*, 255–256
clinical features 255
complications 255
management 256
surgery 256
prognosis 256
cryptococcal meningitis 395*f*
crystal arthropathy 351–352
gout 351–352, 351*f*
pseudogout 118*b*, 352
CT coronary angiography 181
Cullen's sign 20, 87, 263
Curling's ulcer 247
Cushing's reflex 301
Cushing's syndrome 339–341, 340*f*
cyanosis 11–12, 14
central 44
cystic fibrosis 238–239
diagnosis 238
treatment 238–239
cytomegalovirus 395*f*

D

DASHING mnemonic 299*b*
De Musset's sign 15, 207
de Quervain's thyroiditis 325
deafness 7, 26*f*
decubitus ulcers 127
delirium 137, 138*f*
see also confusional states
delirium tremens 137*b*
dementia 137, 138*f*, 312
causes 138–139
see also confusional states
denosumab 329
dermatitis herpetiformis 126
dermatomes 30*f*
dermatomyositis 358–359
dermatophytid reaction 126
detrusor instability 91
dexamethasone suppression test 344
diabetes insipidus 92*f*, 95*f*, 338–339
cranial 338–339, 339*f*
nephrogenic 339, 339*f*
treatment 339
diabetes mellitus 313–320, 343
classification and aetiology 313, 314*f*
clinical features 8*f*, 315, 315*f*
skin manifestations 316, 364
complications 315–316, 315*f*
diagnosis 313–315, 314*f*, 343
emergencies 319–320
diabetic ketoacidosis 319–320
hyperglycaemic hyperosmolar non-ketotic coma 320
hypoglycaemia 319
and ischaemic heart disease 180
management 316–319
diet and lifestyle 317
insulin 318, 318*f*
oral hypoglycaemic agents 317–318
treatment monitoring 343
and surgery 318–319
diabetic ketoacidosis 319–320
diabetic neuropathy 316
diabetic retinopathy 24*f*, 315–316
diagnosis, spot diagnoses 12*f*
diarrhoea
differential diagnosis 72*f*
questions 422

didanosine 395*f*
differential protein clearance 101
digoxin 194, 198
  overdose 400*f*
diltiazem 183, 190, 203
diplopia 299
disability 7
discoid lupus erythematosis 125
disease-modifying anti-rheumatic drugs (DMARDs) 347
disseminated intravascular coagulation 386
dithranol 361
diuretics
  loop 198
  potassium-sparing 203
  thiazide 198, 202
diverticular disease 258
dizziness 7, 161–164, 162*f*
DMARDs *see* disease-modifying anti-rheumatic drugs
documentation, clerking 33–36
dopamine agonists 297
DPP-4 inhibitors 317
Dressler's syndrome 188*f*, 189–190
driving, epilepsy 306
drug overdose/abuse 399–404
  aetiology 399
  complications 401, 401*f*
  epidemiology 399, 400*f*, 401*f*
  examination 399–401
  history 399
  investigations 401
  management 401–402
  psychiatric and social assessment 402
  questions 417, 436–437
  suicide risk 399, 401*f*
drug-induced lupus 354
drug-resistant bacteria 398
dual-energy X-ray absorptiometry (DXA) 329
Duchenne muscular dystrophy 308–309
duodenal ulcer 247
Dupuytren's contractures 13, 20
Duroziez's sign 207
dysarthria 7, 8*f*
dyshidrotic eczema 126
dyspepsia 61–64
  causes 61, 62*f*
  history and examination 61, 62*f*
  investigations 61–63, 62*f*
dysphagia 5, 5*f*
  questions 422
dysphasia 7, 8*f*
dysphonia 7, 8*f*
dyspnoea 4, 5, 43–48
  aggravating/precipitating factors 43
  associated features 43–44
  clinical findings 44*f*
  examination 44–46, 45*f*
  history 43–44
  investigations 46–47, 46*f*
  onset of 43
  questions 419
  severity 43
dysuria 6, 91

E

ECG
  atrial fibrillation 191*f*
  atrial flutter 192*f*
  chest pain 40, 40*f*
  dyspepsia 63
  heart block 194*f*, 195*f*
  hyperkalaemia 287*f*
  infective endocarditis 211
  ischaemic heart disease 181
  NSTEMI 186
  palpitations 52
  pericarditis 209
  pulmonary embolism 228
  pulmonary embolus 40*f*
  STEMI 184, 184*f*
  ventricular fibrillation 193*f*
  ventricular tachycardia 193*f*
echocardiogram
  chest pain 40
  infective endocarditis 211
  ischaemic heart disease 181
economy class syndrome 228
ectopic ACTH syndrome 341
eczema/dermatitis 361–362
  see also specific types
EEG 305
Ehlers-Danlos syndrome 167
Eisenmenger's syndrome 213–214
electrocardiogram *see* ECG
electroencephalogram *see* EEG
electromyogram 160
embolism *see* thromboembolic disorders
emphysema *see* COPD
encephalitis 302
  autoimmune 159*f*
encephalopathy 80, 266, 266*f*
end-stage renal failure 277–278
endocarditis
  culture-negative 212, 212*f*
  infective 211–212, 211*f*
endocrine system 7
  disorders *see* metabolic/endocrine disorders
endoscopy
  anaemia 177
  dyspepsia 63
  haematemesis/melaena 67
  upper GI 41
enoxaparin 187
enteropathic arthropathies 351
entrapment/compression neuropathies 309–310
eosinophilia 59
eosinophilic oesophagitis 246
epidermoid cysts 127
epigastric pain 61
epilepsy 132*f*, 141, 302–306
  aetiology 304
  differential diagnosis 304
  driving and work 306
  investigations 304–305
  precipitants 304
  pregnancy 306
  status epilepticus 306
  sudden unexpected death (SUDEP) 306
  treatment 305–306
ergotamine 294
erysipelas 127
erysipeloid 126
Erysipelothrix insidiosa 126
erythema marginatum 213
erythema migrans 126
erythema multiforme 126, 363
erythema nodosum 127, 363–364
erythrocyte sedimentation rate (ESR) 59
  anaemia 174
erythropoietin 368
essential thrombocythaemia 383–384
essential tremor 297
etanercept 361
evoked potentials 160
examination 11–32
  abdominal 18–22
  breast 31
  cardiovascular system 14–17
  face and body habitus 12
  hands 13–14
  joints 29–30
  limbs 27–29
  lymphadenopathy 31, 31*f*
  neck 31–32
  nervous system 22–27
  preparation for 11
  questions 407, 429
  respiratory system 17–18
  skin 30–31
  spot diagnoses 12*f*
  visual survey 11–12
  see also specific conditions
exercise ECG 181
exercise testing 41
exercise tolerance 4
exfoliative dermatitis 125
extradural haematoma 292–293
exudate 21*f*
eyes
  examination in coma patients 134*f*
  systemic sclerosis 358
  see also entries under visual
ezetimibe 327

F

facial habitus 12, 20
  cardiovascular symptoms 15
  respiratory symptoms 17
facial nerve (VII) 25, 26*f*
facial pain 109–114
  atypical 295
  chronic 111
  differential diagnosis 109, 110*f*
  examination 111–112, 112*f*
  history 109–111
  investigations 112–114, 113*f*
  recurrent episodic 110–111
faecal occult blood test 257
faeces, jaundice 82*f*
familial adenomatous polyposis 257
family history 3
fascioscapulohumeral dystrophy 309
fatigue 3
febuxostat 352
fever *see* pyrexia of unknown origin
fibrates 327
fibrin degradation products 166
fibrinogen 166
figurate erythema 126
finger clubbing *see* clubbing
fingolimod 300
fish oils 327
flapping tremor *see* asterixis
flecainide 195
fluid and electrolyte balance 284–287
fluticasone 221*f*
focal neurological deficit 112
focal (partial) seizures 304
focal segmental glomerulosclerosis 281
folate
  deficiency 172*f*, 175, 175*f*
  replacement 367–368
follicular thyroid carcinoma 326
folliculitis 126
fondaparinux 187
foot drop 159*f*
foot problems in diabetes 316
forced expiratory volume 221
forced vital capacity 221
freckles 125
furuncles (boils) 127

G

gait 28–29
  abnormalities 159*f*
gallbladder disease 261–262
  acute cholecystitis 261–262
  biliary tract cancer 262
  chronic cholecystitis 262
  tumours 262
gallstones 261
γ-hydroxybutyrate 401*f*
gastric carcinoma 66*f*, 249–250
gastric ulcer 247–248
gastrinoma 252
gastritis, erosive 66*f*
gastro-oesophageal reflux disease 245–246
  clinical features 245
  complications 246
  investigations 245
  management 246
gastroduodenal disorders 247–250
gastroduodenitis 247–248
gastroenteritis
  bacterial 259
  viral 260
gastrointestinal disease 5–6, 245–272
  colorectal disease 256–259
  gallbladder disease 261–262
  gastric carcinoma 66*f*, 249–250
  gastroduodenal disorders 247–250
  infective enteritis 259–260
  inflammatory bowel disease 252–256, 253*f*
  irritable bowel syndrome 260
  liver disease 265–272
  non-ulcer dyspepsia 260–261
  oesophageal disorders 245–247
  pancreas 262–265
  questions 411–412, 427, 432–433
  small bowel disorders 250–252
  systemic sclerosis 358
  upper gastrointestinal haemorrhage 248–249
  see also specific systems
gastrointestinal haemorrhage
  lower GI tract 259, 259*f*
  upper GI tract 248–249
gastrointestinal stromal tumour 250
gender-related disease
  alcoholic liver disease 268
  ischaemic heart disease 179
  obstructive sleep apnoea 241
  osteoarthritis 348
genitourinary disease 273–288
  acute kidney injury 273–275
  chronic kidney disease 275–278
  fluid and electrolyte balance 284–287
  glomerular disease 278–281, 278*f*
  questions 412–413, 433–434
  renal calculi 282–283
  urinary tract infection 281–282, 281*f*
  urinary tract malignancies 283–284
genitourinary system 6–7
GET SMASHED mnemonic 263*b*
GI *see* gastrointestinal
giant cell arteritis 355–356
Glasgow coma scale 134*f*, 139, 142
glaucoma 109
glomerular disease 278–281, 278*f*
  ANCA-positive vasculitis 280
  antiglomerular basement membrane disease 280
  clinical features 278–279, 278*f*
  focal segmental glomerulosclerosis 281
  history 279
  IgA nephropathy 280
  investigations 279
  lupus nephritis 280
  management 279–280
  minimal change nephropathy 280
  nephritic syndrome 278
  nephrotic syndrome 278–279
glomerular filtration rate 100
glomerulonephritis
  membranoproliferative 281
  membranous 281
  post-streptococcal 281
  rapidly progressive 280
glossopharyngeal nerve (IX) 26, 26*f*
GLP-1 agonists 318
glucagonoma 252
glucose, fasting 190
glucose-6-phosphate dehydrogenase deficiency 369
glycoprotein IIb/IIIa receptor antagonists 187
goitre 32*f*, 321–322
golimumab 348
Goodpasture's syndrome 280
Gottron's papules 359
gout 117, 351–352, 351*f*
GRACE score 40*b*, 187*f*
Graham Steell murmur 209
granuloma annulare 316
Graves' disease 323
Grey Turner's sign 20, 87, 263
Guillain-Barré syndrome 309
gynaecomastia 20

H

HAART therapy 394
haematemesis 65–70, 85
  differential diagnosis 65, 66*f*
  examination 65–67, 66*f*
  history 65
  investigations 67, 68*f*
  Rockall score 69*f*
haematinics 174
haematological disorders 367–390
  anaemia 66, 171–178, 367–375
  bleeding disorders 384–386
  clinical features 8–9
  disseminated intravascular coagulation 386
  haemolytic uraemic syndrome 388
  leukaemia 375–379
  lymphoma 150*f*, 326, 380–383
  multiple myeloma 379–380, 380*f*
  myelodysplastic syndromes 375
  myeloproliferative disease 383–384

questions 416, 436
thromboembolic disorders 386–388, 387*f*
thrombotic thrombocytopaenic purpura 388–389
haematuria 97–102
differential diagnosis 97–98
examination 100*f*
history 98–99
investigations 99–102, 101*f*
questions 419
haemochromatosis 269–270
haemoglobin 171
synthesis 372*f*
haemolysis 175, 175*f*
haemolytic anaemia 172*f*, 369–370
autoimmune 370
mechanical 370
haemolytic uraemic syndrome 388
haemophilia A 384–385
haemophilia B (Christmas disease) 385
Haemophilus influenzae 226
haemoptysis 44, 53–56
differential diagnosis 53
examination 54, 55*f*
history 53–54
investigations 54–56
questions 425
haemorrhage
lower gastrointestinal 259, 259*f*
splinter 13, 14
subarachnoid 109, 291–292
upper gastrointestinal 248–249
Hallpike manoeuvre 162
hands 18–20
clubbing of fingers *see* clubbing
examination 13–14
cardiovascular symptoms 14
respiratory symptoms 17
questions 424
head thrust test 162
headache syndromes 7, 109–114, 293–295
atypical facial pain 295
chronic headache 111
cluster headache 110, 111, 294
differential diagnosis 109, 110*f*
examination 111–112, 112*f*
history 109–111
intracranial hypertension 294
investigations 112–114, 113*f*
migraine 110, 141, 293–294
progressive 110, 110*f*
questions 421, 427
recurrent episodic headache 110–111
tension-type headache 111, 294
trigeminal neuralgia 111, 294–295
Heaf test 234
haemolytic anaemia 172*f*, 369–370
autoimmune 370
mechanical 370
hearing, altered 7
heart *see* cardiac; cardiovascular
heart block 189, 193–194, 194*f*, 195*f*
heartburn 61
Heberden's nodes 13, 117, 348
Helicobacter pylori 63, 181, 245
hemianopia 23*f*
hemiplegia 159*f*
heparin 165, 186, 187
overdose 400*f*
heparin-like agents 187
hepatitis
acute 265, 265*f*
autoimmune 271
clinical features 268
viral 266–268
hepatitis A 266
hepatitis B 266–267
hepatitis C 267
hepatitis D 267
hepatitis E 267
hepatocellular screen 83
hepatolenticular degeneration 271
hepatomegaly 21*f*
hepatorenal syndrome 284
hernia 88
heroin 401*f*
herpes simplex 126, 362
and HIV/AIDS 395*f*
herpes zoster 126, 362–363
and HIV/AIDS 395*f*
history taking 1–10
bedside manner 1
conclusions 9
family history 3
medications and allergies 2–3
past medical history 2
presenting complaint 2
questions 407, 429
social history 3, 3*f*
systems review 3–9
see also specific conditions
HIV/AIDS 391–396
aetiology 391, 392*f*
epidemiology 391
investigations 392–394, 394*f*
opportunistic infections 395*f*
pathology 391, 392*f*
presentation 391–392, 392*f*, 393*f*, 394*f*
prevention 394–395
prognosis 396
treatment 394, 395*f*
hoarseness 5
Hodgkin's disease 380–382, 381*f*
Holmes-Adie pupil 23
Horner's syndrome 311
hospital acquired (nosocomial) pneumonia 226
Huntington's disease 298
hydralazine 198
hydration 12
hydrocephalus 110
hydroxycarbamide 371
hygiene hypothesis 219
hyperaldosteronism 342
hypercalcaemia 332
causes 332*f*
hyperglycaemic hyperosmolar non-ketotic coma (HONK) 320
hyperkalaemia 275, 277, 286–287, 286*f*, 287*f*
hyperlipidaemia *see* lipid disorders
hypernatraemia 285–286, 286*f*
hyperparathyroidism 332–334
classification and aetiology 333
clinical features 333
investigations 333–334
treatment 334
hyperprolactinaemia 338, 338*f*
hypersensitivity pneumonitis 240*f*
hypertension 103–108, 200–204
aetiology 200
complications 104
definition 103
differential diagnosis 103
essential 103, 200
examination 104, 105*f*, 201, 201*f*
history 103–104, 201
idiopathic intracranial 110
investigations 104–106, 106*f*, 201–202
and ischaemic heart disease 180
malignant 203
management 106–107, 107*f*, 190, 202–203
in pregnancy 203
prognosis 203–204
secondary 103, 201–202
white-coat 202*b*
hyperthyroidism 8*f*, 32*f*, 323–325
skin manifestations 364
see also thyrotoxicosis
hypoalbuminaemia 13*f*
hypocalcaemia, causes 334*f*
hypoglycaemia 132*f*, 319
hypokalaemia 286, 286*f*
hyponatraemia 285, 285*f*
hypoparathyroidism 334–335, 334*f*
hypopituitarism 335–336
hypothalamus-pituitary-adrenal axis 339*f*, 343–344
hypothyroidism 8*f*, 32*f*, 322–323, 322*f*
myxoedema coma 323
palpitations 50
hypoventilation syndromes 241–242
hypovolaemia 66

I

icterus *see* jaundice
IgA nephropathy 280

ileus 22*f*
illegal drugs 401*f*, 402
imaging
  abdominal pain 89
  back pain 123
  bowel habit changes 72–73
  cardiac failure 197
  colorectal cancer 257
  cough/haemoptysis 55
  epilepsy 305
  glomerular disease 279
  haematuria/proteinuria 102
  headache/facial pain 112–114
  joint disease 118–119
  lung cancer 230
  lymphadenopathy/splenomegaly 151
  neurological deficit 159–160
  osteomalacia 331
  pleural effusion 238
  pneumonia 227
  pulmonary embolism 228–229
  respiratory failure 217
  stroke 145, 146*f*
  urinary symptoms 94
  vertigo 164*f*
  see also chest X-ray
immune thrombocytopaenia 385–386
immunology, lymphadenopathy/ splenomegaly 150
impetigo 126, 366
implantable cardioverter/defibrillators 199
incontinence, urinary 7, 91
indigestion 6
infections
  central nervous system 300–302
    abscess 302, 302*f*
    encephalitis 302
    meningitis 109, 114*b*, 300–302
    spinal cord 302
  diabetes mellitus 316
  skin 365–366
  streptococcal 213
  urinary tract 281–282, 281*f*
infectious diseases 391–398
  drug-resistant bacteria 398
  HIV/AIDS 391–396
  malaria 396–398, 397*f*
  questions 417, 436
infective endocarditis 211–212, 211*f*
infective enteritis 259–260
inflammatory bowel disease 252–256, 253*f*
  aetiology and pathogenesis 253
  skin manifestations 364
  see also specific conditions
inflammatory markers 59, 211
infliximab 348, 361
insulin 318, 318*f*
insulinoma 252
intention tremor 14
interstitial lung disease 239–241
  aetiology 239
  clinical features 240
  investigations 240, 240*f*
  management 240
intertrigo 126
intracranial hypertension 294
intracranial pressure, raised 110*f*, 111
  intracranial tumours 307
  meningitis 301
intracranial tumours 306–307, 307*f*
  clinical features 306–307
  investigations 307
  management 307
  prognosis 307
investigations
  questions 408, 429–430
  see also specific conditions
ionotropic therapy 198
ipratropium bromide 222*f*
iron poisoning 400*f*
iron replacement 367
iron-deficiency anaemia 172*f*, 174*b*
  tests for 174–175, 175*f*, 176*f*
  see also anaemia
irritable bowel syndrome 260
ischaemic colitis 259
ischaemic heart disease 179–183
  clinical features 181
  investigations 181–182
  management 182–183
  pathophysiology 180–181
  risk factors 179–180, 180*f*
    modifiable 180
    non-modifiable 179–180
isoniazid 235
isosorbide dinitrate 183
isosorbide mononitrate 183
itching *see* pruritus

J

Jaccoud's arthropathy 353
Janeway lesions 14
jaundice 6, 66, 79–84, 87
  aetiology 82–83
  causes 80*f*
  differential diagnosis 79
  examination 79–81, 81*f*
  history 79
  investigations 81–83, 82*f*
  questions 425
  visual assessment 12
Jo-1 antibodies 360*f*
joint aspiration 118
joint disease 115–120
  differential diagnosis 115, 116*f*
  examination 116–118, 116*f*
  history 115–116
  investigations 118–119
  questions 426
joint position sense, sensory testing 31*f*
joints
  examination 29–30
  hand 13
  swelling 7
  see also musculoskeletal disorders
jugular venous pressure 15, 15*f*, 17, 51
  waveform 16*f*

K

Kallmann's syndrome 22
Kartagener's syndrome 239
Keith-Wagener classification 201*f*
keratoacanthoma 365
Kernig's sign 111, 301*f*
ketamine 401*f*
ketoacidosis 319–320
ketogenic diet 306
kidney
  loop of Henle 91
  palpable 21*f*
Kimmelstiel-Wilson lesions 316
Köbner's phenomenon 360
koilonychia 13, 20
Korotkov sounds 105
Kussmaul respiration 319
Kussmaul's sign 15
kyphoscoliosis 45

L

lactate dehydrogenase 185
Landouzy–Dejerine syndrome 309
Laurence-Moon-Biedl syndrome 23
lead pipe rigidity 27
lead poisoning 374–375
left ventricular assist devices (LVADs) 199
legs *see* lower limbs
lentigo 125
leuconychia 13, 18
leukaemia 375–379
  acute lymphoblastic 375–376
  acute myeloid 376–378, 377*f*
  blood film 150*f*
  chronic lymphocytic 378
  chronic myeloid 378–379
leukopenia 59
leukotriene receptor antagonists 221*f*
levodopa 297
Lhermitte's sign 299
lichen planus 126, 363
lichen simplex chronicus 125
lidocaine 196
limb girdle dystrophy 309
limbs
  examination 27–29
  lower *see* lower limbs
  upper *see* upper limbs
lip pursing 45

lipid disorders 326–328
classification 326
investigations 326–327
management 327–328
see also individual drugs
skin manifestations 365
lipid lowering drugs 183, 186, 187, 190, 327–328
lipoatrophy 316
liver abscess 272
liver disease 265–272
acute hepatitis 265, 265*f*
alcoholic 268–269
autoimmune hepatitis 271
chronic 265–266, 265*f*
haemochromatosis 269–270
hepatolenticular degeneration 271
non-alcoholic steatohepatitis 269
primary biliary cirrhosis 270
primary sclerosing cholangitis 270–271
prothrombin time 67
questions 423
liver function tests
lymphadenopathy/splenomegaly 148
PUO 59
liver tumours 271–272
loin pain 7
long synacthen test 344
loop diuretics 198
Looser's zones 331
loss of consciousness 131–136
differential diagnosis 131
examination 133–134, 133*f*
history 131–133
investigations 134–135
questions 421
risk factors 133
lower gastrointestinal bleeding 259, 259*f*
lower limbs
dermatomes 30*f*
oedema 22*f*
lower urinary tract infection 281
lumbar plexus lesions 154*f*, 157*f*
lumbar puncture 114
neurological deficit 159, 160*f*
lung cancer 229–232
aetiology 229–230, 229*f*
clinical features 230
diagnosis and investigations 230
management 232, 232*f*
occupational 240*f*
pathology 230
pre-operative assessment 232
prognosis 232, 233*f*
TNM staging 231, 231*f*
lungs, collapse 19*f*
lupus nephritis 280
Lyme disease (borreliosis) 365
lymphadenopathy 31, 31*f*, 66, 147–152
abdominal pain 87
differential diagnosis 147–148
examination 149–150, 149*f*
generalized 147, 148, 149–150
history 148
localized 147, 148, 149
lymphocytosis 59
lymphoma 380–383
blood film 150*f*
Hodgkin's disease 380–382, 381*f*
non-Hodgkin's 381*f*, 382–383
thyroid 326

M

magnesium 196
magnesium sulphate 222*f*
malabsorption 250, 250*f*
malaria 396–398
aetiology 396
blood film 150*f*
epidemiology 396
investigations 396
pathology 396, 397*f*
presentation 396, 397*f*
prevention 397–398
prognosis 398
treatment 396–397
Mallory-Weiss tear 66*f*
Mantoux test 234
Marjolin's ulcer 365
MDMA 401*f*
medications 2–3
see also specific drugs
medullary thyroid carcinoma 326
melaena 6, 65–70
differential diagnosis 65, 66*f*
examination 65–67, 66*f*
history 65
investigations 67, 68*f*
Rockall score 69*f*
melanocytic naevus (mole) 125
melanoma 125, 365
melasma 125
membranoproliferative glomerulonephritis 281
membranous glomerulonephritis 281
Ménière's disease 163*f*
meningism 111, 301
meningitis 109, 114*b*, 300–302
causative organisms 300–301
clinical features 301
cryptococcal 395*f*
differential diagnosis 301
investigations 301, 302*f*
predisposing factors 301
treatment 301–302
menstruation 7
mephedrone 401*f*
meralgia paraesthetica 310
mesalazine 255
metabolic syndrome 320–321
metabolic/endocrine disorders 7, 313–344
adrenal glands 339–343, 339*f*
autoimmune polyendocrine syndromes 343
bone disease 328–332
congenital adrenal hyperplasia 343
diabetes mellitus *see* diabetes mellitus
hypercalcaemia 332
hyperparathyroidism 332–334
hypoparathyroidism 334–335, 334*f*
lipid disorders 326–328
metabolic syndrome 320–321
multiple endocrine neoplasia 343
obesity 320–321
pituitary disorders 335–339
questions 414–415, 421, 423, 434–435
thyroid disorders 321–326
metamorphopsia 293
methicillin-resistant *Staphylococcus aureus* 398
methotrexate 347
methyldopa 203
metoclopramide 246
metoprolol 182, 187
microalbuminuria 98*f*, 316
microbiology, lymphadenopathy/ splenomegaly 150–151
micropsia 293
microscopic colitis 259
migraine 110, 293–294
hemiplegic 141
see also headache syndromes
miliaria 126
Miller-Fisher syndrome 159*f*
minimal change nephropathy 280
minoxidil 203
mitoxantrone 300
mitral regurgitation 188*f*, 189, 204–205, 206*f*
mitral stenosis 204, 205*f*
mitral valve prolapse 205
mixed connective tissue disease 359–360, 360*f*
MJTHREADS mnemonic 2*b*
molluscum contagiosum 126
monoamine oxidase B inhibitors 297
monocytosis 59
Moraxella catarrhalis 226
morphoea 358
motor neurone disease 311
motor weakness 299
mouth, examination 20
movement disorders 295–298
Huntington's disease 298
parkinsonism 159*f*, 295–297, 295*f*
Sydenham's chorea 213, 298
tremor *see* tremor

MRSA 398
multifocal motor neuropathy 159*f*
multiple endocrine neoplasia 343
multiple myeloma 379–380, 380*f*
multiple sclerosis 298–300
clinical features 298–299
diagnosis/differential diagnosis 299–300
investigations 300
management 300
pathogenesis 298
prognosis 300
mural thrombus 188*f*
Murphy's sign 88*b*, 261
muscle disorders 307–309
myasthenia gravis 159*f*, 308
myotonic dystrophy 308
muscle power 27, 27*f*, 28*f*
see also motor deficit
muscular dystrophies 308–309
musculoskeletal disorders 345–366
antiphospholipid syndrome 354
clinical features 7, 159*f*
crystal arthropathy 351–352
osteoarthritis 117, 348–349, 349*f*
polymyalgia rheumatica 355
questions 415–416, 420, 435–436
rheumatoid arthritis 116–117, 116*f*, 345–348
spondyloarthropathies 349–351
systemic sclerosis 358
see also specific conditions
myasthenia gravis 159*f*, 308
Mycobacterium avium complex 395*f*
Mycobacterium tuberculosis 232
myelodysplastic syndromes 375
myelofibrosis 384
blood film 150*f*
myeloproliferative disease 383–384
essential thrombocythaemia 383–384
polycythaemia vera 383
primary myelofibrosis 384
myocardial infarction
complications 188–190, 188*f*
NSTEMI 186–190
rehabilitation 190
secondary prevention 190
STEMI 184–186, 184*f*
see also acute coronary syndromes
myoclonic epilepsy 303
myopathies 154*f*
symptoms 157*f*
myotonic dystrophy 308
myxoedema coma 323

N

nails
Beau's lines 13
examination 13
half-and-half 20
koilonychia 13, 20
leuconychia 13, 18
onycholysis 13
yellow 13
natalizumab 300
nausea 6
neck, examination 20, 31–32
necrobiosis lipoidica diabeticorum 316
necrotizing fasciitis 366
nephritic syndrome 278
nephrogenic diabetes insipidus 339, 339*f*
nephrotic syndrome 98*f*, 278–279
nerve roots 28*f*
nervous system
examination 22–27
symptoms 7
neuroendocrine tumours 251–252
see also specific types
neurofibromatosis 364–365
neurological deficit 153–160
autoantibodies 159*f*
differential diagnosis 153, 154*f*
examination 156–158
gait abnormalities 159*f*
history 153–156, 157*f*
investigations 159–160
questions 413–414, 424, 434
neuromuscular junction disorders 154*f*, 157*f*
neuromyelitis optica 159*f*
neutrophilia 59
nicorandil 183
nicotinic acid 327
Nikolsky's sign 126
Nissen's fundoplication procedure 245
nitrates 182–183, 198
'no known drug allergies' (NKDA) 3
nocturia 6, 91
non-alcoholic steatohepatitis 269
non-Hodgkin's lymphoma 381*f*, 382–383
non-nucleoside reverse transcriptase inhibitors 395*f*
non-ST-segment elevation myocardial infarction *see* NSTEMI
non-steroidal anti-inflammatory drugs (NSAIDs)
gout 352
rheumatoid arthritis 346
non-ulcer dyspepsia 260–261
Noonan's syndrome 209
NSAIDs *see* non-steroidal anti-inflammatory drugs
NSTEMI 186–190
diagnosis 186
history 186–187
management 187
inpatient 187–188
risk scoring 186–187, 187*f*
symptoms 186
nuclear imaging, ischaemic heart disease 182
nucleoside reverse transcriptase inhibitors 395*f*
nystagmus 24, 162

O

obesity 320–321
and hypertension 200
obesity hypoventilation syndrome 241
obstructive sleep apnoea 180, 241
obstructive sleep apnoea-hypopnoea syndrome 241
occupational lung disease 240, 240*f*
oculomotor nerve (III) 24–25
oedema 4–5
lower limbs 22*f*
see also swelling
oesophageal cancer 246–247
oesophageal disorders 245–247
achalasia 246
eosinophilic oesophagitis 246
gastro-oesophageal reflux disease 245–246
hiatus hernia 245
oesophageal motility disorders 246
oesophageal varices 249, 265
oesophagitis 66*f*
olfactory nerve (I) 22
oliguria 91
omeprazole 246
Ondine's curse 241–242
onycholysis 13
ophthalmoscopy 23
opiate overdose 400*f*
opportunistic pneumonia 226
optic atrophy 24*f*
optic nerve (II) 23
optic neuritis 299
orthopnoea 4
Osler-Weber-Rendu disease 66
Osler's nodes 14
osmotic diuresis 92*f*
osteoarthritis 117, 348–349, 349*f*
osteomalacia 331
osteopenia 328
osteoporosis 328–329
oxygen therapy 222*f*
COPD 225

P

pacemakers 199
Paget's disease 329–330, 330*f*
extramammary 125
pain
abdominal 5, 85–90
bone 9*f*
epigastric 61
muscular 7
sensory testing 31*f*

pallor 12
palmar erythema 13*f*, 20
palpation 15–16, 16*f*, 20–21
  dyspnoea 45–46
palpitations 4, 49–52, 193
  causes 50, 50*f*
  consequences of 50
  differential diagnosis 49, 50*f*
  examination 50–51, 51*f*
  history 49–50
  investigations 51–52
Pancoast's symptoms 17
pancreatic disease 262–265
  carcinoma 262–263
pancreatitis
  acute 263–264, 264*f*
  chronic 250, 264–265
papillary thyroid carcinoma 326
papilloedema 24*f*
paracetamol overdose 400*f*
paraneoplastic syndromes 159*f*, 230, 231*f*
parathyroid gland
  hyperparathyroidism 332–334
  hypoparathyroidism 334–335, 334*f*
parathyroid hormone 329
parkinsonism 159*f*, 295–297
  clinical features 295–296
  diagnosis 296
  differential diagnosis 295*f*, 296
  management 296–297
paroxysmal nocturnal dyspnoea 4
paroxysmal nocturnal haemoglobinuria 370
paroxysmal supraventricular tachycardia 192
past medical history 2
patent ductus arteriosus 214
patients, visual assessment 11
PCO_2 217
peak expiratory flow rate (PEFR) 220
PEAS mnemonic 1
pemphigus 126
pemphigus vulgaris 363
penile discharge 7
peptic ulcer disease 66*f*, 247–248
percussion 18, 21, 21*f*
  dyspnoea 46
percutaneous coronary intervention 40, 185, 187
pericardial effusion 209–210
pericarditis 188*f*, 189–190, 209–210, 209*f*
  constrictive 209–210
perilymphatic fistula 163*f*
peripheral neuropathies 154*f*, 309
  questions 426
  symptoms 157*f*
peritonism 87, 87*f*
pernicious anaemia 373–374
petechiae 127
Peutz-Jeghers syndrome 66, 257
phaeochromocytoma 342–343
pharyngoscopy 55
Philadelphia chromosome 378–379
photodermatoses 127
Pickwickian syndrome 241
pigmented lesions 12, 125
pink puffers 223
pioglitazone 317
pituitary apoplexy 335
pituitary disorders 335–339
  acromegaly 336–338
  diabetes insipidus 92*f*, 95*f*, 338–339
  hypopituitarism 335–336
  prolactin disorders 338
  tumours 336
pituitary function tests 344
pityriasis rosea 125
pityriasis versicolor 125
plasma viscosity 174
Plasmodium spp. 396, 397*f*
platelet abnormalities 165
platelet function tests 168
pleural effusion 237–238
  aetiology 237
  clinical features 19*f*, 44*f*, 237
  investigations 238
  management 238
pleural fluid aspiration 238
pleuritic chest pain 37
Pneumocystis jirovecii 395*f*
pneumonia 226–227
  aetiology 226
  aspiration 226
  atypical 226
  clinical features 44*f*, 226
  community-acquired (CAP) 226
  diagnosis 227
  hospital acquired (nosocomial) 226
  management 227, 228*f*
  opportunistic 226
  severity 227
pneumothorax 235–236
  clinical features 19*f*, 44*f*, 236
  management 236, 236*f*, 237*f*
polycythaemia vera 383
polydipsia 91, 93
  investigations 95*f*
  psychogenic 92*f*, 95*f*
polymyalgia rheumatica 355
polymyositis 358–359
polyuria 91, 93
  differential diagnosis 92*f*
  investigations 95*f*
pompholyx 126
porphyria cutanea tarda 126
post-streptococcal glomerulonephritis 281
postherpetic neuralgia 111
potassium channel activators 183
potassium
  homeostasis 286
  intake, and hypertension 200
potassium-sparing diuretics 203
praecordium 15
pregnancy
  epilepsy 306
  hypertension 203
presenting complaint 2
  history of 2
primary biliary cirrhosis 270
primary sclerosing cholangitis 270–271
procainamide 195
procyclidine 297
prolactin disorders 338
propranolol 325
prostatic carcinoma 283–284
proteinuria 97–102, 98*f*
  benign 98
  differential diagnosis 98
  examination 100*f*
  history 98–99
  investigations 99–102, 101*f*
  overflow 98
  pathological 98
prothrombin time 168
  liver disease 67
proton pump inhibitors 246
proximal myopathy 159*f*
pruritus 4, 4*f*, 6, 128*f*
pseudobulbar palsy 311
pseudogout 118*b*, 352
pseudomembranous colitis 258–259
Pseudomonas spp.
  drug resistance 398
  P. aeruginosa 226
pseudoxanthoma elasticum 167
psoriasis 125, 360–361
psoriatic arthritis 117, 351
pulmonary embolism 188*f*, 228–229
  clinical features 228
  diagnosis 228–229
  ECG 40*f*
  imaging for 40–41
  management 229
  risk scoring 46*f*, 228, 228*f*
pulmonary fibrosis 19*f*
  clinical findings 44*f*
pulmonary oedema 275
pulmonary rehabilitation 225
pulmonary stenosis 214
pulmonary valve lesions 209
pulse 17
  abdominal pain 87
pulsus paradoxus 14, 17
PUO *see* pyrexia of unknown origin
pupillary reflexes 23
purpura 127
pyoderma gangrenosum 364
pyrazinamide 235
pyrexia 87

pyrexia of unknown origin (PUO) 57–60
 causes 57, 58*f*
 examination 57–58, 58*f*
 history 57
 investigations 58–60
pyruvate kinase deficiency 369
pyuria 91

Q

'question mark' posture 350*f*
Quincke's sign 13, 14, 207

R

rachitic rosary 331
radial nerve palsy 309
radial pulse 14
radioiodine 325
radiotherapy
 acromegaly 338
 colorectal cancer 258
 intracerebral tumours 307
 lung cancer 232
 non-Hodgkin's lymphoma 382
 oesophageal cancer 247
 testicular cancer 284
raloxifene 329
ranitidine 246
rapidly progressive glomerulonephritis 280
rasagiline 297
rasburicase 352
rash 7
Raynaud's phenomenon 357–358
reactive arthritis 118, 350–351
rectal bleeding 6, 6*f*, 85–86
red blood cells
 microcytic 171, 172*f*
 normocytic 171, 172*f*
reflexes 27–28, 29*f*
Refsum's disease 23
relapsing polychondritis 360
relative afferent pupillary defect (RAPD) 23
renal biopsy 279
renal calculi 282–283
renal cell carcinoma 283–284
renal disease
 questions 423, 426
 systemic lupus erythematosus 353
 systemic sclerosis 358
renal osteodystrophy 277, 331–332
respiratory disease 217–244
 ARDS 242
 Aspergillus spp. 241
 asthma 219–221
 bronchiectasis 239
 COPD 221–226
 cystic fibrosis 238–239
 examination 17–18
 hypoventilation syndromes 241–242
 interstitial lung disease 239–241
 lung cancer 229–232
 occupational lung disease 240, 240*f*
 pleural effusion 237–238
 pneumonia 226–227
 pneumothorax 235–236
 pulmonary embolism 188*f*, 228–229
 questions 409–411, 420, 431–432
 sleep-related disorders 241
 symptoms 5, 19*f*
 systemic lupus erythematosus 353
 systemic sclerosis 358
 tuberculosis 54*b*, 232–235
respiratory failure 217–219
 causes 217, 218
 definition 217
 investigations 217–218
 management 218
 prognosis 218–219
 type I 217–218
 type II 218
resting tremor 14
reticulocyte count 174
retinopathy
 diabetic 24*f*, 315–316
 Keith-Wagener classification 201*f*
rheumatic fever 212–213
 Duckett-Jones criteria 212*f*
 skin manifestations 364
rheumatoid arthritis 116–117, 116*f*, 345–348
 clinical features 345, 346*f*, 347*f*
  anaemia 117*b*, 347*f*
 investigations 345–346
 management 346
  biological agents 348
  DMARDs 347
  NSAIDs 346
  steroids 347–348
  surgery 348
 pathological features 345
 prognosis 348
rheumatoid factor 360*f*
rickets 331
rifampicin 235
rigidity in Parkinson's disease 296, 296*f*
riluzole 311
risedronate 330
rituximab 348
Rockall score 69*f*
Romberg's test 28
Roth's spots 15
Rovsing's sign 88*b*

S

salbutamol 222*f*
sarcoidosis 364
scabies 126
sclerodactyly 14
seborrhoeic dermatitis 125, 362
seborrhoeic keratosis 125
seizures *see* epilepsy; and specific conditions
selegiline 297
sensation 28, 29*b*
 testing 31*f*
sensory pathways, spinal cord 30*f*
septic arthritis 118
serology
 PUO 59
 see also specific conditions
shingles 126
 see also herpes zoster
short synacthen test 344
sick sinus syndrome 193
sickle cell anaemia 175*f*, 370–371
sideroblastic anaemia 374
sigmoidoscopy 73
sinus bradycardia 50*f*, 189, 193
sinus tachycardia 50*f*, 191
Sister Mary Joseph's nodule 20
sitagliptin 317
Sjögren's syndrome 359
skin diseases 7, 125–130, 360–364
 acne vulgaris 126, 362
 bullous pemphigoid 126, 363
 differential diagnosis 125–127
 eczema/dermatitis 361–362
 erythema multiforme 126, 363
 erythema nodosum 127, 363–364
 examination 30–31, 128, 129*f*
 figurate erythema 126
 herpes simplex 126, 362
 history 127–128
 infections 365–366
 investigations 129
 lichen planus 126, 363
 pemphigus vulgaris 363
 photodermatoses 127
 psoriasis 125, 360–361
 pyoderma gangrenosum 364
 questions 415–416
 Stevens-Johnson syndrome 127, 363
 systemic disease-related 364–365
  diabetes mellitus 316, 364
  questions 424
  systemic lupus erythematosus 353, 353*f*
  systemic sclerosis 357–358, 357*f*
  see also specific conditions
 toxic epidermal necrolysis 363
 vitiligo 364
skin lesions
 bullous 126
 erosive 127
 maculopapular 127
 papular/nodular 126–127
 petechiae/purpura 127
 pigmented 12, 125

pustular 126
scaly 125–126
ulcerated 127
vesicular 126
weeping/encrusted 126
skin tumours 365
sleep pattern 4
sleep-related disorders 241
small bowel disorders 250–252
bacterial overgrowth 251
chronic pancreatitis 250
coeliac disease 250–251
Crohn's disease 251
malabsorption 250, 250*f*
neuroendocrine tumours 251–252
tropical sprue 251
Whipple's disease 251
smell, altered 7
smoking
and cardiovascular disease 190
cessation 224–225
and COPD 223
and hypertension 200
and ischaemic heart disease 180
and lung cancer 229*f*
social history 3, 3*f*
SOCRATES mnemonic 2*b*, 37, 85
sodium homeostasis 285–286
sodium intake, and hypertension 200
SOFTER TISSUE mnemonic 116*b*
spade-like hands 14
spastic paraplegia 159*f*
speech disturbance 7, 8*f*
spherocytosis, hereditary 369–370
spider naevi 20
spinal cord
disorders 310
compression 310, 310*f*
infections 302
nerve root lesions 154*f*, 157*f*
subacute combined degeneration 310
syringomyelia/syringobulbia 310
sensory pathways 30*f*
spironolactone 198, 266
splenectomy 368
splenomegaly 147–152
differential diagnosis 147–148
examination 149–150, 149*f*, 150*f*
history 148
investigations 150–151
splinter haemorrhage 13, 14
spondyloarthropathies 349–351
ankylosing spondylitis 117–118, 349–350, 350*f*
enteropathic arthropathies 351
psoriatic arthritis 117, 351
reactive arthritis 350–351
spot diagnoses 12*f*
sputum 5, 44, 46*b*
squamous cell carcinoma 365
ST-elevation myocardial infarction *see* STEMI
staphylococcal scalded skin syndrome 127
Staphylococcus aureus 126, 226
methicillin-resistant 398
statins 183, 186, 187, 190, 327
status epilepticus 306
STEMI 184–186, 184*f*
diagnosis 184–185
management 185–186
presentation and symptoms 184, 184*f*
stenting 183
steroids
asthma 221*f*, 222*f*
COPD 225
psoriasis 361
rheumatoid arthritis 347–348
Stevens-Johnson syndrome 127, 363
stiff person syndrome 159*f*
stiffness 7
Stokes-Adams attacks 50, 131, 132
stools, appearance of 6
streptococcal infection 213
Streptococcus pneumoniae 226
streptokinase 185
stress incontinence 91
stridor 44
stroke 141–146, 289–290
aetiology and pathophysiology 289
Bamford classification 142, 145*f*, 289–290
clinical features 289–290
complications 142, 146*f*
definition 289
differential diagnosis 141, 290
examination 141–143, 144*f*
history 141, 143*f*
investigations 143–145, 290, 290*f*
management 290–291
prevention 291, 291*f*
risk factors 143*f*
types and causes 142*f*
strontium ranelate 329
subarachnoid haemorrhage 109, 291–292
subdural haematoma 110, 141, 292, 293*f*
sudden death 188*f*
sudden unexpected death in epilepsy (SUDEP) 306
suicide risk 399, 401*f*
sulfasalazine 347, 350
sulphonylureas 317
sumatriptan 294
supraventricular arrhythmias 189, 191–193
surgery
acromegaly 337
COPD 225
Crohn's disease 256
diabetic patients 318–319
gastroduodenal disorders 248
rheumatoid arthritis 348
splenectomy 368
subtotal thyroidectomy 325
ulcerative colitis 255
swan neck deformity 346*f*
sweats 4
swelling
abdominal 20*f*
ankle 4–5
calf 4–5
joints 7
see also oedema
Sydenham's chorea 213, 298
syncope 4, 131, 132*f*
causes 132*f*
examination 134
see also loss of consciousness
syndrome of inappropriate antidiuretic hormone production (SIADH) 285, 286*f*
syphilis, skin lesions 125
syringomyelia/syringobulbia 310
systemic lupus erythematosus 352–354
clinical features 352–353, 353*f*
drug-induced 354
investigations 354, 354*f*
treatment 354
systemic sclerosis 357–358, 357*f*
systems review 3–9
abdominal swelling 6
cardiovascular symptoms 4–5
gastrointestinal disease 5–6
general symptoms 3–4
genitourinary systems 6–7
haematological symptoms 8–9
metabolic and endocrine symptoms 7
musculoskeletal symptoms 7
neurological symptoms 7
respiratory symptoms 5
skin symptoms 7

T

tazarotene 361
teichopsias 293
temperature, sensory testing 31*f*
temporal arteritis 110, 111, 114
tendons, hand 13
tenesmus 6
tension-type headache 111, 294
testicular cancer 284
tetralogy of Fallot 215
thalassaemia 175*f*, 371–373, 372*f*, 373*f*
theophylline 221*f*
thiazide diuretics 198, 202
thiazolidinediones 317
thigh pain 5
thorax, inspection 18, 19*f*

thrombin time 168
thrombocytopenia 165
thromboembolic disorders 386–388, 387*f*
thrombolytic therapy 185, 290
  contraindications 185*f*
thromboprophylaxis 188
thrombotic microangiopathies 284
thrombotic thrombocytopaenic purpura 388–389
thyroid disorders 321–326, 321*f*
  goitre 32*f*, 321–322
  hyperthyroidism 8*f*, 32*f*, 323–325
  hypothyroidism 8*f*, 32*f*, 322–323, 322*f*
  malignancy 325–326
  subacute (de Quervain's) thyroiditis 325
  thyroid gland enlargement 32*f*
thyroid storm 325
thyrotoxic crisis 325
thyrotoxicosis 323–325
  aetiology 323
  clinical features 323–324, 324*f*
  investigations 324
  management 325
  palpitations 50
  see also hyperthyroidism
tinea corporis 125
tinnitus 7
tissue plasminogen activator 185
TNM classification, lung cancer 231, 231*f*
tocilizumab 348
Todd's paresis 304
tone 27
tonic-clonic seizures 303
torsade de pointes 193
touch, sensory testing 31*f*
toxic epidermal necrolysis 363
toxic lung injury 240*f*
toxoplasmosis 395*f*
trachea 17, 17*f*
transient ischaemic attacks 141–146, 289–290
  see also stroke
transitional cell carcinoma 283
transudate 21*f*
Traube's sign 207
tremor 297–298
  action 14
  asterixis 14, 17, 20
  causes 27*f*, 298*f*
  cerebellar 298
  essential 297
  intention 14
  Parkinson's disease 295–296
  resting 14
Trendelenburg's sign 117
tricuspid regurgitation 207–208, 208*f*
tricyclic antidepressant overdose 400*f*
trigeminal nerve (V) 25, 25*f*
  shingles 111
trigeminal neuralgia 111, 294–295
trigger finger 346*f*
trochlear nerve (IV) 24, 25
Troisier's sign 25, 66
Tropheryma whippelii 251
tropical sprue 251
troponin 39*b*, 184, 186
Trousseau's sign 334
tuberculosis 54*b*, 232–235
  clinical features 234
  control 235
  diagnosis 234–235
  extrapulmonary 234
  management 235
  notification 233*f*
  pathogenesis and disease pattern 233–234
  prophylaxis 235
  pulmonary 233–234
tumour necrosis factor-α inhibitors 348, 350
tumours
  adrenocortical 341
  carcinoid 252
  cerebral 110
  gallbladder 262
  intracranial 306–307, 307*f*
  liver 271–272
  multiple endocrine neoplasia 343
  neuroendocrine 251–252
  pituitary 336
  prostate 283–284
  skin 365
  skin manifestations 364
  thyroid 325–326
tunnel vision 23*f*
two-point discrimination, sensory testing 31*f*

U

ulcerative colitis 253–255, 253*f*
  clinical features 253–254
  complications 254
  investigations and diagnosis 254
  management 254–255, 254*f*
    surgery 255
  prognosis 255
upper gastrointestinal haemorrhage 248–249
upper limbs
  dermatomes 30*f*
  examination 20
upper urinary tract infection 281–282
urea and electrolytes, PUO 59
urge incontinence 91
urinalysis 93, 95*f*, 99–101
  acute kidney injury 273–274
  glomerular disease 279
urinary symptoms 91–96
  differential diagnosis 91, 92*f*
  examination 93, 94*f*
  frequency 6, 91
  hesitancy 6, 91
  history 91–93
  incontinence 7, 91
  investigations 93–95
  questions 425
urinary tract infection 281–282, 281*f*
  clinical features 282
  investigations 282
  lower urinary tract 281
  management 282
  upper urinary tract 281–282
urinary tract malignancies 283–284
  renal cell carcinoma 283–284
urine
  24-h collection 100
  appearance of 6
    haematuria 97–102
    jaundice 82*f*
  protein:creatinine ratio 100–101
  proteinuria 97–102
urticaria 126
ustekinumab 361
UVB radiation therapy 361

V

vaccines
  influenza 199, 225
  tuberculosis 235
vaginal discharge 7
vagus nerve (X) 26, 26*f*
valvular heart disease 204–209
  aortic regurgitation 207, 208*f*
  aortic stenosis 206–207, 207*f*
  mitral regurgitation 188*f*, 189, 204–205, 206*f*
  mitral stenosis 204, 205*f*
  mitral valve prolapse 205
  pulmonary valve lesions 209
  tricuspid regurgitation 207–208, 208*f*
vancomycin-resistant enterococci (VRE) 398
varicella *see* herpes zoster
vascular disorders
  Behçet's disease 357
  giant cell arteritis 355–356
vasculitis 356–357, 356*f*
vasodilators 203
Vaughan Williams classification 195*f*
venous thrombosis *see* thromboembolic disorders
ventricular aneurysm 188*f*
ventricular fibrillation 189, 193, 193*f*
ventricular septal defect (VSD) 188*f*, 189, 213–214

ventricular tachycardia 189, 193, 193*f*
verapamil 183, 190, 194
vertebrobasilar insufficiency 163*f*
vertigo 7, 161–164
  differential diagnosis 161, 162*f*
  examination 162–163, 164*f*
  history 161–162, 163*f*
  investigations 163–164, 164*f*
vessel wall abnormalities 166
vestibular neuronitis 163*f*
vestibulocochlear nerve (VIII) 25–26
vibration, sensory testing 31*f*
vildagliptin 317
VIPoma 252
viral gastroenteritis 260
viral load, PUO 59
Virchow's node 25
vision loss, monocular 23*f*
visual acuity 23
visual assessment
  hydration 12
  jaundice 12
  pallor 12
  pigmentation 12
visual disturbance 7
visual fields 23, 23*f*
visual survey 11–12
  cyanosis 11–12
  patient position and behaviour 11
vital signs 51
vitamin B_{12}
  deficiency 172*f*, 175, 175*f*
  replacement 367
vitamin D
  deficiency *see* osteomalacia
  metabolism 328*f*
  supplements 331
vitamin K deficiency 165
vitiligo 364
vocal fremitus 18, 46
vomiting 6, 85
von Willebrand disease 385
von Willebrand factor 166*b*

W

warfarin 198
  overdose 400*f*
water hammer pulse 207
weakness 7
weight change 4
weight gain, and ischaemic heart disease 180
weight loss 75–78
  differential diagnosis 75, 76*f*
  examination 76–77, 77*f*
  history 75–76
  investigations 77–78
Well's score 228*f*
Wenckebach heart block 194*f*
wheeze 5, 44, 46
Whipple's disease 251
white-coat hypertension 202*b*
Wilson's disease 271

X

xanthoma 13, 14
xerosis 125

Y

yellow nails 13

Z

zidovudine 395*f*
zoledronic acid 330

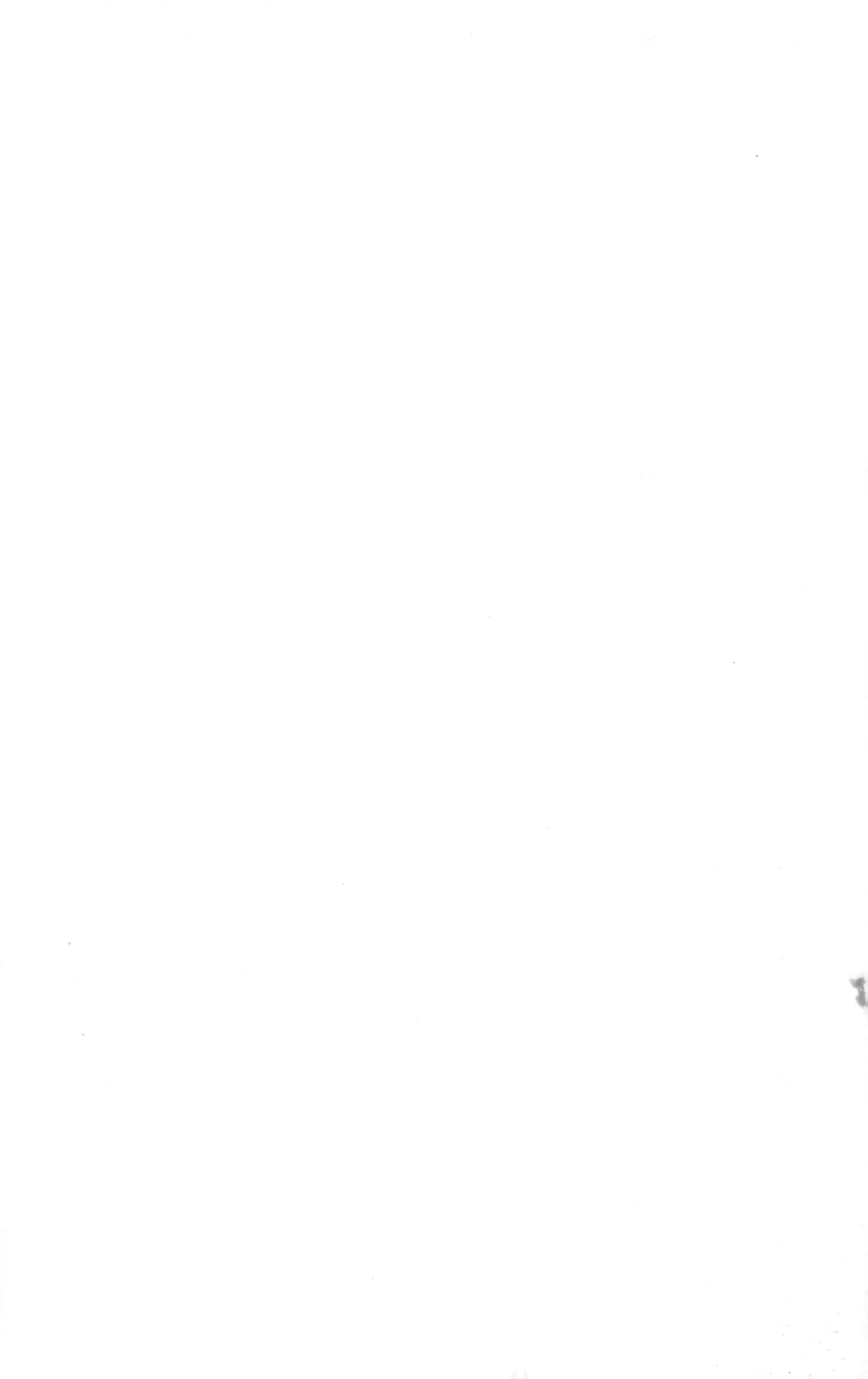